Thieme

Interdisciplinary Management of Orbital Diseases

Textbook and Atlas

Hans-J. Welkoborsky, MD, DDS, PhD
Professor and Chairman
Department of Otorhinolaryngology, Head and Neck Surgery
Nordstadt Clinic
Academic Hospital and Children's Hospital "Auf der Bult"
Hannover, Germany

Burkhard Wiechens, MD, PhD
Professor and Chairman
Department of Ophthalmology
Nordstadt Clinic
Academic Hospital
Hannover, Germany

Michael L. Hinni, MD
Professor and Chairman
Department of Otolaryngology, Head and Neck Surgery
Mayo Clinic
Scottsdale, Arizona, USA

689 illustrations

Thieme
Stuttgart • New York • Delhi • Rio de Janeiro

Library of Congress Cataloging-in-Publication Data is available from the publisher.

Illustrators:
Christine Lackner, Ittlingen, Germany
Markus Voll, Munich, Germany

Cover illustration:
Martina Berge, Stadtbergen, using an image by c Bo Valentino – Fotolia.de

Important note: Medicine is an ever-changing science undergoing continual development. Research and clinical experience are continually expanding our knowledge, in particular our knowledge of proper treatment and drug therapy. Insofar as this book mentions any dosage or application, readers may rest assured that the authors, editors, and publishers have made every effort to ensure that such references are in accordance with **the state of knowledge at the time of production of the book.**

Nevertheless, this does not involve, imply, or express any guarantee or responsibility on the part of the publishers in respect to any dosage instructions and forms of applications stated in the book. **Every user is requested to examine carefully** the manufacturers' leaflets accompanying each drug and to check, if necessary in consultation with a physician or specialist, whether the dosage schedules mentioned therein or the contraindications stated by the manufacturers differ from the statements made in the present book. Such examination is particularly important with drugs that are either rarely used or have been newly released on the market. Every dosage schedule or every form of application used is entirely at the user's own risk and responsibility. The authors and publishers request every user to report to the publishers any discrepancies or inaccuracies noticed. If errors in this work are found after publication, errata will be posted at www.thieme.com on the product description page.

Some of the product names, patents, and registered designs referred to in this book are in fact registered trademarks or proprietary names even though specific reference to this fact is not always made in the text. Therefore, the appearance of a name without designation as proprietary is not to be construed as a representation by the publisher that it is in the public domain.

Thieme Publishers Stuttgart
Rüdigerstrasse 14, 70469 Stuttgart, Germany
+49 [0]711 8931 421, customerservice@thieme.de

Thieme Publishers New York
333 Seventh Avenue, New York, NY 10001 USA
+1 800 782 3488, customerservice@thieme.com

Thieme Publishers Delhi
A-12, Second Floor, Sector-2, Noida-201301
Uttar Pradesh, India
+91 120 45 566 00, customerservice@thieme.in

Thieme Publishers Rio, Thieme Publicações Ltda.
Edifício Rodolpho de Paoli, 25º andar
Av. Nilo Peçanha, 50 – Sala 2508,
Rio de Janeiro 20020-906 Brasil
Tel: +55 21 3172-2297 / +55 21 3172-1896

Cover design: Thieme Publishing Group
Typesetting by Thomson Digital, India

Printed in India by Replika Press Private Ltd.

5 4 3 2 1

ISBN 978-3-13-199421-9

Also available as an e-book:
eISBN 978-3-13-199431-8

MIX
Paper from responsible sources
FSC® C016779

Contents

Videos

Video 3.1: Ophthalmologic examination in patients with orbital diseases.

Video 3.2: Optical coherence tomography of the retina and retinal pigment epithelium. (With permission of Heidelberg Engineering GmbH.)

Video 3.3: Fluorescein and indocyanine green angiography. (With permission of Heidelberg Engineering GmbH.)

Video 3.4: Optical coherence tomography of age-related macular degeneration with pigment epithelial detachment. (With permission of Heidelberg Engineering GmbH.)

Video 3.5: Indocyanine green angiography in age-related macular degeneration. (With permission of Heidelberg Engineering GmbH.)

Video 3.6: Course of an ENT examination in orbital diseases.

Video 5.1: Branch retinal vein occlusion: Fluorescein angiography. (With permission of Heidelberg Engineering GmbH.)

Video 14.1: Construction of a linear accelerator and principle of intensity-modulated radiation therapy. (With permission of Elektra GmbH, Hamburg.)

Video 15.1: Endonasal dacryocystorhinostomy.

Video 18.1: Endonasal endoscopic/microscopic approach to the orbit for excision of a tumor located medially to the optic nerve.

Video 18.2: Transantral approach to the orbit. The excision of a tumor located in the caudal/inferior orbital segment is demonstrated.

Video 18.3: Excision of a tumor located in the laterocranial orbital segment via lateral orbitotomy.

Video 18.4: Anterior orbitotomy with excision of an anteriorly located orbital tumor using a transpalpebral approach.

Video 18.5: Excision of a craniopharyngioma using a subfrontal approach.

Video 18.6: Excision of an extended tumor recurrence (squamous cell carcinoma) of the frontal skin. The patient underwent several previous surgical procedures along with intensive radiotherapy. However, he developed tumor recurrence with diffuse infiltration of the orbit. An orbital exenteration is performed with reconstruction of the forehead skin using a microvascular latissimus dorsi flap and lining of the orbital cavity using split skin.

Preface

Diagnosis and therapy of orbital diseases is an interdisciplinary challenge, in which several specialists are involved, i.e., otorhinolaryngologists, ophthalmologists, oncologists, pediatricians, radio-oncologists, neurosurgeons, anesthesiologists, maxillofacial surgeons, and radiologists. The purpose of this book is to describe this interdisciplinarity and to give an overview on the diagnosis and conservative and surgical treatment of orbital diseases. The work is introduced by a chapter on the topographical and surgical anatomy of the orbit along with a chapter on its pathophysiology. The authors are aware that this book can give only a brief overview on rhinologic and ophthalmologic diseases and must be limited to describe those involving the orbit. It cannot substitute the discipline-specific literature, which is referred to in many chapters. The same applies to the description of surgical approaches to the orbit, which has to be limited to standard surgical procedures.

The editors included their years of experience in this work, gained in numerous interdisciplinary orbit surgery courses, which have been conducted yearly in Hannover, Germany. Some important parts of the text are highlighted in "memorize-boxes." Complimentary videos available on Thieme MediaCenter round up this book.

Such a work is not possible without the help and support of numerous assistants and supporters. The editors want to thank especially: Mrs. C. Kirchhoff, Mr. A. Buchhorn, and Mrs. M. Peter, Institute of Functional and Applied Anatomy, Hannover Medical School, for preparation of the anatomical specimens and photo documentation and for the schematic anatomic illustrations; Dr. Murali Krishnan Varadharajan, Department of Ophthalmology, Nordstadt Clinic, Hannover, for schematic illustrations in Chapters 7.4.4, 15.1, and 16; Dr. Held-Wiechens for her critical review of the ophthalmological chapters; Dr. S. Graß, Department of Otorhinolaryngology, Head and Neck Surgery, Nordstadt Clinic, Hannover, for project coordination; and the residents, fellows, and coworkers of the Department of Ophthalmology, Nordstadt Clinic, for their support. Special thanks to the Department of Ophthalmology, University of Kiel, for provision of some clinical photographs. Furthermore, the editors want to express a special thank to Mr. Stephan Konnry, Thieme Publishers, Stuttgart, for his support. This book could not appear without the help of these people! Thank you all!

Hans-J. Welkoborsky, MD, DDS, PhD
Burkhard Wiechens, MD, PhD
Michael L. Hinni, MD

Contributors

Stephan Behrendt, MD, PhD
Department of Ophthalmology
Rendsburg Clinic
Rendsburg, Germany

Manuel Bernal-Sprekelsen, MD, PhD
Full Professor and Director
Department of Otorhinolaryngology
Hospital Clinic
University of Barcelona
Barcelona, Spain

Hans Christiansen, MD
Professor and Chairman
Department of Radiotherapy
Hannover Medical School
Hannover, Germany

Karel De Leeuw, DDS, MD, MBA, FACS
Consultant
Department Of Otolaryngology
Mayo Clinic
Phoenix, Arizona, USA

Cordula M.C. Deichmueller, MD
Department of Otorhinolaryngology, Head and Neck Surgery
Nordstadt Clinic
Academic Hospital
Hannover, Germany

Harald Essig, Priv.-Doz. Dr. med. Dr. med. dent.
Senior Consultant
Department of Craniomaxillofacial and Oral Surgery
University Hospital Zurich
Zurich, Switzerland

Nils-Claudius Gellrich, MD, DDS, PhD
Professor and Chairman
Department of Maxillofacial Surgery
Hannover Medical School
Hannover, Germany

Sylvia Graß, MD
Department of Otorhinolaryngology, Head and Neck Surgery
Nordstadt Clinic
Hannover, Germany

Robert M. Hermann, MD
Consultant
Center for Radiation Oncology and Therapy
Westerstede, Germany

Michael L. Hinni, MD
Professor and Chairman
Department of Otolaryngology, Head and Neck Surgery
Mayo Clinic
Scottsdale, Arizona, USA

Jan-Peter A.H. Jantzen, MD, PhD, DEAA
Professor and Chairman
Department of Anesthesiology, Intensive Care Medicine, and Pain Management
Academic Teaching Hospital Nordstadt
Hannover, Germany

George J. Kahaly, MD, PhD
Professor of Medicine and Endocrinology/Metabolism
Chief physician, Endocrine Outpatient Clinic
Director, Molecular Thyroid Research Laboratory
Department of Medicine
Johannes Gutenberg University Medical Center
Mainz, Germany

Theresia Kraft, PhD
Professor
Institute of Molecular and Cell Physiology
Hannover Medical School
Hannover, Germany

Devyani Lal, MD
Associate Professor and Consultant, Otolaryngology-Head and Neck Surgery
Consultant, Neurological Surgery
Mayo Clinic
Phoenix, Arizona, USA

Mauricio López-Chacón, MD
Department of Otorhinolaryngology, Head and Neck Surgery
Hospital Clinic
Academic Hospital Barcelona
Barcelona, Spain

Andreas Neumann, MD, PhD
Professor and Chairman
Department of Otorhinolaryngology, Head and Neck Surgery
Lukas Clinic Neuss
Neuss, Germany

Athina Pangalu, MD
Vice Chairman
Department of Neuroradiology
University Hospital Zurich
Zurich, Switzerland

Majeed Rana, MD, DDS
Associate Professor
Department of Craniomaxillofacial Surgery
Hannover Medical School
Hannover, Germany

Prof. Dr. Dr. Martin Rücker
Director
Clinic for Craniomaxillofacial Surgery and Oral Surgery
Center for Dental Medicine
University Hospital Zurich
Zurich, Switzerland

I. Erol Sandalcioglu, MD, PhD
Professor and Chairman
Department of Neurosurgery
Nordstadt Clinic
Academic Hospital
Hannover, Germany

Andreas Schmiedl, MD, PhD
Professor
Institute of Functional and Applied Anatomy
Hannover Medical School
Hannover, Germany

Paul Schumann, Dr. med., Dr. med. dent., PD
Senior Consultant
Department of Oral and Maxillofacial Surgery
University Hospital Zurich
Zurich, Switzerland

Bernd Schwefler, MD
Department of Anesthesiology and Intensive Care Medicine
Nordstadt Clinic
Academic Hospital
Hannover, Germany

Ulrich Sure, MD
Professor and Chairman
Department of Neurosurgery
University Hospital Essen
Essen, Germany

Anton Valavanis, MD
Professor and Chairman
Department of Neuroradiology
University Hospital Zurich
Zurich, Switzerland

Meghana Anika Varde, MS, FEBO, FMRF (Oculoplastics)
Consultant
Department of Ophthalmology
Kantonsspital St. Gallen
St. Gallen, Switzerland

Hans-J. Welkoborsky, MD, DDS, PhD
Professor and Chairman
Department of Otorhinolaryngology, Head and Neck Surgery
Nordstadt Clinic
Academic Hospital and Children's Hospital "Auf der Bult"
Hannover, Germany

Burkhard Wiechens, MD, PhD
Professor and Chairman
Department of Ophthalmology
Nordstadt Clinic
Academic Hospital
Hannover, Germany

Ludwig Wilkens, Prof. Dr.
Head
Institute of Pathology, Klinikum Region Hannover
Klinikum Nordstadt
Hannover, Germany

Chapter 1

Topographical Anatomy of the Orbit

1

1 Topographical Anatomy of the Orbit

A. Schmiedl

1.1 Introduction

The orbit is the bony basis for suspension and positioning of the eyeball (bulb of the eye; bulbus oculi) and its adnexa. Any soft tissue of the visual apparatus is located inside the orbit. It is characterized by much content in a very limited bony compartment, and by particularly thin bony borders toward the paranasal sinuses. It is also a thoroughfare of pathways to and from the face. Due to the presence of numerous blood vessels in this field (i.e., 10 branches of the ophthalmic artery, two large venous vessels along with their afferent vessels), significant hemorrhage can occur during operative procedures. Furthermore, five cranial nerves along with their branches, and vegetative nerve fibers are located inside the orbit, which can be threatened or compromised by surgery.

1.2 Shape, Borders, Orifices, and Topographical Relations

The orbit is located underneath the anterior cranial fossa (fossa cranii anterior, ▶ Fig. 1.1) and is shaped like a four-sided pyramid whose base opens to the face (orbital aditus, ▶ Fig. 1.2). Its axis proceeds from the pyramid basis (anterior) backward medially to the optic nerve canal at to the root of the lesser wing of the sphenoid bone (apex of the pyramid). As the apexes of both orbits are located medially, the longitudinal axis of both orbits are directed exteriorly, and the medial and lateral wall form an angle to each other of about 45° (▶ Fig. 1.1, ▶ Fig. 1.2). The average dimensions of the orbit[1] demonstrate that there is not much space (▶ Table 1.1). The orbit has its largest extension 1 cm behind the anterior orbital rim.[2] The distance between the reverse side of the eyeball and the entrance of the optic nerve canal is about 18 mm.[2]

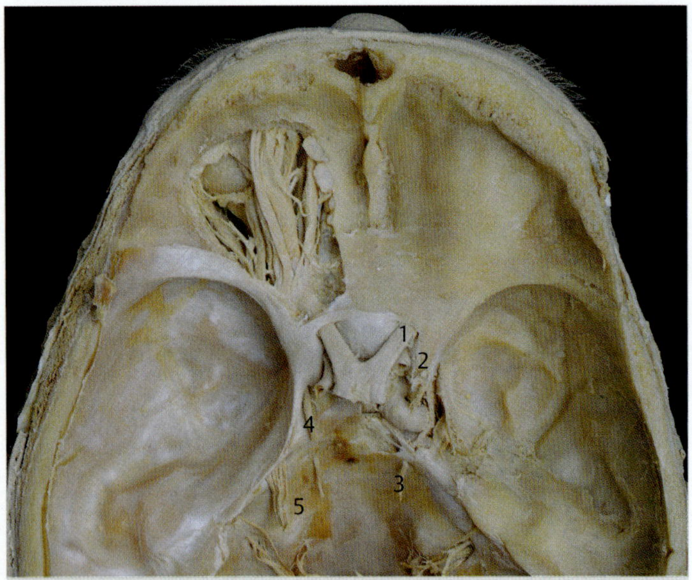

Fig. 1.1 Base of the skull with the orbit, one sided opened. Left: orbital part of the frontal bone, periorbita and adipose body removed. 1, optic nerve; 2, ophthalmic artery; 3, abducens nerve; 4, oculomotor nerve; 5, trigeminal nerve.

1.2.1 Bony Orbital Walls

The orbital aditus is limited by an orbital ridge (orbital margin), which is formed by three bones. The upper orbital ridge (supra-orbital margin) is constituted by the frontal bone; the lower orbital ridge (infra-orbital margin) by the zygomatic bone (laterally) and the maxilla (medially). Altogether the entire bony orbital walls consist of seven different bones (▶ Fig. 1.2).[4,5,6]

The major part of the orbital roof is formed by the concave vaulted orbital part of the frontal bone (▶ Fig. 1.1a). The posterior 1.5-cm wide flattened part of the roof is shaped by the minor wing of the sphenoid bone. Normally both bones are fairly strong and do not fracture following violent trauma to the orbit. Anteriorly in the upper part of the orbit and medially is located a small fossa for the roller cartilage (trochlea), which serves as a fulcrum for the tendon of the superior obliquus muscle (see ▶ Fig. 1.15). The large lacrimal fossa lies anteriorly and laterally in the orbit (▶ Fig. 1.2).

Table 1.1 Dimensions of the orbit[1,3]

Diameter vertical	35 mm
Diameter horizontal	40 mm
Medial wall	45–50 mm (ridge of the lacrimal bone to the superior orbital fissure)
Lateral wall	40 mm (orbital ridge to superior orbital fissure)
Depth	45–55 mm (orbital ridge to orbital apex and orbit nerve canal)
Volume	30 mL

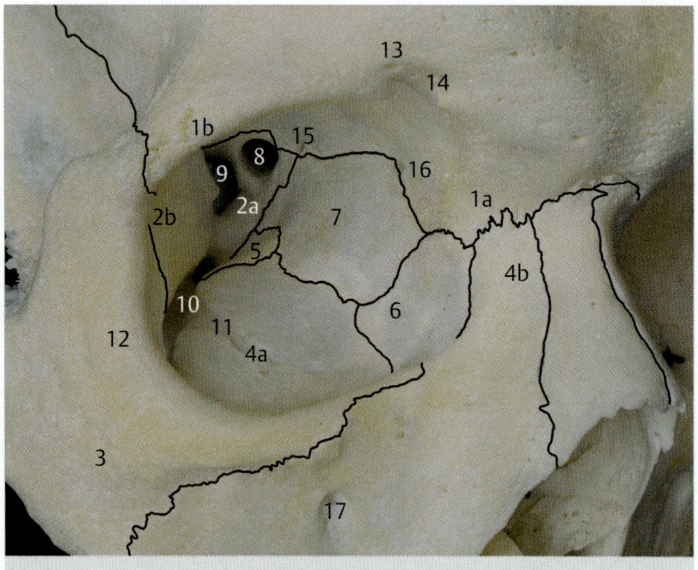

Fig. 1.2 Bony orbit, right. View obliquely from the front. 1a, frontal bone, orbital part; 1b, frontal bone, zygomatic process; 2a, sphenoid bone, lesser wing; 2b, sphenoid bone, greater wing; 3, zygomatic bone; 4a, maxillary bone, orbital surface (facies orbitalis); 4b, maxillary bone, frontal process; 5, palatine bone, orbital process; 6, lacrimal bone;7, ethmoidal bone, orbital lamina; 8, optic canal; 9, supra-orbital fissure; 10, infra-orbital fissure; 11, infra-orbital groove/canal; 12, zygomaticofacial foramen; 13, supra-orbital foramen; 14, frontal incisure; 15, posterior ethmoidal foramen; 16, anterior ethmoidal foramen; 17, infra-orbital foramen.

The major wing of the sphenoid bone forms the major part of the lateral orbital wall. Anteriorly the zygomatic bone and the zygomatic process of the frontal bone are also involved in forming the bony wall. The zygomatic bone thickens caudally, forms the anterior vault of the inferior orbital fissure (▶ Fig. 1.3), and divides the orbit from the subcutaneous adipose tissue of the cheeks.[1] A small protuberance (Whitnall tubercle) is located about 4 to 5 mm behind the lateral orbital ridge.[7] The lateral palpebral ligament, the Lockwood-ligament, and the control band of the lateral rectus muscle (Check ligament) along with parts of the aponeurosis of the superior palpebral levator muscle are connected with the Whitnall-tubercle.[1] The lateral orbital wall is anteriorly fairly thick and protects the orbit from lateral traumatic violence.[1] The posterior part, however, is significantly thinner and can therefore serve as an approach for performing lateral orbitotomy[1] (▶ Fig. 1.3). The temporalis muscle, which fills the temporal fossa underneath the zygomatic arch, is located at the posterior and lateral surface of the lateral orbital wall. Adjacent to the lateral orbital wall is the temporal squama, which forms the lateral wall of the medial cranial fossa. The distance between the lateral border of the orbit, which is suitable for osteotomy, and the border of the medial cranial fossa is only 12 to 13 mm in men, and 7 to 8 mm in women.[8]

The wall that forms the orbital floor is very short, shaped as an equilateral triangle, and consists mainly of the 0.5-mm-thick orbital surface of the maxilla. The orbital surface of the zygomatic bone (lateral anteriorly) and the orbital process of the palatine bone (posteriorly) play minor parts in shaping the orbital floor.

The medial orbital wall is formed by the frontal process of the maxillary bone, by the lacrimal bone, by the minor wing of the sphenoid bone, and by the orbital lamina of the ethmoid bone (synonyms: lamina papyracea; lamina orbitalis). The bony wall that divides the orbit from the posterior ethmoidal cells (cellulae ethmoidales posteriores) is quite thin, only about 0.3 mm thick (▶ Fig. 1.4). However, the honeycomb-like structure of the pneumatized ethmoidal cells has a stabilizing effect, so that fractures occur less in the medial wall than in the slightly thicker orbital floor over the maxillary sinus.[1] On the other hand, the lamina papyracea can easily be affected by inflammations or by tumors of sinogenic origin, and can easily be destroyed during surgical procedures in this area.[1] The orbit is frequently affected by inflammations in the ethmoid cells. The roof of the ethmoid sinus is formed by the bone junction between the orbital lamina of the ethmoid bone and the orbital part of the frontal bone. The anterior cranial fossa along with the frontal lobe of the brain, which is covered by dura, is located above this bone junction. The medial wall exhibits anteriorly a deep cavity (lacrimal sac fossa) that contains the sacculus lacrimalis (lacrimal sac). This cavity is limited anteriorly by the infra-orbital margin and the anterior crista of the maxilla, and posteriorly by the posterior lacrimal crista of the lacrimal bone (▶ Fig. 1.2). The orbital apex is shaped by the sphenoid and the palatine bones.

1.2.2 Orbital Foramina

The bones of the orbital wall contain several foramina that open to the middle cranial fossa, the infratemporal fossa or the pterygopalatine fossa, or to the face and support various different pathways (▶ Table 1.2; ▶ Fig. 1.2).[4,5,6]

The foramen of the **optic nerve canal** (canalis opticus) is located in the orbital apex of the minor wing of the sphenoid bone. The optic nerve canal is separated from the superior orbital fissure by the lower root of the minor wing of the sphenoid bone. This thin bony lamella also limits the optic nerve canal laterally.[1] The ophthalmic artery and the optic nerve pass through the optic nerve canal from the medial cranial fossa into the orbit. The optic nerve enters the orbit with an angle of 45° from the midline (▶ Fig. 1.1). Glioma of the optic nerve and aneurysms of the ophthalmic artery frequently lead to a dilatation of the canal. The **superior orbital fissure** (fissura orbitalis superior) is located beneath the optic nerve canal between the major wing, the minor wing, and the corpus of the sphenoid bone (▶ Fig. 1.1, ▶ Fig. 1.2). The superior orbital fissure is large medially and slim

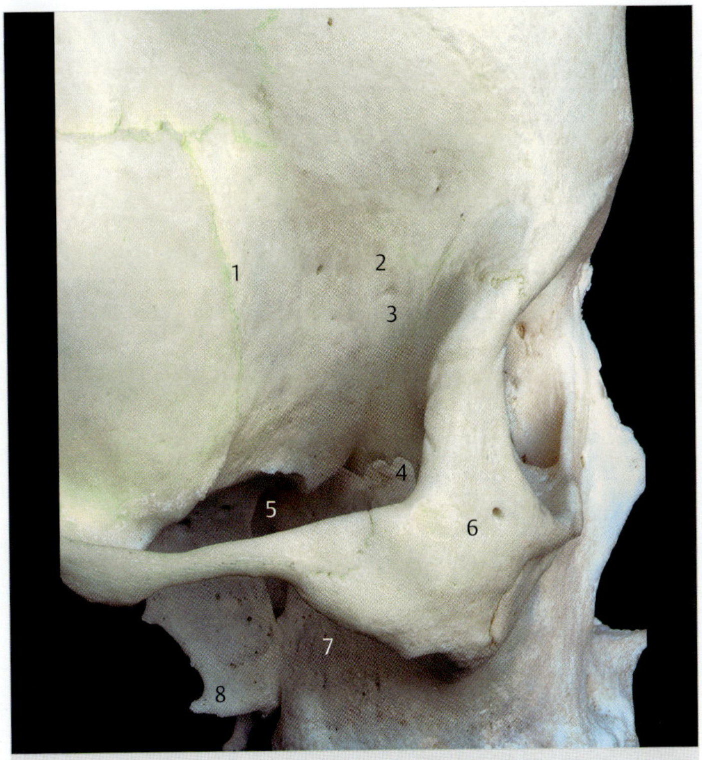

Fig. 1.3 Lateral wall of the orbit. 1, sphenosquamosal suture; 2, greater wing of the sphenoid bone; 3, sphenozygomatic suture; 4, inferior orbital fissure; 5, pterygopalatine fossa; 6, zygomatic bone; 7, infratemporal fossa; 8, pterygoid process.

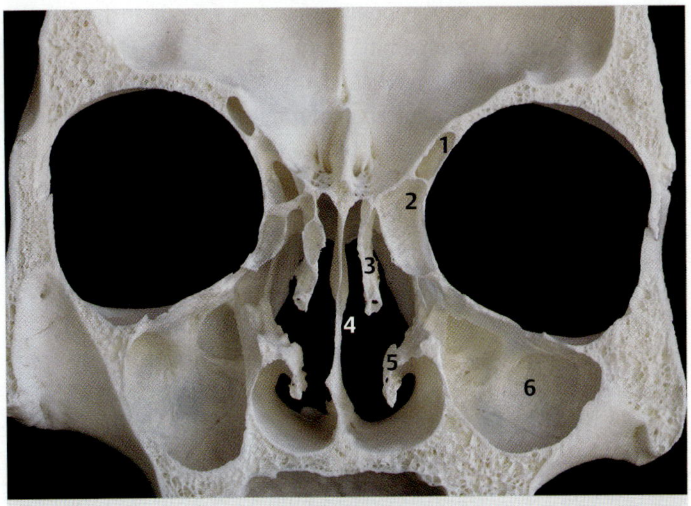

Fig. 1.4 Viscerocranium; frontal saw cut, at the level of the orbit. 1, frontal sinus; 2, ethmoid cells; 3, medial nasal concha; 4, nasal septum; 5, inferior nasal concha; 6, maxillary bone.

Table 1.2 Points of passage for pathways from and to the orbit

Canal	Localization in the orbit and orifice	Bone	Pathway
Optic nerve canal	Posterior upper part of the orbit Medial cranial fossa	Minor wing of the sphenoid bone	Optic nerve; ophthalmic artery
Superior orbital fissure	Posterior upper part of the orbit Medial cranial fossa	Between major wing and minor wing of the sphenoid bone	Oculomotor nerve; trochlear nerve; abducens nerve; ophthalmic nerve; superior ophthalmic vein
Inferior orbital fissure	Posterior lower part of the orbit Infratemporal fossa Pterygopalatine fossa	Between maxilla and major wing of the sphenoid bone	Zygomatic nerve; infra-orbital nerve; inferior ophthalmic vein
Posterior ethmoid foramen	Medial cranial fossa Posterior ethmoid	Between frontal and ethmoid bone	Posterior ethmoid nerve; posterior ethmoid artery
Anterior ethmoid foramen	Medial cranial fossa Anterior ethmoid	Between frontal bone and ethmoid bone	Anterior ethmoid nerve; anterior ethmoid artery
Nasolacrimal canal	Medial Inferior nasal meatus	Maxilla	Nasolacrimal duct
Zygomatico-orbital foramen	Lateral Face	Zygomatic bone	Zygomatico-orbital nerve
Zygomaticofacial foramen			Zygomaticofacial nerve
Frontal foramen Supra-orbital foramen	Frontal region	Frontal bone	Branches of the supra-orbital nerve and supra-orbital artery
Infra-orbital foramen	Face	Maxilla	Infra-orbital nerve; infra-orbital artery

laterally. Parts of the fissure that do not contain pathways are covered with and closed by connective tissue, which can contain smooth muscle cells. The fissure is divided into three sections according to the origin of the intra-orbital muscles: (1) the medial section, which is closed; (2) the oculomotor nerve, the nasociliar nerve, and the abducens nerve pass through the intermediate section, which is framed by the outer eyeball muscles; (3) the superior ophthalmic vein, the frontal nerve, and the lacrimal nerve, along with the trochlear nerve, pass through the narrower lateral section of the fissure (▶ Fig. 1.5).

The **inferior orbital fissure** (fissura orbitalis inferior) is a cleft about 20 mm wide and is located posteriorly between major wing of the sphenoid bone and the maxilla. It maintains the connection between the orbit and the infratemporal fossa and pterygopalatine fossa. It is closed by connective tissue, which contains smooth muscle cells, except at the points of passage for branches of the inferior ophthalmic vein coming from the pterygoid plexus, infra-orbital nerve, zygomatic nerve, and smaller branches of the pterygopalatine ganglion. The inferior orbital fossa extends more anteriorly than the superior orbital fissure, and **terminates 20 mm ahead of the anterior orbital ridge**[1] (▶ Fig. 1.5).

The **posterior ethmoid foramen** (foramen ethmoidale posterius) is located at the posterior upper ridge of the lamina papyracea of the ethmoid bone. This foramen is entered by the posterior ethmoid artery and vein along with the posterior ethmoid nerve, which proceed to the ethmoid cells. The **anterior ethmoid foramen** (foramen ethmoidale anterius) is located at the anterior upper ridge of the orbital lamina. The anterior ethmoid artery and vein along with the anterior ethmoid nerve are leaving the orbit through this foramen. Both foramina are located at the bone junction between the orbital lamina of the ethmoid bone and the orbital part of the frontal bone, approximately 24 to 25 mm dorsal to the anterior ridge of the lacrimal bone[1] (▶ Fig. 1.2).

The supra-orbital margin of the orbital aditus has two variable notches or foramina: the **frontal incisure/foramen**, and the **supra-orbital incisures/foramen**, with branches of the ophthalmic nerve and supra-orbital artery passing through (▶ Fig. 1.2).

The **zygomatico-orbital foramen**, through which the zygomatic nerve enters, is located at the orbital surface of the

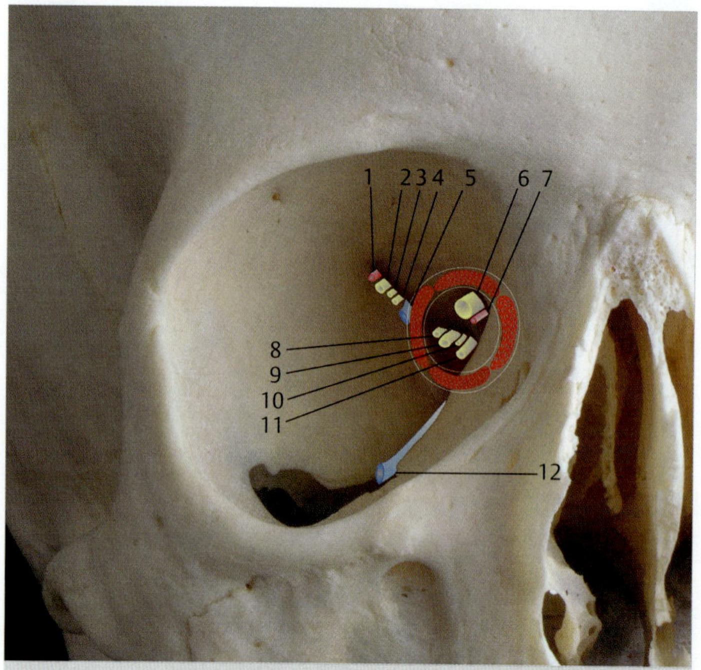

Fig. 1.5 Entry of pathways in the orbit. 1, recurrent meningeal branch; 2, lacrimal nerve; 3, trochlear nerve; 4, frontal nerve; 5, ophthalmic superior vein; 6, optic nerve; 7, ophthalmic artery; 8, oculomotor nerve, superior branch; 9, abducens nerve; 10, nasociliary nerve; 11, oculomotor nerve, lower branch; 12, inferior ophthalmic vein.

zygomatic bone. The canal opens exteriorly into the zygomaticofacial foramen and zygomaticotemporal foramen, through which the correspondingly named sensory terminal branches of the zygomatic nerve along with similar named vessels pass to the temporal region and cheek. These pathways might be injured during lateral orbitotomy, when the temporal muscle is removed.

The posterior part of the orbital floor contains the **infra-orbital sulcus**, which extends anteriorly as the **infra-orbital canal** to the infra-orbital foramen, through which the infra-orbital nerve and the infra-orbital artery reach the face (▸ Fig. 1.2).

1.2.3 Topographic Relations of the Orbit

Due to its topographical position in the head, the orbit has close relations to several areas of the face (▸ Fig. 1.4). The anterior cranial fossa with the frontal lobe of the brain (telencephalon), which is covered by dura, is part of the orbital roof. The orbit has close relations to the medial cranial fossa, which contains the dura-covered temporal lobe of the telencephalon, via the optic nerve canal and superior orbital fissure. The inferior orbital fissure connects the orbit to the pterygopalatine and infratemporal fossae (▸ Fig. 1.3). The orbital floor, the orbital roof, and the medial wall separate the orbit from the paranasal sinuses with distinctly thin bony walls (caudal medially is the maxillary sinus; cranial anteriorly is the frontal sinus; medially is the ethmoid sinus) (▸ Fig. 1.4). However, it should be considered that the paranasal sinuses develop during youth and adolescence and reach their final extension almost in adulthood. Furthermore, the orbit has close relations to the nasal cavity (cavitas nasi) (▸ Fig. 1.4). Inflammations and tumors of the orbit can infiltrate and affect the neighboring regions and vice versa. Close interdisciplinary cooperation is required for considering their management.

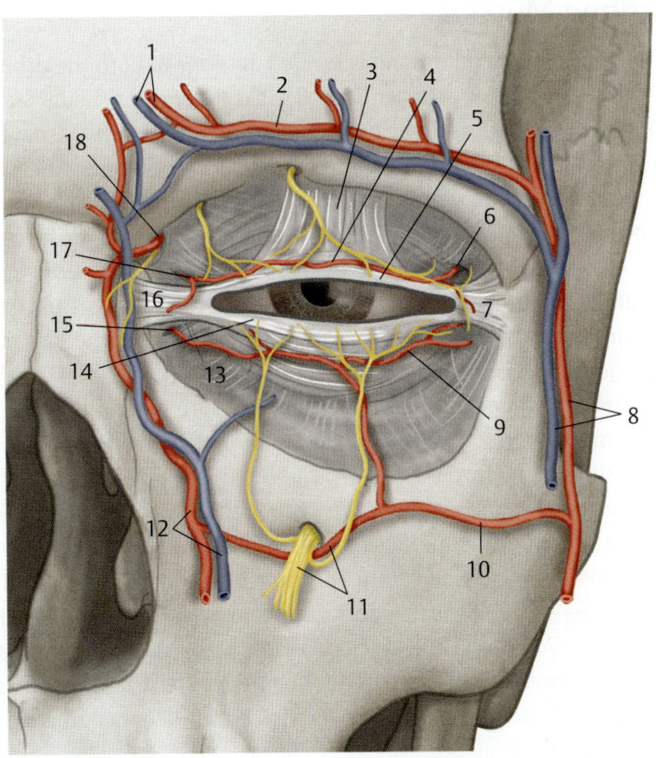

Fig. 1.6 Orbit entrance (aditus orbitalis) with pathways. The periorbital vessel coronary with arteries of the supply area of the internal carotid artery (supra-orbital artery, lateral palpebral arteries of the lacrimal artery, medial palpebral arteries) and of the external carotid artery (facial artery, angular artery, infra-orbital artery). 1, supratrochlear artery, vein, and nerve; 2, supra-orbital artery, vein, and nerve; 3, levator palpebrae superioris muscle; 4, arcus palpebralis superior; 5, upper tarsus; 6, lateral palpebral artery; 7, lateral palpebral ligament; 8, superficial temporal artery and vein; 9, arcus palpebralis inferior; 10, transversal facial artery; 11, infra-orbital nerve and artery; 12, angular artery; 13, orbital septum; 14, lower tarsus; 15, medial palpebral artery; 16, medial palpebral ligament; 17, medial palpebral artery; 18, infratrochlear artery, vein, and nerve.

1.3 Protective Apparatus of the Eye

1.3.1 Orbital Septum

The orbital septum (septum orbitale) (▸ Fig. 1.6) is a thin plate consisting of collagen and elastic connective tissue. It represents a physical barrier against pathogens and stabilizes the postseptal adipose tissue in the orbit.[1] The septum is fixed at the upper and lower orbital ridges, surrounds the eyeball, and extends to the upper lid plate (tarsus). It inserts medially at the lacrimal bone. It joints laterally with the lateral palpebral ligament and the superior levator palpebrae muscle aponeurosis.[1] The septum inserts at the lower lid at the lower ridge of the tarsus. It gets thinner medially, separates from the medial palpebral ligament, and extends at the back side of the smooth superior tarsal muscle behind the lacrimal sac to the lacrimal bone. Preseptally the septum is covered by the orbicularis oculi muscle and the skin.

1.3.2 Eyelids

Macro anatomy and blood supply

The eyebrows, hair-bearing elongated regions of skin that protect the eye from humidity and sweat, are located at the upper orbital rim (▸ Fig. 1.7). The eyelids (palpebrae) are mobile ectodermal folds that enable protection from excess light and dazzle and preserve the cornea from exsiccation, mechanical damage, and—via the opticofacial winking reflex—from foreign body impact on or

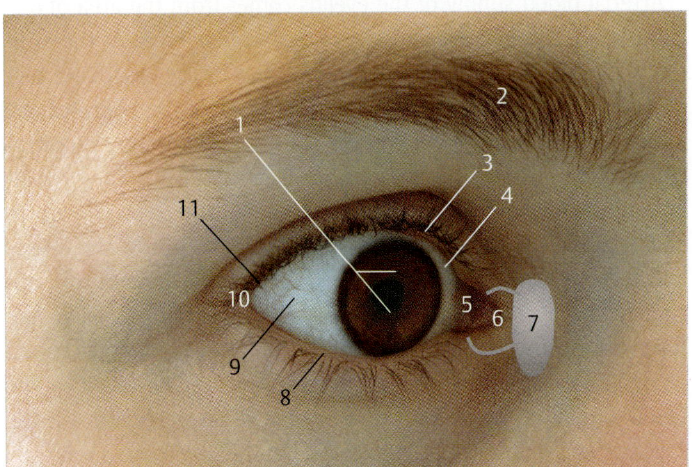

Fig. 1.7 Right eye with the lacrimal apparatus. 1, iris with pupil; 2, eyebrow (supercilium); 3, upper eyelid with eyelashes; 4, angulus medialis oculi; 5, lacrimal caruncle; 6, medial canthus; 7, lacrimal saccule with upper and lower lacrimal channels; 8, lower eyelid; 9, conjunctiva of the bulb; 10, external canthus; 11, angulus lateralis oculi.

into the eye. The lacrimal fluid is dispensed over the cornea with every closure of the eyelid. The eyebrow separates the upper lid from the frontal skin; the zygomatic lid sulcus separates the lower lid from the skin of the cheek. Laterally and medially both lids are connected to each other via the lateral and medial palpebral commissure. Thus both ends of the palpebral fissures (rima palpebrarum) are encircled at the inner and outer canthi. While the lateral canthus (angulus oculi lateralis) is acute-angled, the medial canthus is more roundly shaped and encircles a mucosal island, the lacrimal caruncula (▸ Fig. 1.7). The eyelid skin is very soft, contains only little adipose tissue, and is mobile. Due to the soft structure of the subcutaneous tissue of the eyelids, inflammations, hemorrhage, or fluid retention can lead to significant swelling, so that the palpebral fissure cannot be opened. Due to their rectangular cross-section[1] the margins of the eyelids form an anterior limbus or margin and a posterior limbus (limbus anterior palpebrae; limbus posterior palpebrae). A number of eyelashes (cilia), which are arranged in 3 to 4 rows, originate from the margins of the eyelid between anterior and posterior limbus and spread protectively over the palpebral fissure. The external eyelid surface (facies anterior palpebrae) of both canthi transitions to the posterior surface (facies posterior palpebrae), which is covered by the conjunctiva. The conjunctiva at the reverse side of the eyelids (conjuctiva palpebrae) transitions to the eyeball conjunctiva at its fornix region (fornix conjunctiva superior and inferior). Thus, a pocket is formed, which is called conjunctival sac (saccus conjunctivalis). The conjunctiva at the palpebral fold is called the conjunctiva fornicis. The semi-oval lid plates (tarsi) are the fibrous tissue bases for the eyelids and give them form and stability. A constitutional or age-related relaxation of the orbital septum, which extends into the tarsus, can cause a prolapse of parts of intraorbital adipose tissue with consecutive visible protrusion of the upper lids and impairment of the aesthetic appearance of the eye.[1] The lid plate of the upper lid (superior tarsus) is about 10 mm high; the lid plate of the lower lid (inferior tarsus) is about 5 mm high. Both lid plates are about 25 mm wide and 1 mm thick. They are elastic, suspended with a medial and lateral palpebral ligament on both sides of the orbital aditus[1] (▸ Fig. 1.6). The medial ligament encircles the lacrimal sac.

Arterial blood supply of the eyelids comes from the area of distribution of the internal and external carotid arteries. At the orbital aditus can be found some thin branches of the lacrimal artery as well as from the lacrimal nerve. Branches of the supra-orbital artery and vein along with branches of the supra-orbital, supratrochlear, and infratrochlear nerve course medially. The vessels accomplish a vascular corona anterior to the septum, which encircles the orbital entrance (▸ Fig. 1.6). Branches of the lateral and medial palpebral artery become curved anteriorly of the septum to the eyelids and form the arcus palpebralis superior and inferior for the blood supply of the eyelids and conjunctival tunica (▸ Fig. 1.6). The anterior ciliary arteries are also involved in the blood supply of the conjunctiva. Venous drainage occurs via the superior and inferior ophthalmic veins to the cavernous sinus.

Locomotor System of the Eyelids: Lid Muscles

Two striped and two unstriped (smooth) muscles control the voluntary and involuntary eyelid movements.

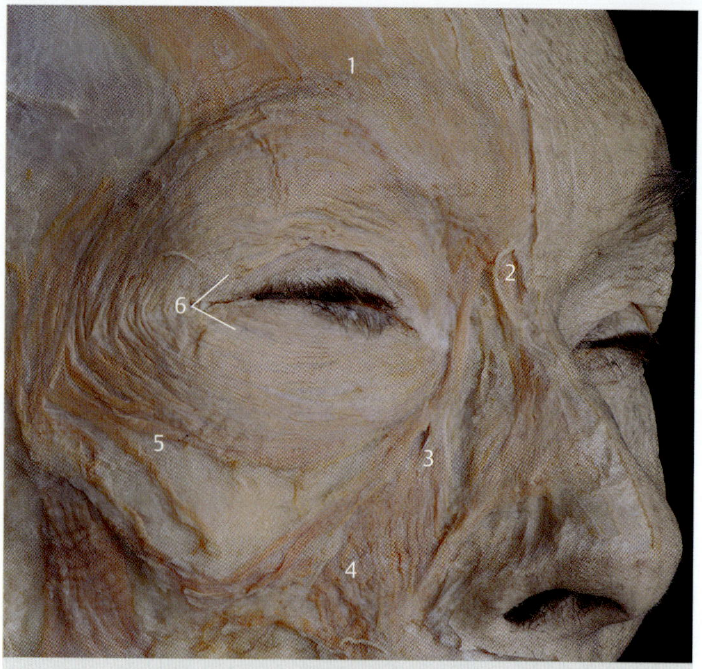

Fig. 1.8 Facial muscles. 1, occipitofrontalis, anterior belly; 2, procerus muscle; 3, levator labii superioris alaeque nasi; 4, levator labii superioris; 5, orbicularis oculi muscle, orbital part; 6, orbicularis oculi muscle, palpebral part.

Striped Muscles

The orbicularis oculi muscle is located anterior to both the orbital septum and the lid plate (▸ Fig. 1.8). It is innervated by the facial nerve. The orbital part of this muscle encircles the orbital margin and effects a voluntary closure of the eye. The external sheet of each eyelid contains muscular tracts of the palpebral part of the orbicularis oculi muscle (Riolan muscle). The lid closure is released by contraction of the palpebral part. It can be performed voluntarily, but in most cases it proceeds involuntarily. The lacrimal part of this muscle, on the other hand, encircles the lacrimal canaliculi and is necessary for lacrimation. Muscle fibers of the levator palpebrae superioris muscle, which are innervated by the oculomotor nerve, course from the minor wing of the sphenoid bone thoroughly through the orbit to the upper lid, where its tendon fans in two layers: one deep layer, which inserts at the upper lid plate, and the superficial layers, which course between the orbicularis muscle fibers into the skin of the lid. Paresis of the orbicularis muscle leads to an incomplete eyelid closure (lagophthalmus). Voluntary eyelid closure in these cases leads to an upward movement of the eyeball when the outer eye muscles are unimpaired—hence, the white sclera is visible (Bell phenomenon).

Unstriped Muscles

Smooth muscles are located in both lid plates, which are innervated by the sympathetic nervous system. The superior tarsal muscle courses from the lower surface of the superior levator palpebrae muscle to the upper rim of the lid plate, the inferior tarsal muscle to the lower lid plate. Both muscles, so-called "Müller eyelid lifting muscle," lead to an extension of the lid plate during contraction.[1]

Palpebral Limbus and Palpebral Glands

The lid rim (palpebral limbus) is blunt-shaped anteriorly and sharp-edged posteriorly. Excretory ducts of large sebaceous glands (sebaceous ciliary glands [Zeis glands]) open to hair funnels of the anterior lid rim for greasing the cilia. Close to the cilia are also located the sudoriferous glands, apocrine sweat glands, (Moll glands). About 30 tubuloalveolar holocrine glands are located in the lamina propria of the upper lid, about 20 of these glands are located in the lower lid (tarsal glands; meibomian glands), which open with their own excretory ducts at the posterior lid rim.[4] Ectropionization of the upper lid exposes the tarsal glands as yellowish spotted lines. Their sebaceous-like secretion is extracted by contraction of the Riolan muscle for lubricating the lid rim and preventing lacrimal overflow. Diseases of the palpebral glands can present as a chalazion, which is characterized by a painless small node in the lid due to an obstruction of the excretory duct of a palpebral gland, or as a hordeolum, which is a painful inflammation of a palpebral gland.

1.3.3 Lacrimal Apparatus

Parts of the lacrimal apparatus, which consists of the lacrimal gland and the lacrimal ducts, are located in the bony orbit. The lacrimal gland is found superior to the lateral canthus in the anterior upper outer orbital quadrant above the eyeball in the frontal bone recess behind the orbital septum (lacrimal gland fossa). The lacrimal gland has dimensions of ca. 20 mm × 12 mm × 5 mm and is divided by the superior levator palpebrae muscle into a larger orbital part and a smaller palpebral part, which lies at the transition zone between conjunctiva and eyelid.[1] However, this division is not complete, as both parts are connected by a parenchymatous bridge dorsal to the muscle. The upper part of the gland is limited anteriorly by the orbital septum and preaponeurotic adipose tissue, dorsally by the intraorbital adipose tissue, and laterally by the frontal bone. The lower part of the lacrimal gland is located underneath the aponeurosis of the superior levator palpebrae muscle in the subaponeurotic Jones space.[1] The palpebral part is medially separated from the conjunctiva by the superior tarsal muscle. Several smaller glands (Krause and Wolfring glands) are distributed over the upper lid conjunctiva. Tear fluid reaches the superior conjunctival fornix via 1 to 5 excretory ducts in the orbital part, and 6 to 8 smaller excretory ducts in the palpebral part. The tear fluid is distributed evenly over the entire cornea by blinking; it runs from temporal to nasal into the medial canthus and collects in the lacrimal lacus, which is located in the inferior conjunctival fornix. The openings of the lacrimal canaliculi are prominent to the lacrimal lacus as upper and lower, ca. 0.25 mm and 0.3 mm, roundish, oval or slitlike lacrimal points.[5] These lacrimal points are located on a small peak at the medial inner surface of the upper and lower lid rims (lacrimal papilla),[4] which are visible when the eyelid is elevated. The tear fluid is cleared from the lacrimal points in the upper and lower lids into the lacrimal sac via upper and lower hooklike curved lacrimal canalicull, ca. 10 mm long (▶ Fig. 1.7). The lacrimal canaliculi course 2 mm vertically and then, after widening (ampulla of the lacrimal canalicula), ca. 8 mm horizontally. The vertical part is surrounded by fibers of the orbicular oculi muscle (pars lacrimalis), the contraction of which facilitates the drainage. In about 70% of cases, a junction occurs of the two canaliculi, which course parallel to the lid rim, into a common canal 1 to 2 mm long, which then terminates in the lacrimal sac, which is limited by both medial crura of the palpebral ligament. A cupula of the lacrimal sac surpasses the upper lacrimal canaliculus by about 3 mm (fornix sacculi lacrimalis).[9]

The lacrimal sac is about 12 mm × 6 mm × 5 mm[3] and lies—covered by the periorbita—in a depression of the medial bony orbital wall (lacrimal sac fossa), which is formed by the posterior lacrimal crista of the lacrimal bone and the anterior lacrimal crista of the maxillary bone (▶ Fig. 1.2). The bone in the lacrimal sac fossa region is significantly thin, so that it is reasonable to perform endonasal lacrimal sac surgery (dacryocystorhinostomy) medially to the sac. Erectile tissue, which is suitable for tear drainage, encircles the lacrimal sac. In case of emotions or foreign bodies penetrating the conjunctival sac, filling of the blood vessels in the cavernous tissue occurs, which leads to congestion of the nasolacrimal duct with subsequent tear drainage over the cheeks.

The ca. 15 mm long and 5 to 6 mm wide nasolacrimal duct is a bony canal that is coated by pseudostratified columnar epithelium with goblet cells. The walls of the canal comprise the maxillary bone, the lacrimal bone, and the inferior nasal concha.[4] This canal courses caudally, laterally and posteriorly and terminates in the inferior nasal meatus. Thus, it projects on a line connecting the medial canthus and the first premolar tooth of the upper jaw. Probing of the nasolacrimal duct is performed in this direction. A reflux of the tear fluid is prevented by multiple mucosal folds with valvelike function. The first valve is the Rosenmüller valve, which is located at the entrance of the lacrimal sac to the common canaliculus; the second valve is the Krause valve, which is located between lacrimal sac and the entrance of the nasolacrimal duct; and finally the Hasner valve develops at the opening of the nasolacrimal duct into the inferior nasal meatus. The Hasner valve has a check function, preventing air penetration into the duct during sneezing.[3] Capillary forces in the canaliculi support tear drainage. Furthermore, a widening of the vertical parts with intensification of a suction effect is caused by lid opening. Every day about 500 mL of tear fluid is produced, which is stimulated by parasympathetic nerve fibers originating in the facial nerve. Lack of lid closure leads to a drying of the cornea, as the tear fluid cannot be distributed equally over the cornea.

In conclusion the tear fluid constitutes a precorneal fluid layer that consists of (1) an outer "oily" mucinous layer, which is produced by the meibomian glands; (2) a waterlike intermediate layer, which is produced by the lacrimal glands; and (3) an inner mucinous layer, produced by the goblet cells in the conjunctival tunica.

1.4 Contents of the Orbit

1.4.1 Classification

According to topographical and functional criteria, the orbit can be divided into several regions, which have also significant relevance for clinical purposes (▶ Fig. 1.9).

The orbital septum divides the merely preseptally located protective apparatus of the eye from the inner orbital content, which is encircled by a layer of connective tissue (periorbita): intraorbital adipose tissue, eyeball, outer eye muscles, lacrimal gland, and several nerve and vascular pathways. The outer eye muscles together with the eyeball form a pyramid-like muscle conus whose apex lies in the deep orbit. Hence it is reasonable to divide the postseptal orbital compartment into spaces and layers:

- Extraconal compartment, upper layer: This is the space between the muscular cone and the orbital roof. The lacrimal gland is located in its temporal upper quadrant.

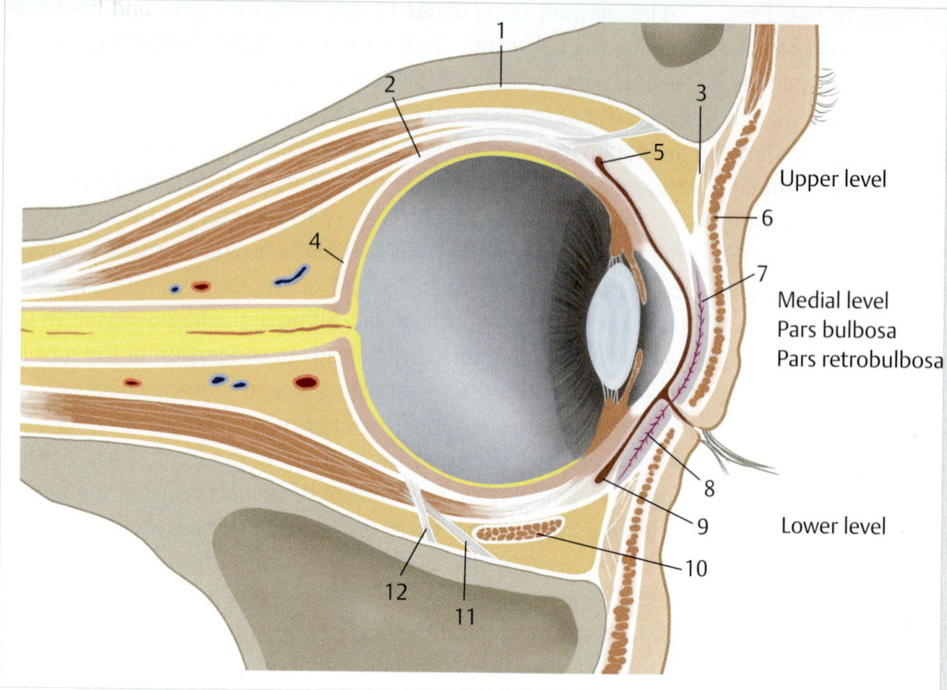

Fig. 1.9 Organization of the orbit. 1, periorbit; 2, spatium episclerale; 3, orbital septum; 4, vagina bulbi, Tenon's capsule; 5, superior conjunctival fornix; 6, orbicularis oculi muscle; 7, superior tarsus; 8, inferior tarsus; 9, inferior conjunctival fornix; 10, inferior obliquus muscle; 11, lacertus of the rectus muscles; 12, retinaculum of the rectus muscles.

- Intraconal compartment, medial layer: This compartment is defined as the space inside the muscle cone, having a bulb part and a retrobulbar part. A slitlike space, called the spatium episclerale, divides the eyeball from a tendonlike thickening of connective tissue, the tenon-capsule (vagina bulbi). Several pathways for nerves and vessels are located In the adipose tissue, in particular those for the outer eye muscles and the eyeball.
- Extraconal compartment, lower layer: This is considered as the space between muscle cone and orbital floor. Several pathways coursing through this space, are entering the orbit in particular via the inferior orbital fissure.

1.4.2 Connective Tissue Structures

Periorbita

The postseptal compartment, which is located behind the orbital septum in the bony orbit, is coated by the periorbita (▸ Fig. 1.9, ▸ Fig. 1.10, ▸ Fig. 1.11). The periorbita transits anteriorly and laterally to the orbital septum. The periorbita consists of a tight, funnel-shaped integument that can easily be ablated and that originates from the periosteum. It is connected rigidly with the bone at the cranial sutures, foramina, fissures, and optic nerve canal, and at the posterior part of the lacrimal bone. It furthermore constitutes the fibrous tendon ring for the origin of most outer eye muscles and is adhered with the dural sheath of the optic nerve.[1] The periorbita is well vascularized and sensitively innervated by branches of the trigeminal nerve. The periorbita protects the inner orbit from periostal hemorrhage and spreading of tumors and infections.[1] It contains smooth muscle cells, particularly in the neighborhood of fissures (i.e., inferior orbital fissure), that are clearly classed as orbital muscle (Müller muscle). These muscle fibers are remnants of a large muscle plate that in many animals serves as a lateral orbital wall with connective tissue instead of bone.[5]

Blockage of the ciliary ganglion causes a failure of the sympathetically innervated smooth muscle cells. Consequently, so-called Horner's syndrome develops, which is characterized by a ptosis (paresis of tarsal muscles), exophthalmos (paresis of the

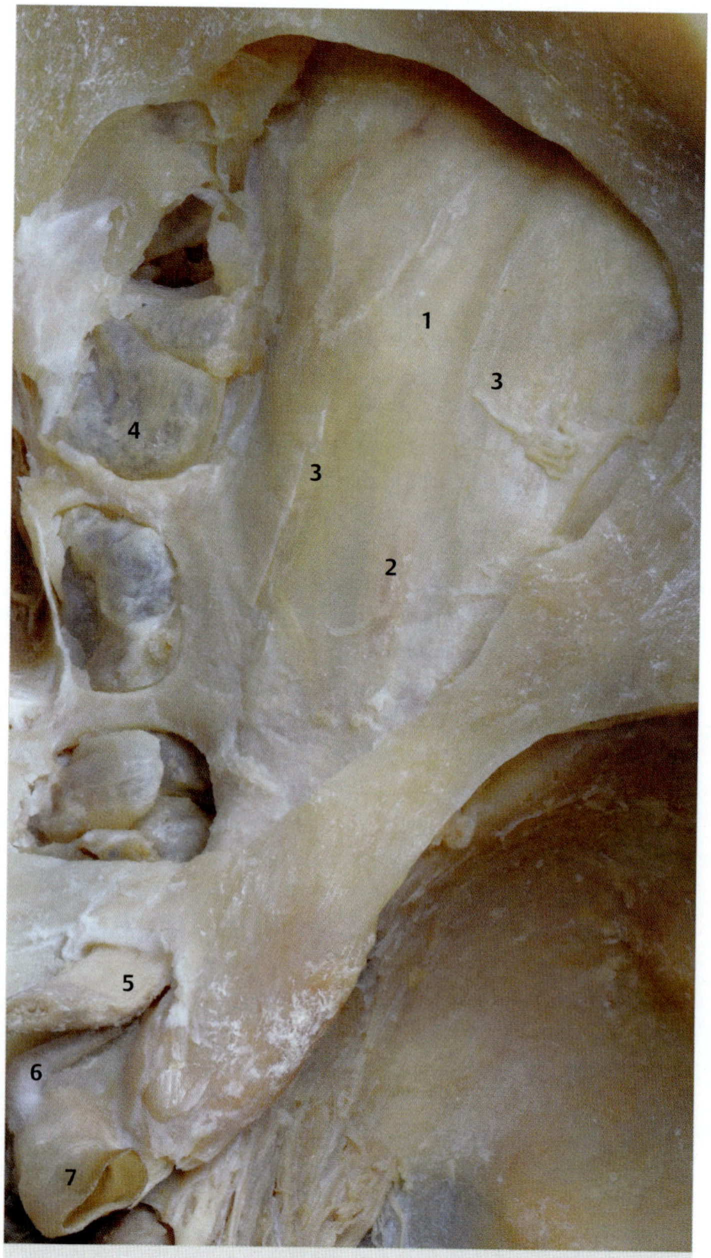

Fig. 1.10 Right orbit: orbital part of the frontal bone has been removed. 1, periorbita; 2, frontal nerve; 3, fat body; 4, ethmoidal cells; 5, optic nerve; 6, ophthalmic artery; 7, internal carotid artery.

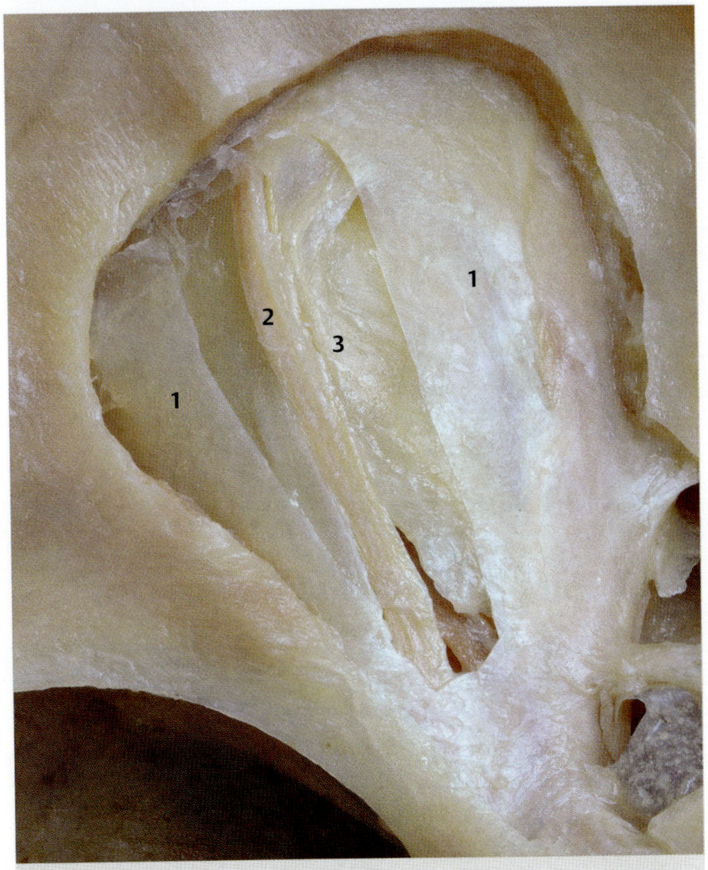

Fig. 1.11 Left orbit, orbital part of the frontal bone; periorbita partly removed. 1, periorbita; 2, frontal nerve; 3, fat body.

orbital muscle in the periorbita), and miosis (paresis of the dilatator muscle of the pupil in the iris).

Corpus Adiposum

The eyeball and outer eye muscles together do not fill the entire orbit. Rather, they are surrounded by adipose tissue that reaches to the periorbita (▶ Fig. 1.9, ▶ Fig. 1.11, ▶ Fig. 1.12a, b). This adipose tissue serves as an elastic pad to support the eyeball and an abutment for eye movements. While the anterior parts of the adipose tissue contain more connective tissue, large adipose flaps are found in the posterior parts. Extrusion of adipose tissue at the orbital aditus is prevented by the orbital septum.

Vagina bulbi

The bulb of the eye (eyeball; bulbus oculi) is separated from the periorbital adipose tissue by fascial sheaths of the eyeball (vagina bulbi = tenon capsule), which is a fascia or tendonlike tight thickening of connective tissue (▶ Fig. 1.9). It begins 2 mm behind the corneal limbus and is connected very tightly with the eyeball, anteriorly at the sclera (close to corneal border) and dorsally at the entrance of the optic nerve. The vagina bulbi divides anteriorly in two sheaths: the inner sheath, which reaches the conjunctiva of the eyeball (conjunctiva bulbi); and the outer sheath, which inserts at the eyelid tarsus. The vagina bulbi is fastened laterally at the periorbita by an upper frontally sited connective tissue plate (retinaculum bulbi superius), and by a horizontal situated lower connective tissue layer retinaculum bulbi inferius) (▶ Fig. 1.9).[4] The vagina bulbi is further perforated by nerves and blood vessels coursing to the eyeball. At the passage points of these pathways the muscle fascia merges with the connective tissue of the tenon capsule.[1] Hence, the vagina bulbi has to follow the eyeball excursions and therefore does not represent a "resting socket" in the classic sense.[5] However, minor movements between eyeball and vagina bulbi are possible by local compression and stretching of the fascia or tendonlike connective tissue. The vagina bulbi can therefore be compared to a tendon sheath.[5]

A sliding space filled with loosely arranged collagen fibers is located between the vagina bulbi and the sclera (spatium episclerale; tenon space, ▶ Fig. 1.9) and represents a shifting cleft for eyeball movements. The outer eye muscle tendons course

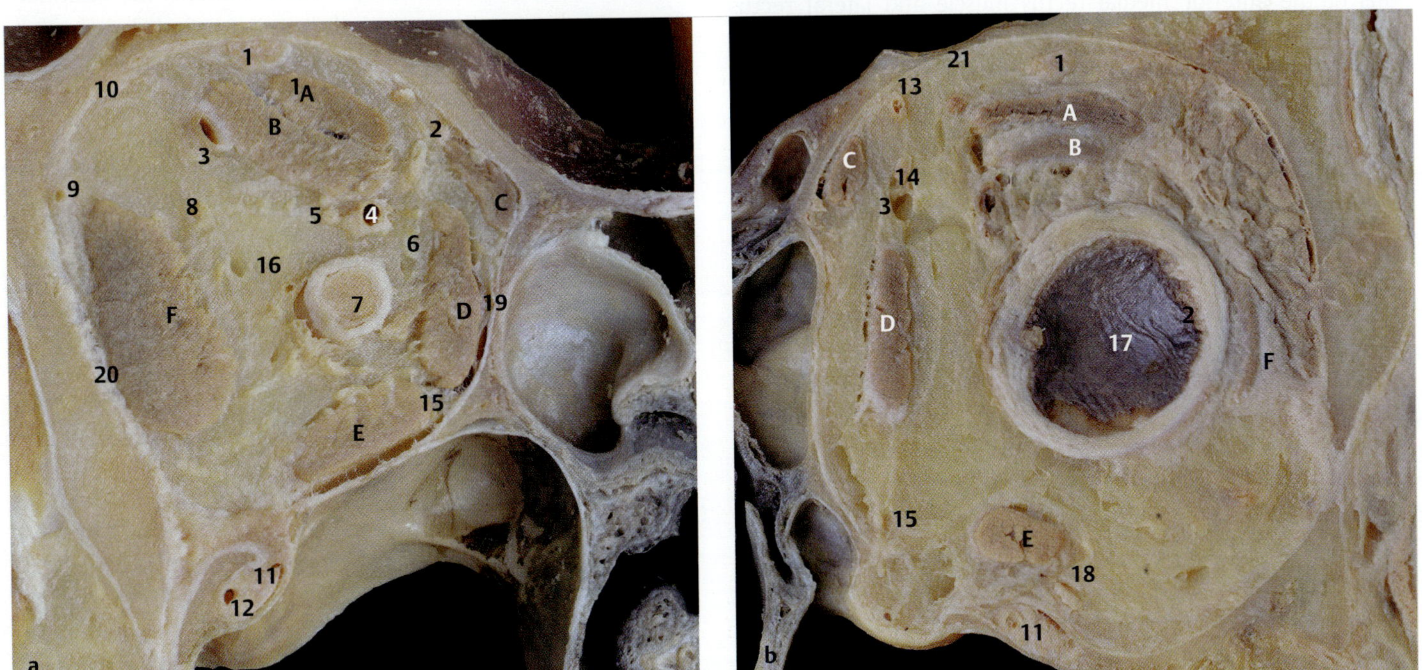

Fig. 1.12 (a) Right orbit, view from behind: Frontal section near the optic nerve. (b) Left orbit, frontal view: Frontal section near the bulb. 1, frontal nerve; 2, trochlear nerve; 3, ophthalmic vein; 4, ophthalmic artery; 5, oculomotor nerve; 6, nasociliary nerve; 7, optic nerve; 8, abducens nerve; 9, lacrimal artery; 10, lacrimal nerve; 11, infra-orbital nerve; 12, infra-orbital artery; 13, supra-orbital artery; 14, supratrochlear nerve; 15, Lockwood's ligament; 16, short posterior ciliary artery; 17, ocular bulb; 18, oculomotor nerve, lower branch; 19, medial retinaculum; 20, lateral retinaculum; 21, periorbita. A, levator palpebrae superioris muscle; B, superior rectus muscle; C, superior oblique muscle; D, medial rectus muscle; E, inferior rectus muscle; F, lateral rectus muscle.

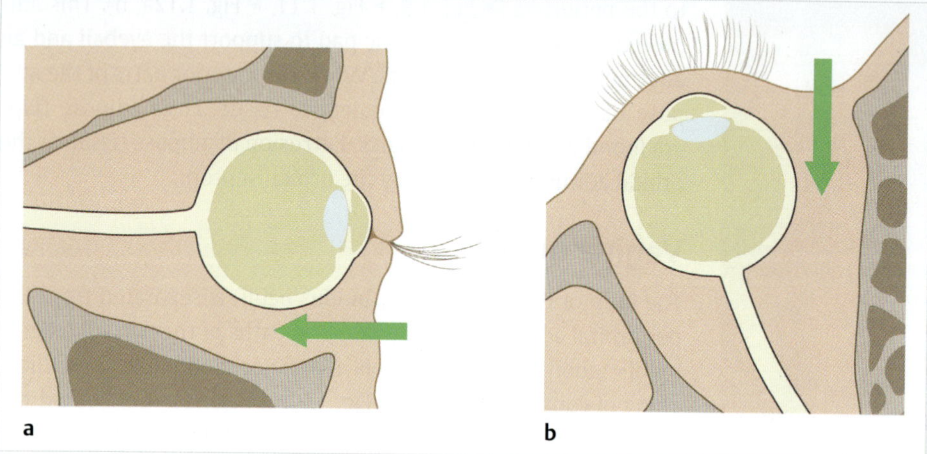

Fig. 1.13 Location of the eyeball in the orbit. **(a)** Sagittal section. **(b)** Horizontal section.

relatively freely to the eyeball. Accordingly, the episcleral space can be used as an approach for tying off the muscle tendons during strabismus surgery. This space can also be used as an approach for eyeball enucleation following severe injuries. In this procedure the eyeball is removed out of the vagina bulbi, like a kernel out of a fruit, while the vagina bulbi is left.[5]

Fibrous Suspension Apparatus

The outer eye muscle fasciae are significantly more tight and robust at the anterior and extraconal part of the muscles compared to the posterior parts and intraconally. Cuffs of connective tissue fix all extraocular muscles at the periorbita retinacula musculorum, ▶ Fig. 1.9).[1] The muscle bellies have an outer orbital stratum and an inner bulbar stratum. While the inner bulbar stratum is fixed with an end-tendon at the sclera, the muscle fibers of the orbital stratum terminate with tendonlike junctions in the periorbita (lacerti musculorum).[1] Prominent fibrous junctions of the anterior medial rectus muscle and lateral rectus muscle to the orbital wall are called medial and lateral check ligaments.[1] While the lateral check ligament is the most strongly developed and inserts at the Whitnall tubercle of the zygomatic bone, at the conjunctival fornix, and at the orbital septum, the medial check ligament inserts anteriorly at the lacrimal bone and orbital septum. The superior rectus muscle fascia and the superior levator palpebral muscle fascia are connected to each other by an intermuscular fascia. Another well-developed check ligament is the Whitnall ligament, which courses cranially and transversally, surrounds the superior levator palpebrae muscle close to its entrance to the upper lid, and finally inserts at the Whitnall tubercle and at the trochlea. Its effect is a limitation of the upper lid elevation. The fasciae of the inferior rectus muscle along with the inferior oblique muscle are also connected to the periorbita with check ligaments.[1] Another ligament is the Lockwood ligament, which courses from the Whitnall tubercle to the medial palpebral ligament and accomplishes a "hammock"-like formation for suspension of the eyeball. It consists of the caudal parts of the bulb retinaculum, the medial palpebral ligament, and the intermuscular connective tissue of the caudal eye muscles.[1] This ligamentous apparatus warrants a stable embedding of the eyeball and keeps it in balance. Tearing of these ligaments due to skull trauma or orbital fractures can cause severe strabismus.[10]

1.4.3 Pars Bulbosa and Bulbus Oculi

The anterior border of the muscle cone is formed by the eyeball. The eyeball, which is slightly irregular in form, is not centered in the orbit because the distance between the eyeball and the upper and lateral orbital walls is smaller than the distance to the medial and inner orbital walls (▶ Fig. 1.13). The eyeball is therefore easily accessible by a lateral surgical approach.

The eyeball axis (axis bulbi) courses from the midline of the cornea (anterior eye pole) to the insertion point of the optic nerve (posterior eye pole). The optic axis, however, courses vertically through the center of curvature of the refractive system towards the central fovea. Thus, eyeball axis and optic axis are not identical.[4] The diameter of the eyeball is about 24 mm (slightly smaller than a table-tennis ball), and it is slightly more curved laterally than dorsally.[1] The median eyeball volume is about 6.5 mL, whereas that of the orbit is about 29.7 mL.[11,12] The interior of the eyeball is divided into two different spaces: the larger posteriorly located compartment contains the gelatinous vitreous body (corpus vitreum); the more anteriorly located compartment contains the eye lens along with the anterior and posterior eye chamber (▶ Fig. 1.14). The vitreous body, along with the aqueous humor, determines the eyeball´s shape. The lens is located in the anterior part of the eyeball and sits in an impression of the vitreous body (fossa hyloidea), which is separated from the latter by an aqueous humor–filled fissure (Berger´s space). The eyeball´s wall consists of three layers (▶ Fig. 1.14).[4,5,6]

Layers of the Eyeball (Eyeball Tunica)

The **outer tunic of the eye bulb** (fibrous layer of eyeball; tunica fibrosa bulbi) contains only a few blood vessels, consists of fibrous connective tissue, and is mechanically stabile. It is nearly spherical and is strained internally by the intraocular pressure (15 mm Hg), and externally by traction of the outer eye muscles.[1] The anterior sixth part of that layer contains the transparent, colorless, refractile cornea, the other parts consist of the opaque whitish sclera, which limits the vitreous body laterally. The watchglasslike cornea is 0.7 mm thick at its edges and 0.5 mm thick in the center. It is significantly more curved than the sclera. With a refractive power of 40 diopters, it provides the main part of the refractive power of the entire eye (65 diopters). The transparency of the cornea is maintained by the regular arrangement of its components in the stroma and by the lack of blood vessels.

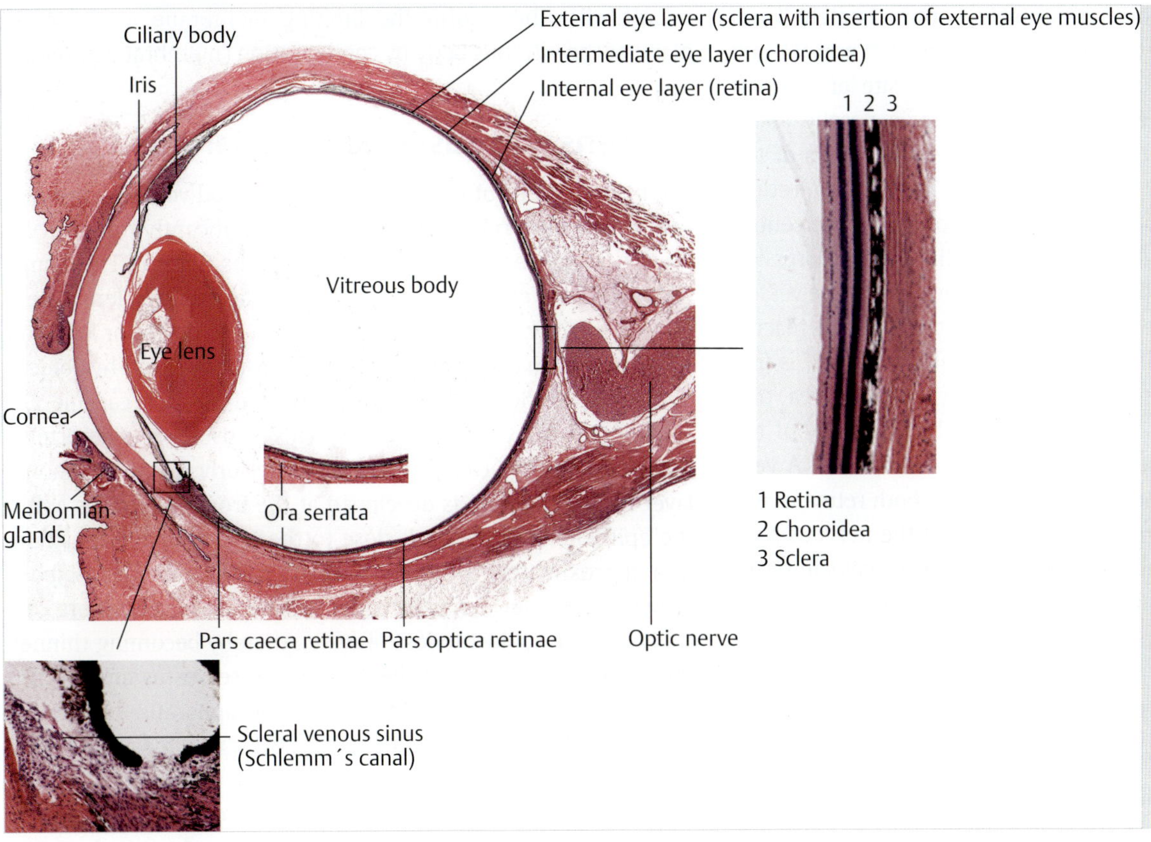

Fig. 1.14 Eyeball (bulbus oculi). H&E staining, sagittal section, macula lutea and optic disc not cut.

Sensory innervation is facilitated by the long ciliary nerves, which are branches from the ophthalmic nerve. The cornea transitions into the sclera and also into the conjunctiva at the corneal limbus. In this area the cornea is thickest at approximately 0.8 mm, whereas the thinnest part (ca. 0.3 mm) is located at the insertion tendons of the outer eye muscles. Blood vessels for nutrition of the sclera are the anterior ciliary arteries, which are branches from the muscular arteries arising out of the ophthalmic artery. Sensory innervation of the sclera is facilitated again by the long ciliary nerves from the ophthalmic nerve. The outer eye muscles can be accessed easily via the limbus—for example, in strabismus surgery.[10]

The **medial tunic of the eye bulb** (vascular layer of eyeball; tunica vasculosa bulbi) is called the uvea and contains blood vessels. This layer consists of the iris, the ciliary corpus, and the choroidea. The pupil, which is generally a circular opening, is located in the center of the anterior half of the eyeball. The anterior surface of the iris does not have a continuous epithelium. Bundles of smooth muscle cells are enclosed in the stroma of the iris. Some of these accomplish contraction of the pupil (pupil sphincter muscle, which is innervated by the parasympathetic nervous system and has a circular course); others provide dilation of the pupil (pupil dilatator muscle, which is innervated by the sympathetic nervous system and has a radiate course). Melanocytes, in greater or lesser numbers and in different arrangements, determine the eye color. The long posterior ciliary arteries along with the anterior ciliary arteries supply the major iris artery circle at the iris basis, and a minor iris artery circle in the stroma of the pupil's edge. Innervation of the iris is by the short ciliary nerves. The iris transitions laterally into the ciliary body. The ciliary body protrudes into the posterior chamber of the eye with some folds (processus ciliares), which form some even smaller plicae (plicae ciliares) (▶ Fig. 1.14). The ciliary body consists mainly of the circular ciliary muscle. The choroidea is well perfused (ca. 85% of the entire blood reaching the eye) and contains all the vessels for the blood supply of the external retinal layers (branches of the ophthalmic artery: short and long ciliary arteries, anterior ciliary arteries), along with nerve fibers from the short and long ciliary nerves. Numerous melanocytes are located in the fibrous stroma. The choroidea is separated from the inner eye tunic by an elastic membrane (Bruch membrane) and participates in maintenance of the intraocular pressure.

The **inner tunic of the eye bulb** (tunica interna bulbi) is called the retina and contains nerve cells. It consists of two separated layers that have different structure in the anterior part of the eyeball at the ciliary body and at the iris from that at the choroidea. The nonvisual retina (pars caeca retinae), which is composed of a two-layered pigmented epithelium and which is insensitive to light, lies anteriorly. The nonvisual part limits a retinal iridical part (pars iridica retinae), which is the posterior plate of the iris (ciliary retinal part of the ciliary body), and transitions abruptly into the light-sensitive optic part of the retina (pars optica retinae). This region is called the ora serrata due to its serrated border in the transit zone. Blood supply is maintained by the anterior ciliary arteries; there is no sensory or autonomous innervation. The optic part of the retina is composed of two layers and covers the posterior part of the eyeball. The outer pigmented layer is called the pigmented stratum. Here pigment epithelial cells are connected to each other by tight junctions and adhere very tightly to a basal lamina of the Bruch's membrane (blood–retina barrier). The first three neurons of the visual pathway are located at the inner layer close to the vitreous body (stratum nervosum); light-sensitive parts of the photoreceptors are orientated toward the pigmented epithelium. The axons of the third neuron converge to a prominence (optic nerve papilla) at the optic nerve discus (diameter 1.6 mm). The nerve fibers turn at right-angles at this papilla and develop into the optic nerve. As no photoreceptors are located in this area, the optic nerve papilla presents as a blind spot during perimetry, approximately 3 mm medial to the posterior eye pole, and 4 mm medial and 0.1 mm below the macula lutea, which represents the site of sharpest sightedness. The distance to the ora serrata is nasally about 27 mm and temporally about 31 mm.[4] Hence, the radius of the discus is greater nasally than temporally. The central retinal artery, a branch of the ophthalmic artery, along with the central retinal vein, passes through the optic nerve discus in a depression (excavatio disci). Numerous smaller end branches of these vessels pass radially approximately 3 to 4 mm temporally to the macula lutea, which is 3 mm in diameter.[3] The macula lutea itself is free of blood vessels and has in the center a cavity (central fovea) that is endowed mainly with retinal cones. The blood supply of the central fovea is maintained by vessels of the choroidea. A very narrow gap persists for the whole life between both retina layers, with the possibility of a retinal detachment of the nervous stratum (except the ora serrata and the optic nerve discus). In terms of origin and organization the retina is a protruded part of the diencephalon.[4,5,6]

Eyeball Compartments

Three different fluid-containing compartments can be distinguished within the eyeball (▶ Table 1.3; ▶ Fig. 1.14).

The eye chambers contain the aqueous humor, which is released by the nonpigmented epithelium of the ciliary part of the retina (pars ciliaris retinae) and which resembles the blood plasma in its composition. It serves for nutrition of the lens and parts of the cornea, and sustains the maintenance of the intraocular pressure (ca. 15 mm Hg).[5] Drainage occurs over the iridocorneal angle into the scleral venous sinus (Schlemm canal) (▶ Fig. 1.14). Anterior to the Schlemm canal are located the Fontana compartments, through which pass the cornoscleral trabecular meshwork and which expand during contraction of the ciliary muscle, facilitating drainage of the aqueous humor. The Schlemm canal is circular and is connected to the episcleral veins. Disturbance of aqueous humor drainage leads to a significant increase of intraocular pressure (cataract) with consequent hazard to the optic nerve at its exit point and therefore considerable risk of blindness.

The vitreous body (corpus vitreum) consists of 99% water and has a significant content of water-binding hyaluronic acids, which are released by the nonpigmented epithelium covering the ciliary bod, and produce to a high viscosity of the inner vitreous body contents.[4] The watery phase is crossed by collagenous microfibrils; these form the limiting membrane at the outer plane of the vitreous body by condensation (membrana vitrea).

Table 1.3 Borders and contents of eye chambers[4,5,6]

Chamber	Borders	Volume
Anterior eye chamber	Ventrally: cornea	200 µL
	Dorsally: front of the iris; lens	
	Laterally: iridocorneal angle	
Posterior eye chamber	Ventrally: back of the iris	100 µL
	Medially: lens	
	Dorsally: vitreous body	
	Laterally: ciliary body	
Vitreous body	Ventrally: lens; ciliary body	4 mL
	Dorsally: vitreous body	
	Laterally: retina	

Eye Lens and Suspension Apparatus

The biconvex lens of the eye has neither blood vessels nor innervation. The posterior part of the lens is significantly more curved (radius 6 mm) than the anterior part (radius 11 mm). The diameter at the lens equator is 9 mm.[4] While the anterior lens pole is located directly behind the pupil and iris, the posterior lens pole is situated in an depression of the vitreous body (fossa hyaloidea). The lens is enclosed by a dense carbohydrate-rich capsule and surrounded by aqueous humor. This capsule is significantly thicker anteriorly (10–19 mm) than posteriorly (5 mm).[4] A monolayer lens epithelium is developed at the front of the lens, while the epithelium at the back close to the lens equator transitions into approximately 8-mm-long lens fibrils as a result of bipolar growth. The older denucleated lens fibrils are located more centrally and are subject to loss of water, thereby becoming thinner; they form the nucleus of the lens, which serves as an insertion point for younger fibrils. The suspension apparatus of the lens consists of 8 to 12-mm-thick zonular fibrils, which originate from the basal membrane of the nonpigmented epithelium covering the ciliary body. They pass through the posterior eye chamber to the lens equator and insert at the front and back of the lens capsule. The zonula fibrils hold the lens in position behind the iris and stabilize it in the center behind the pupil. Contraction of the ciliary muscle, which is innervated by the parasympathetic nervous system, leads to an increase of the muscle belly and consequent relaxation of zonula fibers with rounding of the lens; this enables short-distance accommodation. Relaxation of the muscle leads to applanation of the elastic fibers located in the lens and antagonizes eye accommodation. The blood supply of the lens is provided by the anterior ciliary arteries and the long posterior ciliary arteries.

1.4.4 Topography and Function of Outer Eye Muscles

The presence of a shifting cleft between the fascial sheath of the eyeball (vagina bulbi) and the sclera (▶ Fig. 1.9) enables the eyeball to perform upward and downward movements. Nasal and temporal movements and minor rotation are also possible. The insertion tendons of the outer eye muscles pass through the episcleral space and insert on the sclera behind the corneal limbus. Any outer eye muscles except the inclined inferior and superior oblique muscles originate from a tendon circuit (anulus of Zinn = anulus tendineus communis),[1] which is located at the orbital apex (▶ Fig. 1.15). This tubelike collagenous circuit surrounds the optic nerve canal, encircles the superior orbital fissure, and leads to a division of the orbit into an intraconal part and an upper and a lower extraconal compartment (▶ Fig. 1.9, ▶ Fig. 1.16). Pathways entering the orbit course either within the muscle cone or outside the tendon circuit (▶ Fig. 1.5, ▶ Fig. 1.16).

The muscle cone is formed by the four straight outer eye muscles, which pass through the adipose tissue. These muscles reach the bulb through gaps in the Tenon capsule and insert at its anterior quadrant in characteristic pattern (▶ Fig. 1.9, ▶ Fig. 1.15, ▶ Fig. 1.16, ▶ Fig. 1.17). The imaginary connecting line of the four

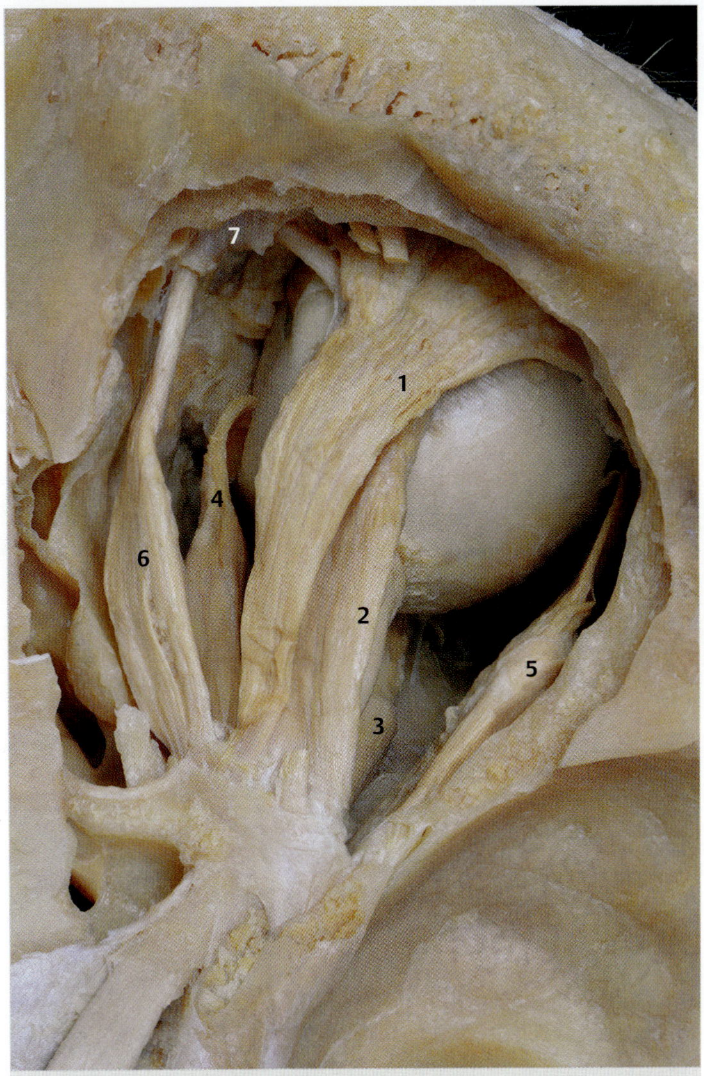

Fig. 1.15 Outer eye muscles. 1, levator palpebrae superior; 2, rectus superior; 3, rectus inferior; 4, rectus medialis; 5, rectus lateralis; 6, obliquus superior; 7, oblique inferior.

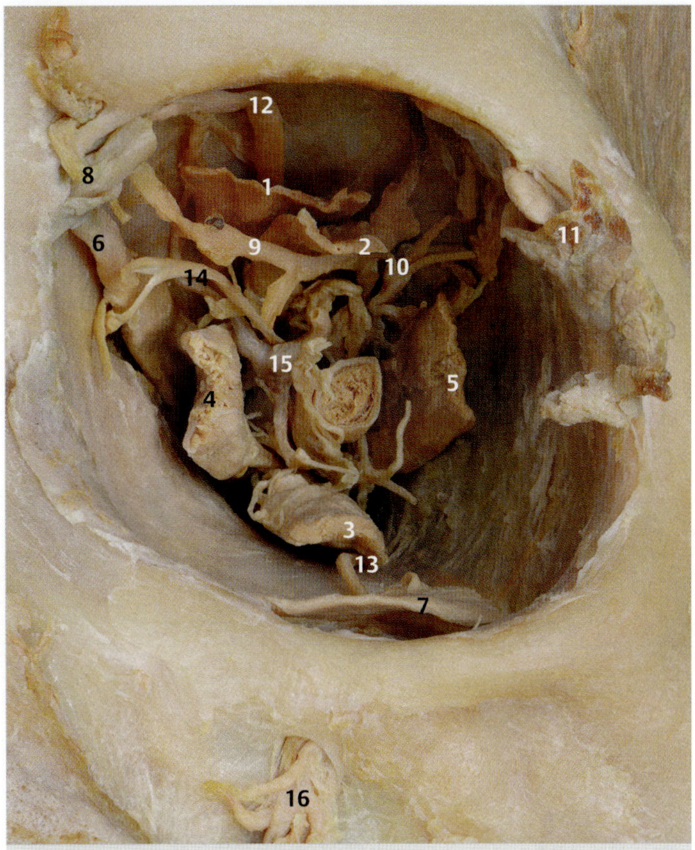

Fig. 1.16 Left orbit with outer eye muscles. 1, levator palpebrae superior; 2, rectus superior; 3, rectus inferior; 4, rectus medialis; 5, rectus lateralis; 6, obliquus superior; 7, oblique inferior; 8, trochlea musculi obliqui superioris; 9, ophthalmic vein; 10, lacrimal artery and nerve; 11, lacrimal gland; 12, frontal nerve; 13, oculomotor nerve, lower branch; 14, nasociliary nerve; 15, ophthalmic artery; 16, infraorbital artery and nerve.

muscular attachments is called Tillaux's spiral.[10] Frontobasal approach to the orbit displays first the **levator palpebrae superioris muscle**, which is the most superiorly located muscle in the orbit and innervated by the oculomotor nerve. It originates at the minor wing of the sphenoid bone and courses to the superior tarsus. The **superior rectus muscle** is located underneath the levator palpebrae superioris muscle and originates at the upper rim of the tendon anulus, the periosteum of the optic nerve canal, and the dural sheath of the optic nerve. It courses to the anterior eyeball in an angle of about 25° to the optic axis. Its insertion point lies approximately 7 mm behind the corneal limbus.[4] It serves as a vertical motor and essentially elevates the optic axis with the eyeball rotated upward to the sky (the “religious muscle”).[4] The **inferior rectus muscle** is the second vertical motor. It originates from the caudal rim of the commune tendon anulus, passes the orbital floor, and courses also in an angle of 25° to the optic axis through the vagina bulbi to the caudal anterior part of the eyeball, where it inserts with a 8.8-mm-wide tendon at the sclera, 7 mm behind the corneal limbus.[3] Its main function is infraduction of the eyeball (the “capuchin muscle”).[4] Both vertical motors are innervated by the superior and inferior branches of the oculomotor nerve; the blood supply is maintained by muscular branches of the ophthalmic artery. The **medial rectus muscle** is innervated by the inferior branch of the oculomotor nerve and has the largest site of origin at the medial rim of the tendon circuit. It runs as a horizontal motor medially alongside the orbital part of the ethmoid bone to the medial part of the anterior eyeball, where it inserts at the sclera approximately 5.7 mm behind the corneal limbus. It acts as a strong adductor.[4] The lateral rectus muscle is the second horizontal motor and courses from the tendon circuit laterally through the vagina bulbi toward the eyeball, where it inserts at the sclera approximately 7 mm behind the corneal limbus.[4] In contrast to the other outer eye muscles it arises from the anulus of Zinn with an upper and a lower tendon. It is a pure abductor and is innervated by the abducens nerve (see ▸ Fig. 1.20a).

Rotary motions of the eyeball are effected by the oblique eye muscles: the superior oblique muscle, and the inferior oblique muscle. The thin **superior oblique muscle** originates at the upper rim of the tendon circuit or at the sphenoid bone corpus medial to the tendon circuit, and runs anteriorly above the medial rectus muscle between orbital roof and medial orbital wall. It goes into a roundish tendon ca. 1 cm ahead of a U-shaped fibrocartilage sponge (superior oblique muscle trochlea) (▸ Fig. 1.15, ▸ Fig. 1.16). The tendon crosses the trochlea and is then turned posteriorly downward and laterally with an angle of 50° (▸ Fig. 1.15). After passing through the Tenon capsule, its tendon crosses under the distal edge of the superior rectus muscle

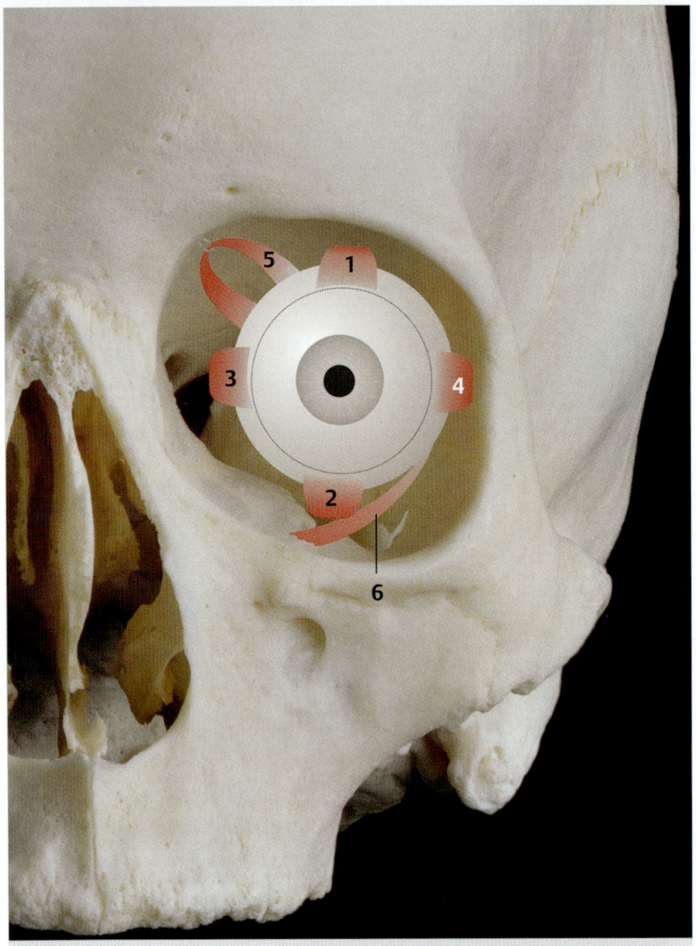

Fig. 1.17 Eyeball with attachment of the outer eye muscles. 1, levator palpebrae superior; 2, rectus superior; 3, rectus inferior; 4, rectus medialis; 5, rectus lateralis; 6, obliquus superior.

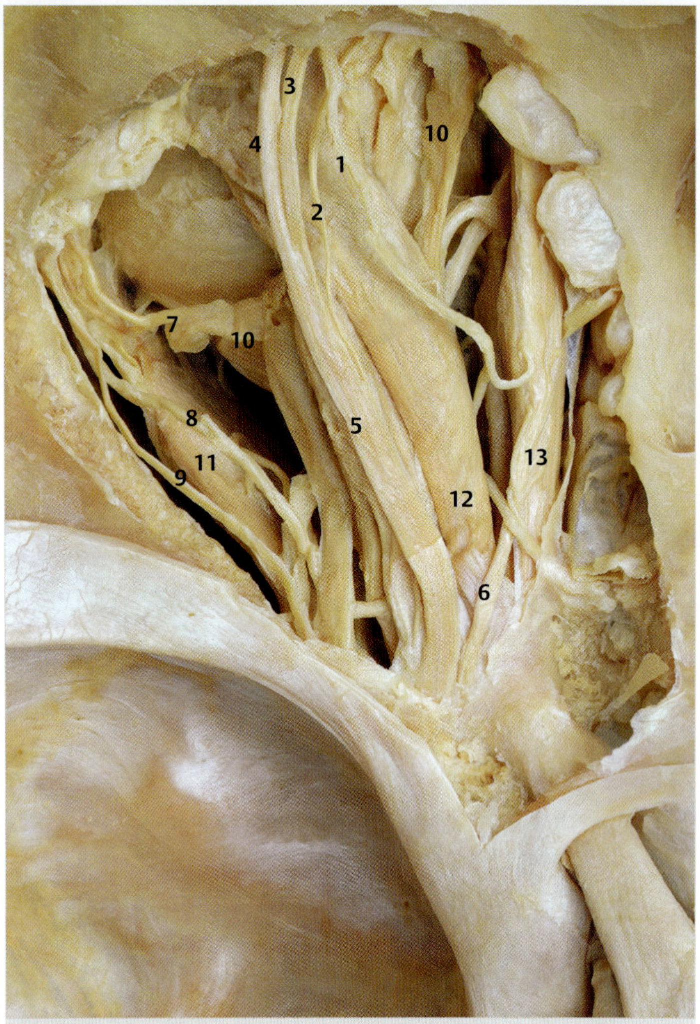

Fig. 1.18 Left orbit, frontobasal access, upper floor. 1, m. levator palpebrae superioris; 2, m. rectus superior; 3, m. rectus inferior; 4, m. rectus medialis; 5, m. rectus lateralis; 6, m. obliquus superior; 7, m. obliquus inferior; 8, trochlea m. obliqui superioris; 9, ophthalmic vein; 10, lacrimal artery and nerve; 11, lacrimal gland; 12, frontal nerve; 13, inferior branch of the oculomotor nerve; 14, n. nasociliaris; 15, a. ophthalmica; 16, a., n. infraorbitalis.

(▶ Fig. 1.15), and inserts obliquely at the sclera of the outer posterior quadrant of the eyeball, approximately 11 to 19 mm from the corneal limbus. The superior oblique muscle is innervated by the trochlear nerve and carries out infraduction, abduction, and internal rotation of the eye. The **inferior oblique muscle** arises from the anterior ridge of the orbit. It runs from the maxillary bone close lateral of the entrance of the nasolacrimal duct at the infra-orbital ridge posteriorly and laterally to the eyeball (▶ Fig. 1.15, ▶ Fig. 1.16). Thus it proceeds on the lower side of the eyeball between inferior rectus muscle and orbital floor. Because its tendon is only a few millimeters long, the muscle fibers course very close to the eyeball. It then inserts at the posterior quadrant of the bulb behind the superior oblique muscle, approximately 5 to 7 mm from the entrance of the optic nerve.[4] Furthermore, the insertion point is located ca. 2 mm below and lateral of the macula lutea. The inferior oblique muscle receives innervation by the inferior branches of the oculomotor nerve and leads to abduction, elevation and external rotation of the eyeball.

1.5 Topography of Pathways Located Postseptally

1.5.1 Topographic Relations to the Common Anular Tendon of Zinn

According to their position the pathways entering the orbit are lying in different relation with the common anular tendon, or common tendinous ring (▶ Fig. 1.5). The frontal nerve, lacrimal nerve, and trochlear nerve, along with the superior ophthalmic vein, run above the anulus. Pathways underneath the anulus are the inferior ophthalmic vein, the infra-orbital artery, the zygomatic nerve. Pathways within the anulus and therefore within the muscle cone are the optic nerve, the ophthalmic artery, the nasociliar nerve, oculomotor nerve, and abducens nerve.

1.5.2 Extraconal Pathways in the Upper Compartment

Several pathways course in the upper compartment between the superior palpebral muscle and the periorbita to the frontal region, the lacrimal gland, and superior oblique muscle (▶ Fig. 1.18).

Nerves and Arteries

The ophthalmic nerve, which is a sensitive nerve, divides within the superior orbital fissure into the frontal and lacrimal nerves, which course above the anulus, and into the nasociliar nerve, running through the anulus (▶ Fig. 1.5). The **frontal nerve**, innervating sensitively the frontal skin, the skin of the upper lid, and the frontal sinus mucosa, courses closely underneath the periorbita on the levator palpebrae superioris muscle and divides into the **supra-orbital nerve** (with its medial and lateral branches) and the **supratrochlear nerve** (▶ Fig. 1.18). The **lateral branch** leaves the orbit through the supra-orbital foramen or supra-orbital notch accompanied by the supra-orbital artery, which comes from the medial compartment. The **medial branch** courses through the frontal foramen or frontal notch to the frontal skin, accompanied by the **supratrochlear artery** (= terminal branch of the ophthalmic artery), which is located medially to the supra-orbital artery. The supratrochlear nerve runs also to the medial orbital rim above the trochlea of the superior oblique muscle through the frontal notch and reaches the skin of the medial canthus (▶ Fig. 1.16). The sensitive **lacrimal nerve** reaches the lacrimal gland together with the **lacrimal artery**, which is the first branch of the ophthalmic artery, rising from the medial compartment. This nerve divides at the posterior surface of the lacrimal gland into two branches: The upper branch goes through the lacrimal gland to the lateral canthus. The lower branch joins at the eyeball level with a thin nerve branch, which goes along with the zygomatic nerve, rises at the lateral orbital ridge, and contains postganglionic parasympathetic and sympathetic fibers for the lacrimal gland (▶ Fig. 1.19).

The **trochlear nerve** runs from lateral to medial after entering the upper compartment to the superior oblique muscle. It crosses the origin of the superior palpebral levator muscle medially to the frontal nerve, and reaches the muscle belly at the lateral rim of the first muscle third (▶ Fig. 1.18).

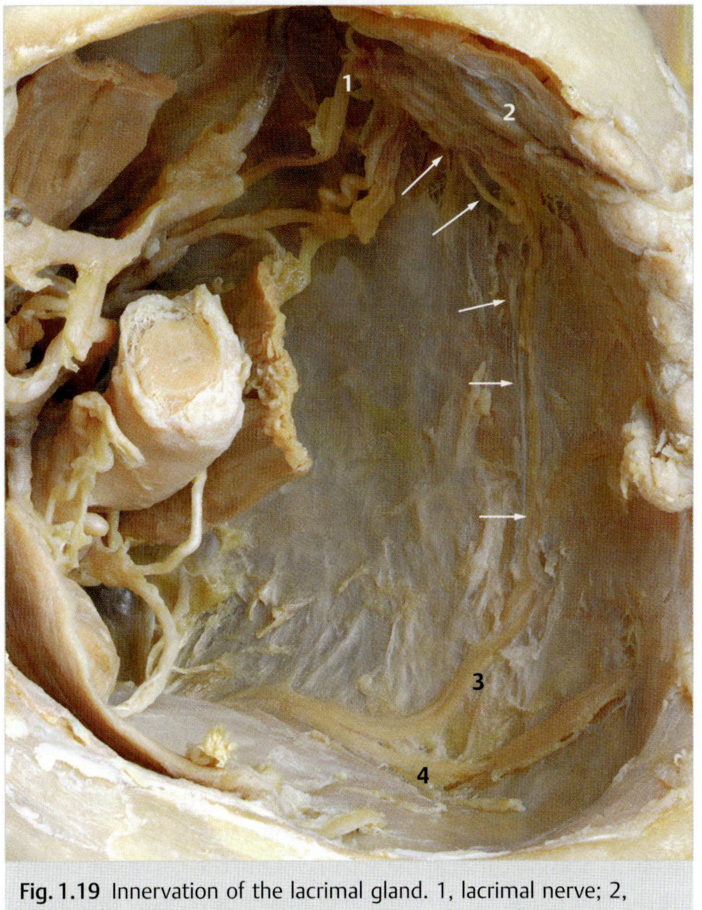

Fig. 1.19 Innervation of the lacrimal gland. 1, lacrimal nerve; 2, lacrimal gland; 3, ramus communicans nervi lacrimalis cum nervo zygomatico; 4, zygomatic nerve.

Veins

The supra-orbital vein courses together with the supra-orbital artery medially, and the lacrimal vein together with the homonymous artery laterally to the levator palpebrae superioris muscle (▶ Fig. 1.1, ▶ Fig. 1.18).

1.5.3 Intraconal Pathways (Medial Compartment)

The eyeball is located in the medial compartment of the orbit. The retro-bulbar intraconal space contains numerous pathways for supplying the outer eye muscles and the eyeball, and pathways that use the orbit as transit routes for sensitive innervation of the frontal sinus, ethmoid sinuses, and nasal cavity. The ciliary ganglion is also located in this compartment at the lateral surface of the optic nerve. The medial orbital compartment is encircled by the outer eye muscle cone and is limited anteriorly by the eyeball. The pathways enter this compartment within the tendon circuit via the optic nerve canal (optic nerve; ophthalmic artery) and the superior orbital fissure (oculomotor nerve, abducens nerve, nasociliary nerve).

Nerves

The **optic nerve** represents a part of the diencephalon. Basically the nerve section from the optic nerve discus to the optic chiasm is called the optic nerve. It contains central glia cells, mainly oligondendrocytes, which are responsible for the development of the myelin sheath. It is furthermore surrounded by meninges, which constitute a "splinting" of the nerve. Cerebrospinal fluid surrounds the nerve axons and communicates with the cerebrospinal fluid of the subdural space of the brainstem, which can lead to acute respiratory arrest following retrobulbar injections. Topographically the optic nerve can be divided in three segments: the canalicular part (5–9 mm), the orbital part (25 mm), and the ocular part (1–2 mm).[1]

The **canalicular part of the optic nerve** is located in the optic nerve canal, and with a length of 5 to 9 mm is fairly short. The optic nerve canal can be divided into three sections: the orbital part, the optic canal waist, and the intracranial part. The optic canal waist has a transverse diameter of 4.4 mm and a vertical diameter of 4.7 mm and represents the narrowest position of the canal.[2] In rare cases the optic nerve canal can have the configuration of a number "8" because of an apparent bipartition that leads to an independent ophthalmic artery canal.[2] The dural sheath in the optic nerve canal is adherent with the canal periosteum.[3]

The **intra-orbital part of the optic nerve** is completely embedded in the orbital adipose tissue (▶ Fig. 1.12a). With a length approximately 30 mm greater than the direct distance between eyeball and optic nerve canal, it takes a slightly meandering course, which enables the nerve to follow the eyeball movements without any damage.

The ca. 1.5-mm-thick **ocular part of the optic nerve** is unmyelinated as it enters the eyeball. It can be divided into three sections: the scleral, the choroidal, and the retinal sections. The point of passage of the optic nerve axons through the sclera is shaped as a cribriform plate (cribriform lamina). When leaving the sclera the oligodendrocytes develop a myelin sheath, which increases the nerve's diameter to 3 to 4 mm.[4]

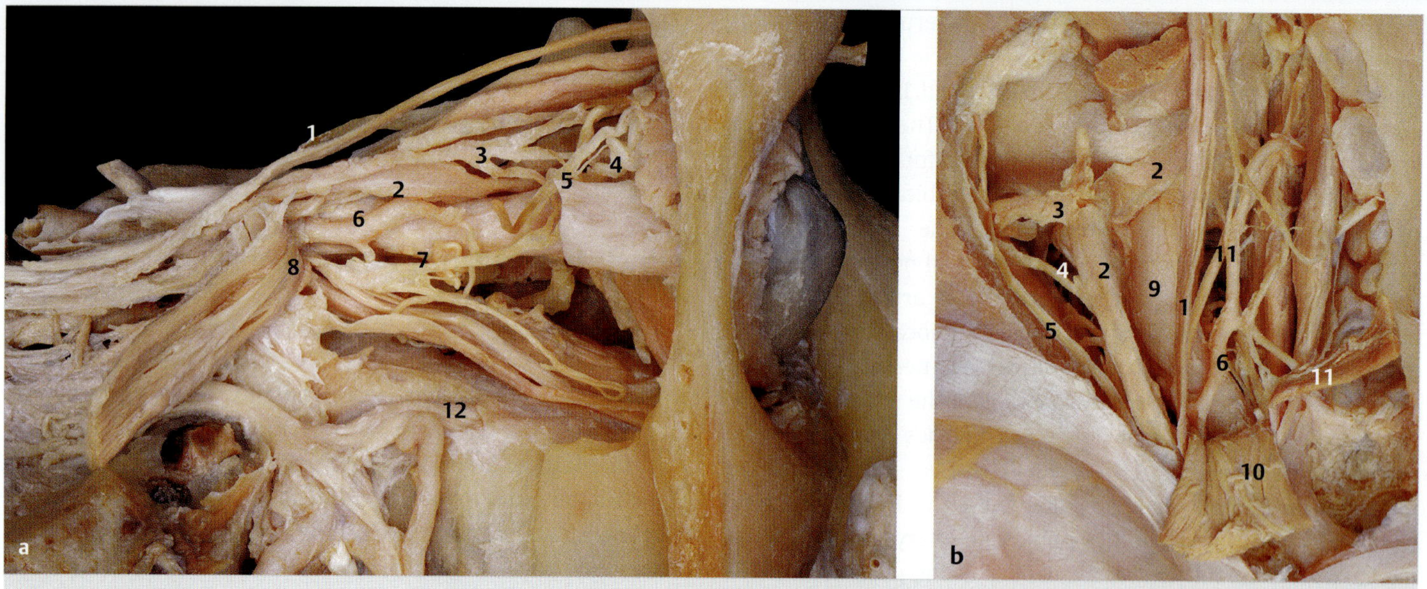

Fig. 1.20 **(a)** Orbit, lateral access, ciliary ganglion. **(b)** Pathways in the middle floor, frontobasal access. 1, frontal nerve; 2, upper ophthalmic vein; 3, lacrimal vein; 4, lacrimal artery; 5, lacrimal nerve; 6, ophthalmic artery; 7, ciliary ganglion; 8, abducens nerve; 9, optic nerve; 10, oculomotor nerve; 11, nasociliary nerve; 12, infra-orbital artery, vein, and nerve.

The **oculomotor nerve** passes from the cavernous sinus wall through the medial angle of the superior orbital fissure and divides within the common tendineus ring (common anular tendon) in a superior and an inferior branch. Both branches are divided by the nasociliary nerve.[1] The superior branch contains somatomotoric fibers for the superior rectus muscle and the superior palpebral levator muscle. It courses intraconally approximately 15 mm below the orbital roof.[1] The inferior branch contains somatomotoric fibers for the medial rectus muscle, inferior rectus muscle, and inferior oblique muscle after releasing preganglionic parasympathetic fibers. These are switched in the ciliary ganglion, which is located in the adipose tissue lateral to the optic nerve, approximately 1 cm distal to the orbital apex and ca. 15 to 20 mm behind the eyeball[1] (▶ Fig. 1.20a). Preganglionic parasympathetic fibers of the oculomotor nerve are switched to postganglionic fibers in this ganglion. The sensitive **nasociliary nerve** is a branch of the ophthalmic nerve. It enters the orbit within the anular tendon, accompanies the ophthalmic artery, crosses the optic nerve together with the artery, and is then located between the superior oblique muscle and the medial rectus muscle (▶ Fig. 1.20b). The nasociliary nerve emits a few branches: (1) Two **long ciliary nerves** course lateral to the optic nerve into the sclera for sensitive innervation of the choroidea, the ciliary corpus, the iris, and the cornea. (2) One **communicating branch with the ciliary ganglion**; 15 to 20 **short ciliary nerves** come out of this branch, which course above and underneath the optic nerve to the eyeball, containing parasympathetic axons (switched from preganglionic to postganglionic fibers in the ciliary ganglion) for innervating the ciliary and sphincter pupillary muscles, along with postganglionic sympathetic fibers for the dilator pupillae muscle, and sensitive fibers originating in the eyeball.[13]

The **posterior and anterior ethmoidal nerves** run together with the correspondingly named arteries to the medial orbital wall and leave the orbit through the posterior and anterior ethmoidal foramina, respectively (see Chapter 1.3). They are responsible for the sensitive innervation of the nasal cavity, ethmoid sinuses, and the dorsum of the nose.[11] The **infratrochlear nerve** is the terminal branch of the nasociliary nerve. It courses underneath the trochlea for the superior oblique muscle tendon to the skin of the medial canthus for sensitive innervation of the skin along with the lacrimal sac, the conjunctiva above the lacrimal caruncle, and the upper- and lower lid via palpebral branches.

The **abducens nerve** enters the medial orbital compartment underneath the oculomotor nerve within the tendon circuit through the superior orbital fissure after crossing the lumen of the cavernous sinus (▶ Fig. 1.1). It reaches the lateral rectus muscle medially, courses along the muscle belly, and finally penetrates the muscle (▶ Fig. 1.20a).[1]

Ophthalmic Artery and Its Branches

The **ophthalmic artery** comes from the internal carotid artery and enters the intraconal compartment laterally and underneath the optic nerve through the optic nerve canal. It then divides in ca. 10 branches. The circulation area of this artery comprises the eyeball, the eye muscles, the lacrimal gland, the eye lids, and the facial skin surrounding the eyes, along with a part of the paranasal sinuses and nasal cavity.

The ophthalmic artery courses from lateral to medial shortly after entering the orbit and crosses over (in 85–90% of cases) or crosses under (in 10–15% of cases) the optic nerve.[9] The **central retinal artery** is the first branch of the ophthalmic artery, which is relatively thin and is released almost before crossing the optic nerve. It accompanies the optic nerve and enters the nerve medially from underneath approximately 10 mm before the eyeball, reaches the retina within the optic nerve, and divides then in the area of the optic nerve discus into four branches. An arterial network from the central retinal artery extends below the pial layer maintaining the blood supply of the optic nerve.[1,13]

The **short posterior ciliary arteries** (10–15) are other branches of the ophthalmic artery, accompanying the optic nerve below it, passing through the sclera close to the nerve, and reaching the choroidea. Their terminal branches develop to the greater arterial circle of the iris. The long posterior ciliary arteries course laterally and medially along the nerve and pass the sclera also at

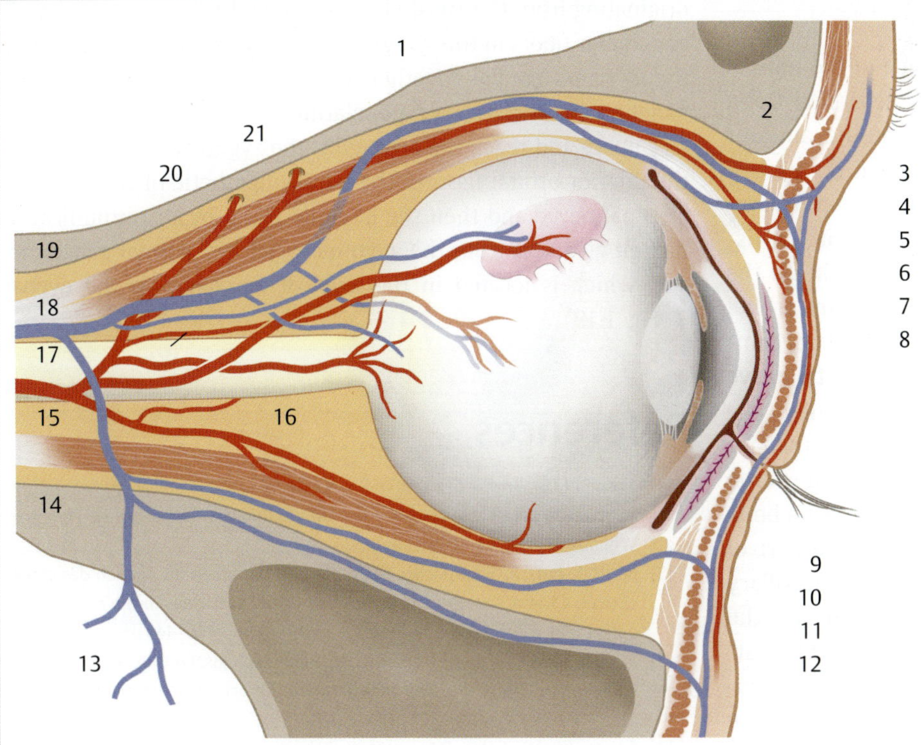

Fig. 1.21 Arteries and veins in the orbit 1, upper ophthalmic vein; 2, supra-orbital artery; 3, supratrochlear artery; 4, supra-orbital vein; 5, nasofrontal vein; 6, dorsal nasal artery; 7, medial palpebral artery; 8, angular artery; 9, angular vein; 10, lower ophthalmic vein; 11, facial vein; 12, infra-orbital vein; 13, plexus venosus pterygoideus; 14, anterior ciliary artery; 15, muscular arteries; 16, central retinae artery; 17, ophthalmic artery; 18, lacrimal artery; 19, short posterior ciliary arteries; 20, posterior ethmoid artery; 21, anterior ethmoidal artery.

the posterior edge of the eyeball to provide the blood supply of the ciliary corpus and greater arterial circle of the iris.[9]

The **lacrimal artery** arises from the ophthalmic artery anterior to the crossing with the optic nerve. Accompanied by the lacrimal nerve it runs into the upper compartment, and courses at the upper edge of the lateral rectus muscle to the lacrimal gland. The lacrimal artery releases zygomatic branches, passing through the zygomaticotemporal and zygomaticofacial foramina to the temporal fossa and zygomatic region, which maintain the blood supply of the lateral parts of the upper and lower lids via its terminal branches, the lateral palpebral arteries (▸ Fig. 1.6). It is noteworthy that the lacrimal artery sends the recurrent meningeal branch back intracranially through the superior orbital fissure.

The **supra-orbital artery** is released by the ophthalmic artery directly behind their over- or under-crossing of the optic nerve. The supra-orbital artery courses with the similar named vein at the medial rim of the levator palpebrae superioris muscle into the upper compartment and reaches below the orbital roof the supra-orbital notch for the blood supply of the frontal skin and the frontal mimic muscles.

The ophthalmic artery then turns medially and runs together with the nasociliary nerve underneath the superior oblique nerve to the medial orbital wall. It releases the **anterior and posterior ethmoidal arteries**, which cross the medial rectus muscle and leave the orbit through the correspondingly named foramen (▸ Fig. 1.21). Numerous muscular arteries are also released by the ophthalmic artery during its course through the orbit, which reach the outer eye muscles medially. Additionally, these muscular arteries release some anterior ciliary arteries, which also course to the greater arterial circle of the iris.

The ophthalmic artery divides into its three terminal branches at the medial anterior orbital rim: (1) The **medial palpebral arteries** develop underneath the trochlea of the superior oblique muscle, coursing behind the lacrimal sacculus caudally to the upper and lower lids (▸ Fig. 1.6). They form the superior and inferior palpebral arches, together with the lacrimal artery (▸ Fig. 1.6). (2) The **supratrochlear artery** is the second terminal branch of the ophthalmic artery. It courses medial to the supra-orbital artery through the frontal notch to the frontal region. (3) The **dorsal nasal artery** is the third terminal branch leaving the orbit between the trochlea of the superior oblique muscle and the medial palpebral ligament and anastomoses with the angular artery out of the facial artery.

Veins

The course and afferent vessels of the valveless **superior ophthalmic vein** correspond to those of the ophthalmic artery and its branches.[13] The vein arises from a venous plexus behind the upper lid at the medial surface of the eyeball, which is connected via the **nasofrontal vein** either with the angular vein or with the **supra-orbital vein**.[13,14] The supra-orbital vein runs above the nasofrontal vein and courses underneath the tendon of the superior oblique muscle. Both veins unite behind the muscle to the superior ophthalmic vein.[14] It courses underneath the superior rectus muscle from medial anterior to lateral posterior, crosses the optic nerve, reaches the upper orbital compartment, and passes then beyond the tendinous ring through the superior orbital fissure where it joints into the cavernous sinus.[13,14] The superior ophthalmic vein collects the blood from the palpebral veins, the ethmoid veins, the lacrimal veins, and the eyeball veins (i.e., vorticose veins [posterior ciliary veins]; ciliary veins; central retinal vein).

1.5.4 Extraconal Pathways (Lower Compartment)

Pathways supplying the temporal skin, the medial part of the face, and the mucosa of the upper jaw teeth and also for the inferior oblique muscle are located in the lower orbital compartment.

Nerves and Arteries

The lower orbital compartment is located outside of the muscle cone between the inferior rectus muscle and the orbital floor. The inferior oblique muscle, which originates at the anterior medial orbital ridge and inserts at the sclera behind the eyeball equator, is located in this very narrow space. This space is connected to the pterygopalatine fossa over the inferior orbital fissure (▶ Fig. 1.3), in which the **maxillary nerve** comes in via the foramen rotundum and splits into its branches: The infra-orbital nerve and the zygomatic nerve. Both enter the lower orbital compartment by the inferior orbital fissure.[14] The **infra-orbital nerve** is accompanied by the **infra-orbital artery** and vein, enters the infra-orbital canal and sulcus (▶ Fig. 1.20a), and reaches the face skin underneath the eye (▶ Fig. 1.16). The **zygomatic nerve** courses to the lateral orbital wall (▶ Fig. 1.19) and reaches a bony canal via the zygomatico-orbital foramen of the orbital part of the zygomatic bone. Both terminal branches of the maxillary nerve pass through the zygomaticotemporal foramen and the zygomaticofacial foramen for the sensitive innervation of the lateral face region. Furthermore the inferior ramus of the oculomotor nerve courses through the lower orbital compartment to the inferior oblique muscle (▶ Fig. 1.16).

Veins

The valveless **inferior ophthalmic vein** is also located in the lower orbital compartment. It arises behind the lower lid at the transition zone from the lateral orbital wall to the orbital floor, and collects the blood from the lower eye muscles of the eyelids, from the lacrimal gland, and from the choroid of the eyeball. It opens into the superior ophthalmic vein and therefore also into the cavernous sinus. It goes also through the inferior orbital fissure and connects with the pterygoid venous plexus, collecting the blood from the circulation area of the maxillary artery (▶ Fig. 1.21).

1.5.5 Secretory, Parasympathetic Innervation of the Lacrimal Gland

The vegetative pterygopalatine ganglion is located in the pterygopalatine fossa, which is connected to the orbit via the inferior orbital fissure. Preganglionic secretory (parasympathetic) fibers originating from the facial nerve are switched from pre- to postganglionar fibers in this ganglion. The postganglionic parasympathetic fibers course together with sympathetic fibers of two ganglionic branches (pterygopalatine nerves) back to the maxillary nerve and reach the orbit with the zygomatic nerve through the inferior orbital fissure. The parasympathetic fibers reach the lacrimal nerve and then the lacrimal gland by a communicating branch given off from the zygomatic nerve (lacrimal anastomosis), which is located in the level of or cranial to the eyeball (▶ Fig. 1.19).

References

[1] Sherman DD, Burkat CN, Lemke BN. Anatomy and its clinical applications. In: Tasman W, Jaeger EA, eds. Duane's Ophthalmology. Philadelphia: Lippincott Williams & Wilkins; 2006:chapter 21

[2] Berlis A, Putz R, Schumacher M. Maße und Varianten im Bereich des canalis opticus. CT und Anatomie. [Measurements and variations in the region of the optic canal. CT and anatomy]. Radiologie. 1992; 32:436–440

[3] Watzek G. Vergleichende anatomisch-röntgenologische Untersuchungen der knöchernen Orbita und des Neurokraniums. Fortschr Kieferorthop. 1978;39 (4):265–273

[4] Graumann W, Sasse D, CompactLehrbuch Anatomie/Sinnessysteme, Haut, ZNS, Periphere Leitungsbahnen. Vol. 4. Stuttgart: Schattauer; 2005

[5] Lippert H. Lehrbuch der Anatomie. 8th ed. München, Jena: Urban & Fischer; 2011

[6] Schünke M, Schulte E, Schumacher U. Prometheus, Lernatlas der Anatomie. Kopf, Hals und Neuroanatomie. 2nd ed. Stuttgart: Thieme; 2009

[7] Whitnall SE. On a tubercle on the malar bone, and on the lateral attachments of the tarsal plates. J Anat Physiol. 1911; 45(Pt 4):426–432

[8] Simonton JT, Garber F, Ahl N. Margins of safety in lateral orbitotomy. Arch Ophthalmol. 1977; 95(7):1229–1231

[9] Lippert H, Pabst R. Arterial Variations in Man. München: JF Bergmann; 1985

[10] Kaufmann H. Strabismus. 3rd ed. Stuttgart: Thieme; 2003

[11] Bylkl JR, Jakobiec A. Embryology and anatomy of the orbit and lacrimal system. In: Tasman W, Jaeger EA, eds. Duane's Ophthalmology. Philadelphia: Lippincott Williams & Wilkins; 2007:chapter 32

[12] Whitnall SE. Anatomy of the Orbit. London: Oxford University Press; 1932

[13] Kirsch J, May CA, Lorke D, et al. Taschenlehrbuch Anatomie. Stuttgart: Thieme; 2011

[14] Sesemann E. Die Orbitalvenen des Menschen und ihr Zusammenhang mit den oberflächlichen Venen des Kopfes. In: Reichert CB, Du Bois-Reymond, eds. Archiv für Anatomie, Physiologie und wissenschaftliche Medicin. Leipzig: von Veit et Comp; 1869:154–174

[15] Liu GT. The trigeminal nerve and its central connections. In: Miller NR, Newman NJ, eds. Walsh and Hoyt's Clinical Neuro-ophthalmology. 6th ed. Philadelphia: Lippincott Williams & Wilkins; 2005:1233–1274

Chapter 2

Pathophysiological Aspects of the Orbit

2

2 Pathophysiological Aspects of the Orbit

H.-J. Welkoborsky and T. Kraft

2.1 Introduction

Pathophysiological phenomena play a decisive role in the understanding of the diseases of the orbit and its inner structures. The difficulty here is that there does not exist just a single pathophysiology. There are, rather, many different pathomechanisms, which lead individually or in combination to different pathophysiologies and which are important to the understanding of clinical symptoms of orbital diseases. In this chapter, some important pathophysiological processes are described that in their interactions contribute to orbital diseases. The effects of these processes on the optic nerve with consequent loss of vision are especially considered. The consequences of increased intraorbital pressure and also the pathophysiology of Graves's ophthalmopathy will not be addressed: both of these are dealt with in other specific chapters (see Chapter 7 and Chapter 17).

2.2 The Orbit as a Closed Bony Compartment

The orbit consists of several bony structures. The orbital content is extensively surrounded by a bony shell, which while it gives protection against external incidences on the other hand means that increase of intraorbital pressure can only be very slightly mitigated. There is only the aditus orbitalis through which the orbital structures can expand in order to reduce the pressure. An increase of the intraorbital—especially the retrobulbar—pressure leads to an anterior displacement of the eye bulb, but the resulting decrease in the pressure is very limited. An increase of intraorbital pressure presents a hazard to the optic nerve, although the nerve itself with its axons is usually not damaged by increased pressure. The damage and functional impairment that can be observed arises more from compression of the vessels that supply the dural sheath with blood, and from compression of the nutritive vessels of the nerve itself, with consequent ischemia. As well as this, traction forces act on muscles and the optic nerve following an anterior displacement of the eye bulb. Both aspects will be discussed later in more detail.

Anatomically the optic nerve can be divided into four sections (▶ Fig. 2.1):

- An intraocular section at the sclera nerve crossover.
- An intraorbital section.
- An intracanalicular section.
- An intracranial/chiasmal section.

The hazardous potential for the optic nerve differs considerably between the sections. A fairly resistant layer of connective tissue is located at the crossover from the sclera to the optic nerve, which decreases its elasticity. Intense rotations of the eye bulb may cause axon damage in this transition zone and can lead to avulsion trauma or to axonotmesis.[1,2] The potential risk for injury of the optic nerve is relatively low in the intraorbital section, partly because its course is slightly curved, which protects the nerve from traction forces when the eye bulb is dislocated anteriorly, and partly because the nerve is covered by fat tissue in this segment, which acts as a pressure pad and, together with the cerebrospinal fluid, protects the nerve. The optic nerve canal is the narrowest site in the nerve course: the anulus of Zinn is located in this area at the aditus of the nerve canal, which is the starting point for the inner orbital muscles and which has only little elasticity. In this bony channel the nerve cannot compensate increased pressure. It is additionally at risk from avulsion injuries due to skull base fractures, which can pass through the orbit apex and through the optic nerve canal. Injuries of the optic nerve in its intracranial and chiasmal part are rare. In this area the effects of skull base tumors, inflammatory diseases of the central nervous system, or ischemia and tumors of the brain, which can lead to visual impairment, are more important.

There are basically four pathomechanisms, which can be distinguished according to damage to the intraorbital structures and the optic nerve:

- Orbital trauma.
- Inflammation with infiltration of the nerve.
- Tumors.
- Increase of the intraorbital pressure, for example, due to acute hemorrhage into the orbit or due to Graves's ophthalmopathy.

These various pathomechanisms lead clinically to functional impairment, which may manifest in a disturbance of eye bulb motility or—more frequently—in loss of vision.

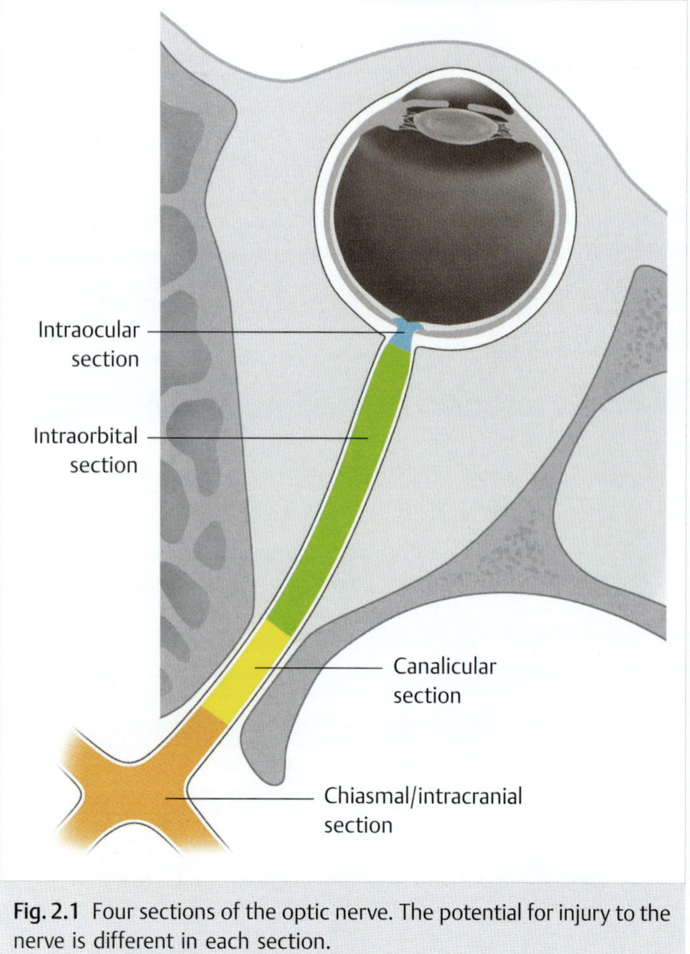

Fig. 2.1 Four sections of the optic nerve. The potential for injury to the nerve is different in each section.

2.3 Intraorbital Inflammation

Inflammation can affect the structures of the inner orbit in two different ways: as an acute inflammation, or as a chronic inflammation that is often generated by autoimmune processes that can lead, for example, to demyelinization of nerve fibers in cases of disseminated encephalomyelitis.[3,4] The optic nerve represents an extension of the diencephalon. Its axons are surrounded by oligodendroglia, which increases the velocity of nerve conduction but hampers nerve regeneration following severe inflammation or trauma. This anatomical feature is the reason why diseases of the central nervous system can spread to the optic nerve.[5,6]

The orbital complication of acute sinusitis is a classic example of an inflammation that can spread to the optic nerve, with resulting blindness (see Chapter 6). In stage III or IV of the disease, diffuse spread of the inflammation into the internal orbital structures can occur with consequent orbital phlegmon, which can lead to an acute neuritis of the optic nerve. The nerve axons can be directly affected by the inflammatory processes. However, this is less likely, because the nerve is covered by a dural sheath: it is rather more likely in the first instance that the meninges surrounding the nerve and their nutritive blood vessels are affected by acute inflammation.[7]

Bacterial inflammations result in a number of highly complex reactions of the affected tissue. These pathogen–host cell interactions can be caused by the bacteria themselves as agents (direct adherence) as well as by toxins expressed by the bacteria (endotoxins)[8] (▶ Fig. 2.2). Which of these mechanisms predominates depends very much on the bacteria. For example, the pore-forming exotoxin S. aureus α-toxin is expressed by *Staphylococcus aureus*. At the target cell this toxin leads to the formation of a pore ca. 1 nm in size by interaction with lipid chains and other integral membrane proteins. This pore represents a hydrophilic canal, which allows an ion flow.[7,9] Consequently, disturbance of the barrier function of the cell membrane occurs; in addition there is activation of particular signal pathways, which will be detailed later in this chapter. As a result, vasoactive substances are expressed by the toxin-exposed endothelial cells, such as prostacyclin (PGI_2) and nitric oxide (▶ Fig. 2.2), which dilate blood vessels. Calcium ions (Ca^{2+}) play a key role in some of this expression.[7] Activation of the complement cascade occurs parallel to these events. Activated endothelial cells also lose their anticoagulative function, which leads to increased blood clotting.[9] The bacterium *Streptococcus pneumonia*, which is most frequently identified in orbital complications of acute sinusitis, also expresses an exotoxin (pneumolysin) that has quite similar effects.

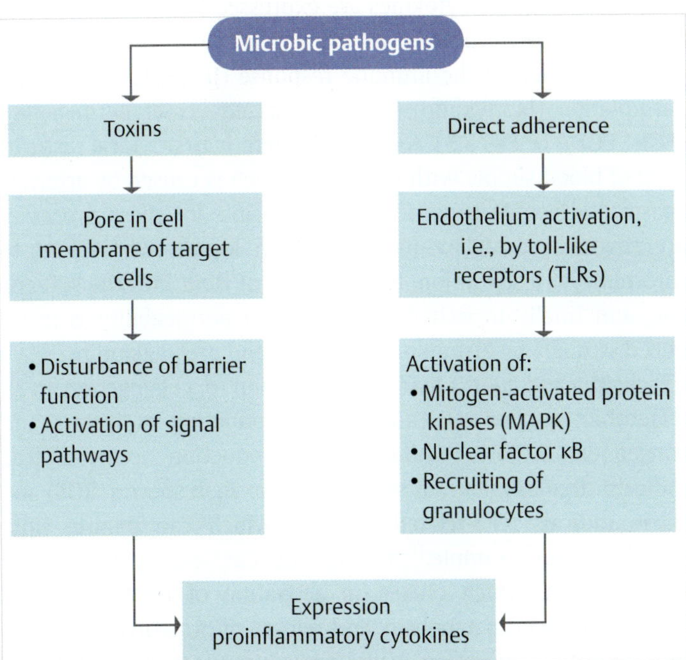

Fig. 2.2 Scheme of pathophysiological events when host cells are affected by microbial pathogens. Cell reactions can be triggered by expression of toxins as well as by direct adherence.

The vascular endothelium of the dura and of the nerve's nutritive vessels plays a fundamental role in the process of an inflammatory reaction. The gathering of bacteria on endothelial cells leads to attachment of the pathogen (adherence). Some surface structures of the pathogen are involved in this process, which imitate endogenous ligands on the endothelial cells. For example, *Staphylococcus aureus* binds to fibronectin on endothelial cells and to extracellular matrix proteins (e.g., vitronectin; elastin).[9] The inhibition of the β_2-integrin-mediated recruitment of inflammatory cells, such as neutrophil granulocytes, is a result of the effects of bacterial adhesion molecules[9,10] (▶ Fig. 2.2).

Bacteria carry molecular structures on their surface (such as lipopolysaccharides, LPS) that can be recognized by the host cells via receptors. Common representatives of these receptors are the toll-like receptors (TLR), which have been intensively investigated and play an essential role in the recognition of microorganisms.[11] An upregulation of TLR, particularly of TLR-2 and TLR-4, activates signal pathways in which tyrosine kinases, mitogen activated protein kinases (MAPK), and transcription factors (e.g., nuclear factor κB [NF-κB]) are involved,[9,11,12] leading to recruitment of granulocytes and expression of proinflammatory cytokines (e.g., tumor necrosis factor α). Activation of NF-κB can be caused by bacteria, cytokines, or chemical or physical stimuli. It is normally present inactively in the cytosol of the cell but following activation it reaches the nucleus, where it contributes to the expression of different genes, which are called "early response genes".[8,12]

Toll-like receptor-mediated activation of host cells by microbial pathogens also lead to stimulation of GTP-binding Rho-proteins (e.g., RhoA).[11,13] Among other things, Rho proteins regulate functions of cell contraction and cell migration, of phagocytosis, and activity of transcription factors.[9] Along with NF-κB, the p38 mitogen activated protein kinase (p38MAPK), which controls angiogenetic processes as well as proliferation, migration, and cell permeability, serves as a central control unit in acute inflammatory processes.[9,12,14]

Contact with a microbial pathogen leads first to an unspecific immune response, which is dominated by phagocytosing leukocytes (polymorphonuclear granulocytes; macrophages). Activation of leukocytes can be divided into different stages: (1) the "rolling" stage (in which the cells "roll" at the endothelial surface), (2) tight adhesion to endothelial cells, and (3) transmigration into subendothelial tissue.[9] Several biokines are involved in these processes:

- Integrins, particularly of group β. As well as cell-to-cell interaction they mediate important functions of the cell–matrix-interaction, and are of particular importance in both acute and chronic inflammations, such as in middle ear cholesteatoma.[15]

Table 2.1 Overview on the most important cytokines involved in an acute inflammatory reaction

Cytokine	Site of expression	Important function
NF-κB	Macrophages Endothelial cells	• Important transcription factor Regulation of several genes: • Adhesion molecules • Cytokine (TNF-α; IL-1β) • Cyclooxygenase 2
Histamine	Mast cells basophile Granulocytes	• Release of inflammatory mediators • Activation of NF-κB • Increase in vessel permeability
IL-1β	Monocytes	• Transduction, cyclooxygenase 2 • increased production of PGE_2
IL-2	T-helper cells	• Proliferation and differentiation of B- & T-lymphocytes • Production of interferon and TNF • Stimulation of NK-cells
IL-6	Endothelial cells Macrophages	• Activator of acute-phase proteins • Stimulation of lymphocytes • Activation of MAP-kinase signal pathway
IL-12	Monocytes Macrophages	• Activates cellular defense Supports T-killer cells
TNF-α	Macrophages	• Activates transcription factor NF-κB • Stimulation of phagocytes • Supports migration of granulocytes
TGF-β	Macrophages Endothelial cells	• Influences cell proliferation • Anti-inflammatory effects
Bradykinin	Endothelial cells	• Mediator of inflammation • Vasodilation • Chemotactic effects on leukocytes
Prostaglandins (PGE_3; PGI_2)	Endothelial cells Macrophages (from arachidonic acid metabolism)	• Increase of vessel permeability

- Adhesion factors such as E-selectin, P-selectin, intercellular adhesion molecules (ICAM-1 and ICAM-2), which act as ligands for β-integrins, as well as the vascular cell adhesion molecule (CD106 = VCAM), which controls the rolling and adherence of leukocytes on the endothelial surface.

The pathophysiological processes described above, along with products of stimulated granulocytes (oxygen radicals; proteases) constitute a disturbance of endothelial barriers, with increased permeability.[16] Blood plasma extravasated into the tissue and corpuscular blood constituents lead to edema but can also lead to exacerbation of the inflammation. Hypoxia or acidosis of the tissue caused, for example, by edema can also impede the regular metabolism and can therefore contribute to a progression of the pathological process. The vascular endothelial growth factor (VEGF), which can also initiate processes of angiogenesis, might play a key role in edema formation.[9,12]

The severity of clinical inflammation symptoms—edema and blood vessel constriction, later blood vessel dilatation—is considerably influenced by this endothelial activation.[9]

Leukocytes (polymorphonuclear granulocytes; macrophages) that migrate into the tissue begin to phagocytose bacteria. Attachment of complement system factors at the bacterial wall predisposes to this process (opsonization). Several specific immunoglobulins that activate the complement system are involved in this. Opsonized bacteria are recognized as "foreign bodies" by the phagocytes and ingested by endocytosis.[9] *Pneumococcus* has a polysaccharide capsule that prevents complement attachment. For phagocytosis, interleukin-6 (IL-6) is expressed by macrophages.

In a subsequent step or in parallel to this, there is expression of several cytokines, particularly of interleukins 1β, 2, 6, 12 (IL-1β, IL-2, IL-6, IL-12), tumor necrosis factor α (TNF-α), transforming growth factor β (TGF-β), interferons, fibrinogen, bradykinin, and cytokines arising from arachidonic acid metabolism (prostaglandins, particularly PGE_2; prostacyclins, particularly PGI_2) (▶ Table 2.1). These cytokines are expressed by endothelial cells, by macrophages or polymorphonuclear granulocytes, and lead to an accentuation of the immune response (IL-1β, IL-2, IL-12), to vasodilation (bradykinin), or to increased vessel permeability (PGI_2; PGE_2) (▶ Fig. 2.3). As a result, there is first a local disturbance of blood supply with ischemia, which is caused by arteriole spasm and venule constriction. Responsible for these processes are several prostaglandins, along with kinins, which lead to thrombocyte aggregation, to exudation of fluid into the soft tissue, and finally to ischemia. Increase in permeability is influenced strongly by histamine, serotonin, and prostaglandins.[9,12,14]

Ischemia and edema lead to hypoxia and to a changeover to an anaerobic metabolism, causing overproduction of lactate and consequent acidosis.[17] Additionally, production occurs of free radicals—free oxygen radicals (reactive oxygen species, ROS) and nitric radicals (NO-related species)—which can oxidize lipid structures, for example.[16] Finally, the Ca^{2+}-pump of the cells breaks down, which causes an activation of lipolysis and of arachidonic acid metabolism, and release of proteolytic enzymes and of excitatory amino acids (e.g. glutamate; aspartate). The anterograde and retrograde transport, which is an energy consuming process, is stopped. All of these processes have considerable influence on the axons, which cannot maintain their function.[10]

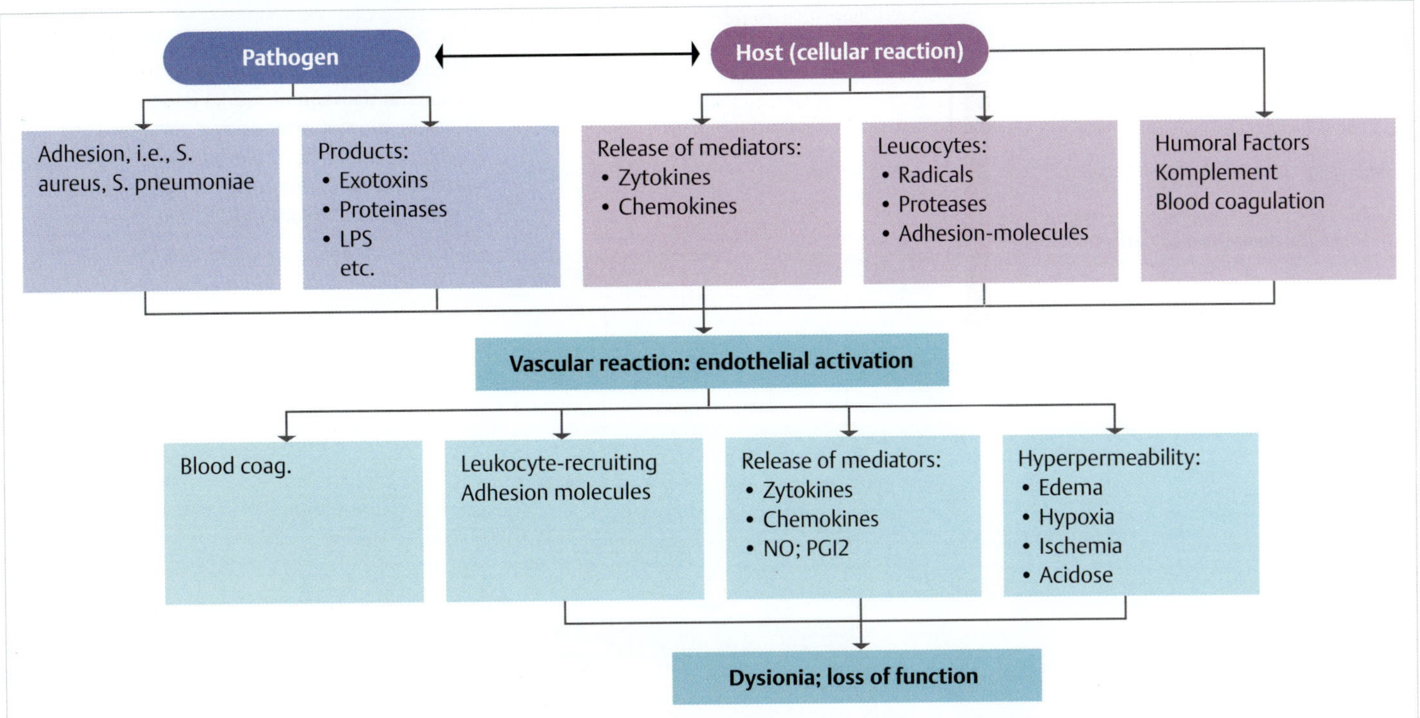

Fig. 2.3 Scheme of the interaction between pathogens (microbial pathogen) and host cells. There is either a cellular reaction mediated by leukocytes or a vascular reaction based on endothelial activation. Release of inflammatory biokines and hyperpermeability result in edema, ischemia, acidosis, and loss of function.

In conclusion, these complex processes lead to cell swelling, edema, and to ischemia, which may cause depolarization and electrical disturbance of the axons.[18] The clinical consequence is an impairment of visual acuity up to amaurosis, which is reversible in the first hours but certainly is irreversible after a period of 8 to 24 hours. From these facts it must be considered that treatment of phlegmonous orbital inflammation including removal of the septic focus should be performed as soon as possible and as an emergency procedure.

In summary, reaction of the optic nerve sheath following an inflammatory stimulus is a highly complex process, which can be differentiated into stages:

1. An unspecific immune reaction following activation of endothelial cells with rolling, adherence, and transmigration of polymorphonuclear granulocytes and macrophages.
2. A specific immune reaction mediated by immunoglobulins. Several cytokines are involved in the inflammatory reaction, with NF-κB being the central transcription factor for gene expression of cytokines and prostaglandins. Edema and local ischemia, which can lead to a function loss of the nerve, are the consequences of the inflammatory reaction.

2.4 Increased Intraorbital Pressure

Increased intraorbital pressure can have several causes:

- Overproduction or diminished reabsorption of aqueous humor, e.g., in glaucoma.
- Orbital tumors or disturbed reabsorption of cerebrospinal fluid.
- Adipose tissue proliferation or hypertrophy of intraorbital muscles, e.g. in Graves's orbitopathy.
- Intraorbital hemorrhage, e.g. iatrogenic following functional endonasal sinus surgery.
- Accidents and bony fractures of the bony orbital walls.

Here we detail the consequences of increased intraorbital pressure due to injury or hemorrhage.

Injuries (i.e., penetrating foreign body) with hemorrhage into the orbit lead to a rapid increase of pressure. According to Circovic et al. frontal penetrating foreign bodies can induce intraorbital pressure of more than 300 mm Hg, which regularly produces pressure damage of the optic nerve, with the transition zone between the sclera and the optic nerve being the site of predilection ("optic nerve knob").[1,2]

Apart from this excessive and very rapid increase in pressure, the nerve is jeopardized by some injuries that produce slow but considerable increase in pressure, for example, due to hemorrhage.[18] Normally the intraorbital pressure is about 4 mm Hg, clearly below the intraocular pressure of 10 to 21 mm Hg.[19,20] The blood pressure in the central vein, which drains the majority of the blood from the retina and optic nerve, is normally some 4 mm Hg above the intraocular pressure. The maintenance of this pressure gradient is essential for venous drainage.[21] Intraorbital and intraocular pressure undergo some daily variation, but they remain fairly constant within a small range. Hemorrhage into the orbit leads to a considerable increase of intraorbital pressure. The eye bulb and the optic nerve can alleviate this pressure increase to only very limited extent anteriorly. Furthermore, the suspension apparatus of the eye bulb at the intraorbital muscles plus the eyelids and the corneal septum restrain the pressure drainage.[22] As a consequence an orbital compartment syndrome occurs. The optic nerve is especially threatened in its transition zone from the sclera to the intraorbital compartment of the nerve and at the apex region (Zinn's common tendinous ring).[23,24,25] Increase of intraorbital pressure at the sclera–nerve transition zone and at the optic nerve knob induces microglial activation, which leads to an acute inflammatory reaction of the retina with expression of cytokines, particularly interleukin-1 (IL-1) and tumor necrosis factor α (TNF-α), with consequent destruction and loss of retinal ganglion cells.[26,27]

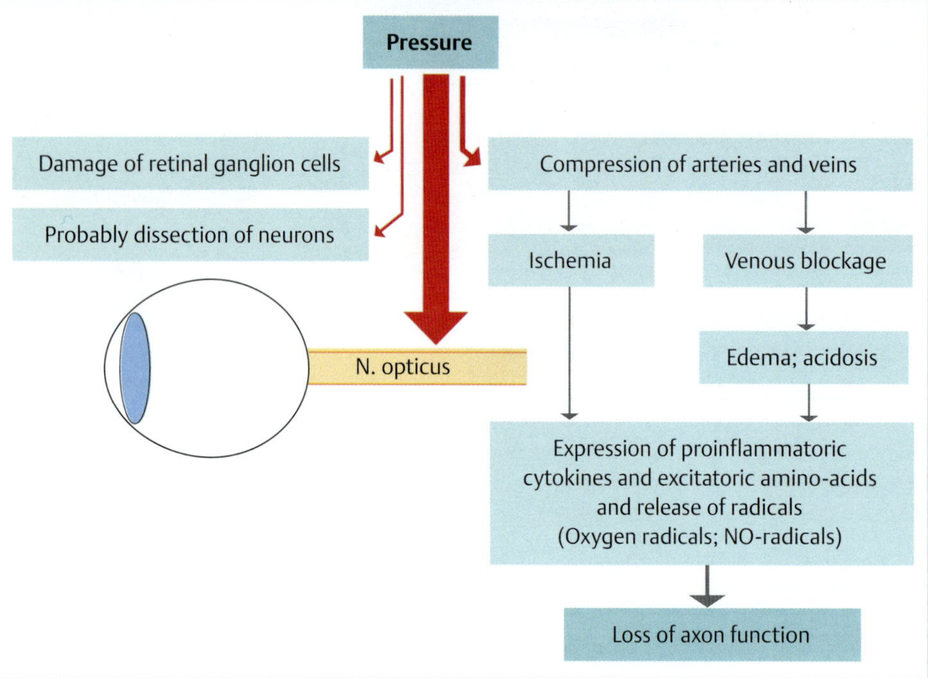

Fig. 2.4 Scheme of pathophysiological events following pinching of the optic nerve, which results in damage of retinal ganglion cells. Compression of arteries and veins leads to ischemia and venous blockage with consequent edema, acidosis, expression of proinflammatory cytokines, and release of radicals.

Direct pressure damage of the optic nerve proximal to the eye bulb can only be expected with excessive pressure increase and due to hemorrhage in the optic nerve canal,[1,2] because the optic nerve itself is fairly well protected by the surrounding dura, cerebrospinal fluid, and adipose tissue, which serve as a kind of pressure pad and mitigate the influence of pressure.

Compression of nutritive and draining vessels of the optic nerve and of its surrounding dura is the second, and probably much more important, pathogenetic mechanism that is induced by an increase of intraorbital pressure. It leads to a circulation deficit and ultimately to ischemia and to venous stasis.[25]

Ischemia and venous stasis lead to a disruption of the supply of high-energy phosphate (ATP), so that anaerobic glycolysis must increasingly be used for its synthesis. This process produces lactate, which induces acidosis in the tissue. Normally the intra- and extracellular ionic gradients are adjusted by ATP-dependent pump systems. Ischemia leads to a release of excitatory amino acids, particularly glutamate (excitoxicity), which causes an influx of calcium into the neurons. This calcium overload induces production and release of reactive oxygen species and nitric oxide, which leads to cell damage by activation of lipoxygenase. This produces a chain reaction with cell necrosis and apoptosis as its end point following the release of additional excitatory amino acids and production of radicals.[28] Breakdown of active ionic pump systems in the cells induces an exchange of ions. The flow of ions into the cells is followed by that of water, which leads to a swelling of the cells and the surrounding tissue (edema) and makes the ischemia worse. Parallel to this, expression of an array of cytokines occurs, similar to the cascades that have been described in detail in Chapter 2.3 (▸ Fig. 2.4).

The processes described might be reversible over a period of some hours. According to investigations in animals by Gellrich et al[29] there is a clear correlation between the number of damaged neurons and the time for which an increase of pressure continues: in the albino rat an increase of intraorbital pressure for 60 minutes reduced healthy neurons by 14.5%, whereas an increase of pressure for 90 minutes reduced them by almost 48.3%. A similar correlation was demonstrated between degenerated retinal ganglion cells and the length of time following the injury.[26]

In conclusion, increase of intraorbital pressure can damage the optic nerve by two different pathogenetic mechanisms:

1. Damage to and destruction of neurons and retinal ganglion cells and activation of microglial cells by the direct effect of pressure on the nerve. This can be expected in cases of excessive and rapid increase of intraorbital pressure (e.g., penetration of a large foreign body at high velocity into the orbit), with the sclera–nerve transition zone and orbital apex being sites of predilection for this damage.
2. Indirect damage by compression-related disruption of blood supply in the arterioles and impairment of venous drainage, with consequent ischemia, edema, acidosis, release of radicals and excitatory amino acids, and expression of proinflammatory cytokines. These processes and the damage caused by them are reversible over a period of some hours.

2.5 Pathophysiology of Orbital Trauma

Traumatic lesions of the orbit can arise from direct or indirect trauma. In direct trauma the bony orbit or the inner orbit is injured, for example, by anterior sharp traumatic violence such as the penetration of a foreign body. Indirect injuries affect the orbit and its inner structures by bone transmission.[30] Avulsion trauma of intraorbital nerves must be distinguished from both of these types of injuries and is described separately.

2.5.1 Direct and Indirect Orbital Trauma

Direct trauma of the orbit is caused, for example, by incision wounds, gunshot wounds, or penetration of a foreign body, events that normally deliver traumatic violence from anteriorly. Sharp objects can lead to a complete cutting of nerves and muscles and also to a perforating eye bulb injury. According to the computer simulations by Circovic et al, inertial forces of 5g, translational accelerations of > 1 m/s^2, increase of intraorbital pressure to > 300 mm Hg, and rotatory accelerations of > 500 degrees/s^2 can occur when a foreign body penetrates the orbit. These leads to torsion of the eye bulb with flexion and avulsion of the nerve's axons in the area of the sclera–nerve transition.[1,2]

Four percent to 5% of all craniocerebral traumas are accompanied by indirect injury of the orbit and optic nerve. Other cranial nerves, which are quite frequently involved and injured in craniocerebral trauma, are the oculomotor nerve and the abducens nerve.[30] In these cases the energy usually is transferred by bone conduction. A bony fracture occurs when the energy exceeds the elasticity of the bony walls. The bone often fractures at its weakest point or in the skull base.

Several pathophysiological processes in the optic nerve and retina can be induced by indirect orbital trauma—nerve sheath hematoma, intraretinal and subretinal hematoma, nerve torsion, and destruction of axons.[31,32] Nerve damage can be divided into neurapraxia, axonotmesis, and neurotmesis. Neurapraxia is characterized by nerve contusion, which leaves axons and nerve sheaths intact. Axonotmesis refers to interruption of the axons while the nerve sheath and the surrounding tissue remains uninjured. Neurotmesis is defined as complete cutting of the nerve and its sheaths; an example of this is the avulsion trauma of the optic nerve (see Chapter 2.5.2).

Pathophysiologically a hematoma of the nerve sheath of the optic nerve leads to the processes described in Chapter 2.4: hematoma causes ischemia, disturbance of the ionic metabolism, edema, and expression of proinflammatory cytokines, which can exacerbate the tissue damage.[33] Hematoma or avulsion trauma of the retina and optic nerve head induce microglia cell activation, which causes an acute inflammatory response in the retina with loss of retinal ganglion cells. Detachment of retinal ganglion cells or disruption of axons can also occur.

Due to its anatomy, the optic nerve has only a very limited capacity for regeneration, so that the injuries described result in most cases in irreversible loss of function after a period of some hours. There are currently under way animal studies investigating drugs to support nerve regeneration (e.g., with brain-derived neurotrophic factor), but to date these substances are not available for clinical application.[34]

Injuries of the retina and optic nerve often lead to a loss of retinal ganglion cells. This process is irreversible, due to microglial activation and the resulting inflammatory reaction. Retinal ganglion cells have only a limited regeneration potential. Animal experimental studies published in 2014 investigated the possibilities for treating these pathophysiological processes on a molecular level. The results of an intravitreal injection of a Rho-GTPase blocker or medication with the growth factor simvastatin are encouraging, but clinical application in humans is currently not feasible.[27,35,36]

The optic nerve and its surrounding sheaths have a capability for limited compensation of traction forces due to the fact that the nerve does not have a straight course through the orbit but a slightly curved one. Extensive traction forces, such as due to a retrobulbar inflammation or severe retrobulbar hemorrhage, result in a pressure load on the nerve along with an anterior displacement of the eyeball. Consequently, the dural sheath of the nerve is strained with disruption of small blood vessels, edema, and ischemia. If the nerve itself is affected by the traction forces, disruption of the nerve and neurotmesis can occur, which result in an irreversible loss of function.[37]

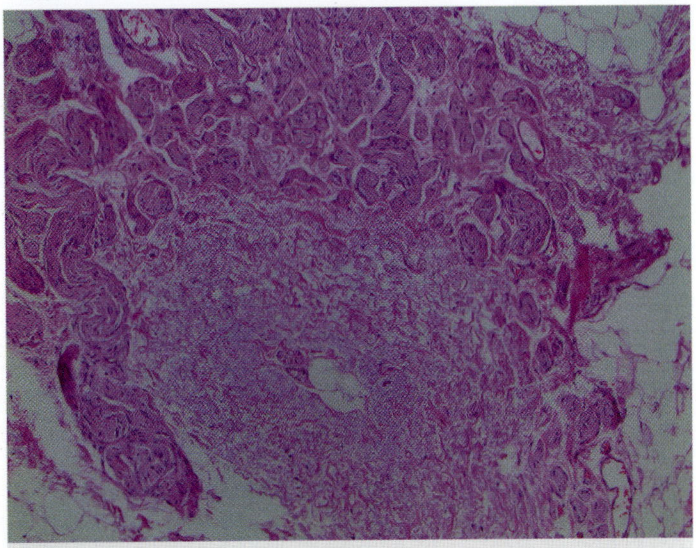

Fig. 2.5 Histologic picture of a dissected nerve. A thickening in the proximal nerve stump occurs which is due to a hyperplasia of myelin sheaths and nerve cells along with fibrous scar tissue.

2.5.2 Avulsion Trauma of the Optic Nerve

Avulsion trauma of the optic nerve can occur during massive rotation of the eye bulb at the sclera–orbit- transition zone, or in case of a fracture passing through the optic nerve canal with dislocation of bony fragments. Additionally, comminuted fractures in the optic nerve canal can lead to bony debris penetrating the optic nerve, which results in an axonotmesis or complete neurotmesis with irreversible loss of function. The optic nerve, which is a part of the diencephalon, does not have the capability for regeneration. Histologically, in the first hours following complete cutting of the nerve, edema of the proximal nerve stump occurs with parallel degeneration of retinal ganglion cells. Some days posttraumatically, hyperplasia and proliferation of glial tissue can be observed, followed by apoptosis of ganglion cells and axons. Degeneration of optic nerve fibers reaches its maximum 7 days posttraumatically, and after 4 weeks scarred metaplasia of the nerve stumps is completed (▶ Fig. 2.5). Most recent studies investigating the regeneration potential of retinal ganglion cells and optic nerve axons aim to improve proliferation and reinsertion of the axons by medication with growth factors.[38]

References

[1] Cirovic S, Bhola RM, Hose DR, et al. Computer modelling study of the mechanism of optic nerve injury in blunt trauma. Br J Ophthalmol. 2006; 90(6): 778–783

[2] Cirovic S, Bhola RM, Hose DR, Howard IC, Lawford PV, Parsons MA. A computational study of the passive mechanisms of eye restraint during head impact trauma. Comput Methods Biomech Biomed Engin. 2005; 8(1):1–6

[3] Moshkelgosha S, So PW, Deasy N, Diaz-Cano S, Banga JP. Cutting edge: retrobulbar inflammation, adipogenesis, and acute orbital congestion in a preclinical female mouse model of Graves' orbitopathy induced by thyrotropin receptor plasmid-in vivo electroporation. Endocrinology. 2013; 154(9):3008–3015

[4] Maier K, Merkler D, Gerber J, et al. Multiple neuroprotective mechanisms of minocycline in autoimmune CNS inflammation. Neurobiol Dis. 2007; 25(3): 514–525

[5] Elamin M, Alderazi Y, Mullins G, Farrell MA, O'Connell S, Counihan TJ. Perineuritis in acute lyme neuroborreliosis. Muscle Nerve. 2009; 39(6):851–854

[6] Kuwabara S, Yuki N. Axonal Guillain-Barré syndrome: concepts and controversies. Lancet Neurol. 2013; 12(12):1180–1188

[7] Chiu IM, Heesters BA, Ghasemlou N, et al. Bacteria activate sensory neurons that modulate pain and inflammation. Nature. 2013; 501(7465):52–57

[8] Toosy AT, Mason DF, Miller DH. Optic neuritis. Lancet Neurol. 2014; 13(1):83–99

[9] Hippenstiel S. Endothel und Entzündung—Pathomechanismen der bakteriellen Endothelaktivierung [Habilitationsschrift]. Berlin: University of Berlin; 2003

[10] Henderson AP, Altmann DR, Trip SA, et al. Early factors associated with axonal loss after optic neuritis. Ann Neurol. 2011; 70(6):955–963

[11] Hamprecht A. Genetische Polymorphismen in Toll-like-Rezeptoren, rheumatoide Arthritis und Höhe von Rheumafaktoren im Serum [Inaugural dissertation]. Berlin: University of Berlin; 2005

[12] Riechelmann H. Cellular and molecular mechanisms in environmental and occupational inhalation toxicology. In: Schultz-Coulon HJ, ed. Environmental and Occupational Health Disorders. Niebüll: Videel Verlag; 2004:12–30

[13] Teusch N, Lombardo E, Eddleston J, Knaus UG. The low molecular weight GTPase RhoA and atypical protein kinase Czeta are required for TLR2-mediated gene transcription. J Immunol. 2004; 173(1):507–514

[14] Nahirnyj A, Livne-Bar I, Guo X, Sivak JM. ROS detoxification and proinflammatory cytokines are linked by p38 MAPK signaling in a model of mature astrocyte activation. PLoS One. 2013; 8(12):e83049

[15] Welkoborsky HJ, Jacob RS, Hinni ML. Comparative analysis of the epithelium stroma interaction of acquired middle ear cholesteatoma in children and adults. Eur Arch Otorhinolaryngol. 2007; 264(8):841–848

[16] Dahiya P, Kamal R, Gupta R, Bhardwaj R, Chaudhary K, Kaur S. Reactive oxygen species in periodontitis. J Indian Soc Periodontol. 2013; 17(4):411–416

[17] Kempski O. Pathologische Neurophysiologie. In: Jantzen JP, Löffler W, eds. Neuroanaesthesie. Stuttgart: Thieme; 2000:90–104

[18] Rose GE, Verity DH. Acute presentation of vascular disease within the orbit-a descriptive synopsis of mechanisms. Eye (Lond). 2013; 27(3):299–307

[19] Berthout A, Vignal C, Jacomet PV, Galatoire O, Morax S. [Intraorbital pressure measured before, during, and after surgical decompression in Graves' orbitopathy]. J Fr Ophtalmol. 2010; 33(9):623–629

[20] Brinker T, Lüdemann W, von Rautenfeld DB, Brassel F, Becker H, Samii M. Breakdown of the meningeal barrier surrounding the intraorbital optic nerve after experimental subarachnoid hemorrhage. Am J Ophthalmol. 1997; 124 (3):373–380

[21] Hartmann K, Meyer-Schwickerath R. Measurement of venous outflow pressure in the central retinal vein to evaluate intraorbital pressure in Graves' ophthalmopathy: a preliminary report. Strabismus. 2000; 8(3):187–193

[22] Otto AJ, Koornneef L, Mourits MP, Deen-van Leeuwen L. Retrobulbar pressures measured during surgical decompression of the orbit. Br J Ophthalmol. 1996; 80(12):1042–1045

[23] Gauden AJ, Hardy T, Mack HG, Danesh-Meyer HV, Kaye AH. Orbital compartment syndrome following aneurysm surgery. J Clin Neurosci. 2012; 19(7): 1032–1036

[24] Lima V, Burt B, Leibovitch I, Prabhakaran V, Goldberg RA, Selva D. Orbital compartment syndrome: the ophthalmic surgical emergency. Surv Ophthalmol. 2009; 54(4):441–449

[25] Carrim ZI, Anderson IW, Kyle PM. Traumatic orbital compartment syndrome: importance of prompt recognition and management. Eur J Emerg Med. 2007; 14(3):174–176

[26] Gellrich NC, Schimming R, Zerfowski M, Eysel UT. Quantification of histological changes after calibrated crush of the intraorbital optic nerve in rats. Br J Ophthalmol. 2002; 86(2):233–237

[27] Wu N, Yu J, Chen S, et al. α-Crystallin protects RGC survival and inhibits microglial activation after optic nerve crush. Life Sci. 2014; 94(1):17–23

[28] Lau A, Tymianski M. Glutamate receptors, neurotoxicity and neurodegeneration. Pflugers Arch. 2010; 460(2):525–542

[29] Gellrich NC, Schramm A, Rustemeyer J, Schön R, Theodor Eysel U. Quantification of the neurodegenerative impact on the visual system following sudden retrobulbar expanding lesions - an experimental model. J Craniomaxillofac Surg. 2002; 30(4):230–236

[30] Sharma B, Gupta R, Anand R, Ingle R. Ocular manifestations of head injury and incidence of post-traumatic ocular motor nerve involvement in cases of head injury: a clinical review. Int Ophthalmol. 2014; 34(4):893–900

[31] Azari AA, Kanavi MR, Saipe NB, Potter HD, Albert DM, Stier MA. Shaken adult syndrome: report of 2 cases. JAMA Ophthalmol. 2013; 131(11): 1468–1470

[32] Wang J, Fox MA, Povlishock JT. Diffuse traumatic axonal injury in the optic nerve does not elicit retinal ganglion cell loss. J Neuropathol Exp Neurol. 2013; 72(8):768–781

[33] Welkoborsky HJ, Möbius H, Bauer L, Wiechens B. Traumatische Optikusneuropathie. Langzeitergebnisse nach endonasaler mikrochirurgischer Dekompression des N. opticus. [Traumatic optic nerve neuropathy. Longterm results following microsurgical optic nerve decompression]. HNO. 2011; 59(10):997–1004

[34] Weber AJ, Harman CD. BDNF treatment and extended recovery from optic nerve trauma in the cat. Invest Ophthalmol Vis Sci. 2013; 54(10):6594–6604

[35] Drummond ES, Rodger J, Penrose M, Robertson D, Hu Y, Harvey AR. Effects of intravitreal injection of a Rho-GTPase inhibitor (BA-210), or CNTF combined with an analogue of cAMP, on the dendritic morphology of regenerating retinal ganglion cells. Restor Neurol Neurosci. 2014; 32(3):391–402

[36] Morishita S, Oku H, Horie T, et al. Systemic simvastatin rescues retinal ganglion cells from optic nerve injury possibly through suppression of astroglial NF-κB activation. PLoS One. 2014; 9(1):e84387

[37] Park CH, Jee DH, La TY. A case of odontogenic orbital cellulitis causing blindness by severe tension orbit. J Korean Med Sci. 2013; 28(2):340–343

[38] Zuo L, Khan RS, Lee V, Dine K, Wu W, Shindler KS. SIRT1 promotes RGC survival and delays loss of function following optic nerve crush. Invest Ophthalmol Vis Sci. 2013; 54(7):5097–5102

Chapter 3

Clinical Examination in Patients with Orbital Diseases

3 Clinical Examination in Patients with Orbital Diseases

3.1 Ophthalmologic Examinations

B. Wiechens and S. Behrendt

3.1.1 Introduction

Broad knowledge about orbital disorders has been accumulated in the literature over the last decades. To date more than 170 diseases of the orbit have been defined.[1,2,3,4,5,6] Despite the multiplicity of etiologies, the ophthalmologic symptoms in orbital diseases are mainly characterized by few key symptoms, exophthalmos being the most important one,[7] followed by restrictions to the visual functions (visual acuity, visual field), ocular motility problems (double vision), and further symptoms when the anterior segment of the eye is involved (e.g., pain, epiphora, redness).

Ocular symptoms in orbital diseases are often unspecific. As a result there is a wide variety of possible explanations when the patient first presents to an ophthalmologist. To permit an efficient, cost-effective, and less demanding diagnostic work-up, it is efficacious to follow a step-by-step approach, whereby it is possible to exclude a large number of possible orbital disorders. It is advisable to proceed gradually from basic to advanced diagnostic tests. Patients with orbital disorders often present to an ophthalmologist first. Thus, ophthalmological diagnostics may play a key role in the investigation of the patient. Systemic diseases, which make an ophthalmologic or orbital involvement likely, make a brief ophthalmologic history, even by nonophthalmologists, and refer to an ophthalmologist mandatory. This is where interdisciplinary collaboration is of great importance. However, one should ensure that the specialist to whom the patient first presented, for the time being, "holds the reins" until a final therapeutic decision has been made.[8,9] Only in the later course of the diagnostic work-up and, above all, of the therapeutic plan can the onus be passed to other specialists to take charge (Video 3.1).

3.1.2 Case History

An accurate recording of the patient´s history will gather significant information that will determine further diagnostic investigation and work-up. It is important to gain information on the following symptoms:

- Nature of complaints
  - Main complaint
  - Pain (spontaneous, during eye movements, upon pressing)
  - Diplopia
  - Visual impairment
  - Visual field defects
  - Lid reddening, lid swelling, asymmetry of palpebral fissure
  - Chemosis, conjunctival injection
  - Periorbital swelling and redness
  - Proptosis (Valsalva maneuver), pulsating exophthalmos
  - Crepitation of the eye lid skin on pressure
  - Headache (type and course)
  - Accompanying neurologic symptoms
  - Pain or feeling of pressure in the area of the paranasal sinuses
  - Sensory deficits such as paresthesia in the area of the teeth (most importantly in the upper jaw)
  - Olfactory deficits
  - Audible bruits
- Beginning and course of the symptoms
  - Progression rate
    - Acute (e.g., inflammations)
    - Subacute (e.g., Graves's orbitopathy)
    - Chronic (e.g., tumors)
  - Increase or decrease of the complaints or triggering factors
  - Is this a first incidence or a recurrence?
  - Has an investigation already been carried out for similar symptoms?
- Possible etiology
  - Age of the patients: children in particular are affected by inflammations, injuries and certain tumors; in middle age there is predomination of Graves's ophthalmopathy; while in older patients tumors are more likely.[10]
  - Preceding trauma
  - Operations (e.g., paranasal sinuses or neurosurgical interventions)
  - Allergies
  - General diseases such as hyperthyroidism, other endocrinal or tumorous (e.g., malignant) diseases
  - Drug history to exclude toxic side effects from medication
- Previous examinations
  - Is it the first presentation or have previous examinations already been made on the current problems? Are the findings are available? Names of the other treating physicians should be acquired and documented.
  - If indeterminate findings or symptoms have existed for some time, patients should be asked to bring old photographs that may give a clue how long the current finding may have already existed.
- Family history

3.1.3 Inspection

Before a more advanced examination is carried out, the first procedure should be the inspection of the patient, preferably in an erect position. The examination room should be sufficiently well illuminated; a penlight can be used to augment ambient lighting but the examiner has to make sure not to blur the patient as it might interfere with the ensuing visual acuity testing. When carrying out the inspection, attention should be paid to findings such as facial anomalies or asymmetries, signs of inflammation or injuries, hematomas, or other(s). Always compare one eye with the other and determine whether they are symmetrical in size and position. Given that one eye is normal, unilateral eye pathologies are much more easily recognized. When a difference is observed, it is essential to determine which side exhibits the abnormality.

In cases with unilateral proptosis or eyelid swelling with occlusion of the palpebral fissure, close attention has to be paid to properly examine the eye and the extraocular motility (e.g., limited extraocular motility in orbital cellulitis).

The eyeballs should be checked to see if they are in the same plane as the eyebrows and maxillae. In orbital diseases the key symptom is exophthalmos. The best way to assess proptosis is by looking from behind over the shoulder of the patient or from the front after pulling up the upper eyelids and asking the patient to look down. It is very important to exclude pseudoexophthalmos (e.g., in severe myopia or an enlarged palpebral fissure) or enophthalmos of the other eye.

During the inspection, attention should also be paid to a possible malposition of the affected eye in primary position (looking straight). In this position the upper eyelid covers the upper portion of the cornea. An axial anterior displacement of the eye usually indicates an intraconal disease process, such as cavernous hemangioma. However, if additional lateral displacement is present, an extraconal disease has to be ruled out. In general, the localization of the disease process should usually be sought on the opposite side of the displacement (▶ Fig. 3.1): If there is an inferior and medial displacement of the eye then a pathologic process in the temporal upper orbital space, such as a disorder of the lacrimal gland, has to be suspected. If there is an inferior and temporal displacement of the eye, a process in the upper nasal orbital space, such as a mucocele, should be excluded.

When carrying out the inspection, possible pulsations of the eye should be ruled out. These can best be identified by looking from the lateral side and by examining with a magnifying glass.

The relative height and the position of the two lid margins as well as the surface of the eyelids are observed for pathologic changes. The facial skin in the vicinity of the orbit has to be checked. In inflammatory diseases, such as orbital cellulitis, marked swelling of the eyelids can occur (see ▶ Fig. 6.3). These changes have to be differentiated from local lid inflammation (e.g., chalazion or hordeolum). Lid mobility can be affected in Graves's orbitopathy (e.g., upper lid retraction = Dalrymple's sign), after oculomotor nerve damage, or after trauma (ptosis).

If the patient states that there has been an acute trauma previous to the presentation, one should look for signs of injury, which sometimes can be very subtle, such as small wounds and orbital hematomas (▶ Fig. 3.2).

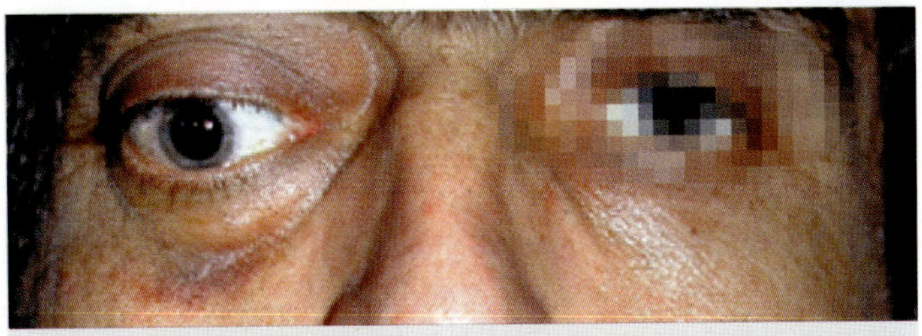

Fig. 3.1 Patient with a traumatic orbital hematoma causing an inferotemporal displacement of the eye globe.

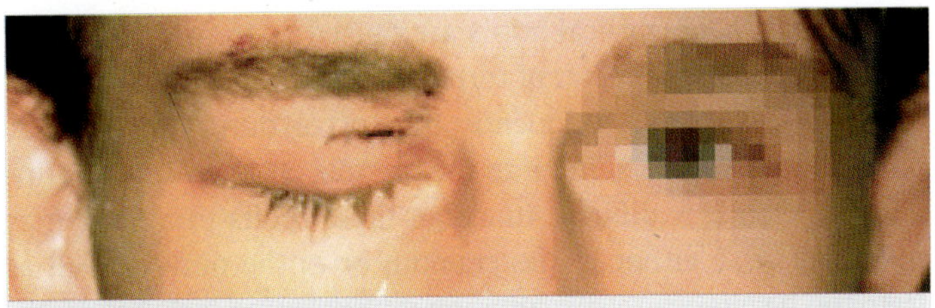

Fig. 3.2 Patient with a traumatic ptosis and a small wound in the upper lid caused by a foreign body injury on the right eye.

During the inspection, signs of generalized diseases with possible involvement of the orbit can be disclosed such as café au lait spots in patients with neurofibromatosis.

3.1.4 Palpation

After the inspection, palpation of the periorbital regions should be carried out. As a rule, the palpation is started on the unaffected side in order to better assess pathological findings.

Space-occupying processes in the anterior orbit or in the eyelids, such as lacrimal gland processes or dermoid cysts, can often be palpated subcutaneously. Attention is paid to consistency, color, shape (well-defined or diffuse), margins, pain, and movability.

Changes to the bony orbital rim caused by fractures or bone defects caused by malignant tumors are likewise palpable. Fractures of the medial orbital wall (lamina papyracea) can lead to orbital and lid emphysema, which becomes noticeable through a typical crepitation upon pressure to the lid tissue. Sometimes pulsations can be felt or seen in pathologic vascular processes.

The paranasal sinuses should be examined for pain over the cheek and radiating to frontal region or teeth, increasing with straining or bending down. Regional painful lymph nodes can point to an acute inflammation, whereas painless lymph node enlargement occurs more frequently in chronic processes, for example, with tumors. Pain sensation or numbness in the cutaneous distribution (dermatomes) of V_1, V_2 and V_3 is tested by touching the skin at the nerve exits of the sensory branches of the trigeminal nerve.

Ocular diseases should always be excluded if the patient complains of pain sensation in the (peri)orbital region. These encompass intraocular inflammations, ocular surface problems (e.g., sicca syndrome), asthenopia due to uncorrected refractive errors, and elevated intraocular pressure in glaucoma. The latter can be tested by a simple method, which is done bimanually with careful pressure of both index fingers on the closed upper eye lid, comparing the two sides (▶ Fig. 3.3).

3.1.5 Visual Acuity Test

Any disease process in the orbit can lead either to direct impact on the optic nerve (e.g., compression through tumor growth; posttraumatically) or to indirect nerve damage (e.g., through inflammatory mediators or perfusion disorders),

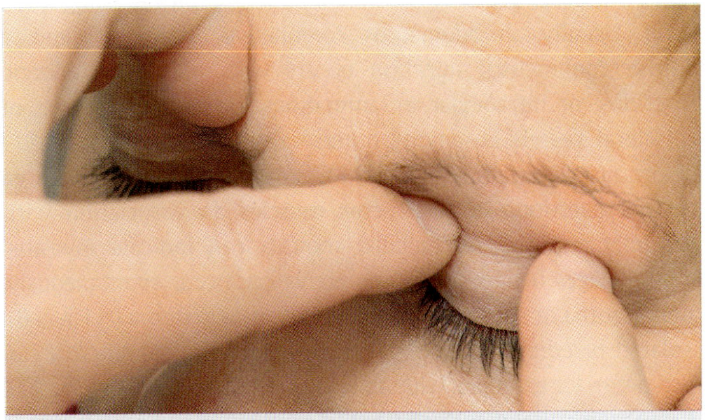

Fig. 3.3 Bimanual palpation to estimate the intraocular pressure. Note that this examination must always be performed on both eyes.

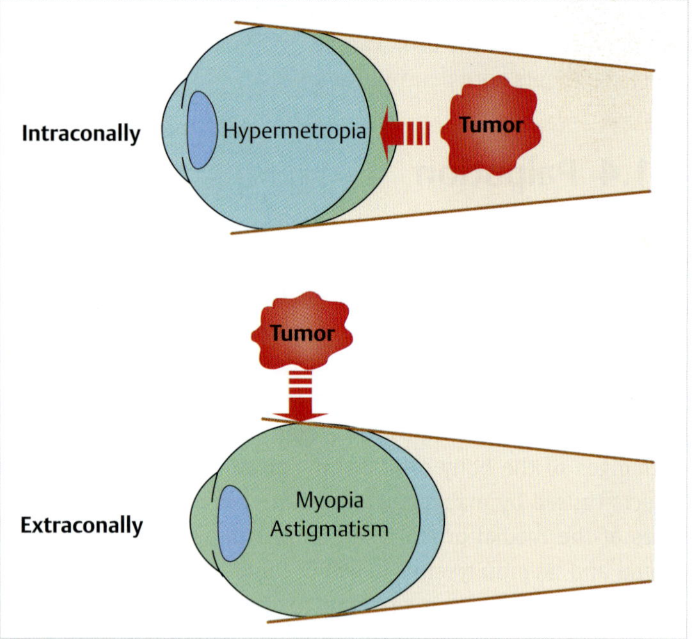

Fig. 3.4 Mechanism of refractive change in an eye due to intraorbital tumor formation.

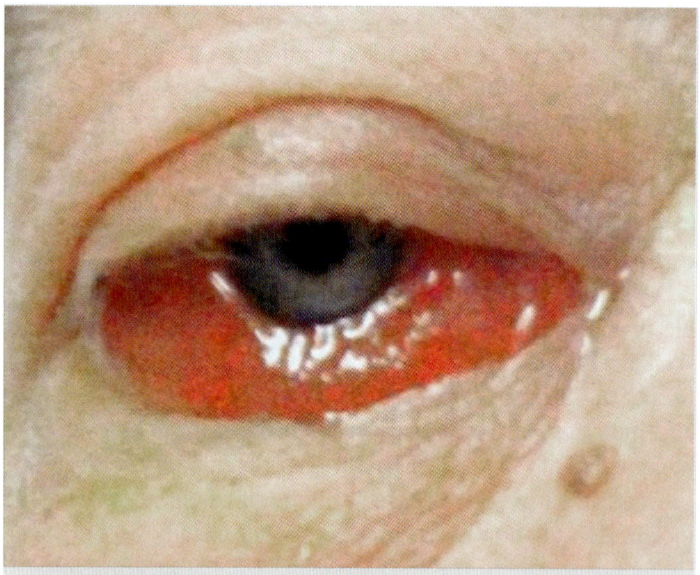

Fig. 3.5 Dilatation of conjunctival blood vessels and congestion of episceral veins in a patient with an internal carotid artery–cavernous sinus-fistula.

which often result in impairment of visual acuity and/or disturbances in the visual field. Space-occupying lesions in the orbit can cause direct compression of the eye globe. Under certain circumstances this can lead to a significant refractive changes. The resulting refractive errors can give hints to the localization of the orbital mass (▶ Fig. 3.4): An intraconal process—for example, a cavernous hemangioma—leads to a shortening of the eye globe due to axial pressure and thus to hyperopia. In contrast, an extraconally located tumor—for example, processes in the lacrimal gland or a mucocele—leads to lateral compression of the eye globe, which can result in myopia, astigmatism, or a combination of both. For this reason, orbital pathologies have to be excluded in any patient, who presents with an unexplained refractive change.

3.1.6 Slit-lamp Biomicroscopy of the Anterior Segment of the Eye

Although many pathologic findings of the anterior segment of the eye—such as of the cornea or of the conjunctiva—can be distinguished with the naked eye, definitive results and classification of diseases are only possible biomicroscopically using a slit lamp. Usually an edematous conjunctiva (chemosis) and/or diffuse conjunctival injection occurs with infections, allergic reactions, or intraocular inflammations. Isolated congestion of episcleral vessels is—among others—a typical sign for carotid–cavernous sinus fistula (▶ Fig. 3.5). Isolated injection in the area of the insertions of the rectus muscles, in association with painfully restricted extraocular motility can indicate myositis. Hemorrhages beneath the conjunctiva can occur spontaneously, after trauma or subsequent to retrobulbar hematoma (▶ Fig. 3.6). Isolated bleeding into the lymph vessels of the conjunctiva can also occur, for example, with an orbital lymphangioma (▶ Fig. 3.7). A localized, salmon-colored patched swelling of the conjunctiva is typical for lymphoma (MALT lymphoma). This typical finding gives a hint for a conclusive diagnosis at the first examination.

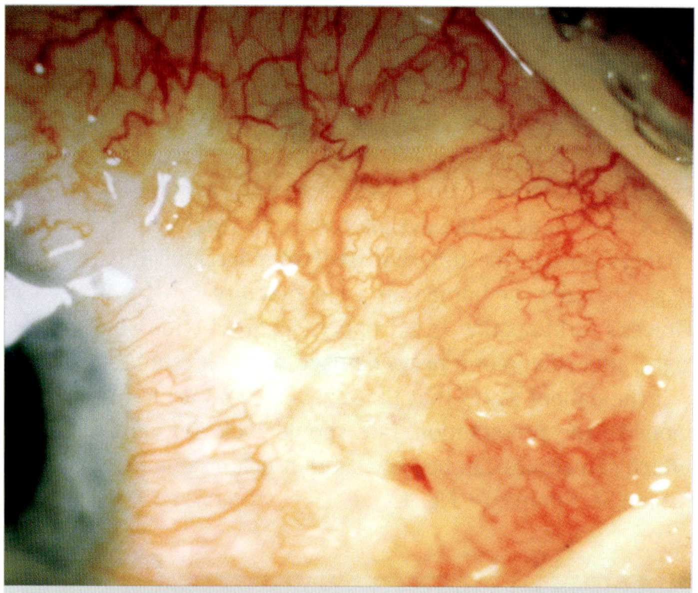

Fig. 3.6 Significant conjunctival chemosis and intraconjunctival hemorrhage.

Lower and upper lid hematoma (monocle hematoma) is common finding after lid or orbital trauma (▶ Fig. 16.2). In these cases an intraorbital hematoma always has to be excluded.

3.1.7 Auscultation

Cranial, orbital or cervical bruits are caused by transferred vibrations, which are the result of turbulences in intra- or extracranial blood vessels.[11] Most frequently they occur during the systolic phase, but can also extend into the diastole or be present continuously. Often it is difficult to assign these bruits to an origin as they may arise either in the cranium or in the neck as well as from the heart. Orbital auscultation is a screening technique indicated in patients with tinnitus, pulsatile exophthalmos, persistent conjunctival injection unresponsive to therapeutic efforts,

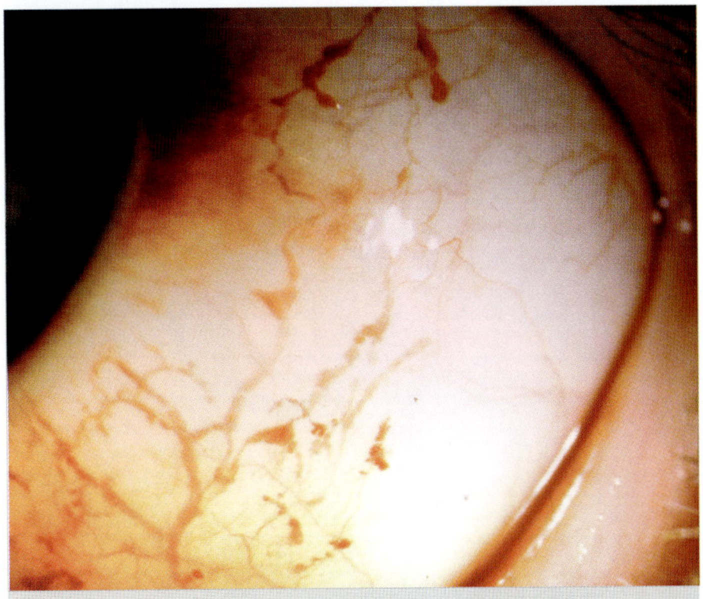

Fig. 3.7 Hemorrhagic conjunctival lymph vessels.

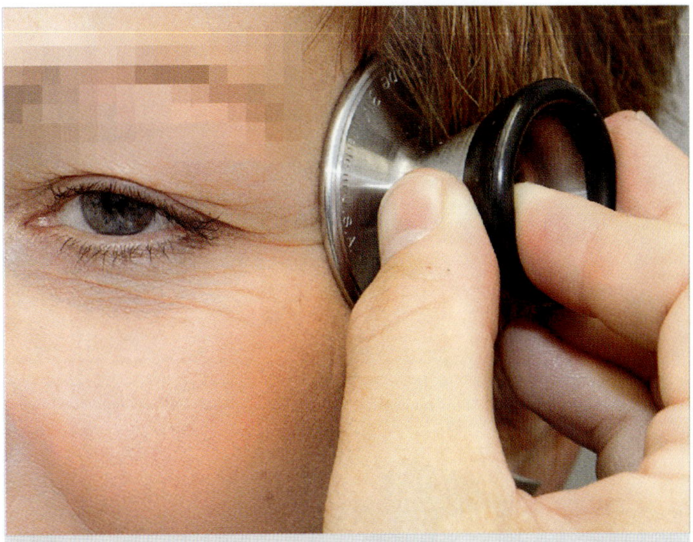

Fig. 3.8 Auscultation of the orbit.

headache, and neurologic disorders. It is performed by gently placing the stethoscope over the closed eyes and should include the zygomatic and lateral regions as well as the skull (▶ Fig. 3.8). In order to correlate the acoustic phenomena with cardiac activity, the radial pulse is palpated simultaneously. Bruits or noises may be crucial in guiding further diagnostic evaluation. A pulse-synchronous "machine noise" over the orbit is pathognomonic for a carotid–cavernous sinus fistula. Pulse-synchronous noises can also occur in orbital/cerebral AV malformations, in intracranial space-occupying masses with raised intracranial pressure, as well as in other diseases such as vascularized tumors and bone defects (e.g., sphenoid wing aplasia in neurofibromatosis). However, these conditions are very rare.[12]

3.1.8 Exophthalmometry

One of the key symptoms of most orbital diseases is *exophthalmos*. *Enophthalmos* is encountered less frequently (e.g., in cirrhotic breast carcinoma metastasis). As facial asymmetries, osseous malformations, anomalies of the palpebral fissure, or pseudoexophthalmos (e.g., in high myopia) can mimic exophthalmos, objective measurement of the proptosis is crucial. Exophthalmometry is an important means to objectively identify clinically suspected exophthalmos and plays an important role in follow-up examinations to assess the clinical course. There are various devices available (e.g., Hertel exophthalmometer, Luedde or Naugle exophthalmometer), the Hertel exophthalmometrer being the most widely used (▶ Fig. 3.9). The extent of an axial forward displacement of the eyeball can be objectively determined using this device. The distance between the corneal apex and the orbital rim is measured at the level of the zygomaticofrontal suture. Values under 15 mm and above 20 mm as well as a difference between the eyes exceeding 2 mm are significant and make further investigation mandatory. The actual exophthalmometer readings as well as the interorbital distance are important parameters to be documented for monitoring purposes. Conclusions about the actual course of the proptosis can only be drawn if the correct interorbital distance is set in repeated measurements. More recent developments in this field are digital exophthalmometry[13] and Hertel exophthalmometry without contact to the orbital rim.[14]

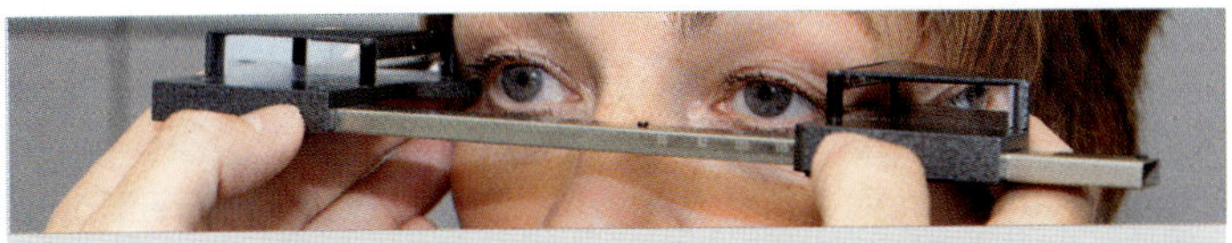

Fig. 3.9 Hertel exophthalmometry.

Normal exophthalmometry values vary significantly depending on age, sex, and ethnic origin. In a meta-analysis of different studies, Rootman stated that black people usually have higher average values than whites, whereas people of Asian origin stand between the two.[5] Analyses of exophthalmometry values suggest that they increase with age[5]: thus, in children between 5 and 7 years of age, the average values range from 12.6 mm (girls) to 13.7 mm (boys), but in 8- to 10-year old children they are from 14.1 mm (girls) to 13.7 mm (boys). In the adult group the average values rise to 16 mm for men and 16.5 mm for women.

3.1.9 Tonometry

Palpation of the intraocular pressure (as described in Chapter 3.1.4) is only used if no other instruments are available. By comparing both sides differences in intraocular pressure can be revealed and in some cases increased intraocular pressure can be concluded. However, various tonometers are available to determine the intraocular pressure accurately, such as the Goldmann or Schiøtz tonometers, the noncontact tonometer, the I-Care tonometer, or the Perkins hand-held applanation tonometer, the most common being the Goldmann tonometer. In contrast to Schiøtz impression tonometry, which nowadays is not routinely used, almost no intraocular fluid is displaced so that Goldmann tonometry provides more reliable values. Local anesthetic drops containing fluorescein must be applied before starting the measurement. The amount of force required to flatten a 3.06-mm diameter circle of the anesthetized cornea (▶ Fig. 3.10) is measured with the patient in an erect position. The intraocular pressure can be read directly on the calibrated dial of the tonometer after the mires (semicircles) in the prism of the tonometer head have been properly aligned.

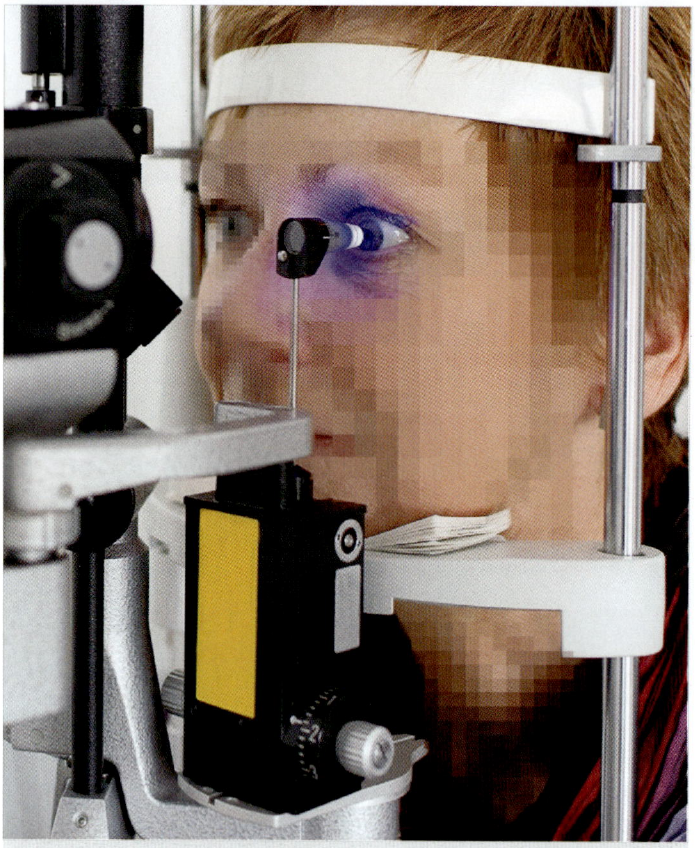

Fig. 3.10 Applanation tonometry with the Goldmann tonometer.

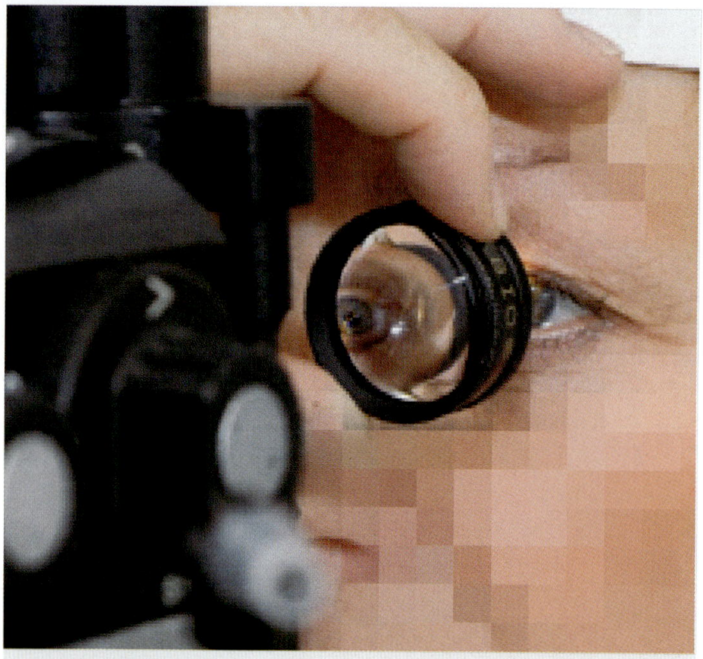

Fig. 3.11 Opthalmoscopy of the central ocular fundus using a Volk lens.

Changes in intraocular pressure related to orbital disease occurs mainly in Graves's disease, arteriovenous shunts, trauma, and orbital neoplasia. In Graves's orbitopathy, the intraocular pressure is commonly elevated because of intraorbital inflammation and edema. In upgaze the globe is often squeezed between the rectus superior muscle and the fibrotic rectus inferior muscle. This results in a temporary elevation of the intraocular pressure which rapidly returns to normal after looking straight ahead again. This is why the intraocular pressure should be measured and documented in upgaze and downgaze as well as in the primary position.

Elevated intraocular pressure can also be correlated with thrombosis of the superior ophthalmic vein or a carotid–cavernous sinus fistula.

Increased intraocular pressure secondary to orbital diseases has to be differentiated from glaucoma of ocular origin such as primary open-angle glaucoma. A careful patient history has to be taken in order to identify pre-existing glaucoma.

Reduced intraocular pressure occurs after intraocular inflammations with ciliary body involvement and ocular phthisis. If ocular hypotony after trauma is noted, penetrating/perforating injury of the eye (open or closed) has to be ruled out.

3.1.10 Motility Testing

Motility disorders can be of mechanical origin (e.g., with entrapment of the inferior rectus muscle in orbital floor fracture), inflammatory origin (e.g., with myositis), or paretic origin (e.g., as the result of nerve lesion following trauma, compression, or inflammation).[15] Palsies can occur after injury to a single nerve (such as traumatic palsy of the trochlear nerve or abducens nerve), after primary nerve damage (e.g., with a neurinoma), or after a combination of various cranial nerve injuries (such as in superior orbital fissure or orbital apex syndrome). Thus patients may complain of a variety of visual problems, such as diplopia, blurred vision, visual confusion, oscillopsia, or tilted images accompanied by vertigo.

Whereas double vision can arise very early in acute diseases, it may develop quite late in slowly expanding processes (mucoceles, etc.), as over time even significant globe dislocations can be compensated. The extent of the double vision depends on the direction of gaze, on the location of the process, and on the nature of the disturbance to the nerves or muscles. The displacement of the eye by a tumor can cause double vision already in straightforward gaze, whereas paretic double vision usually occurs when looking in the direction of the primary action of the eye muscle (noncomitant strabismus: for example, abduction in abducens nerve palsy).

Motility disorders can also occur as complications after orbital surgery. If these are caused by postsurgical hemorrhage or swelling, they frequently decrease spontaneously over time. Subsequent strabismus following surgical interventions (e.g., optic nerve decompression in Graves's orbitopathy) is not uncommon. Thus, patients should be informed preoperatively about the potential risk of restriction of ocular motility and disturbing symptoms. However, postoperative double vision may be regarded as evidence that orbital decompression has been successful. Because ocular motor disorders are not uncommon in the population and may already be present, an ocular motility examination should always be obtained prior to surgery.

3.1.11 Ophthalmoscopy

If an orbital disease is suspected, ophthalmoscopy should be carried out after the pupil has been pharmacologically dilated. Even nonophthalmologists can examine the posterior fundus by means of a direct ophthalmoscope. A major drawback is the poor visibility of the peripheral fundus. Ophthalmologists prefer binophthalmoscopic funduscopy by means of an indirect ophthalmoscope, a contact lens, or a handheld lens (e.g., Volk lens + 78 diopters) (▶ Fig. 3.11).

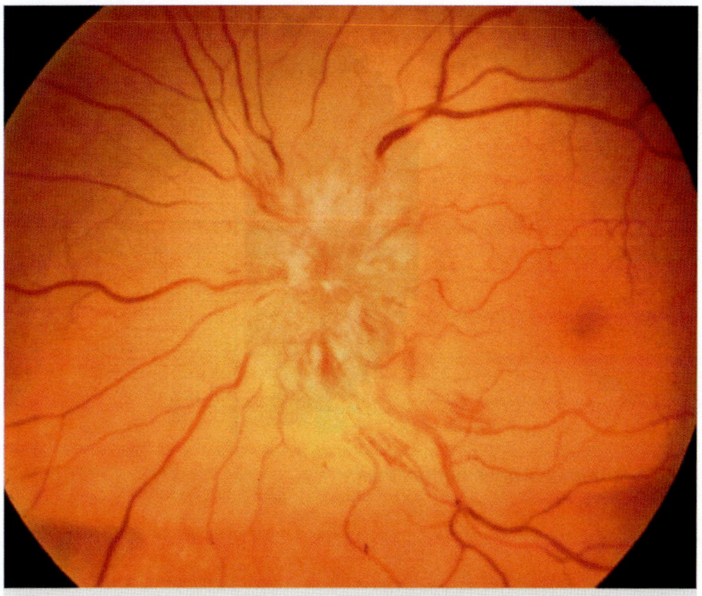

Fig. 3.12 Papilledema with optic disc hemorrhages and retinal vascular tortuosity.

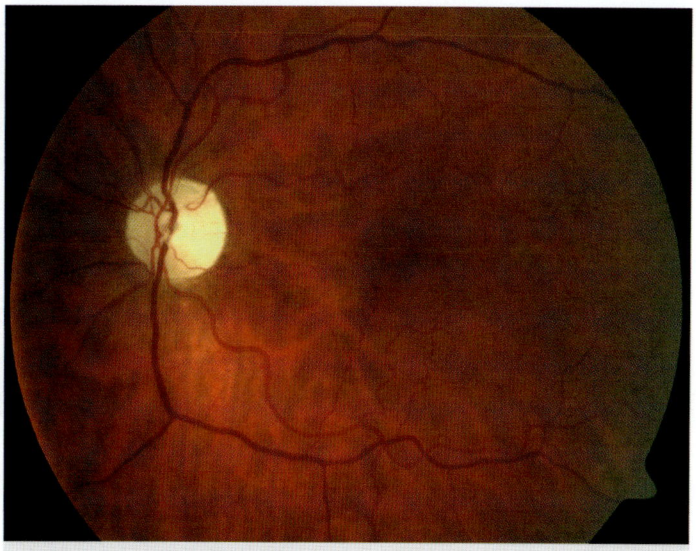

Fig. 3.13 Optic disc atrophy.

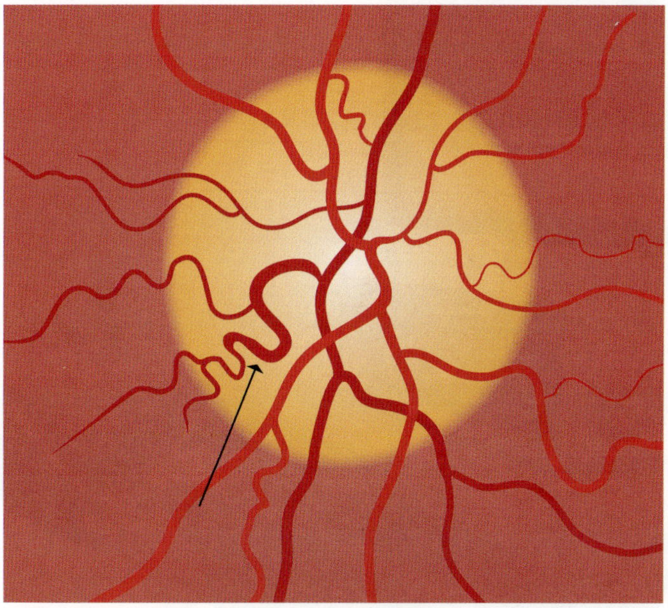

Fig. 3.14 Opticociliary shunt vessel (*arrow*) in a patient with optic nerve sheath meningioma.

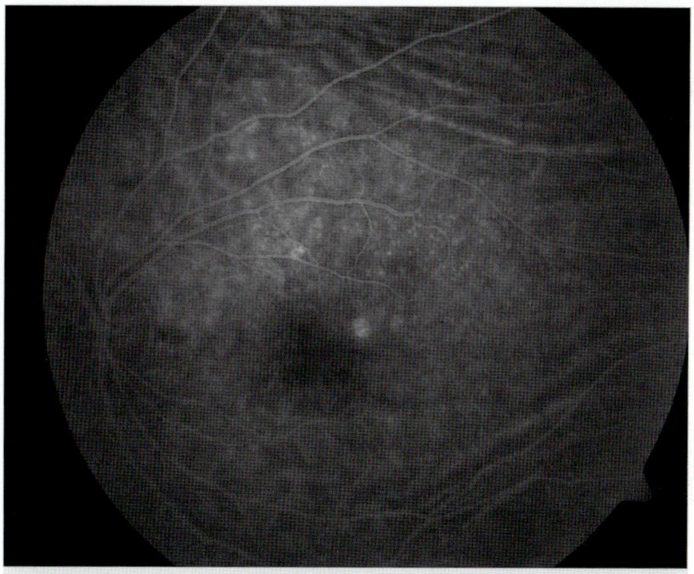

Fig. 3.15 Retinal and choroidal folds.

Funduscopic findings can give clues for orbital diseases.[16] Inflammatory or neoplastic processes can cause optic disc edema by direct compression or venous congestion (orbital papilledema, ▶ Fig. 3.12). Long-lasting compression of the optic nerve or the optic disc can result in optic atrophy (▶ Fig. 3.13). Opticociliary shunt vessels can be pathognomonic for optic nerve sheath meningioma (▶ Fig. 3.14). Venous drainage obstruction is often associated with congestion of the retinal veins. Mass-induced globe indentation may cause chorioretinal folds that are visible in funduscopy (▶ Fig. 3.15). Likewise, primary intraocular tumors with subsequent infiltration of the orbit can be discovered by ophthalmoscopy (e.g.. malignant melanoma of the choroid, retinoblastoma).

Those optic disc changes that cannot be attributed to ocular or systemic diseases, necessitate further diagnostic tests in order to exclude orbital or intracerebral disorders. Likewise chorioretinal folds, which cannot be explained by an eye disease, require exclusion of orbital disease.

3.1.12 Perimetry

Apart from impaired visual acuity, visual field defects are typical symptoms of optic nerve damage. They can occur in optic nerve compression by inflammatory disease, tumors, after trauma of the optic canal, or by swelling of extraocular muscles in Graves's orbitopathy.

Advanced visual field defects already can be disclosed by using confrontation perimetry, a technique in which the examiner compares his or her own visual field with that of the patient. Better and more precise, however, are Goldmann or computed perimetry. With these perimetric techniques even fairly small defects can be detected (▶ Fig. 3.16).

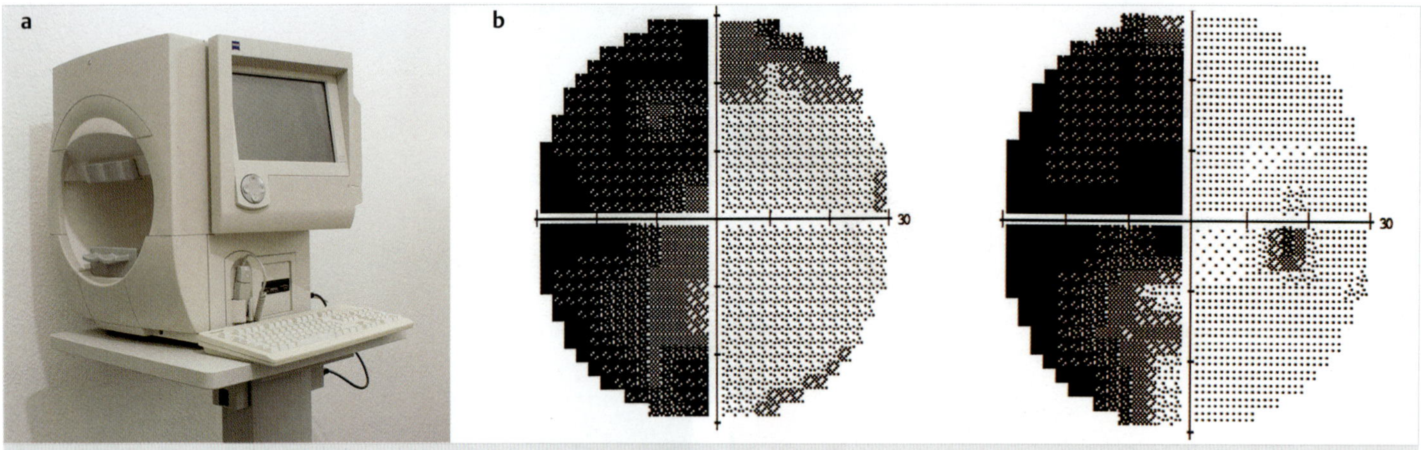

Fig. 3.16 **(a)** Modern perimetry device. **(b)** Perimetric findings in a patient with left homonymous hemianopia.

Only in the minority of cases are visual field defects disease-specific. However, the severity of visual field defects varies significantly depending on the nature of the damage to the optic nerve. Lesions such as optic nerve sheath meningioma that interrupt the papillomacular bundle produce a cecocentral scotoma and sometimes peripheral field defects, whereas a tumor-induced papilledema can cause an enlarged blind spot; with advanced atrophy peripheral visual field defects can occur.

When interpreting perimetric findings one should bear in mind that computed perimetry in particular requires a high degree of patient compliance. Thus a first "pathologic" perimetric tests should always be repeated as poor cooperation of the patient may lead to visual field defects that do not correspond to actual clinical findings. To avoid misinterpretation of the results of perimetry, an underlying eye disease (such as glaucoma, preceding vascular occlusion, preceding history of laser coagulations, maculopathies, opacification of optic media, sicca syndrome, etc.) that might have an impact on the evaluation of perimetric findings should always be excluded.

3.1.13 Pupil Examination

Pupil testing has a key role in ocular examination and should be incorporated in every comprehensive examination. Even in unconscious patients conclusions can be drawn about the function of the optic nerve and the subjacent neurologic structures (pupillary reflex pathway).

Results of a normal pupil examination can be documented using the acronyms PERRLA (pupils equal, round, reacting to light, and accommodation) and no RAPD (relative afferent pupillary defect).

The direct and consensual pupillary reaction should be tested in either eye as well as the convergence reaction in order to exclude possible lesions affecting the pupillary reflex pathway. Lesions of the optic nerve can be assessed by the *swinging light test*. This comparative test is helpful in separating visual deterioration due to pathologies in the optic media from those of severe retinal or optic nerve disorders. To perform this test the patient is asked to look into the distance. The examiner sits to the side of the patient to avoid accommodation of the patient and swings a dimmed light back and forth in front of the two pupils. A convergence reaction produced by fixating the examination lamp should be avoided as this can lead to false results of the test. After initial constriction of the pupil in the consensual pupillary reaction, a paradoxical widening of the pupil occurs when the direct pupillary reaction is tested on the affected side, indicative of optic nerve damage.

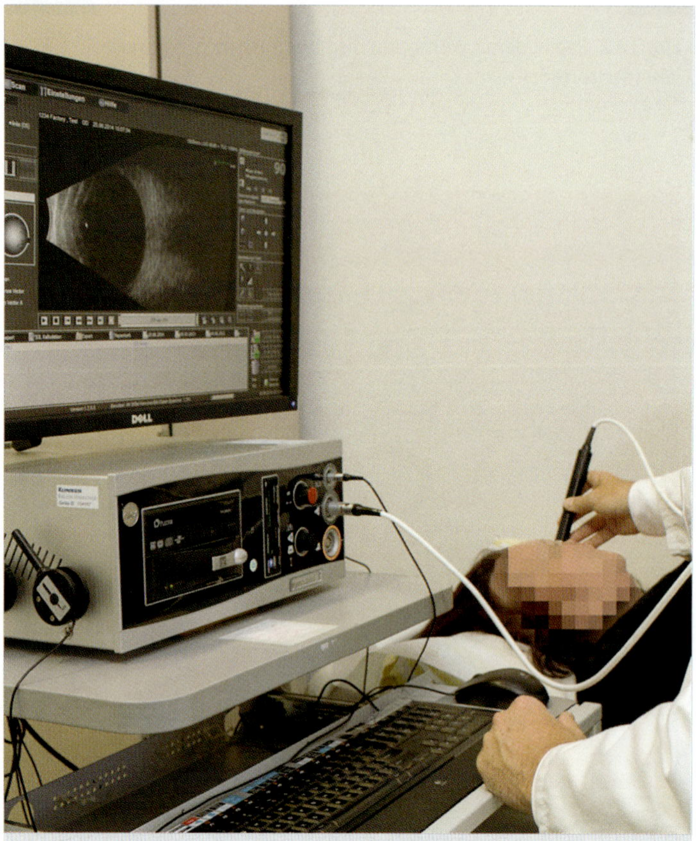

Fig. 3.17 Ultrasonography of the eye and orbit.

3.1.14 Ocular and Orbital Echography

Echography plays an important role in primary diagnostics and follow-up examinations of ocular diseases and the anterior orbital space (▶ Fig. 3.17), but it should be kept in mind, that ultrasound sonography of the orbital apex is not possible. Therefore, computed tomography and magnetic resonance imaging far outweigh the conclusiveness of ultrasound sonography of the entire orbit and the adjacent anatomical structures.[17,18,19,20] Nevertheless, due its minimal stress for the patient, low cost, and wide availability, echography is an important means in the diagnostics of many

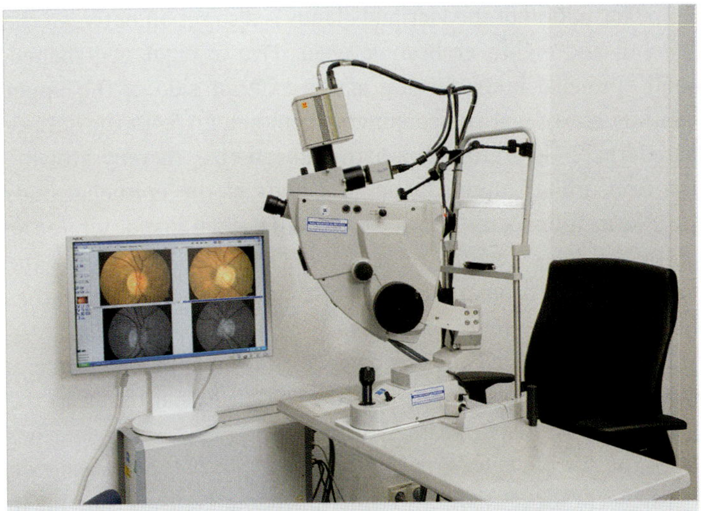

Fig. 3.18 Fluorescence angiography.

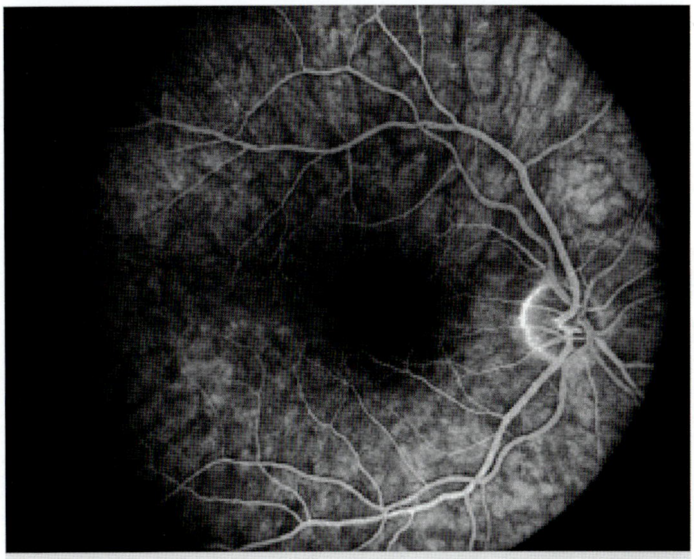

Fig. 3.19 Fluorescence angiogram.

orbital disorders. With the combination of standardized A-mode echography, which permits tissue diagnostics to a certain extent, and B-mode echography, it is frequently possible to obtain diagnostic clues to specific ocular and orbital disorders.[21,22,23]

Color-coded duplex sonography allows the evaluation of hemodynamic findings of orbital vessels.[24] Ultrasound biomicroscopy can be helpful in investigating processes of the anterior segment of the eye (e.g., ciliary body melanoma) with secondary involvement of the orbit. High-frequency transducers (50–100 MHz) allow high resolution of ocular structures but only a minimal depth of penetration. Thus this technique is not suitable for diagnosis in the orbit.

3.1.15 Fluorescein and Indocyanine Green Angiography; Spectral Domain Optical Coherence Tomography

Fluorescein (FAG) and indocyanine green (ICG) angiography can be performed (▶ Fig. 3.18; ▶ Fig. 3.19, Video 3.2, Video 3.3, Video 3.4, Video 3.5) to investigate pathological processes in the anterior segment of the eye (conjunctiva, sclera, iris) as well as in disorders of the ocular fundus (retinal and choroidal disorders). Spectral domain optical coherence tomography (SD-OCT) can be used to examine ocular disorders of the anterior segment of the eye and—more frequently—of the macular region, though OCT plays a minor role in the primary diagnosis of orbital diseases.

For advanced diagnostic imaging (angiography, computed tomography, and magnetic resonance imaging, PET) refer to Chapter 4.

3.1.16 Visual Evoked Potentials (VEP)

Using evoked potentials, the response of the central nervous system to an external stimulus is registered in an EEG-like procedure. Responses to the stimulus are differentiated from other brain activity by sampling and averaging. The stimulus for visual evoked potentials (VEP) is a repeated flash of light (for children or persons with very low visual acuity) or an alternating black and white checkerboard pattern.

Characteristic waveforms manifest as sequential surface-positive and surface-negative potentials. Time delays (or latencies) and amplitudes of particular waves are measured to allow signal processing evaluation in the optic nerve and in the visual cortex. Anomalies of VEP may present as changes in latency, amplitude, topography, and waveform. These anomalies may indicate visual pathway dysfunction, such as compression, toxic damage, inflammation, or vascular abnormalities.

Although VEP provide valuable additional information about the extent and the course of a visual dysfunction, the information is unspecific and usually does not allow any definitive pathogenetic assignment.[25,26] In any case, other ocular or retinal disorders have to be excluded. In the absence of disorders of the retina.

3.1.17 Biopsy

If a final diagnosis has not been reached after application of all noninvasive diagnostic procedures described above, a tissue biopsy must be obtained. Performing a biopsy requires a sufficient conclusive (if possible) preoperative diagnostic imaging such as MRI, CT, etc. In localized orbital lesions, a combined diagnostic and therapeutic approach is preferable. If possible, a complete removal of the pathologic process during the first operation may be advantageous, which could be best achieved by frozen section analysis. An interdisciplinary operation should be planned depending on the nature and extent of the disease. Fine needle aspiration biopsy for cytopathologic examination is controversial because of lesser diagnostic accuracy compared with histological examinations and the potential risk of cell seeding.

3.2 ENT Examinations

S. Graß and H.-J. Welkoborsky

3.2.1 Embryology of the Orbit and the Eye and of Its Related Adnexa

The orbit presents itself as a bony compartment in which numerous cranial bones are involved (cf. Chapter 1.2). The roof of the orbit is composed of the orbital fascia of the frontal bone and—in the dorsal part—the lesser wing of the sphenoid bone. The front of the medial wall is formed by the lacrimal bone and the back by the orbital lamina of the ethmoid bone. The zygomatic bone and the greater wing of the sphenoid bone form the lateral wall. Parts of the maxillary bone, the zygomatic bone, and the palatine bone compose the orbital floor. These bones are of mesenchymal origin. Two months into the embryonic development, the initiation of a bone formation in the basal part of the mesenchyme surrounding the developing brain starts, forming both the frontal end of the notochord and the parachordal cartilage. Geminate prechordal cartilage develops in front of the notochord. A protuberance of the ectodermal oral cavity roof (Rathke's pouch) between the two streaks reaches to the base of the brain, forming the anterior pituitary.[27] Cartilaginous nasal capsules develop in front of the prechordal cartilage. The fusing of these complexes generates the cartilaginous skull base, the so called primordial cranium. Endochondral ossification leads to the transformation of the primordial cranium into (among others) the ethmoidal bone, the lower turbinate, and the sphenoid bone with the exception of its greater wing.

Direct ossification of the connective tissue of other osseous structures in the orbit leads to the formation of membrane bones (intramembranous ossification) including large parts of the frontal bone, the lacrimal bone, the zygomatic bone and the maxillary bone.[27,28] Since the process of ossification of the orbit is not terminated at birth, ossification zones are still traceable in adults and are usually palpable in clinical examinations in cases of diastasis. Ectodermal (neuroectoderm and surface ectoderm) as well as mesodermal structures are part of the eyeball and optic nerve primordium.[29] The eyeball primordium is already visible in a 22-day-old embryo in the form of the optic groove. Both optic grooves present themselves as furrows on either side of the neural folds at the cranial end of the neural tube. They are transformed into the neuroectoderm of the forebrain (prosencephalon) and proceed to the surface ectoderm where they develop optic vesicles.[30] Subsequently, the surface ectoderm thickens to become the lens placode.[30] In the 27-day-old embryo the optic stalk, which will later transform into the optic nerve, is already detectable. In course of the development of the lens vesicle, the optic vesicles bulge to form bilayered optic cups with the neuroectoderm entering here. Its inner plate eventually differentiates into the neural retina, while the outer plate transforms into the retinal pigment epithelium.[31] The entire developing complex of the eye is surrounded by mesenchyme, which subsequently builds the osseous walls of the orbit as well as other structures. In the fifth embryonic week the mesenchyme of the optic cup transforms into the vitreous body.[28,30] In week 6, the anterior and posterior closing of the optic cup starts at the equator, and the ends of the optic fissure merge completely in week 7.

The eyelids develop in week 7 from two skin folds consisting of the surface epithelium and mesectoderm.[28] On the exterior the epidermis and the eyelashes develop, while on the interior the palpebral parts of the conjunctival epidermis are formed. The mesoderm also transforms into the muscular structure of the eyelids, especially the levator palpebrae muscles. Meanwhile, the orbicular eye muscle is generated from the second pharyngeal arch, explaining its innervation through the facial nerve. Scattered, persistent squamous cells can be the reason for dermoid cysts in the lateral part of the upper eyelid.

The formation of the lacrimal glands is also set off between the seventh and eighth embryonic week. Five to eight peg-shaped, solid epithelial buds develop at the exterior side of the upper canthus, starting at the conjunctival epithelium from the surface ectoderm.[29] They grow in length and arborize, thereby growing into the orbital mesenchyme. The ends of the epithelial buds transform into secreting cauda of the lacrimal gland, while the epithelial ducts become excretory ducts. Approximately by the end of the third postpartum month, the lacrimal gland reaches its final form and function.

The excretory lacrimal glands develop from epithelial tissue. A solid epithelial cord grows into the mesenchymal tissue in the passage of the nasolacrimal furrow. This gland soon detaches from the surface ectoderm and develops into two piston-shaped epithelial branches that grow onto the medial canthus. Starting in the third embryonic month, the epithelial branches transform into canals to form the lacrimal canaliculi.[32]

Originating from the nasal cavities, at the same time another epithelial bud starts to canalize and grow toward the upper lacrimal glands. Fusion of the bud and the lacrimal glands occurs in the sixth embryonic month. From this moment onwards, the lacrimal glands form an open connection between the eyelids and the nasal cavities—the nasolacrimal duct.[32]

3.2.2 Patient's History

ENT examination starts with thorough medical history taking, which should include reference to the following:

- Complaints
  - Pains?
  - Painful bulb motility?
  - Diplopia? In which direction?
  - Visual field constraints?
  - Lacrimation?
  - Swelling/reddening?
  - Eyelid motility?
- Onset of complaints
  - Size progression?
  - Growth rate?
  - First occurrence?
- Possible reasons
  - Trauma?
  - Infection?
  - Allergic reaction? Known allergies?
- Previous examinations
  - Radiological diagnostics?
  - Previously induced or completed therapeutic measures?
- Preexisting condition
  - Thyroid disease?
  - Eye disease?
  - Tumor?
  - Medication?
  - Previous surgeries?

3.2.3 Clinical Examination

The following illustration of an ENT examination is focused primarily on the orbit and its surrounding structures (Video 3.6).

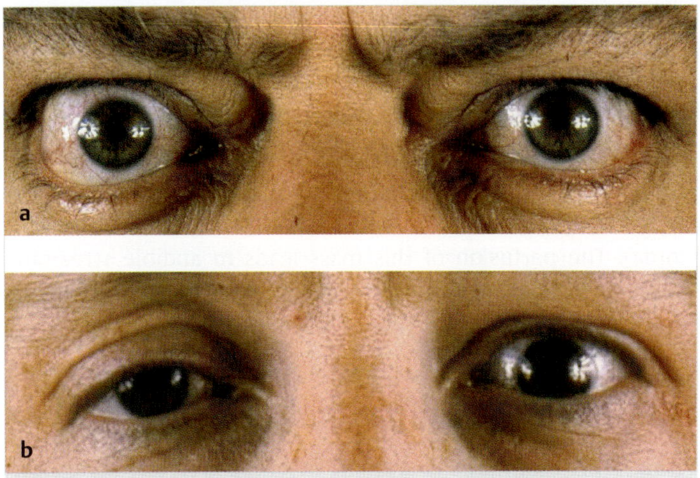

Fig. 3.20 Bulbar protrusion due to (a) hyperthyreosis and (b) malignant sinus tumor on the left with infiltration of the orbit.

Inspection

Inspection is the initial examination step. Patients should be seated and—if applicable—take off their glasses. At first, the examiner should obtain an overall impression of the patient and check the facial area for signs of inflammation, hematoma, injuries, lesions, and deformations. Alterations of the eye including displacements, swelling and reddening, or increased lacrimation are of special significance. Nasal secretion can be a sign of rhinitis or sinusitis. Unilateral secretion can hint at liquorrhea or tumor. Hemorrhagic nasal secretion in particular can be caused by tumor growth.

An assessment of the bulbar positioning follows. Anterior bulging of the eyeball is referred to as exophthalmos (▶ Fig. 3.20); posterior displacement of the eyeball is called enophthalmos. In addition, patients should be checked for a deviation of the eyeball from the horizontal line. The elevation of one pupil in comparison to the other is described as bulbar protrusion, the opposite—a lowered pupil—is described as bulbar depression. According to the location of the eye bulb, palpebral positioning can alter as well. Patients with pronounced exophthalmos may exhibit restricted eye lid closure in such a way that parts of the sclera remains visible (Dalrymple's sign). A displaced lid fold is a typical sign of lid swelling.

Palpation

Inspection is followed by palpation, which is always carried out bimanually to allow a comparison of both sides. Using thumb and index finger, an increase of the inner eye pressure can be estimated by gently placing one finger in the closed eye and carefully applying resilient pressure on the bulb. This also allows for a differentiation between a soft eye lid edema and a pressure-sensitive swelling and a hematoma.

The continuity of the facial skull bones (infra-orbital rim, orbital roof, lateral orbital rim, zygomatic arch, etc.) can be evaluated by bimanual palpation, which hence provides information regarding suspected fractures. Palpable diastases, crepitation, or bone gaps indicate a fracture (▶ Fig. 3.21).[33] On the other hand, palpable intact continuity of a bone is not sufficient to exclude a fracture.

Sensory Evaluation

Sensory checks are essential, especially in patients presenting fractures. The supra-orbital nerve is a branch of the ophthalmic nerve that exits the supra-orbital foramen at the orbital roof. It innervates the skin of the forehead and the upper eyelids.

The infra-orbital nerve is an end-branch of the maxillary nerve. Passing through the infra-orbital foramen, it arborizes in the cheek skin, which it also innervates (sensory), as it does the teeth of the upper jaw.

A two-point-discrimination method can be useful to assess a sensory disorder. Using this method, the distance between the tips of calipers carefully applied to the skin is measured. In cases in which the distance or two-point barrier is abnormally high on one side compared to the other side a sensory disorder might be present. Alternatively, a cotton bud can be used to identify a sensory disorder. Here, the examiner swipes a swab over each side of the patient's face, with the patient providing a comparative evaluation.

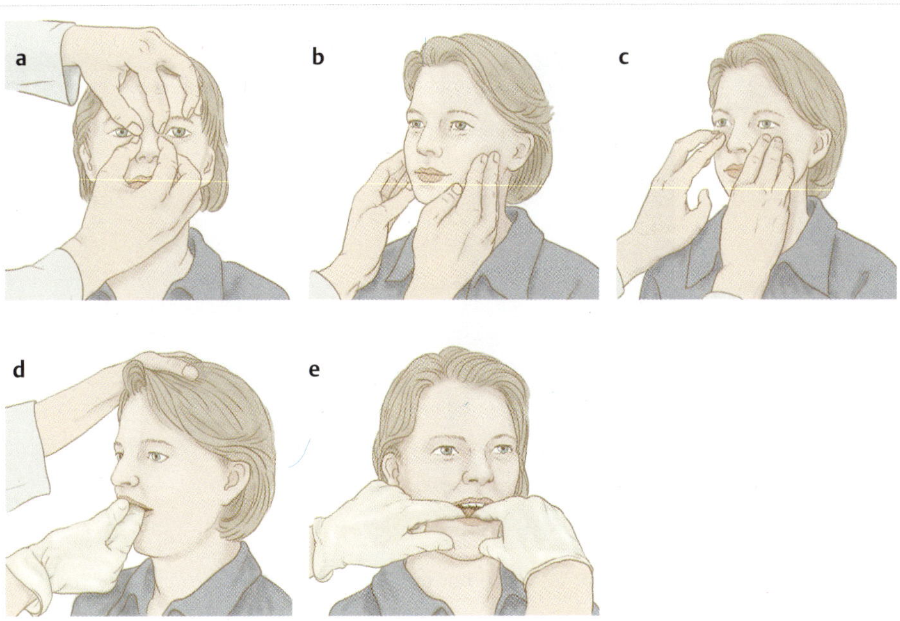

Fig. 3.21 Clinical examination of a patient with cranial trauma. (a–c) Bimanual palpation of the nasal pyramid (a), the zygomatic area (b), and the infra-orbital rim. Noted are contour defects (diastases), bone gaps, and crepitation of bone fragments. (d) Bimanual examination of the upper jaw for abnormal motility. One hand is fixed on the skull while the other hand moves the upper jaw on the frontal teeth. (e) Manual palpation of the lower jaw and the chin region.

3

Clinical Functionality Testing

In the course of clinical functionality testing, a patient's ability to actively open their eyes is checked. If this is not possible, the examiner has to passively open the eye for evaluation. This is followed by assessment of bulbar motility. The patient is asked to monocularly rotate the eye, following the finger of the examiner, while keeping the head fixed and to report on potential diplopia. The examiner moves the finger slowly horizontally upward (supraduction) and downward (infraduction), axially to the patient's nose (adduction) and to his temporal region (abduction), as well as diagonally in all directions (cf. Chapter 3.1). A motility disorder of the extraocular muscles or of the respective nerves can be determined through this examination (▸ Fig. 3.22).[33]

In patients presenting with trauma in the head and neck area, the oral fissure has to be examined as well. The patient should be asked to open the mouth as wide as possible to allow detection of a potential motility disorder. A facial bone fracture (e.g., zygomatic arch fracture, maxillary fracture) may lead to occlusal disturbances (cf. Chapter 8).[33]

In some rare cases, auscultation of the orbit can provide a hint. This is especially true, for example, in AV fistula, vascular malformations (e.g., carotid cavernous fistula (▸ Fig. 3.5) or hemangioma). The perfusion of this mass leads to audible streaming sounds. Auscultation is performed with a common stethoscope that is placed on the closed eye to examine the bulb.

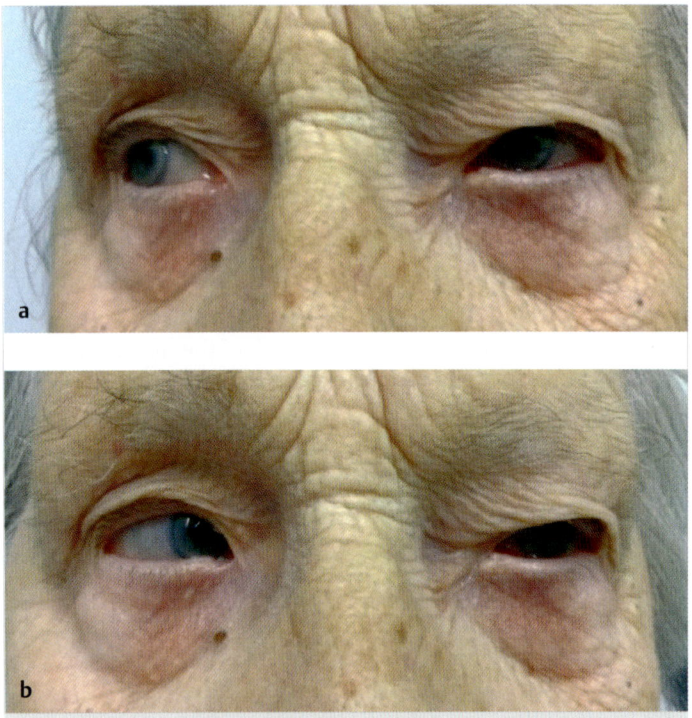

Fig. 3.22 (a, b) Motility disorder of the left eye due to a maxillary sinus carcinoma growing into the orbit (left). The left bulb remains in a center-position during abduction and adduction.

Clinical ENT Examinations

Visual ENT examinations are part of every ENT test series. Initially, the oral cavity and oropharynx are examined. A tongue depressor is used to caudally fixate the tongue in order to expose the palate, palatal arch and uvula as well as—if possible—the tonsils and laryngopharynx. Tumors of the paranasal sinuses or the orbit presenting extensive growth can also appear endorally if they perforate the maxillary sinuses as part of the maxilla (▸ Fig. 3.23).[34]

Afterwards, an anterior rhinoscopy is performed using headlamp and speculum. In this, deviations from the regular anatomy of the inner nose can be evaluated just as can the texture of the nasal mucosa as well as endonasal secretions (where applicable) and pathological lesions. The nasal septum separates the right nasal cavity from the left and can present pathologic deviations with cartilaginous or bony groins and spurs. Within the nose, three cavernous bodies, the turbinates, are located on top of each other at the lateral nasal wall. They are referred to as the inferior, medial, and superior nasal conchae, bordering the lower, middle, and upper nasal meatus.[34] Lesions of the maxillary or ethmoidal sinus spreading to the orbit are at times visible within the nose (▸ Fig. 3.24).

Endoscopic Examination of the Nasal Cavity

Endoscopy is needed for a more thorough assessment of endonasal findings. First, the mucous membrane has to be decongested by means of an α-sympathomimetic drug (e.g., 0.1% xylometazoline hydrochloride solution). A reliable method is

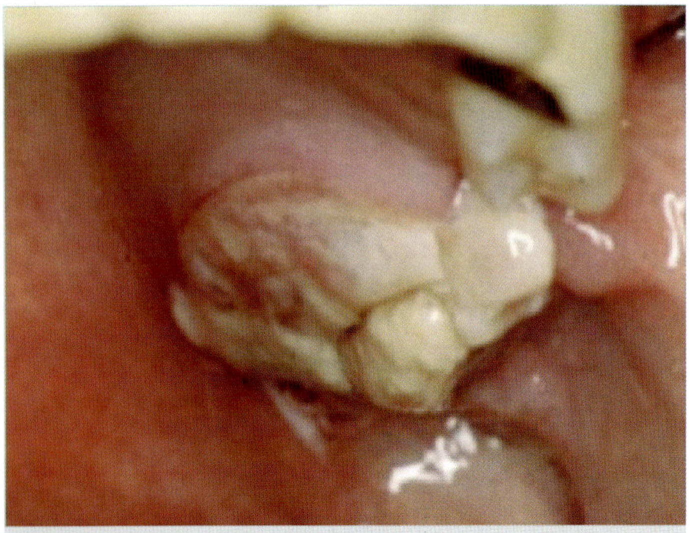

Fig. 3.23 Perforation of the oral cavity by a maxillary sinus carcinoma.

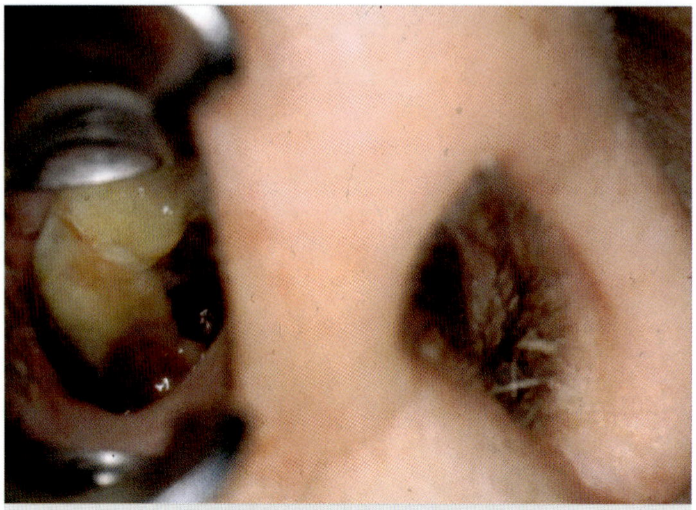

Fig. 3.24 Visible tumor growth within the nose.

detumescence by application with a spray nozzle. Alternatively, nasal spray liquid can be applied within the nose using a swab. The mucous membrane should be anesthetized with one puff of xylocaine pump-spray (10 mg lidocaine) to reduce pain during the endoscopy. When assessing the lateral nasal wall as well as protrusions from the maxillary sinus or orbital roof the use of a 30° angle lens is recommended. The endoscope is gently inserted into the inferior meatus. Here, the ostium of the nasolacrimal duct should be visible. Inspection of the middle meatus follows: to do this, the endoscope is placed under the middle turbinate where the ostium of the maxillary sinus can be seen (▶ Fig. 3.25). Secretions originating in the maxillary sinus or protruding tumors are often visible at this point. Protrusions from the orbit into the nasal cavity can also be identified in the middle and in the upper nasal passage (▶ Fig. 3.26).[34]

3.2.4 Instrument-Based Diagnostics

Ultrasonography

A-mode (amplitude mode) ultrasonography allows an assessment of the superficial frontal and maxillary sinuses. It can be distinguished whether the sinuses are filled with liquid or air, and whether they are displaced by tissues, such as tumor, or by mucosal swelling.[35,36]

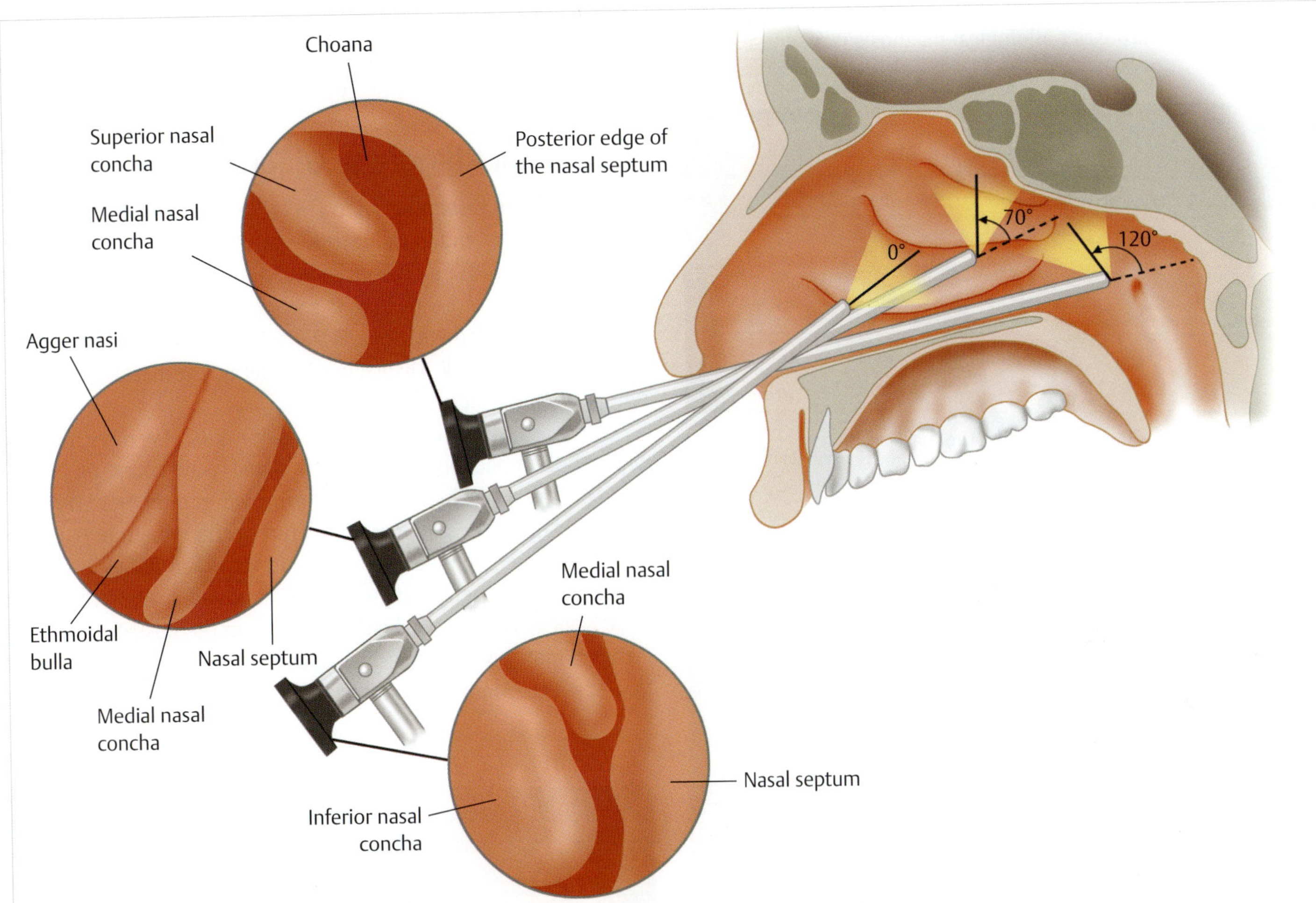

Fig. 3.25 Endoscopic nasal findings.

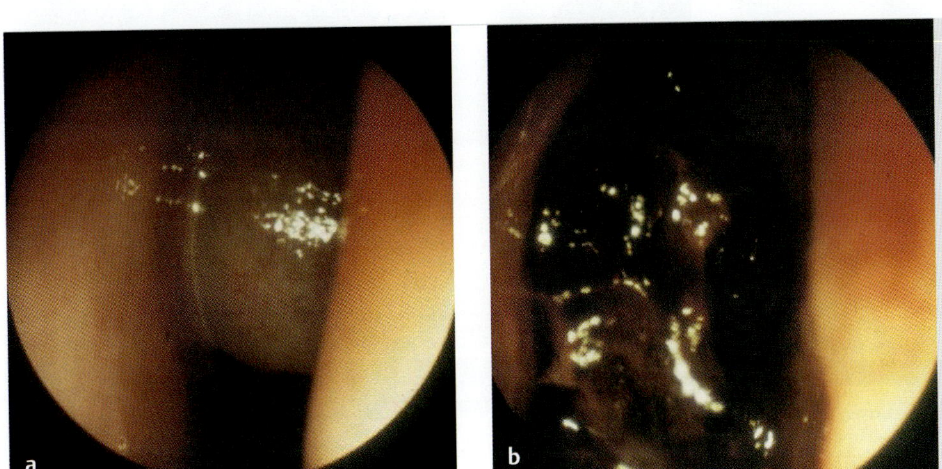

Fig. 3.26 Endoscopic and endonasal findings in **(a)** nasal polyps and **(b)** adenocarcinoma of the ethmoid cells.

With B-mode (brightness mode) ultrasonography the frontal and maxillary sinuses and infra-orbital soft tissue changes, such as tumors and swellings of the muscles and the lacrimal gland, as well as fractures of the facial bones, can be presented (▶ Fig. 3.27).

For fractures, ultrasonography can be used in cases of nasal fractures, orbital wall fractures, maxillary fractures, zygomatic arch fractures, and fractures of the frontal walls of the frontal and maxillary sinuses. Ultrasound is strongly reflected by bone, so that the sonographic image of bones is displayed as a hyperechoic structure. Fractures are shown as discontinuities of the bone structure (cf. Chapter 8).[35,36]

Radiological Diagnosis

For a more precise evaluation of fractures and especially for documentation purposes radiological diagnosis is essential. With conventional radiography (of the nose laterally, waters' view, handle-pot) fractures of the nasal bone, the zygomatic arch, and the infra-orbital rim can be assessed (▶ Fig. 3.28), but for accurate evaluation of complex midface fractures thin-slice computed tomography (CT) imaging of the paranasal sinuses in two planes (axial and coronal) is necessary. This provides information on bony rims, fractures, acute and chronic inflammation, and pathological lesions of the parabasal sinuses and orbit (▶ Fig. 3.29). Furthermore, eye muscles, bulb and retrobulbar tissues can be inspected (cf. Chapter 4).[37]

Magnetic resonance imaging (MRI) is indicated for the evaluation of soft tissue. The high soft tissue contrast allows the assessment of tumor growth, inflammatory infiltration, and abscess formation, which appear dark (hypointense) in T1-weighted images and light (hyperintense) in T2-weighted images (▶ Fig. 3.30). The lack of radiation exposure is another significant advantage of MRI over CT diagnostics (see Chapter 4).[37]

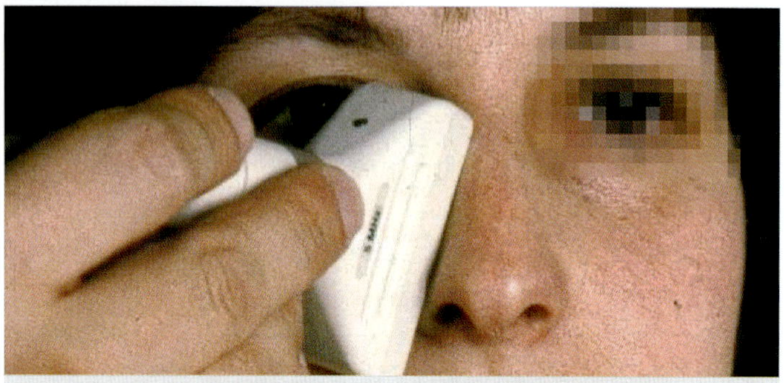

Fig. 3.27 B-mode ultrasonography of the maxillary sinus.

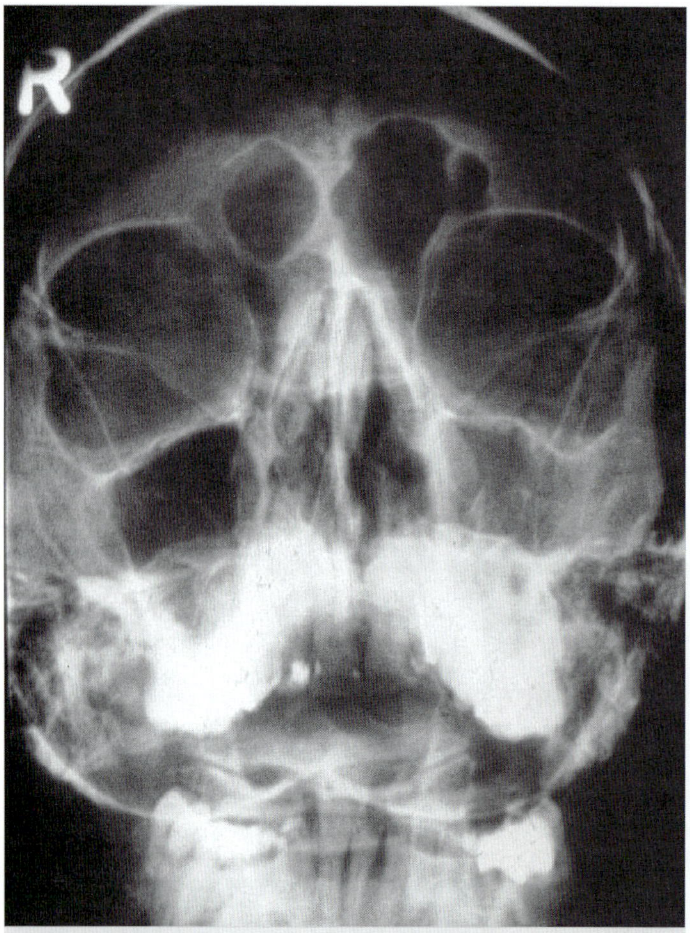

Fig. 3.28 Conventional X-ray of the paranasal sinuses om in maxillary sinusitis on the left.

Functional Rhinology Diagnostics

Active anterior rhinomanometry is a measurement method for determining the endonasal airflow (in mL/s) of each side of the nose while breathing. The pressure difference between nostril and choana (posterior nostril) is recorded in a diagram. In turns, one nostril is sealed with an adapter while breathing is continued through a face mask. Displacing lesions in the nasal cavity can reduce airflow volume.[34]

During acoustic rhinometry the anatomy of the inner nose is depicted by reflection of an acoustic signal (echo sounding principle). For this, a clicking sound is transmitted into the nose through a nasal adapter. The endonasal structures reflect the sound, which in turn is picked up by a microphone to record an individual curve of the nasal geometry. This identifies confined spaces within the nasal cavities and shows their distance from the nostrils.[34]

Olfactometry is used to assess olfaction. The olfactory mucosa is located on the lamina cribrosa of the ethmoid bone, which is found

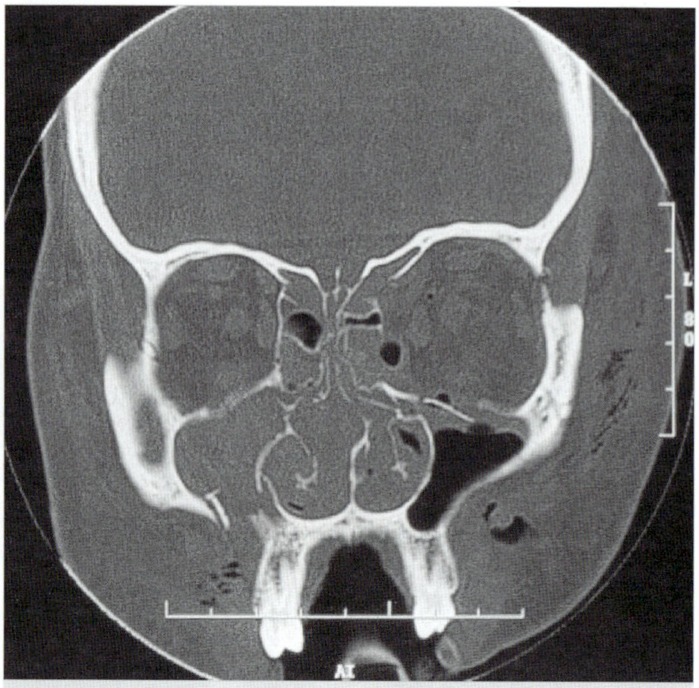

Fig. 3.29 CT scan (coronal) of paranasal sinuses in a midface fracture.

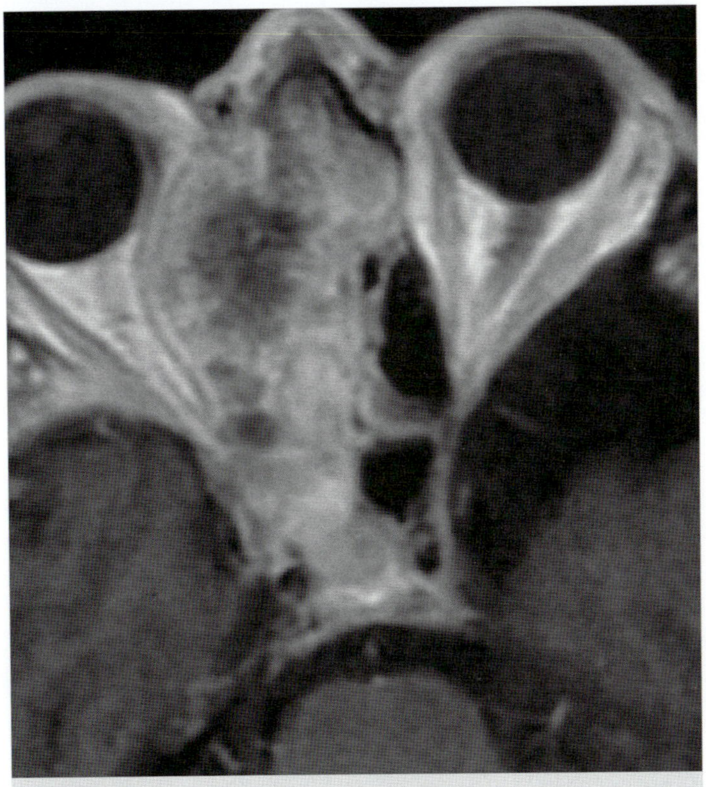

Fig. 3.30 MRI scan of an adenocarcinoma of the ethmoid cells.

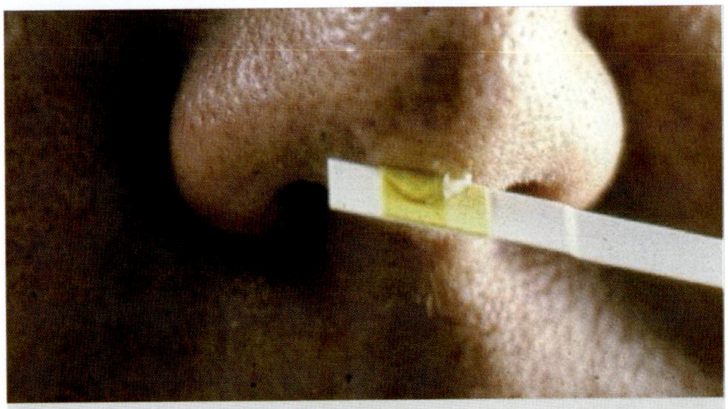

Fig. 3.31 Glucose strip testing.

in the upper turbinate. Olfactory nerve fibers pass through the cribriform plate into the cranial cavity and form the olfactory bulb. From here, the information is sent to the olfactory cortex. Olfactometry distinguishes subjective from objective odor testing. For the subjective odor test the patient is presented with 12 different fragrances, for example, in the form of "Sniffin' Sticks," on each side individually. Patients are asked to name the fragrances using a selection card. As part of the objective test, olfactory evoked potentials (OEPs) are derived from the olfactory tract. Since this method is rather complex, it is only rarely used in clinical practice.[34]

Laboratory Diagnostics

A supplementary blood test can be very useful in orbital diseases. Increase in inflammatory markers (ESR, CRP, leukocytes), for example, is indicative for an infectious cause of an acute orbital swelling, such as orbital complications of an acute sinusitis. Pathologically altered thyroid function (TSH, T_4, T_3 in peripheral blood) and positive thyroid autoantibodies (TSH-receptor-antibodies [TRAb], thyroid-peroxidase antibodies [TPOAb], thyroglobulin antibodies [TgAb]) can be present, for example, in an endocrine orbitopathy as part of Graves's disease or Hashimoto's thyroiditis (cf. Chapter 7).

Violations of the skull base by fractures or tumor growth may lead to laceration of the cerebral membrane and to leakage of cerebrospinal fluid (CSF) from the nose (rhinoliquorrhea) or from the ear (otoliquorrhea). The leakage of liquid from the nose via the eustachian tube in a lateral skull base fracture is called indirect rhinoliquorrhea. Various tests can distinguish CSF from nasal secretions and blood. For liquor diagnostics, the secretion has to be collected in a tube. The glucose test is a strip test that determines the sugar content of the collected liquid. Since liquor has a higher glucose content (35–70 mg%) than nasal secretion, a rough distinction is quickly possible (▶ Fig. 3.31). Complex immunoelectrophoresis can also detect the protein β_2-transferrin, which occurs only in CSF and is thus specific for cerebrospinal fluid. The biochemical evidence of increased β-trace-protein (prostaglandin-D-synthase) in the secretion is also a evidence for a CSF leak since its concentration in CSF is about 30 times higher than in blood.[34]

Electrodiagnostics of Motor Nerves

Nerve damage and severity can be assessed as well as the prognosis using electrodiagnostics. The facial nerve is of particular interest for ENT examinations in case of facial nerve paralysis.

Nerve excitability testing (NET) is an indirect test for excitability of the affected nerves. Electrical stimuli (of 1 millisecond duration) are applied transcutaneously on both sides with increasing strength. The threshold current is the level at which the corresponding muscle contracts for the first time. A side difference of under 3.5 mA indicates good recovery; anything higher than 3.5 mA hints at a poor prognosis. Because of delayed axonal degeneration, testing is not possible sooner than 4 days after the nerve damage.[38]

Electroneurography (ENOG) is used to measure nerve function and nerve conduction velocity. Electrodes are applied at two points to trigger stimulation with short pulses (0.2 millisecond duration). This leads to depolarization of the nerve and the transmission of action potentials via the axons. Since the impulse is triggered at two different points, the nerve conduction velocity can be calculated on the basis of distance and latency. The amplitude gives in turn a rough indication of the number of axons and, in cases of paresis, of axon degeneration (▶ Fig. 3.32).[38]

Electromyography (EMG) facilitates the recording of spontaneous or arbitrary triggered muscle action potentials using intramuscular needle electrodes.[38]

Nerve conduction velocity from the central core areas of the nerve to the periphery (muscles) can be measured using transcranial muscle stimulation. A magnetic field coil can be applied to the head, for example, in a retroauricular position, in order to record the nerve response in the corresponding muscle using needle electrodes. An indication of the degree of damage and the prognosis can be derived on the basis of the measured amplitude and latency (▶ Fig. 3.33).[38]

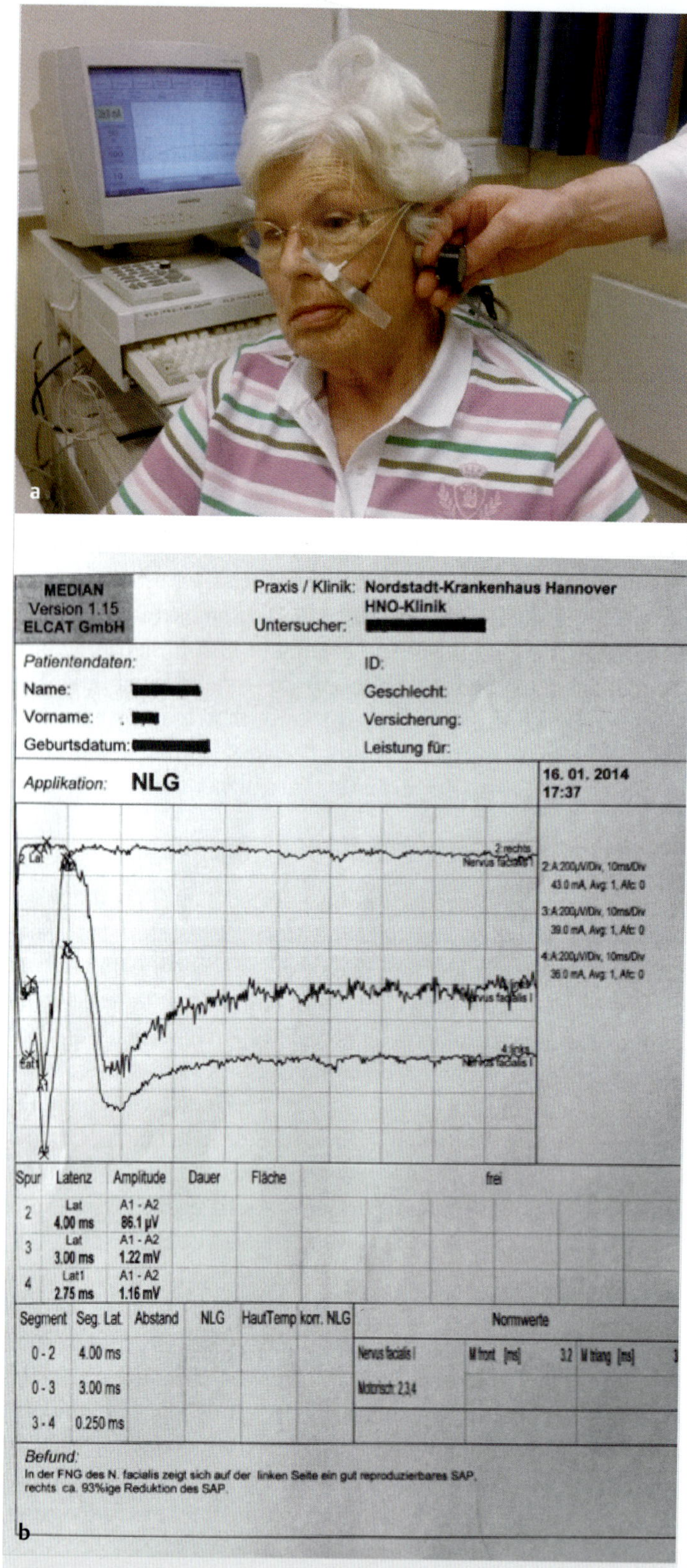

Fig. 3.32 Neurography of the facial nerve in a patient with a right-sided facial nerve paralysis. (a) Equipment for facial nerve neurography. (b) Acquired data and display of results in a plot. The amplitude differences between the left and right sides reveal an axonal degeneration of 93% of axons on the affected right side.

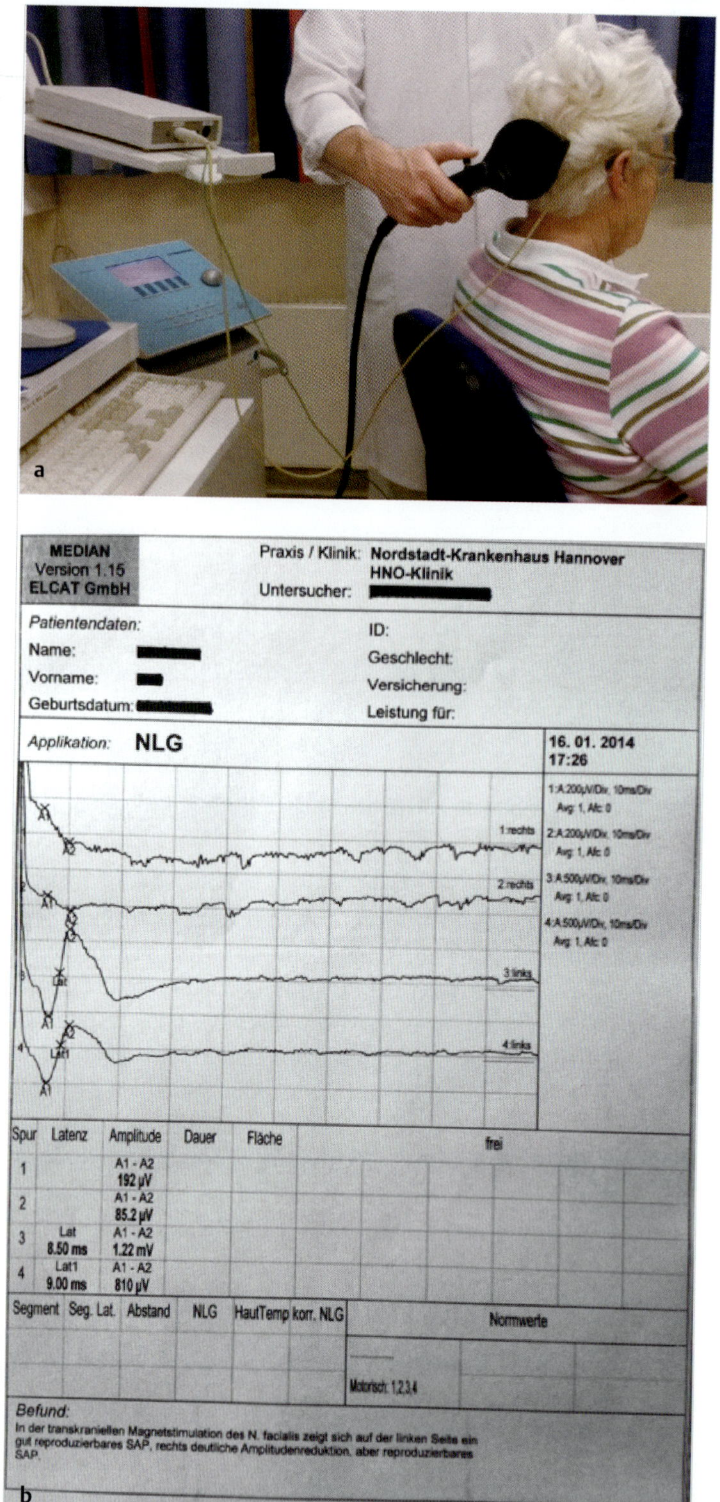

Fig. 3.33 Transcranial magnetic stimulation of the facial nerve in a patient with right-sided facial nerve paralysis. (a) Equipment for transcranial magnetic stimulation of the facial nerve. (b) Acquired data and display of results in a plot. A compound action potential is evoked on the affected right side but it is reduced by 90% compared to that evoked from the unaffected left-sided nerve.

References

[1] Duke-Elder SS. System of Ophthalmology. Vol XIII. Part II. London: Kimpton; 1974:773–1227

[2] Henderson JW, Farrow GM. Orbital Tumors. 3rd ed. New York: Raven; 1994

[3] Jakobiec FA, Font RL. Orbit. In: Spencer WH, ed. Ophthalmic Pathology. An Atlas and Textbook. 4th ed. Philadelphia, PA: Saunders; 1996:2438–2933

[4] Jones IS, Jakobiec FA. Diseases of the Orbit. Hagerstown, MD: Harper & Row; 1979

[5] Rootman J. Diseases of the Orbit: A Multidisciplinary Approach. Philadelphia, PA: Lippincott; 1988

[6] Shields JA. Diagnosis and Management of Orbital Tumors. Philadelphia, PA: Saunders; 1989

[7] Rochels R. Rationelle Diagnostik beim Leitsymptom “Exophthalmus”. In: Lund OE, Waubke TN, eds. Okuläre Symptome: Strategie der Untersuchung. Stuttgart: Enke; 1987:221–234

[8] Guthoff RF. Erkrankungen der Orbita–Die Rolle des Augenarztes als Netzwerk Koordinator. Klin Monatsbl Augenheilkd. 2004; 221(11):891–892

[9] Guthoff R. Orbitachirurgie unter besonderer Berücksichtigung rekronstruktiver Gesichtspunkte. 22nd Internationaler Kongress der Deutschen Ophthalmochirurgen, Nürnberg; 2009

[10] Behrendt S, Rochels R. Erkrankungen der Orbita—Trauma, Entzündung, Tumor —aus der Sicht des Ophthalmologen. Sitzungsbericht der Dtsch. Gesellschaft für Hals-, Nasen- Ohrenheilkunde, Kopf- und Halschirigie. Berlin Heidelberg New York: Springer; 1998:1–22

[11] Kurtz KJ. Bruits and hums of the head and neck. In: Walker HK, Hall WD, Hurst JW, eds. Clinical Methods: The History, Physical, and Laboratory Examinations. 3rd ed. Boston, MA: Butterworths; 1990:101–106

[12] Gallego DF, Rivas-Grajales AM, Gallego CJ. Ocular auscultation: a review. Int J Med Students. 2015;3(2):45–49

[13] Jankauskiene J, Jarusaitiene D. Estimating proptosis by digitalized exophthalmometry in children and teenagers with thyroid diseases. Schol J Med. 2012; 2(4):51–56

[14] Kratky V, Hurwitz JJ. Hertel exophthalmometry without orbital rim contact. Ophthalmology. 1994; 101(5):931–937

[15] Kaufmann H, et al. Strabismus. 2nd ed. Stuttgart: Enke; 1994

[16] De La Paz MA, Boniuk M. Fundus manifestations of orbital disease and treatment of orbital disease. Surv Ophthalmol. 1995; 40(1):3–21

[17] Bilaniuk LT, Zimmermann RA, Newton TH. Magnetic resonance imaging: orbital pathology. In: Newton TH, Bilaniuk LT, eds. Radiology of the Eye and Orbit. New York: Raven; 1990:5.1–5.84

[18] Char DH, Unsöld R, Sobel DF, Salvolini U, Newton TH. Computed tomography: ocular and orbital pathology. In: Newton TH, Bilaniuk LT, eds. Radiology of the Eye and Orbit. New York: Raven; 1990:9.1–9.64

[19] DePotter P, Shields JA, Shields CL. MRI of the Eye and Orbit. Philadelphia, PA: Lippincott; 1995

[20] Hammerschlag SB, Hesselink JR, Weber AL. Computed Tomography of the Eye and Orbit. Norwalk, VA: Appleton; 1983

[21] Byrne SF, Green RL. Ultrasound of the Eye and Orbit. St. Louis, MO: Mosby; 1992

[22] Ossoinig KC. Echography of the eye, orbit and periorbital region. In: Arger PH, ed. Orbit Roentgenology. New York: Wiley; 1977:224–296

[23] Rochels R. Ultraschalldiagnostik in der Augenheilkunde: Lehrbuch und Atlas. Landsberg: Ecomed; 1986

[24] Lieb WE, Flaharty PM, Ho A, Sergott RC. Color Doppler imaging of the eye and orbit. A synopsis of a 400 case experience. Acta Ophthalmol Suppl. 1992; 204 (204):50–54

[25] Alexandridis E, Krastel K. Elektrodiagnostik in der Ophthalmologie. 2nd ed. Berlin, Heidelberg, New York: Springer; 1997

[26] Heckenliveley JR, Arden GB. Principles and Practice of Clinical Electrophysiology of Vision. St. Louis, MO: Mosby; 1991

[27] Waldeyer A. Anatomie des Menschen. Part 2. 13th ed. Berlin: de Gruyter; 1975:25ff

[28] Augustin A. Augenheilkunde. 3rd ed. Heidelberg: Springer; 2007:1123ff

[29] Moore K, Persaud TVN. Lehrbuch und Atlas der Entwicklungsgeschichte des Menschen. Stuttgart: Schattauer; 1996:121ff

[30] Wright KW. Textbook of Ophthalmology. Philadelphia, PA: Williams & Wilkins; 1997: 24ff

[31] Markowski J. Die Embryologische Entwicklung des Bulbus oculi und seiner Adnexe [Inaugural Dissertation]. Graz, Austria, University of Graz; 2009:11ff

[32] Francois J, Hollwich F. Augenheilkunde in Klinik und Praxis. Vol 1. Stuttgart: Thieme; 1977

[33] Welkoborsky H-J. Traumatologie. In: Strutz J, Mann W, eds. Praxis der HNO-Heilkunde, Kopf- und Halschirurgie. 2nd ed. Stuttgart: Thieme; 2010:798–300

[34] Hosemann W, Kühnel T. Untersuchung der Nase und des Pharynx. In: Strutz J, Mann W, eds. Praxis der HNO-Heilkunde, Kopf- und Halschirurgie. 2nd ed. Stuttgart: Thieme; 2010:70–89

[35] Jecker P. Ultraschalluntersuchung bei Erkrankungen der Nasennebenhöhlen, der Gesichtsweichteile, der Orbita und der knöchernen Strukturen des Gesichts. In: Welkoborsky H-J, Jecker P, Maurer J, Mann WJ. Ultraschalldiagnostik Kopf – Hals. Stuttgart: Thieme; 2013:121–130

[36] Welkoborsky H-J. Physikalische Grundlagen der Ultraschalldiagnostik. In: Welkoborsky H-J, Jecker P, Maurer J, Mann WJ. Ultraschalldiagnostik Kopf – Hals. Stuttgart: Thieme; 2013:121–130

[37] Vogl TJ, Weisser P. Radiologische Diagnostik. In: Strutz J, Mann W, eds. Praxis der HNO-Heilkunde, Kopf- und Halschirurgie. 2nd ed. Stuttgart: Thieme; 2010:197ff

[38] Strutz J. Untersuchung der motorischen Hirnnerven. In: Strutz J, Mann W, eds. Praxis der HNO-Heilkunde, Kopf- und Halschirurgie. 2nd ed. Stuttgart: Thieme; 2010:128–137

Suggested Further Reading

Weber R, Keerl R, Rochels R, Schick B, Draf W, Kahle G. Checklists for the differential diagnosis of orbital affections. Orbit. 1997; 16(1):11–24

3

Chapter 4

Imaging of the Orbit

4

4 Imaging of the Orbit

4.1 Introduction

In addition to evaluation of clinical symptoms, the use of imaging techniques is crucial for diagnosing inflammatory, tumorous, and traumatic orbital diseases. The following imaging techniques are available for this:

- Conventional radiography.
- Computed tomography (CT).
- Magnet resonance imaging (MRI).
- Positron emission tomography (PET).
- Ultrasound examination.

4.2 Conventional Radiography

A. Pangalu and A. Valavanis

Conventional radiography of the orbit can be performed with a survey radiograph of the paranasal sinuses in an occipitomental view (paranasal sinus radiograph OM), which is the so-called "Waters projection." A lateral picture can be performed additionally. The optic nerve canal can be visualized by a "Rhese projection," but, to date, this is of minor importance.[1]

Because of minor thickness of the bony orbital walls, especially of the orbital floor (▸ Fig. 4.1), discontinuities of bony structures are difficult to visualize by conventional radiographic techniques. This is why conventional radiographs are becoming less used in trauma cases. Their use is limited particularly to postoperative position control following reposition of bony fragments and osteosynthesis (▸ Fig. 4.2), or in localization of foreign bodies in the orbit (▸ Fig. 4.3). Small glass splinters from clear glass are not visible in a radiograph; with a wavelength of 10 picometers to 1 nanometer, the electromagnetic radiation is not absorbed or reflected by glass.

4.3 Computed Tomography (CT)

A. Pangalu and A. Valavanis

With modern multislice or spiral CT scanners, volume data sets can be captured, from which sections in any planes and in any thickness can be computed. Usually axial, coronal, and sagittal pictures with a thickness of 2 mm are produced. Because of the high radiosensitivity of the eye lens, modern low-dose examination protocols are used for the orbit to achieve maximal picture quality with minimal radiation exposure.

4.3.1 Radiological Anatomy

For bony orbital structures, orbital pathways, and intraorbital muscles, refer to Chapter 1 (▸ Fig. 4.4, ▸ Fig. 4.5).

4.3.2 Orbital Trauma

For evaluation of an acute orbital trauma CT scans are crucial and are regarded as imaging technique of first choice. With the ability to visualize both bony and soft tissue structures, they enable rapid and accurate diagnosis of bony and soft tissue injuries (e.g., eyeball hematoma [▸ Fig. 4.6], eyeball rupture [▸ Fig. 4.7], retrobulbar hematoma, peribulbar hematoma, incarceration of outer eye muscles, prolapse of orbital adipose tissue, orbital emphysema).

The short examination time for upset of the data set is of great advantage in evaluation of this frequently restless and agitated cohort of patients who have to be handled. Three-dimensional imaging is possible with 3D reconstruction, which is crucial when contemplating surgical procedures.

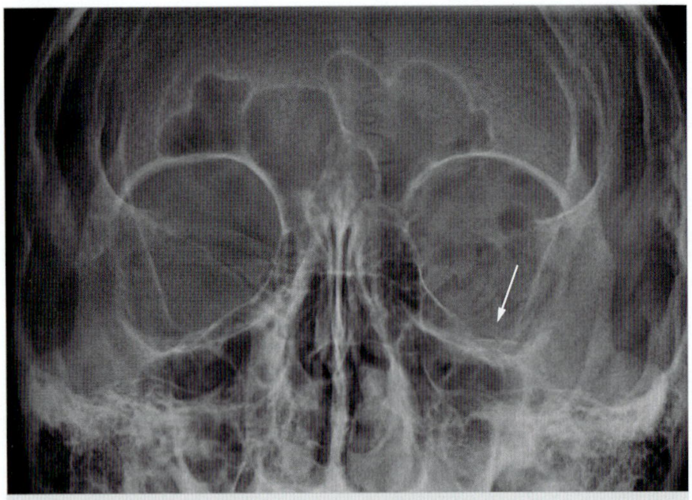

Fig. 4.1 Orbital floor fracture on the left side. Discontinuity of the left bony orbital floor (*arrow*).

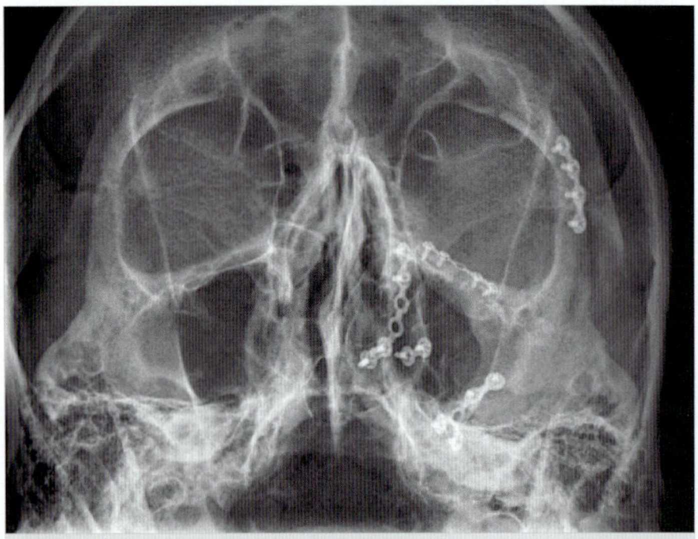

Fig. 4.2 Position control following repositioning and miniplate osteosynthesis. Correct position of the lateral orbital wall and orbital floor.

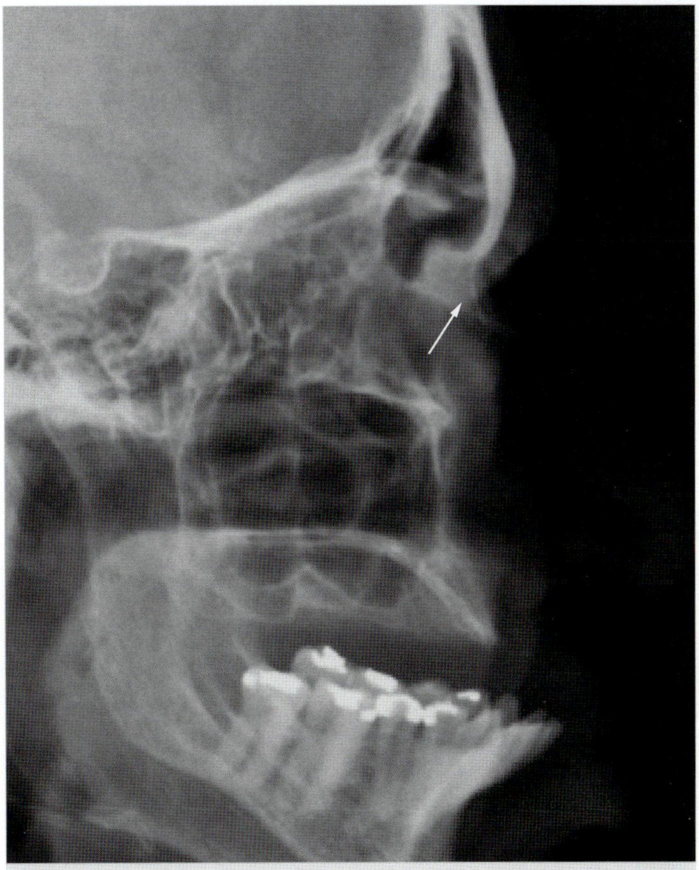

Fig. 4.3 Surgical instrument (needle) in the periorbita. Lateral projections can be useful in radiopaque foreign body localization (*arrow*).

Orbital fractures are fractures of the bony orbital walls that can extend to the orbital apex, with consequent incarceration of muscles, adipose tissue, or nerves. They can occur in isolation or in combination with midface or skull base fractures. Hence, they can affect either only a part of the orbit or the entire orbit,[2] which can lead to a prolapse of orbital content through the fracture line into the maxillary sinus (see Chapter 8)[3] (▶ Fig. 4.8, ▶ Fig. 4.9).

Le Fort III fractures (centrolateral midface fractures) (▶ Fig. 4.10) are characterized by splintering of the entire midface skeleton including the bony nose from the skull base. The fracture line runs through the lateral orbital wall, orbital floor, medial orbital wall, and nasofrontal suture to the opposite side and through the zygomatic arches.

CT scans provide crucial information regarding the course of the optic nerve and probable injuries in patients in whom the nerve's function cannot be clinically evaluated (▶ Fig. 4.11).

4.3.3 Tumors

Magnet resonance imaging (MRI), which will be discussed in detail later, is generally superior to CT in the evaluation of orbital tumors. However, in cases of orbital tumors infiltrating the periosteum and/or adjacent bony orbital structures, CT scans can provide significant diagnostic information. Frequent tumorous lesions involving the bony orbital walls and wings of the sphenoid bones are osteomas (▶ Fig. 4.12), malignant tumors (▶ Fig. 4.13), fibrous dysplasia (▶ Fig. 4.14), and especially sphenoid wing meningioma.[4]

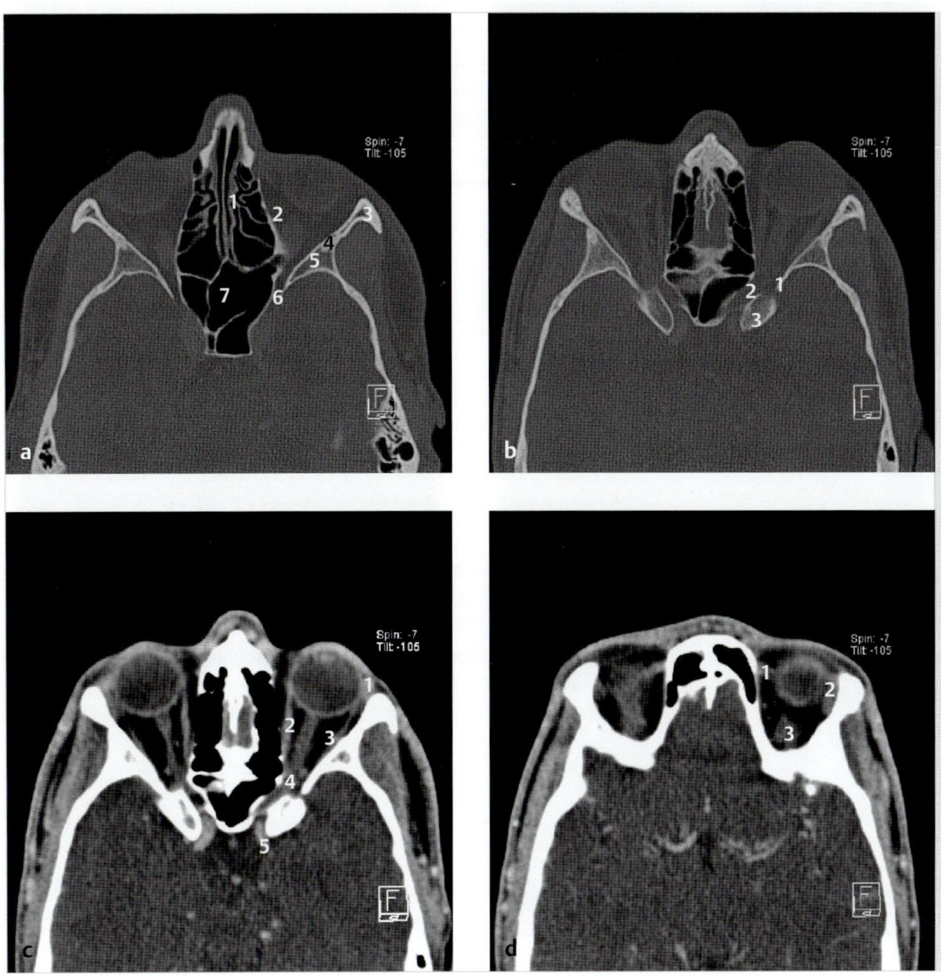

Fig. 4.4 Radiological anatomy of the orbit. **(a, b)** Axial CT scans in bone window. **(c, d)** Axial CT scans in soft tissue window. **(a)** 1, ethmoid; 2, lamina papyracea (orbital lamina); 3, zygomatic bone; 4, sphenozygomatic suture; 5, greater wing of the sphenoid bone; 6, inferior orbital fissure; 7, sphenoid sinus. **(b)** 1, superior orbital fissure; 2, optic canal; 3, anterior clinoid process. **(c)** 1, lacrimal gland; 2, medial rectus muscle; 3, lateral rectus muscle; 4, optic nerve; 5, internal carotid artery. **(d)** 1, tendon of superior oblique muscle; 2, lacrimal gland; 3, superior rectus muscle.

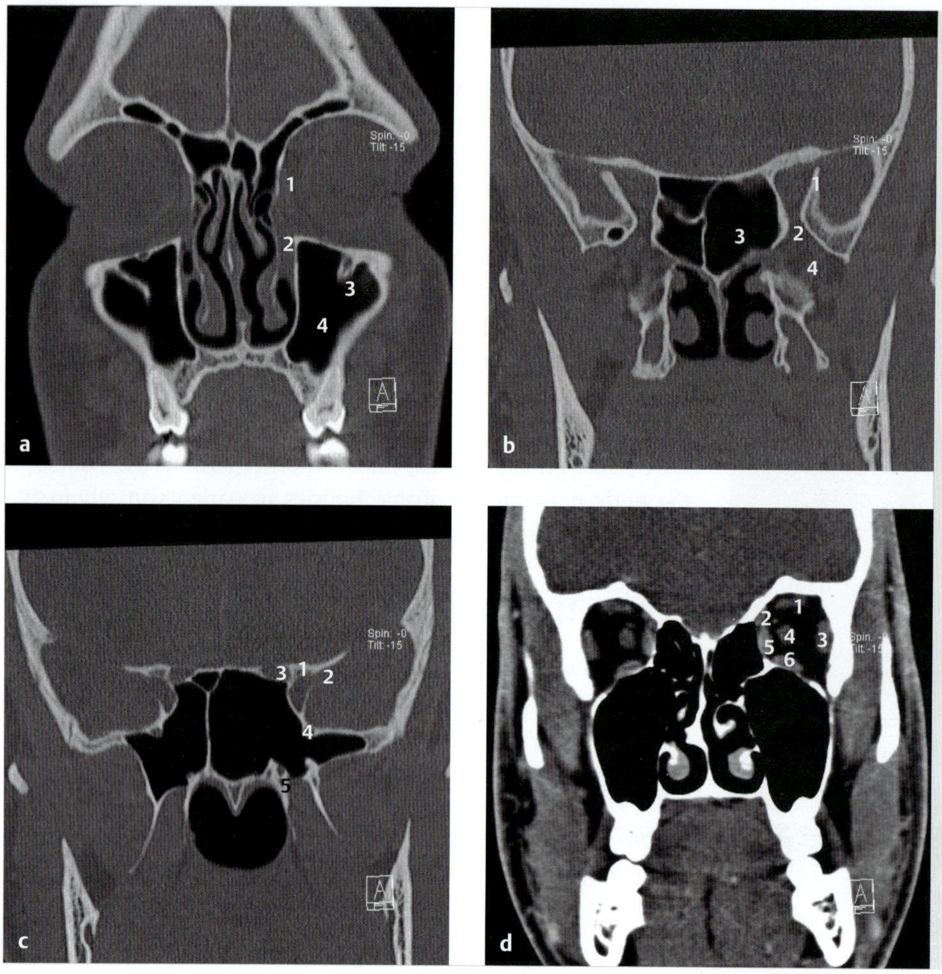

Fig. 4.5 Radiological anatomy of the orbit. **(a, b, c)** Coronal CT scans in bone window. **(d)** Coronal contrast-enhanced CT scan in soft tissue window. **(a)** 1, fossa of lacrimal sac; 2, nasolacrimal duct; 3, infraorbital canal; 4, maxillary sinus. **(b)** 1, superior orbital fissure; 2, inferior orbital fissure; 3, sphenoid sinus; 4, pterygopalatine fossa. **(c)** 1, lesser wing of sphenoid bone; 2, superior orbital fissure; 3, optic canal; 4, foramen rotundum; 5, pterygoid canal. **(d)** 1, superior rectus muscle; 2, superior oblique muscle; 3, lateral rectus muscle; 4, optic nerve; 5, medial rectus muscle; 6, inferior rectus muscle.

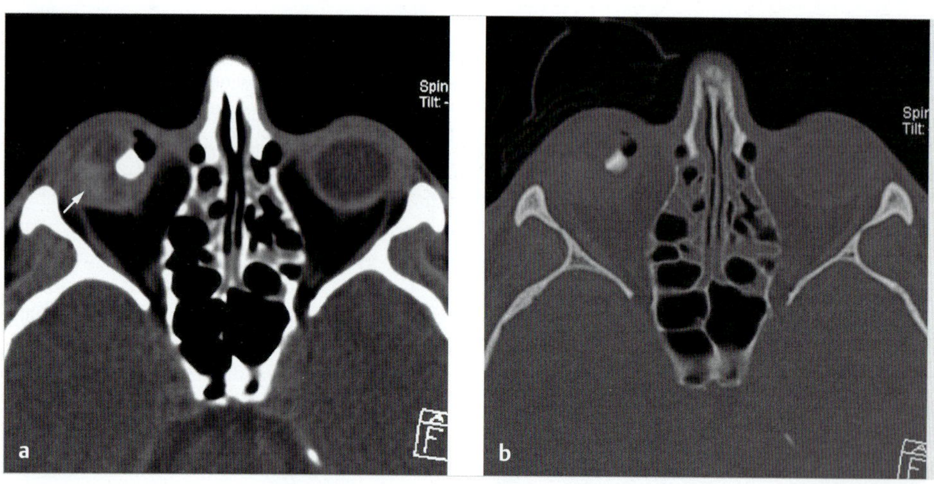

Fig. 4.6 Eye bulb perforation with hematoma. **(a)** Noncontrast axial CT scan shows an eyeball perforation along with an intraocular foreign body (glass splinter) and intraocular hematoma (*arrow*). **(b)** Axial CT scan in bony window allows differentiation between air that has penetrated into the orbit and the more dense fat.

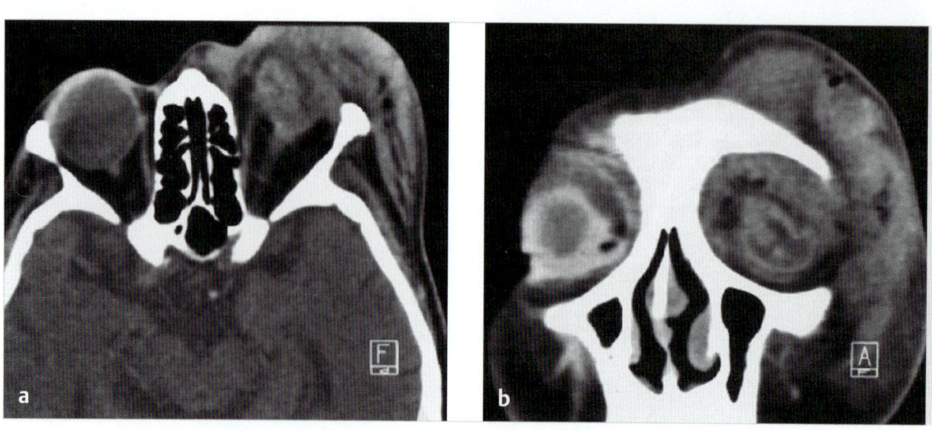

Fig. 4.7 Eyeball rupture. Noncontrast axial CT scan **(a)** and coronal CT scan **(b)** visualize the unrounded shape of the eyeball along with extensive periorbital hematoma.

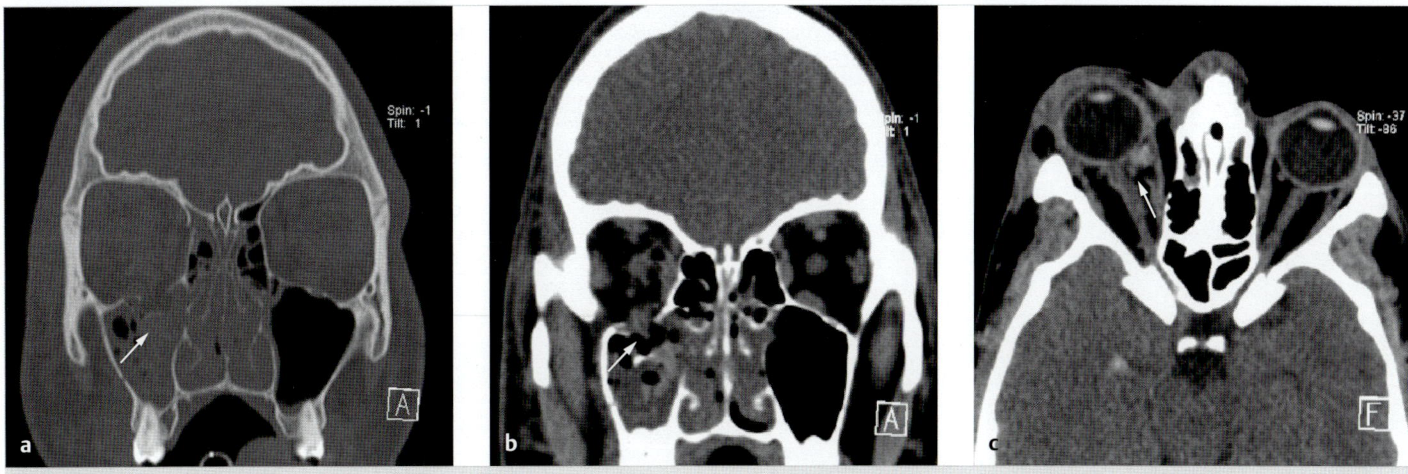

Fig. 4.8 Orbital floor fracture (blow-out fracture). **(a)** Coronal CT scan in bone window shows the fracture of the orbital floor with dislocation of orbital adipose tissue and a larger bony fragment of the orbital floor (*arrow*) into the maxillary sinus. **(b)** Noncontrast coronal CT scan in soft tissue window displays a displacement of the inferior rectus muscle (*arrow*) through the fracture line along with its incarceration. Hematoma in the maxillary sinus. **(c)** Noncontrast axial CT scan additionally shows a retrobulbar hematoma (*arrow*).

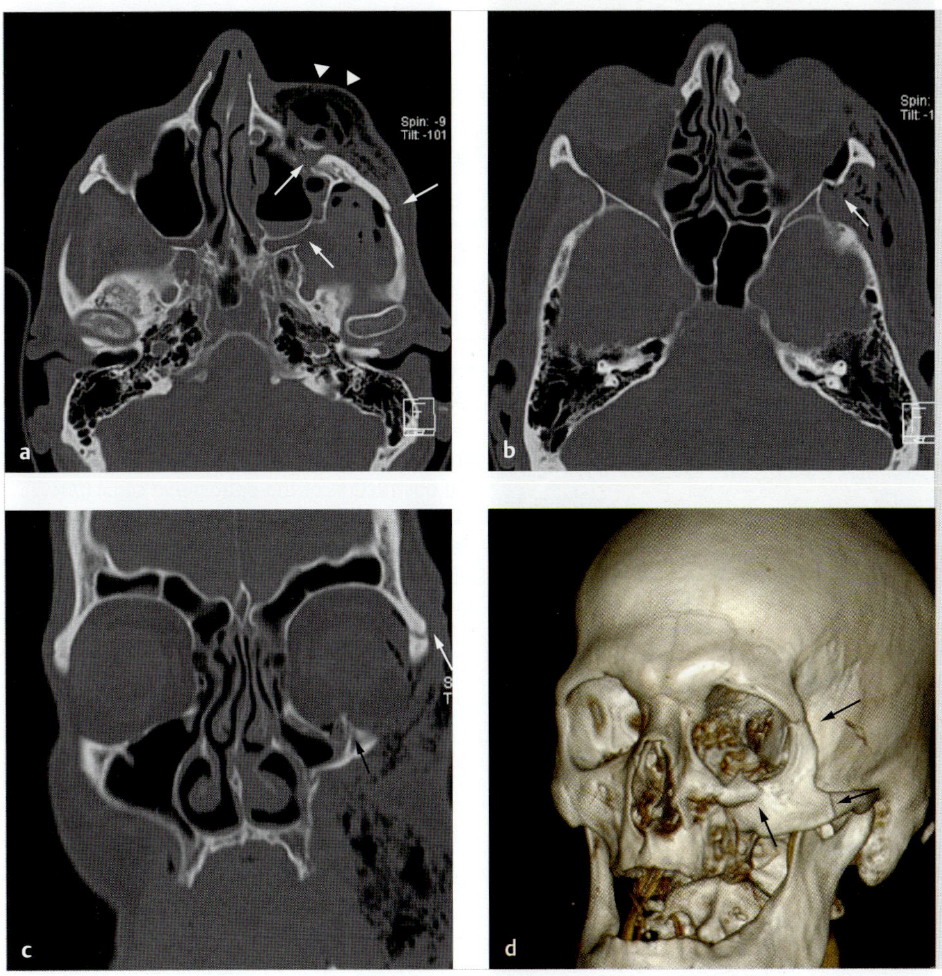

Fig. 4.9 Fracture of the zygomatic bone (so-called "tripod-fracture"). **(a)** Axial CT scan shows a zygomatic arch fracture (*arrow*), and fracture of the lateral (*arrow*) and anterior bony walls of the maxillary sinus (*arrow*). Soft tissue emphysema (*arrowheads*). **(b)** Axial plane through the orbit, showing a dislocation of the bony lateral wall fragments (*arrow*), and a periorbital emphysema. **(c)** Coronal plane to demonstrate a dislocation of orbital floor fragments. The infraorbital canal is also involved (*black arrow*). The frontozygomatic suture is burst (*white arrow*). **(d)** 3D reconstruction: fractures of the inferior and lateral orbital wall along with the zygomatic arch (*arrows*).

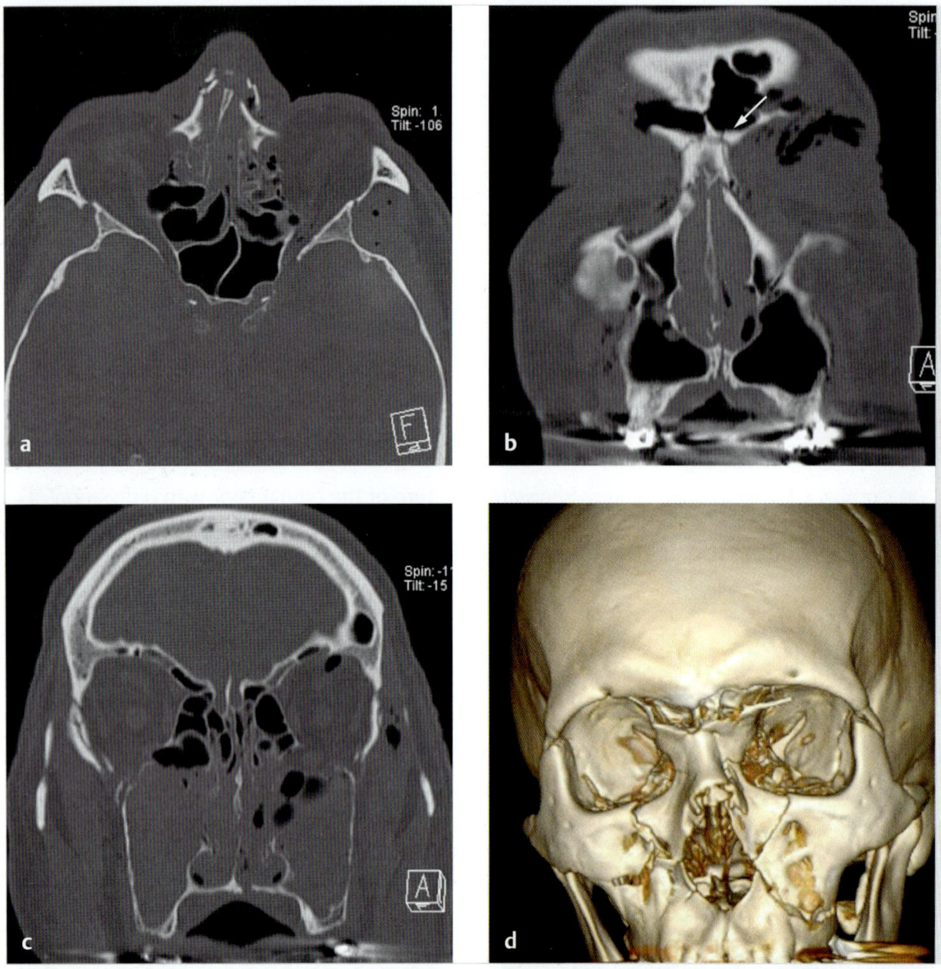

Fig. 4.10 Le Fort III fracture. **(a)** Axial CT scan shows a fracture line coursing through the lateral orbital wall and orbital lamina on both sides, and involving the nose and nasal septum. **(b, c)** Coronal CT scans show the fracture line crossing the root of the nose and the orbital floor bilaterally. **(d)** 3D-reconstruction of the CT in the same patient.

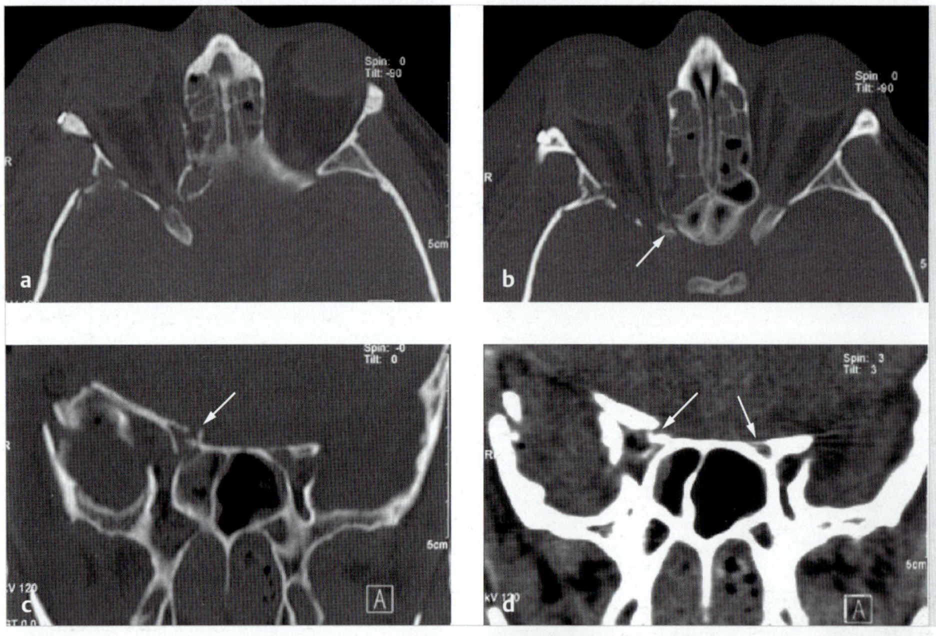

Fig. 4.11 Injury of the optic nerve. **(a)** Axial CT scan in bone window showing a right-sided fracture of the minor and major wings of the sphenoid bone. **(b)** Compression of the optic nerve canal due to a bony fragment (*arrow*). **(c)** Coronal CT scan elucidates both the fracture and the obstruction of the optic nerve canal (*arrow*). **(d)** Noncontrast soft tissue coronal CT scan demonstrates the unaffected optic nerve on the left side (*arrow*) and the nerve compression on the right side (*arrow*).

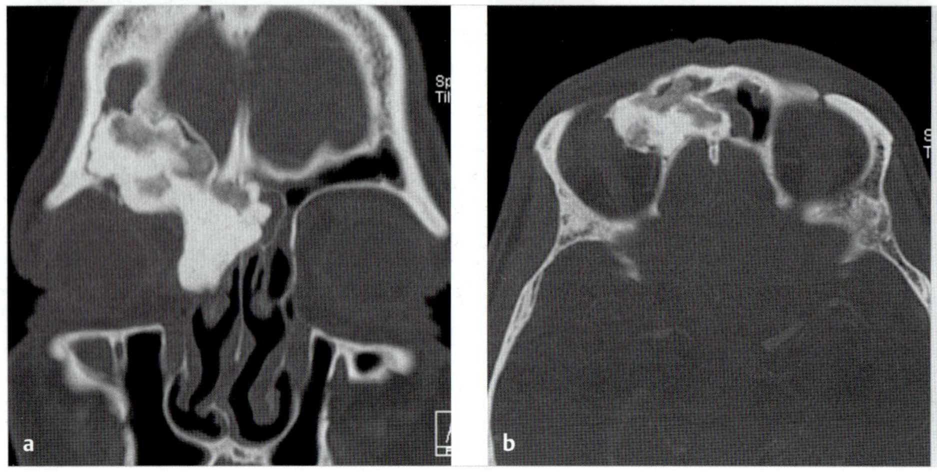

Fig. 4.12 Frontal sinus osteoma. Coronal **(a)** and axial **(b)** CT scans show a right frontal sinus osteoma extending into the orbit. Note characteristic areas of different density inside the tumor, and the downward displacement of the eyeball.

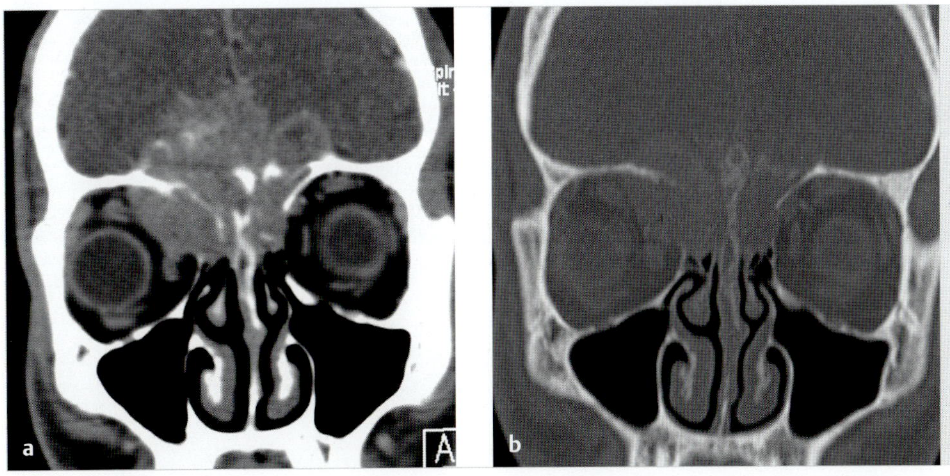

Fig. 4.13 Ewing sarcoma. **(a)** Contrast coronal CT in soft tissue window demonstrates a huge mass in the skull base area, extending intracranially and into the periorbita. **(b)** Coronal CT scan in bone window shows bilateral osteolytic destruction of the anterior skull base and the medial orbital walls.

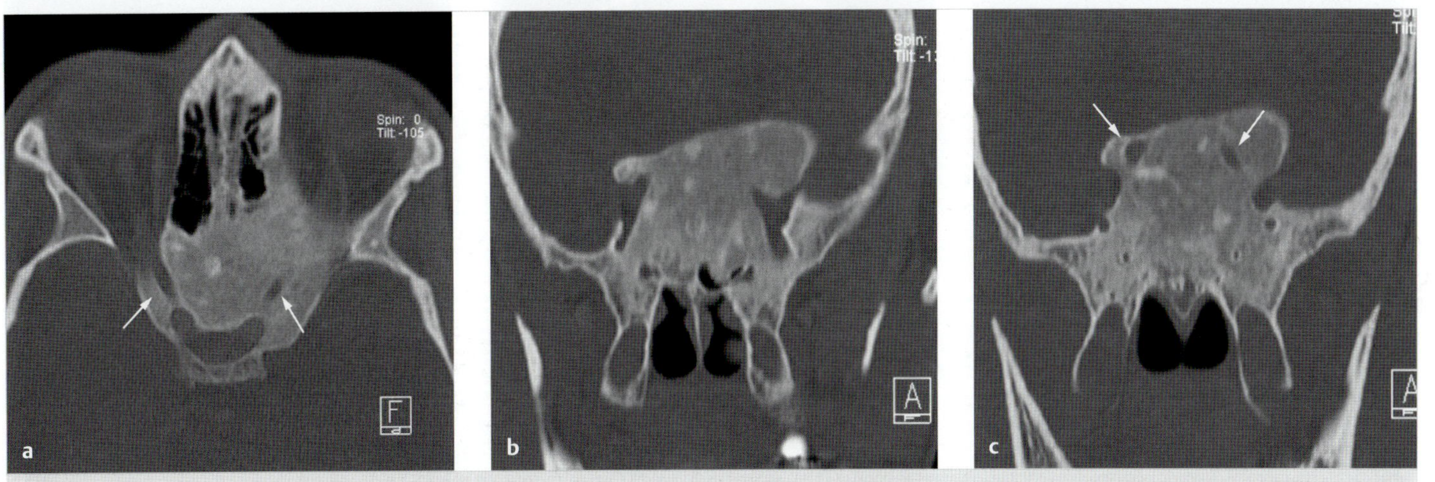

Fig. 4.14 Fibrous dysplasia. Axial **(a)** and coronal **(b, c)** CT scans show an extensive ground-glass appearance of altered bone. The optic nerve canal (*arrows*) is bilaterally surrounded and compressed by the mass.

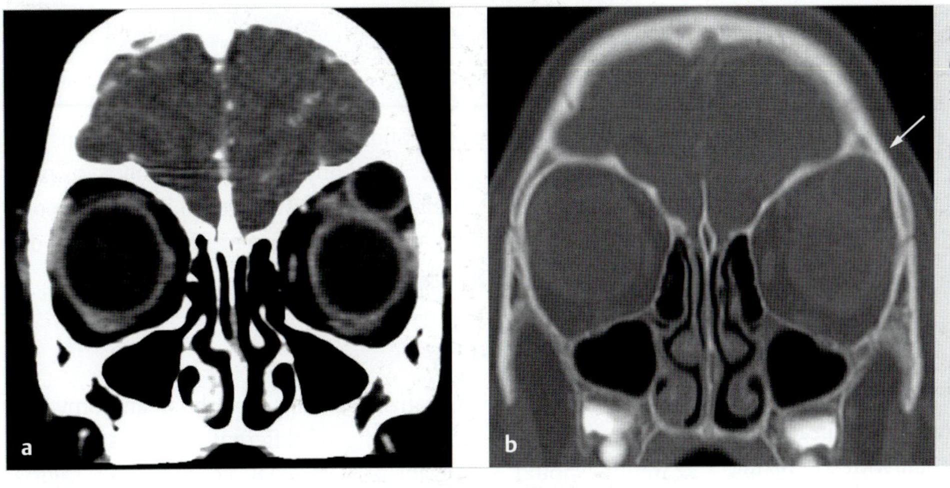

Fig. 4.15 Dermoid of the left orbit. **(a)** Contrast coronal CT in soft tissue window shows a superior laterally located lesion with sharp margins, centrally hypodense with peripheral ring-shaped contrast enhancement. **(b)** Coronal CT scan in bone window shows erosion of the adjacent bone (*arrow*), which is a sign of a longer-lasting lesion.

Osteoma (< 1 per cent of all orbital tumors) frequently originates in the bones of the paranasal sinuses, whereas primary osteoma of the bony orbital walls is less frequent. Surgical resection is required only in cases with clinical symptoms.[4]

Fibrous dysplasia is a benign developmental disorder of the bone affecting most frequently the orbital roof. It grows slowly, but the optic nerve canal is commonly involved. In case of clinical complaints, such as deterioration of visual acuity, decompression of the optic nerve is indicated.

Dermoid cysts (▶ Fig. 4.15) are the most frequent cystic lesions in the orbit. They represent congenital lesions that manifest in childhood and early adolescence.[4] Dermoids contain fat and occasionally calcifications. Inflammation or rupture of these lesions can occur.

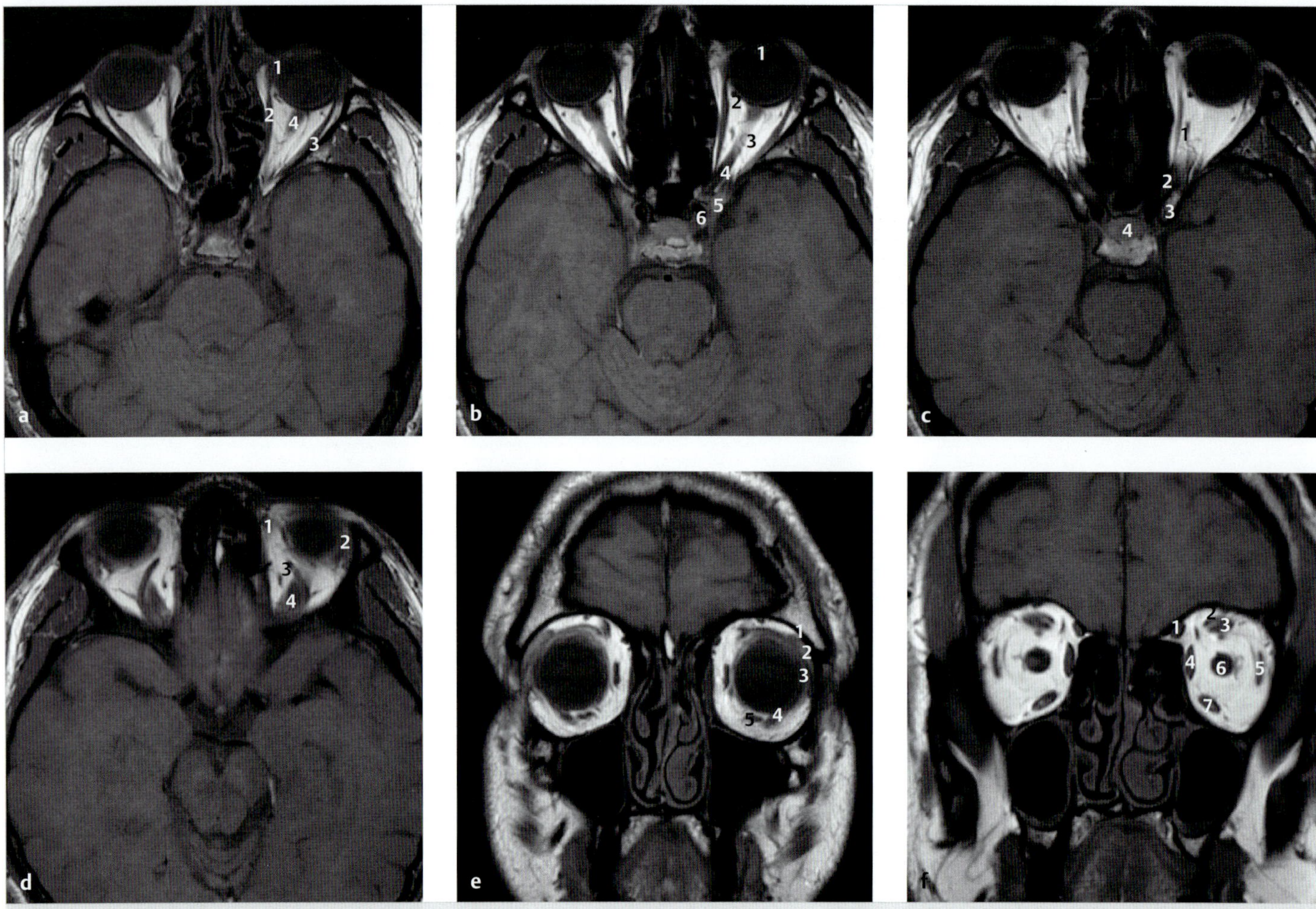

Fig. 4.16 (a–d) Axial nonenhanced T1 W MR images without fat suppression. **(e, f)** Coronal nonenhanced T1 W MR images without fat suppression. **(a)** 1, orbital septum; 2, medial rectus muscle; 3, lateral rectus muscle; 4, optic nerve. **(b)** 1, lens; 2, posterior ciliary artery; 3, ophthalmic artery; 4, optic nerve; 5, cavernous sinus; 6, internal carotid artery. **(c)** 1, ophthalmic artery; 2, optic nerve; 3, anterior clinoid process; 4, hypophysis. **(d)** 1, trochlea; 2, lacrimal gland; 3, superior ophthalmic vein; 4, superior rectus muscle. **(e)** 1, lacrimal gland-orbital part; 2, aponeurosis of levator palpebrae superior; 3, lacrimal gland palpebral part; 4, inferior oblique muscle; 5, inferior rectus muscle. **(f)** 1, superior oblique muscle; 2, levator palpebrae superior muscle; 3, superior rectus muscle; 4, medial rectus muscle; 5, lateral rectus muscle; 6, optic nerve; 7, inferior rectus muscle.

4.4 Magnet Resonance Imaging (MRI)

A. Pangalu and A. Valavanis

During this century the diagnostic use of CT scans has increasingly been replaced by MRI scanning, especially for diagnostic clarification of retrobulbar pathologies. Because of MRI's better soft tissue contrast, both the visualization and the anatomical localization of orbital lesions is significantly more precisely than with CT. Taking account of the different signal intensities using different sequences some narrowing of differential diagnosis is possible with MRI. The lack of radiation exposure is another advantage of this technique. The topographical resolution can be significantly improved by using special orbit coils but excellent image quality and topographical resolution can also be achieved with the head coil of the newest MRI machines. For high image quality, it is crucial to avoid eye movements by the patient so as not to produce movement artifacts. Due to the relatively small orbital volume and small pathological structures, thin image slices of about 2.5 to 3.0 mm are required. Basically T1 W and T2 W sequences are captured. It is advantageous to perform T1 W sequences with fat suppression following application of contrast agents, to suppress the significantly bright fat signal and allow visualization of small lesions that take up contrast agents. The bony cortical substance displays hypointensity (dark) in all sequences. The eyeball appears hypointense in T1 W sequences and hyperintense in T2 W sequences due to the fluid inside the organ.

4.4.1 Anatomy

MRI is suitable for visualizing details of orbital anatomy. For demarcation of the topography of different orbital structures, scanning should be performed in axial, coronal, and sagittal planes (▸ Fig. 4.16, ▸ Fig. 4.17).

4.4.2 Inflammatory Diseases

There is a wide spectrum of inflammatory diseases affecting the orbit, including infectious diseases, idiopathic orbital inflammatory disease (pseudotumors), optic nerve neuritis, and dysthyroid endocrine orbitopathy (Graves's disease). Together they represent more than 50% of all orbital lesions.[5]

Most acute orbital infections originate in the paranasal sinuses. However, orbital infections can also develop from infections of the face and pharynx, and can also be caused by a trauma or a foreign body. A proportion of them develop secondarily following

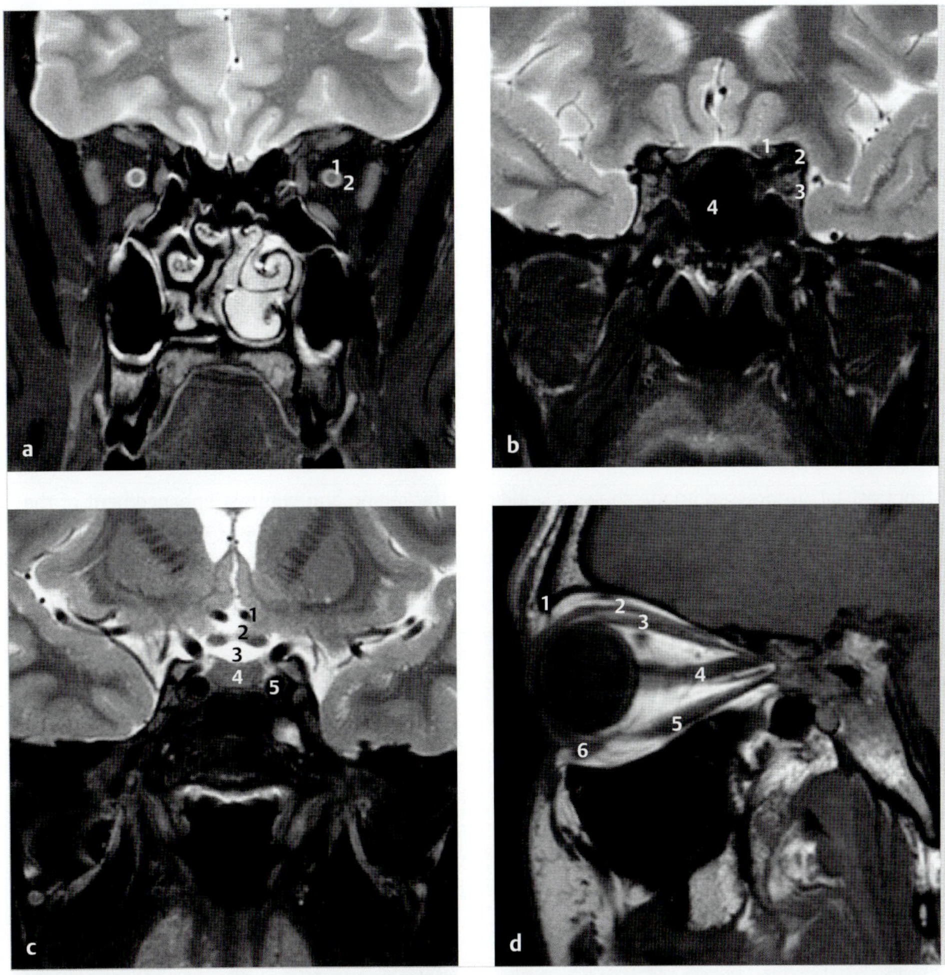

Fig. 4.17 **(a–c)** Coronal T2 W images with fat suppression. **(d)** Sagittal nonenhanced T1 W image without fat suppression. **(a)** 1, optic nerve; 2, optic sheath. **(b)** 1, optic nerve; 2, anterior clinoid process; 3, cavernous sinus; 4, sphenoid sinus. **(c)** 1, anterior cerebral artery; 2, optic chiasm; 3, suprasellar cistern; 4, hypophysis; 5, internal carotid artery. **(d)** 1, orbital septum; 2, levator palpebrae superior muscle; 3, superior rectus muscle; 4, optic nerve; 5, inferior rectus muscle; 6, inferior oblique muscle.

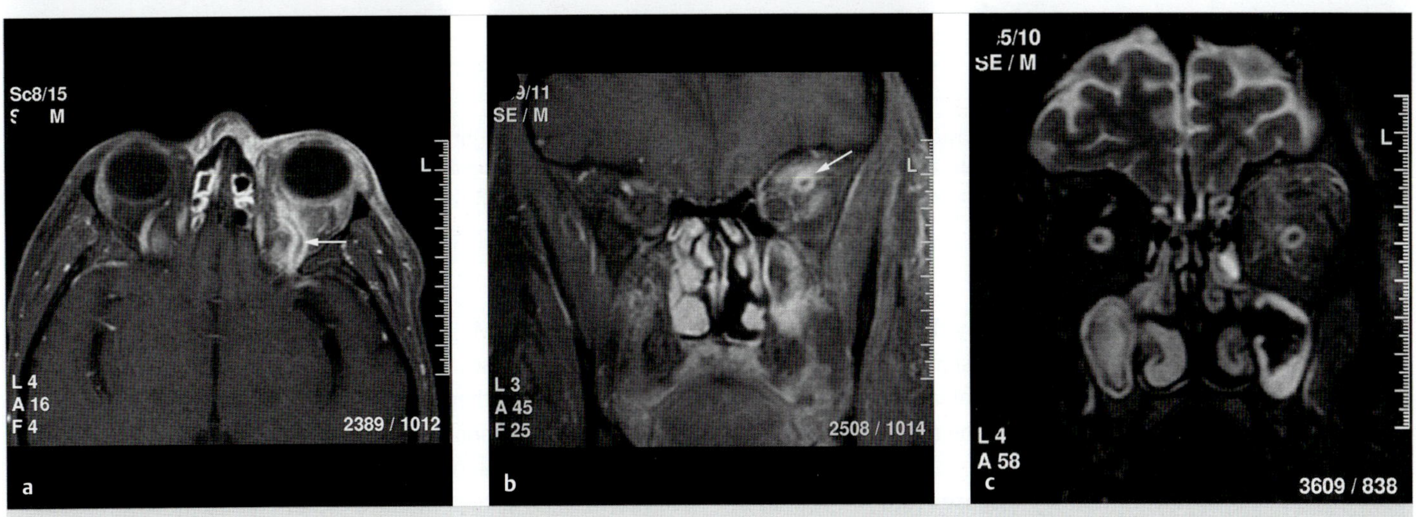

Fig. 4.18 Orbital phlegmon and superior ophthalmic vein thrombosis. **(a)** Contrast-enhanced T1 W image with fat suppression demonstrating diffuse contrast enhancement in the intraconal space. Enhancement is visible also in the walls of the thrombosed superior ophthalmic vein (*arrow*), whereas the vein's lumen is spared. **(b)** The thrombosed superior ophthalmic vein can be recognized as a roundish structure (*arrow*) superolateral to the optic nerve in the coronal T1 W image. **(c)** In contrast to the right side, the retrobulbar adipose tissue on the left side shows a hyperintense signal due to inflammatory infiltration and edema in the coronal T2 W images with fat suppression. Note the swollen mucosa and obliteration of the maxillary sinuses on both sides and of the ethmoid cells.

septicemia.[6] Orbital cellulitis can be classified in five stages of orbital involvement[7]:

1. Inflammatory edema.
2. Subperiosteal phlegmon and subperiosteal abscess.
3. Orbital cellulitis.
4. Orbital abscess.
5. Ophthalmic vein and cavernous sinus thrombosis (▶ Fig. 4.18).

Graves's orbitopathy (▶ Fig. 4.19) is an autoimmune disease and the most frequent cause of bilateral exophthalmos (see Chapter 7). The disease is characterized by a thickening of extraocular muscles, commonly the muscle bellies, and sparing of the muscles' tendons. Muscle thickening is caused by an infiltration of lymphocytes, plasma cells, and mast cells and by deposition of hydrophilic mucopolysaccharides, with the inferior rectus muscle

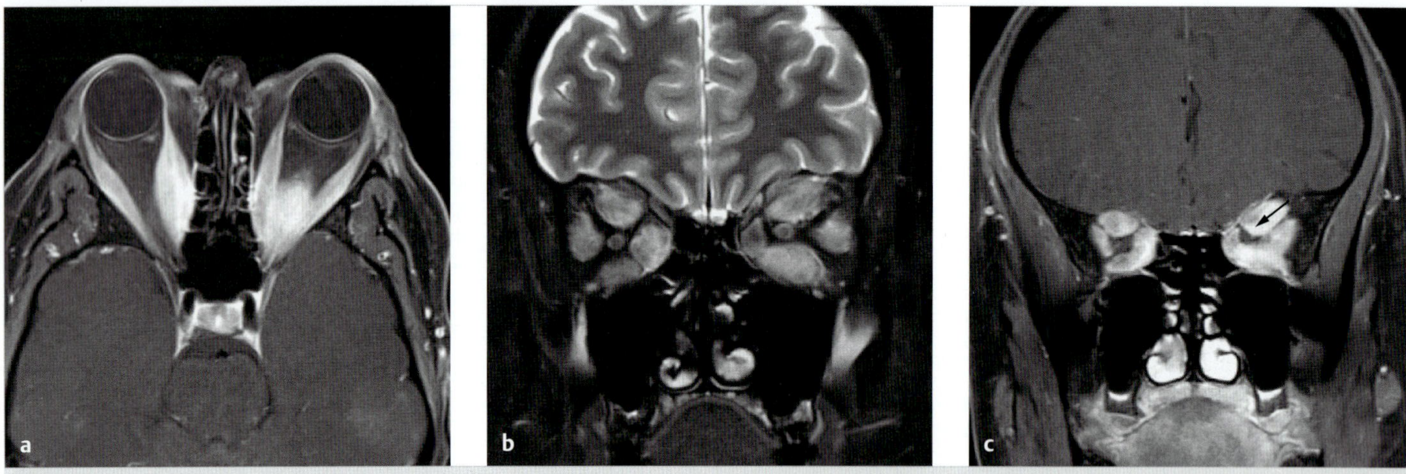

Fig. 4.19 Graves's orbitopathy. **(a)** Axial, T1 W postcontrast fat-suppressed image shows a significant thickening and contrast enhancement of the muscle bellies of any extraocular muscle. **(b)** Coronal fat-suppressed T2 W image shows hyperintense signal of the affected muscles, **(c)** Coronal postcontrast fat-suppressed T1 W image shows that considerable muscle thickening leads to a compression of the optic nerve in the orbital apex (*arrow*).

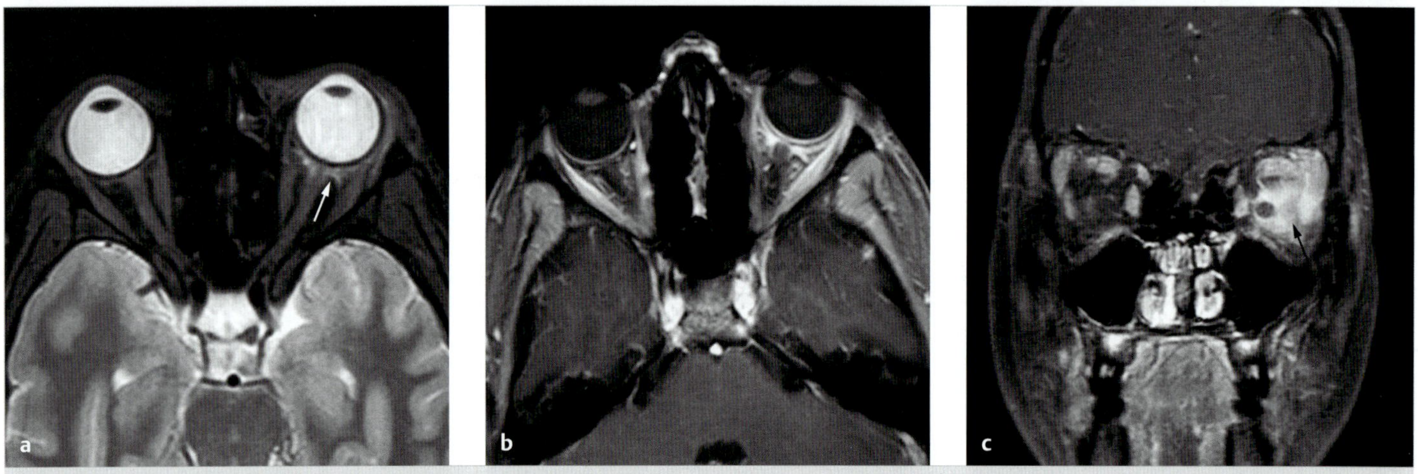

Fig. 4.20 Anterior orbital inflammation with posterior scleritis. A 24-year-old woman with pain, slight proptosis, and lid swelling on the left side. **(a)** A hyperintensity in the retrobulbar adipose tissue adjacent to the sclera is shown by an axial fat-suppressed T2 W image (*white arrow*). **(b, c)** Contrast administration leads to significant contrast enhancement of the posterior sclera and retrobulbar fat tissue in axial **(b)** and coronal **(c)** fat-suppressed T1 W images (*black arrow*).

being most frequently affected, followed by the medial, superior, and lateral rectus muscles. Other clinical signs are thickening of the lacrimal gland, proliferation of orbital adipose tissue, and stretching of the optic nerve. Myositis is the most important differential diagnosis.

Idiopathic orbital inflammatory disease (IOID) (▶ Fig. 4.20) represents a heterogeneous group of unspecific inflammations of the orbital tissues for which no specific, systemic or local causes can be determined.[8,9] The disease was first described by Birch-Hirschfeld as orbital pseudotumor.[10] Histopathologically a mixed infiltration by immature T lymphocytes, granulocytes, plasma cells, histiocytes, and macrophages occurs, accompanied by fibrosis.[11] The course of the disease can be acute, subacute, or chronic.

Six sites of inflammation can be distinguished: anterior orbital inflammation, diffuse orbital inflammation, apical posterior orbital inflammation, lacrimal inflammation, orbital myositis, and perineuritis. The main clinical symptoms are pain, diplopia, and vision loss. A rapid improvement after application of glucocorticoids is typical in this disease.

An acute inflammatory process of the optic nerve is termed **optic nerve neuritis** (▶ Fig. 4.21), which is most commonly due to multiple sclerosis (MS).[12] Optic nerve neuritis can also be caused by numerous diseases other than MS, e.g., autoimmune diseases (systemic lupus erythematosus), post- and parainfectiously during herpes infections, mononucleosis, rubella, toxoplasmosis, syphilis, borreliosis, or granulomatous diseases. Optic nerve neuritis is characterized by a hyperintense signal and swelling of the nerve in T2 W images. Contrast enhancement of the nerve develops after application of a contrast agent (▶ Fig. 4.21a–c).

4.4.3 Tumors

Although they are responsible for at least 25% of all orbital diseases, orbital tumors are rare. Primary and secondary tumors can be distinguished. While primary orbital tumors originate from different tissues in the orbital compartments, secondary tumors develop by infiltration of the orbit from the adjacent organs or as metastases. The topographical association of intraorbital tumors with a particular compartment is advantageous for diagnostic purposes.

The most frequent primary intraocular malignant tumor in adults is the **primary orbital melanoma**. Ninety percent of all melanomas develop in the choroidea.[13] With progressive growth

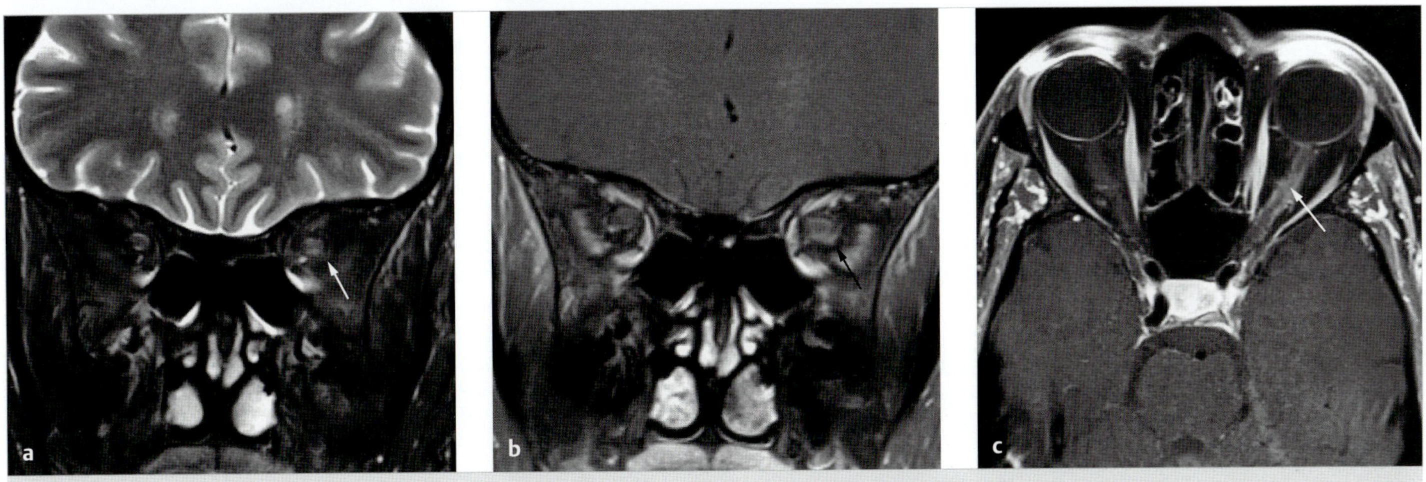

Fig. 4.21 Left optic nerve neuritis in a patient with multiple sclerosis. **(a)** Coronal fat-suppressed T2 W image shows swelling and hyperintense signal changes of the left optic nerve (*white arrow*). **(b)** Significant contrast enhancement of the left optic nerve after contrast administration in a coronal fat-suppressed T1 W image (*black arrow*). **(c)** Contrast enhancement of the entire left optic nerve in axial fat-suppressed T1 W images (*white arrow*).

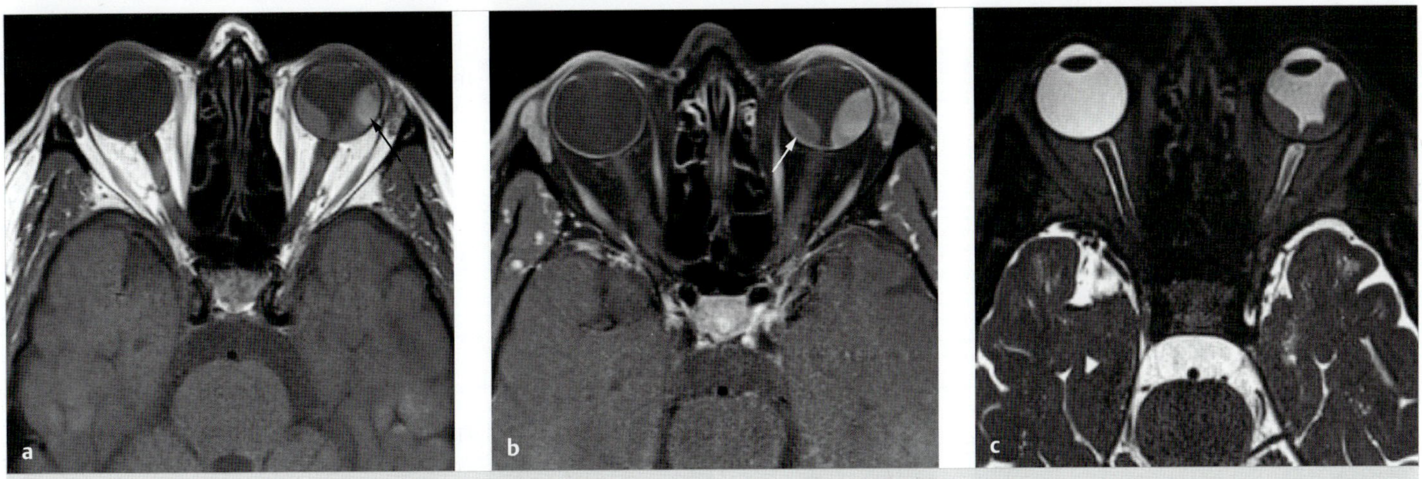

Fig. 4.22 Primary malignant melanoma. **(a)** The tumor displays a hyperintense signal (*arrow*) in an axial noncontrast T1 W image. A retinal detachment is seen medially. **(b)** Axial postcontrast fat-suppressed T1 W image shows contrast enhancement of the tumor but no enhancement in the area of the retinal detachment (*arrow*). **(c)** Melanoma: hypointense signal in an axial T2 W image.

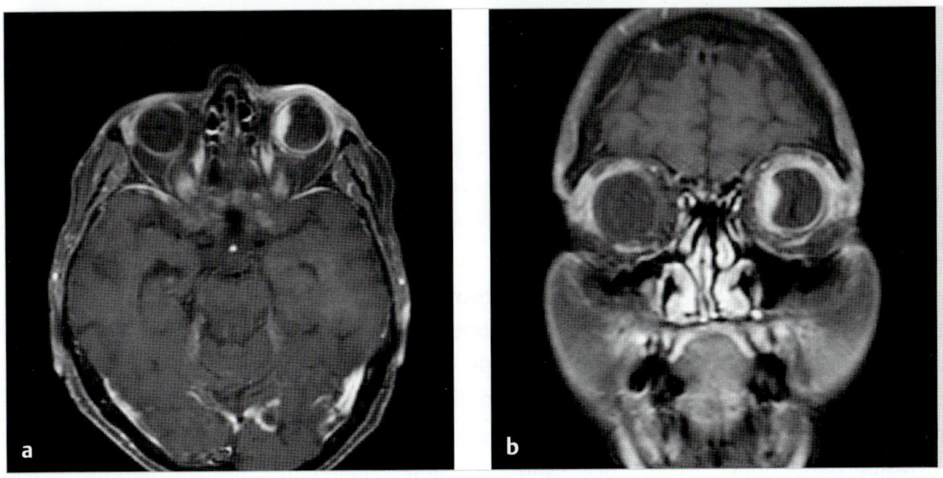

Fig. 4.23 Uveal metastasis of a breast cancer. Axial **(a)** and coronal **(b)** postcontrast fat-suppressed T1 W images show choroidal metastasis of a breast cancer, medially on the left.

they penetrate the Bruch's membrane and develop their characteristic fungiform shape (▶ Fig. 4.22). Melanin displays as hyperintensity in T1 W images and hypointensity in T2 W images.

Breast cancer and lung cancer are the most frequent causes for **intraocular metastases** (▶ Fig. 4.23), which can affect both the retina and the choroidea.[14]

Glioma and meningioma are **neoplasias** arising directly from the optic nerve or the nerve sheath. Nearly all **optic nerve gliomas** (▶ Fig. 4.24) are juvenile pilocytic astrocytoma occurring in children younger than 8 years of age. They are associated to neurofibromatosis type 1 (NF-1); 20% of all NF-1 children develop optic nerve glioma.[15,16]

Perioptic meningioma (▶ Fig. 4.25) arise from cap cells of the arachnoid surrounding the optic nerve in the orbit or optic canal. Primary meningiomas are less frequent than secondary, originating intracranially and invading into the orbit.

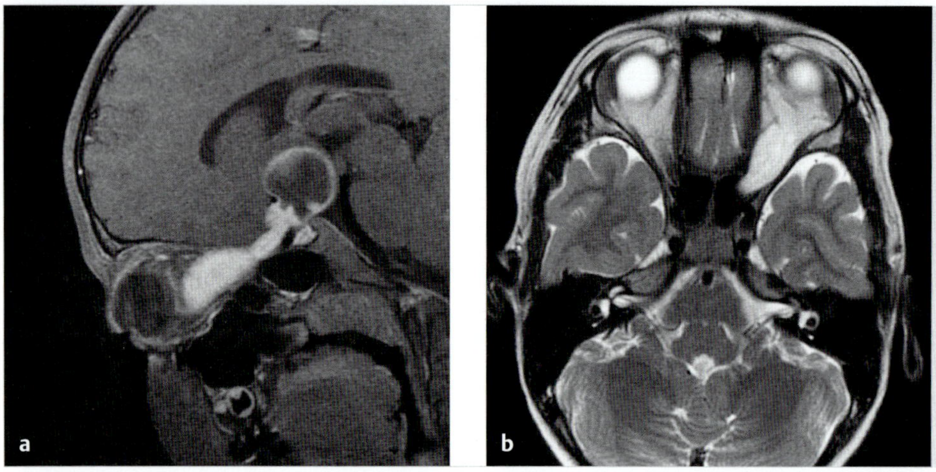

Fig. 4.24 Pilocytic astrocytoma in a patient with NF-1. **(a)** Sagittal T1 W images demonstrate thickening, fusiform enlargement, and contrast enhancement of the left optic nerve. The optic chiasm is affected by the cystic part of the glioma. **(b)** The optic nerve displays hyperintensity and is dilated in axial T2 W images, with inability to distinguish between nerve and subarachnoid space.

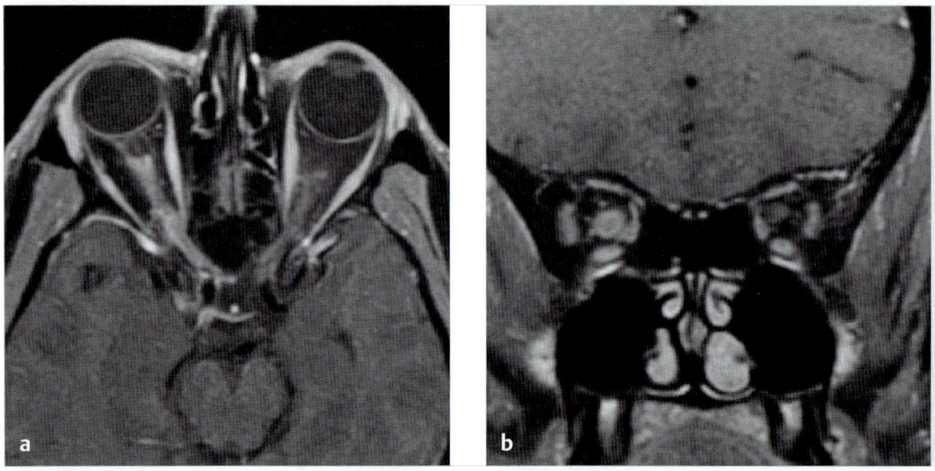

Fig. 4.25 Perioptic meningioma. The figure shows axial **(a)** and coronal **(b)** postcontrast fat-suppressed T1 W images. There is a significant contrast enhancement along the optic nerve sheath on the right side with lack of enhancement of the nerve itself, which appears as a hypointense structure (so-called "tram-track sign"). The contrast enhancement extends into the intracanalicular part of the optic nerve.

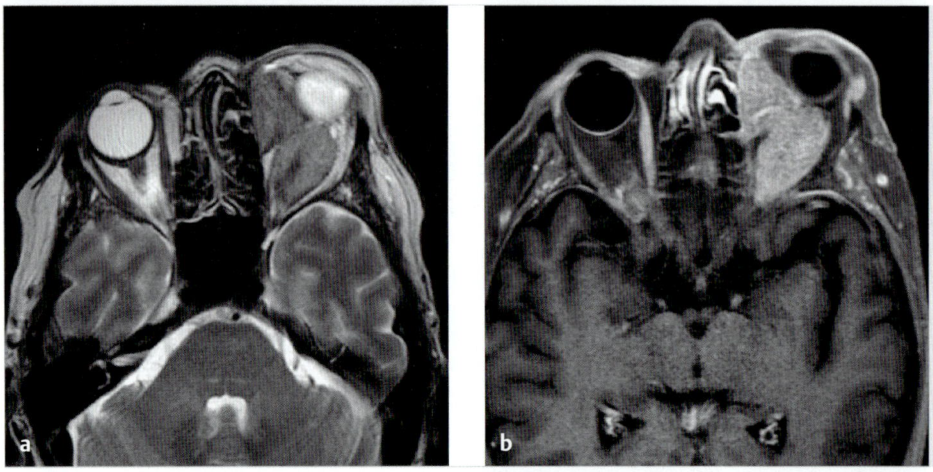

Fig. 4.26 Malignant MALT lymphoma of the orbit. **(a)** T2 W image shows a large hypointense mass, located intra- and extraconally. **(b)** Contrast-enhanced T1 W axial image with fat suppression. Here the mass significantly takes up the contrast agent and surrounds the optic nerve.

With a frequency of 67 to 90% of all lymphoproliferative orbital masses, and 24% of all orbital tumors, **malignant lymphoma** is the most frequent orbital tumor in patients older than 65 years.[17] These masses can represent either an orbital manifestation of a systemic lymphoma or a tumor, arising primarily in the orbit. The most frequent orbital lymphoma is the MALT lymphoma (▶ Fig. 4.26), a subtype of malignant non-Hodgkin's lymphoma.

Cavernous hemangioma (▶ Fig. 4.27) represents the most frequent benign tumor condition in the orbit. It occurs commonly in middle-aged adults and shows no gender preference.[18] Radiologically it presents as a circumscribed ovoid or roundish mass with sharp borders, located lateral in the intraconal compartment.[19] However, it can also occur in the entire orbit. Cavernous hemangioma usually has a slowly progressive growth pattern with no tendency for spontaneous remission.

Lacrimal gland tumors are relatively rare with a rate of 5 to 7% of all orbital masses.[18,20] The most frequent epithelial tumor of the lacrimal glands is the **benign pleomorphic adenoma** (▶ Fig. 4.28). A complete tumor resection without injury of the tumor's pseudocapsule is mandatory to reduce the risk of tumor recurrence and probable malignant transformation.[21] The **adenoid cystic carcinoma** represents the most frequent *malignant* epithelial tumor of the lacrimal glands.

Cholesterol granulomas (▶ Fig. 4.29) are tumors of the subperiostal compartment, usually appearing secondarily following a trauma, an operation, or inflammation. The superior temporal space of the orbit is the most common site of this tumor. The tumor shows an expansive growth pattern due to recurrent bleeding and causes bone erosions.

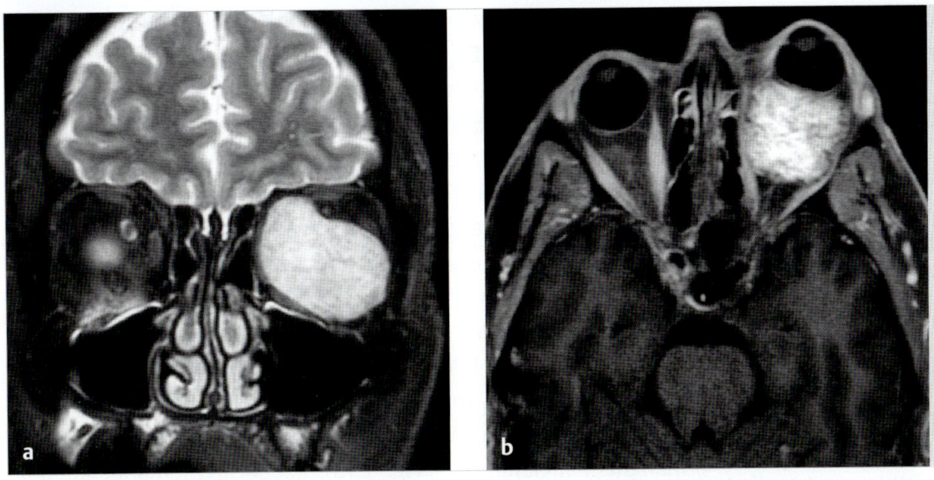

Fig. 4.27 Cavernous hemangioma. **(a)** The tumor displays as an intraconally located circumscribed hyperintense mass in a coronal T2 W image. **(b)** The hemangioma depicts a significant contrast enhancement in the axial T1 W image after contrast administration and fat suppression. Note the compression and anterior displacement of the eyeball.

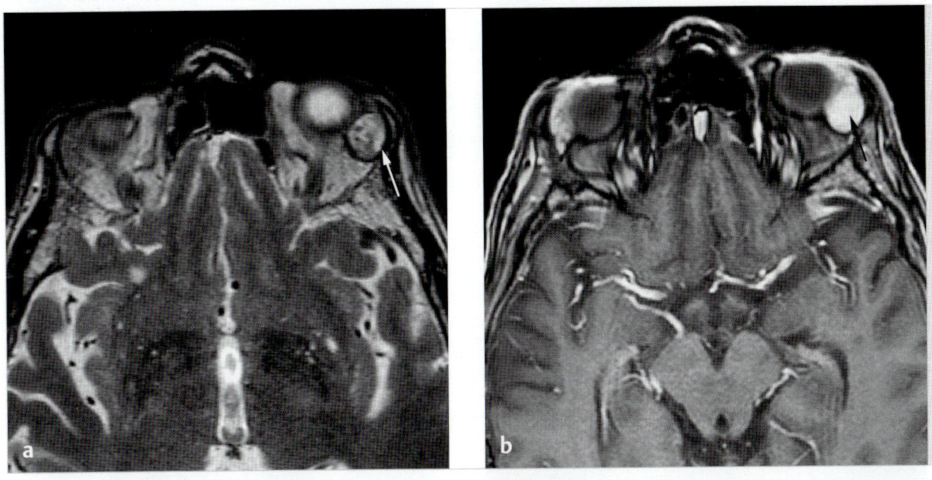

Fig. 4.28 Pleomorphic adenoma of the lacrimal gland. **(a)** Axial T2 W image shows an inhomogeneous hyperintense mass with a hypointense capsule located in the extraconal space in the lacrimal gland (*arrow*). **(b)** The lesion shows markedly homogenous contrast enhancement (*arrow*) in a T1 W image.

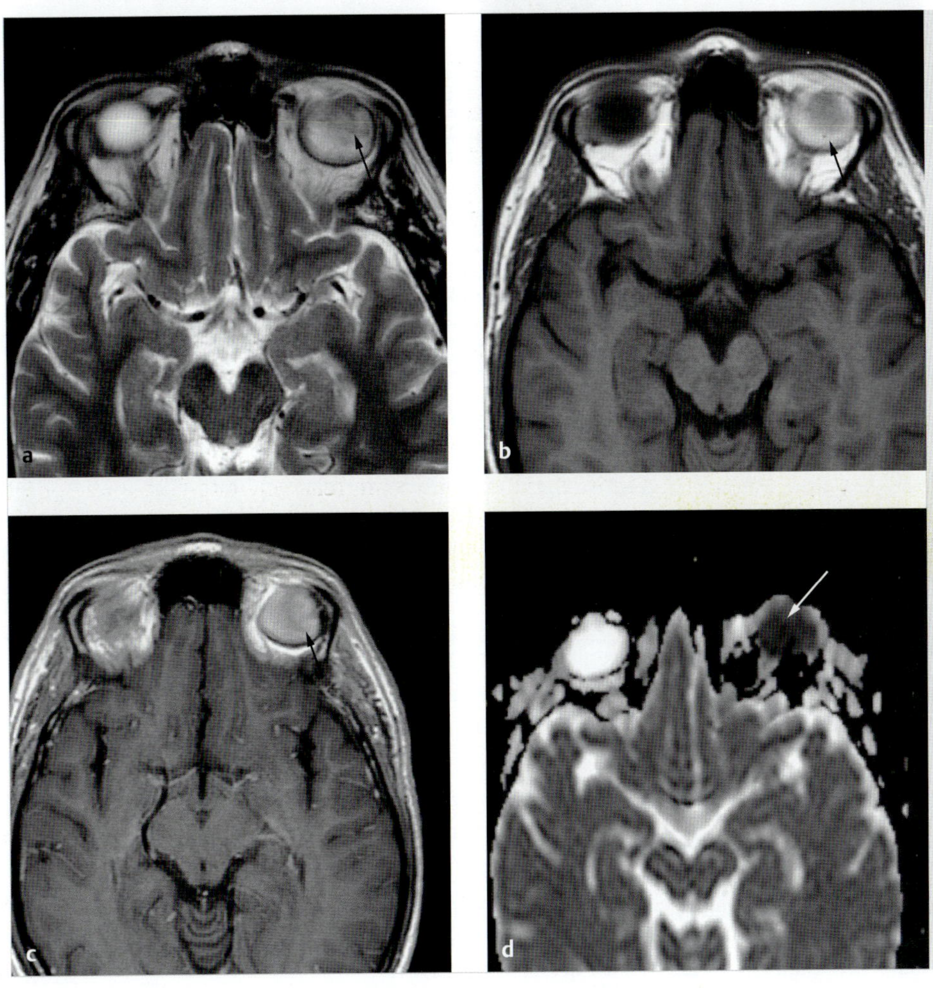

Fig. 4.29 Cholesterol granuloma in the left orbit. The cholesterol granuloma shows an hyperintense signal in both, T2 W **(a)** and nonenhanced T1 W **(b)** images. Lack of contrast enhancement **(c)** in an enhanced T1 W image, and diffusion restriction in diffusion- weighted image **(d)** (hypointense signal) (*arrow*).

4.5 Positron Emission Tomography (PET)

A. Pangalu and A. Valavanis

Positron emission tomography (PET) is a nuclear medicine functional imaging technique that visualizes the distribution and emission of a radionuclide tracer that has been intravenously injected; it can therefore detect specific biochemical and physiological functions. Radiopharmaceuticals (radiotracers) are compounds whose molecules are marked with a radionuclide. The most commonly used nuclide in PET scanning is the radioactive isotope fluorine 18 (^{18}F). To date, FDG PET (PET scans with ^{18}F-fluorodeoxyglucose [FDG; fludeoxyglucose F 18]) in combination with CT scans is widely used in tumor diagnosis and in tumor staging for detecting lymph node or distant metastases. However, the usually tiny regions of pathologic tissue in the orbit are hard to evaluate with PET scans. To make it more difficult, several inflammatory diseases, e.g., idiopathic orbital inflammatory disease (IOID),[22,23] and also some normal tissues, e.g., extraocular muscles, exhibit increased FDG uptake. Nevertheless FDG PET imaging is preferable to alternative options such as CT or MRI, as it provides information on the tumor metabolism and early tumor response to a therapy, and evaluation of asymptomatic residual lesions. FDG PET is also sensitive in detecting and investigating small, distant metastases that would otherwise not be detected early. The FDG uptake in benign orbital tumors is comparable to that in the normal contralateral tissue. Malignant tumors (e.g., malignant lymphoma [▶ Fig. 4.30; ▶ Fig. 4.31], malignant melanoma [▶ Fig. 4.32], adenocarcinoma, or adenoid cystic carcinoma), however, usually exhibit significantly increased FDG uptake.[24] The *standardized uptake value* (SUV) quantifies regional radioactive concentration in particular

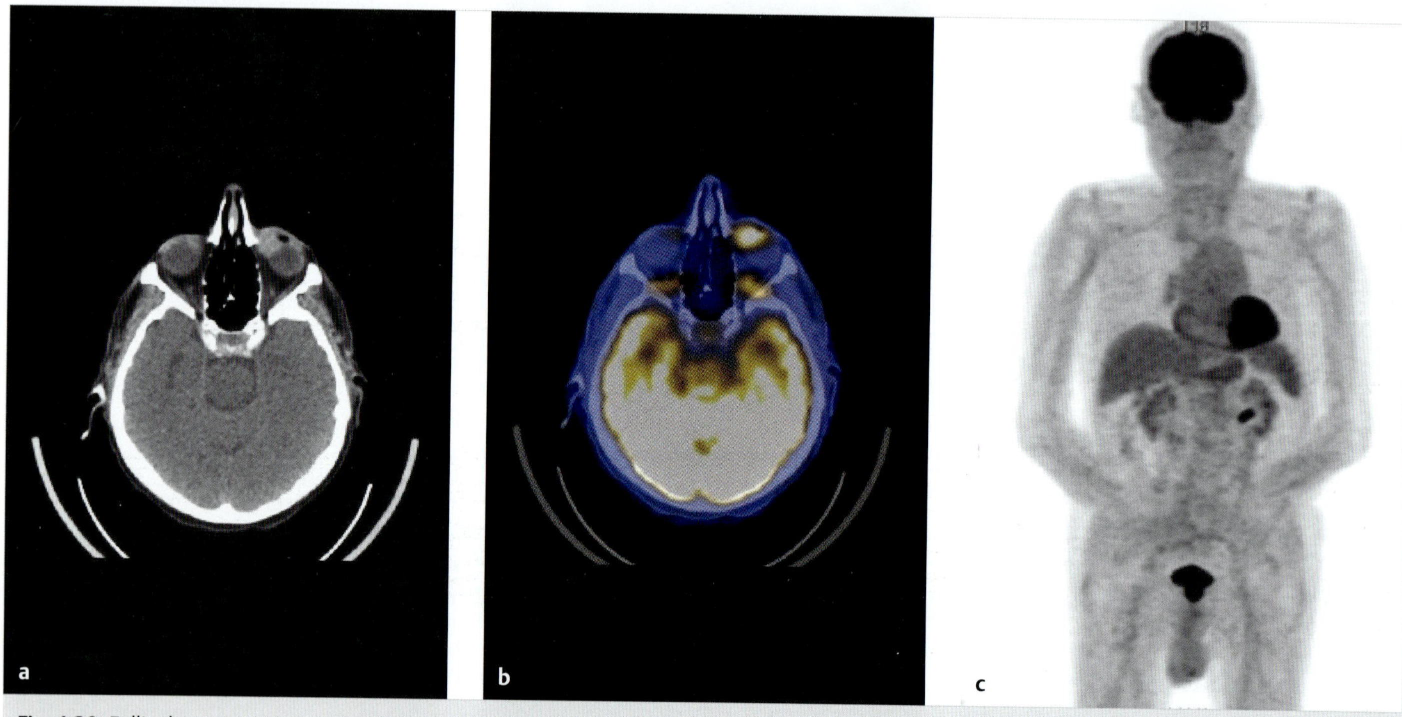

Fig. 4.30 Follicular non-Hodgkin's lymphoma. An 88-year-old man after irradiation of a follicular non-Hodgkin's lymphoma in the axilla one year previously. Tumor recurrence in the left orbit, which has been histologically confirmed. **(a, b)** Corresponding PET/CT images show a hyperdense lesion in the left orbit with increased metabolic activity (SUV_{max} = 6.6). **(c)** No extraorbital manifestations are detectable.

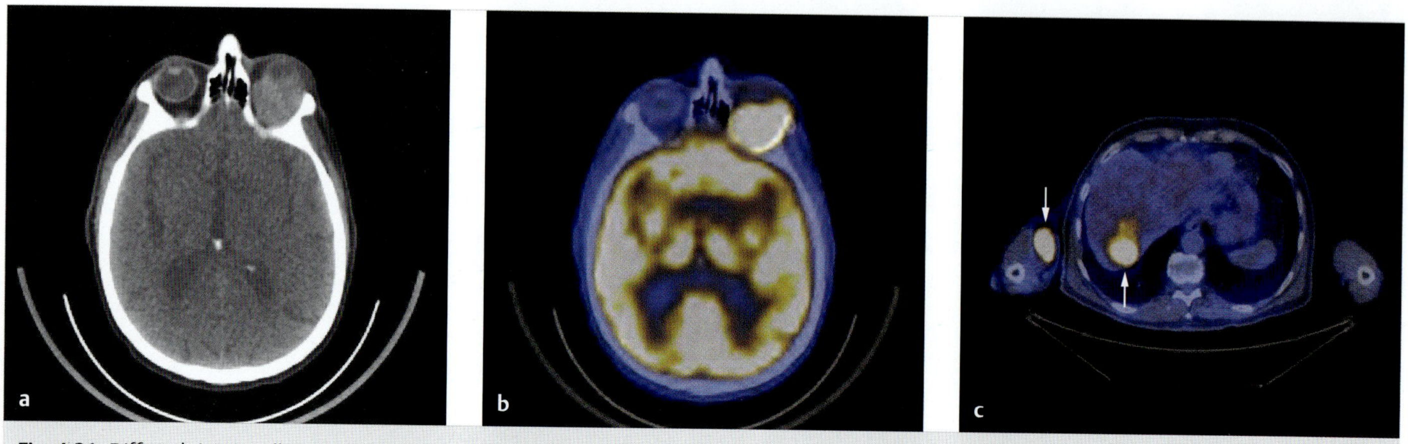

Fig. 4.31 Diffuse large B-cell non-Hodgkin's lymphoma. **(a, b)** A left-sided hyperdense retro-orbital mass is demonstrated by PET/CT with markedly increased metabolic activity (SUV_{max} = 19.7). The lymphoma was histologically confirmed. **(c)** Additional hypermetabolic extranodal manifestations of the lymphoma in the right medial upper arm and in liver segment VII (*arrows*) are detected by PET/CT.

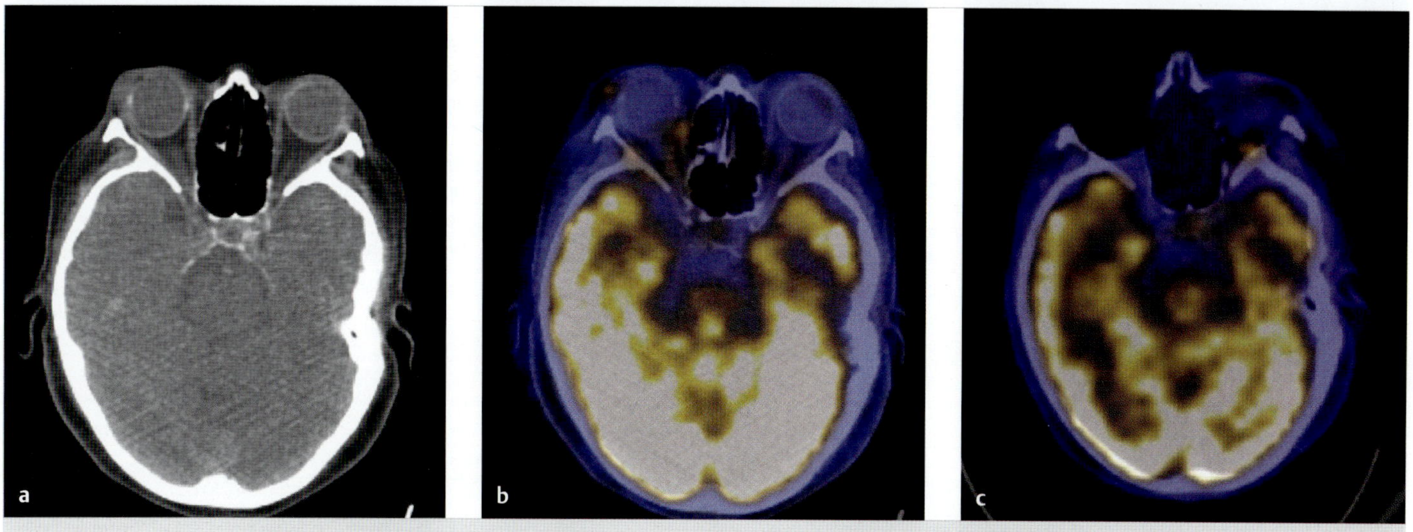

Fig. 4.32 Malignant melanoma of the conjunctiva on the right side. (a, b) PET/CT was initially performed for tumor staging and shows a soft tissue lesion at the right-sided canthus with focal minor increase of metabolic activity ($SUV_{max} = 3.5$). There is no evidence for lymph node or distant metastases. (c) Follow-up PET/CT scan after orbital exenteration shows no evidence of local tumor recurrence or of distant metastases.

tissues. It is used, for example, when FDG is applied as tracer for quantification of the glucose metabolism in a tumor.

4.6 Interventional Neuroradiology of Orbital Diseases

A. Pangalu and A. Valavanis

Endovascular therapy comes into play for therapy of first choice of orbital vascular lesions or as a preoperative procedure. Precise knowledge of the vascularization of the orbit and mastering of the superselective microcatheterization of the ophthalmic artery and its branches, as also the branches of the external carotid artery, is an absolute prerequisite for performing these procedures.

There are several main indications for endovascular treatment:

- Arteriovenous malformations of the orbit and the upper and lower lids.
- Carotid artery–cavernous sinus fistulas with venous drainage via the superior ophthalmic vein.
- Venous malformations in the extraconal space.
- Infantile capillary hemangioma of the upper lid, to avoid an amblyopia.

Arteriovenous malformations of the orbit (▶ Fig. 4.33) are very rare lesions, which occur most likely congenitally. They can be localized inside the orbit and/or periorbitally. A very rare combination of intracerebral arteriovenous malformations and retinal malformations occurs with the Wyborn–Mason syndrome. Arteriovenous malformations are characterized by a nidus, which is a convolution of pathologic vessels with arteriovenous shunts, along with their dilated feeding arteries and draining veins. In most cases the feeding arteries originate in the ophthalmic artery or in branches of the external carotid artery (e.g., internal maxillary artery).

Carotid artery–cavernous sinus fistulas (▶ Fig. 4.34) can occur either posttraumatically following an injury of the internal carotid artery or, less frequently, spontaneously. In the latter case a rupture of the internal carotid artery due either to an aneurysm or to alterations of the vessel's wall in patients with osteogenesis imperfecta or Ehlers–Danlos syndrome is commonly causative.

The clinical symptoms are characterized by upper-eyelid edema, pulsatile exophthalmos, chemosis, vision loss, and pulsatile noise that can be auscultated. Endovascular embolization with closure of the fistula by a balloon or by coils, or a combination of both, is the therapy of first choice.

Lymphangiomas (lymphatic–venous malformations) occur most frequently in children and youths. They usually do not have any capsule structures, show a diffuse growth pattern, and are composed of connective tissue lacunar spaces, which can contain blood or serous fluid. In the first two decades they are progressive, with increase of extension. Lymphangiomas are most commonly multilobular in shape and located extraconally (▶ Fig. 4.35).

Capillary hemangiomas are usually congenital or develop in the first year of life. An initial increase of the lesion is common. However, a decrease in volume or a complete regression occurs in most cases. Hemangiomas can have an arterial blood supply and a tendency to bleeding. It is recommended to wait for the involution of the lesion before contemplating any other therapeutic procedures (▶ Fig. 4.36).

4.7 Ultrasonography of the Orbit

H.-J. Welkoborsky

The sustained increase in demand for precise imaging of the orbit to investigate even very small structures in thin slices has led to wide application of CT and/or MRI (see Chapters 4.3–4.5). Nowadays CT and/or MRI scans are regarded as the "gold standard" for imaging of the orbit. The two techniques are used in complementary fashion as CT and MRI are sensitive to different tissue properties, and images obtained with the two techniques differ markedly. Ultrasound examinations, in contrast, are of only of minor importance. However, ultrasound imaging is more sensitive than CT and/or MRI, particularly for examining superficial soft tissue diseases or tumors of the anterior orbit or lacrimal glands, and can therefore give valuable diagnostic

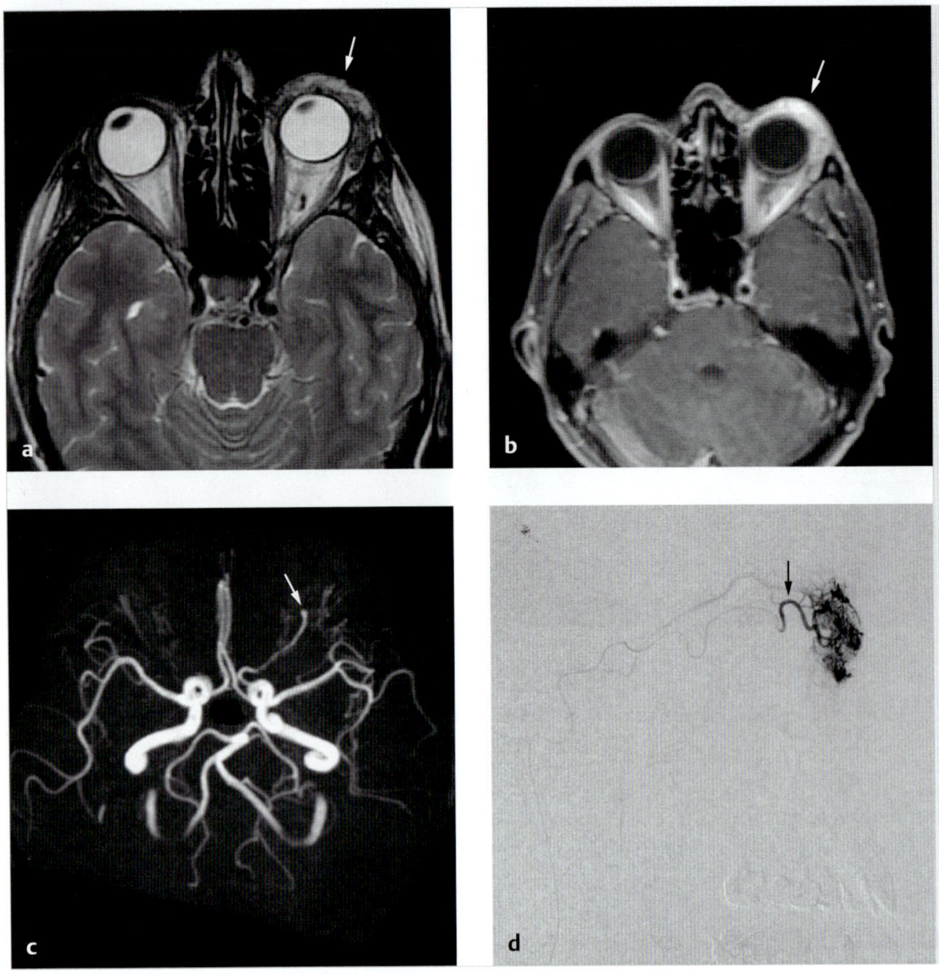

Fig. 4.33 Arteriovenous malformation of the left upper lid. **(a)** AxialT2 W image shows a vascular mass in the left-sided upper lid (*arrow*). **(b)**Axial contrast-enhanced T1 W image shows significant intralesional contrast enhancement (*arrow*). **(c)** The markedly dilated ipsilateral ophthalmic artery (*arrow*) is displayed by time-of-flight (TOF) MR angiography. **(d)** An arteriovenous malformation in the left-sided upper lid with the ophthalmic artery as feeding artery (*arrow*) is confirmed by superselective angiography (DSA) of the ophthalmic artery.

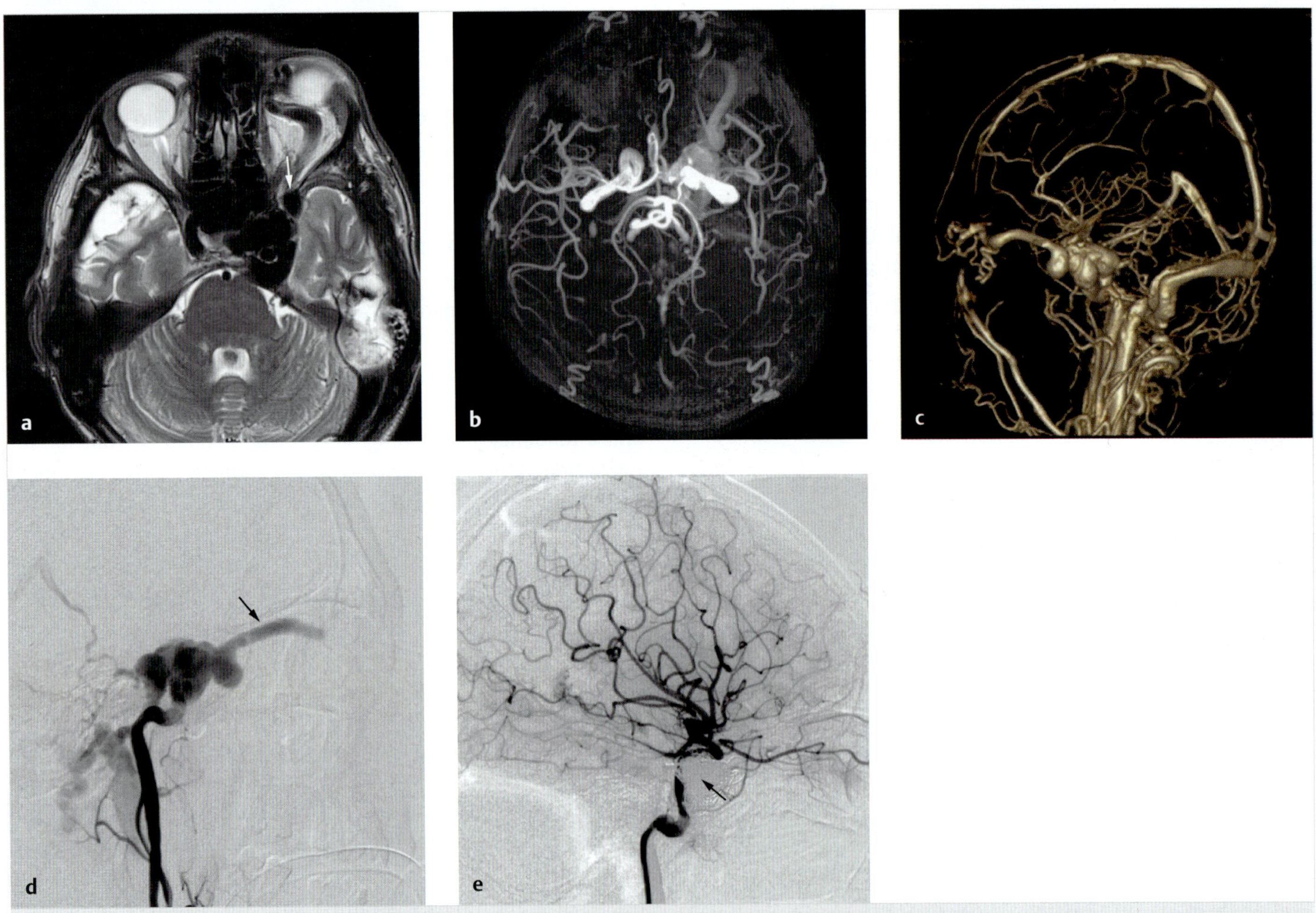

Fig. 4.34 Posttraumatic carotid cavernous fistula (CCF) in a 25-year-old patient who developed an exophthalmos accompanied by chemosis and a pulsatile noise. **(a)** A significantly dilated left-sided superior ophthalmic vein is displayed by the axial T2 W image. The left cavernous sinus is filled with significantly dilated vessels (*arrow*). Cortical contusions are visible on both sides. **(b)** The significantly dilated left-sided superior ophthalmic vein and cavernous sinus are visualized by MR angiography. **(c)** 3D angiography of the fistula. **(d)** Digital subtraction angiography of the fistula before embolization. Venous filling of the cavernous sinus and superior orbital vein is shown already in the arterial phase of the examination (*arrow*). **(e)** Control angiography after embolization and closure of the large fistula with coils (*arrow*) reveals lack of venous structures in the arterial phase of the examination and normal filling of the cerebral hemisphere.

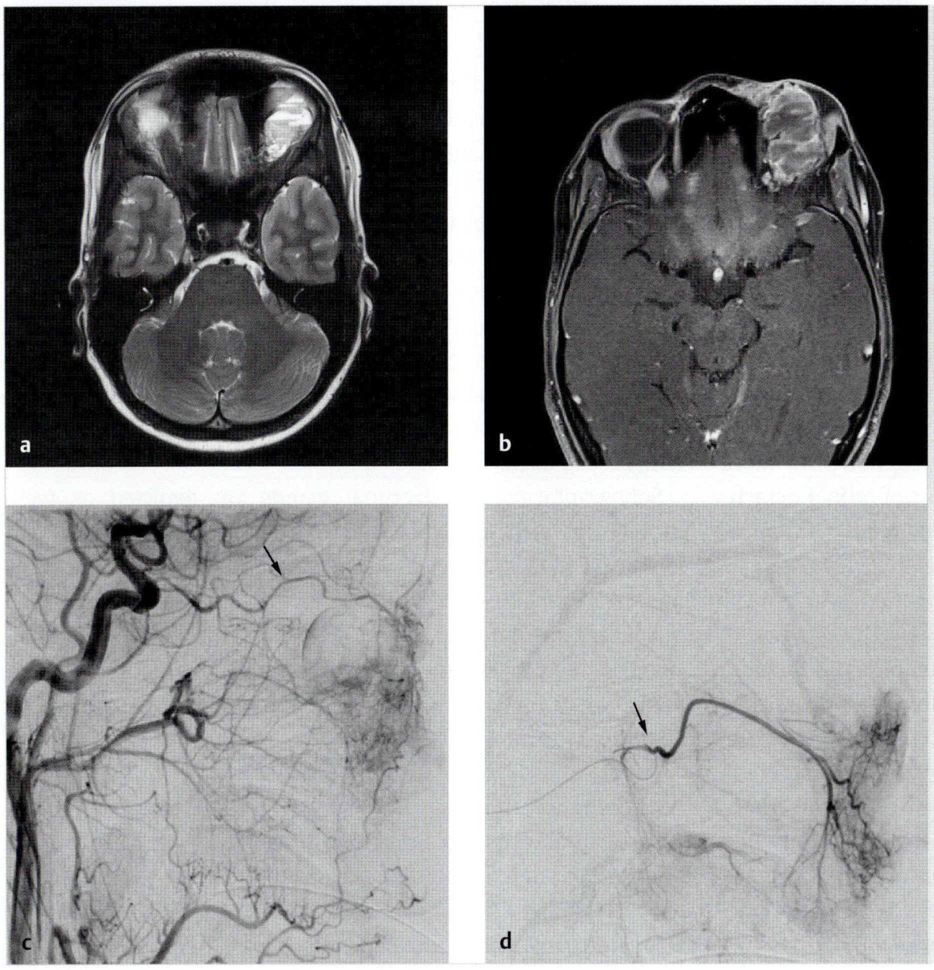

Fig. 4.35 Lymphangioma. (a) Axial T2 W image shows a lymphangioma with characteristic fluid levels in the lymph-filled sinuses. (b) A multilobular lymphangioma with extraconal and intraconal extension is shown in this axial T1 W image with fat suppression after administration of a contrast agent. (c) Preoperative embolization. The arterial blood supply is sustained by distal palpebral branches of the ophthalmic artery (*arrow*) along with orbital branches of the infraorbital artery and internal maxillary artery. (d) Superselective distal catheterization of the infraorbital artery and embolization with poly (vinyl alcohol) (*arrow*).

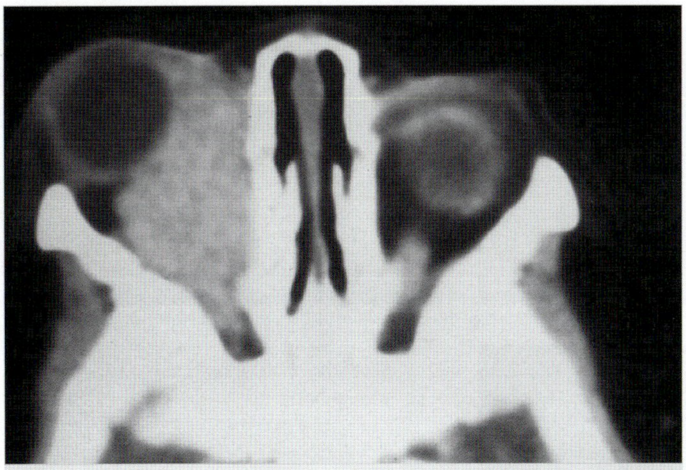

Fig. 4.36 Capillary hemangioma of the right orbit. Contrast-enhanced axial CT scan of a 13-month-old child shows a capillary hemangioma that extends into the intraconal and extraconal space and into the inferior orbital fissure. Considerable exophthalmos.

information. In these cases ultrasound is complementary to other imaging techniques applied.[25] Another indication for ultrasound is its application in patients in whom no exposure to ionizing radiation should occur (children; pregnant women). The purpose of this section is to demonstrate some typical ultrasound findings, particularly in some frequent diseases of the orbit and its adnexa.

4.7.1 Technical Conditions for Orbital Ultrasound

Ultrasound examinations of the orbit are preferably performed with the patient in a sitting or lying position, with small multifrequency ultrasound transducers of appropriate frequency in the 7 to 12 MHz band. For precise imaging the ultrasound transducer is covered with a gel and set up onto the closed eye. This transducer position is appropriate for investigating superficial anatomical structures, such as eyelids, lacrimal glands, and bony orbital rims.[26,27] The eyeball can be used as a water-filled adapter that improves contrast for examining the deeper parts of the orbit.[28] In that way it is possible to investigate the insertion zones of the extraocular muscles, the retrobulbar adipose tissue, and the eyeball layers, along with the anterior parts of the optic nerve.[29,30] However, the orbital apex and adjacent structures usually evade sonographic evaluation.

4.7.2 Ultrasound Anatomy

Sonographically the eye lids display as tiny bandlike hyperechoic structures. Small nodular lesions, e.g., tumors of the eyelids, can be detected. Ultrasound with very high-resolution transducers is–like ultrasonography of the skin–suitable for investigating the infiltration depth of malignant tumors, such as basal cell carcinomas of the eyelids, which might have consequences when contemplating the therapeutic procedures.[31] The cornea displays as a hypoechoic sickle-shaped structure in the dorsal part of the eyeball, which is commonly surrounded by a slightly more hyperechoic limbus, caused by an impedance gap between skin and cornea. The anterior eye chamber is located behind the cornea. The lens, the iris, and the ciliary body can be identified more dorsally (▶ Fig. 4.37a).

The normal vitreous body displays sonographically as an anechoic structure with dorsal enhancement. The sclera, choroidea, and retina can be visualized at its dorsal border. However, ultrasonography usually does not allow certain differentiation of these structures in nonpathogenic conditions.[30] Ultrasound transducers operating with very high frequency are more sensitive and offer better visualization of the eye bulb layers. Using these transducers and reducing the distal amplification (time compensated gain, TCG), the choroidea appears slightly more hypoechoic than the retina or sclera.[28] In cases of retinal detachment, however, the retina displays as a separated membrane, which is easily visible in the ultrasound image.[29]

The optic nerve papilla can usually be identified by a protrusion in the dorsal border of the eyeball. Moving the ultrasound transducer and variation of the sound direction provides the possibility to identify the optic nerve, which displays as a band-like hypo-echoic structure with a thickness of 4–5 mm dorsally of the eye bulb center[28] (▶ Fig. 4.37b). The optic nerve is surrounded by a dural sheath and cerebrospinal fluid, which causes an impedance gap and provides better contrast between the nerve and adjacent more hyperechoic adipose tissue. Measurement of the nerve's diameter in patients with demyelinating diseases provides important information about the severity and possible deterioration of the disease.[32,33] The extraocular eye muscles display as bandlike or spindle-shaped hypoechoic structures, which are surrounded by the hyperechoic adipose tissue and exhibit longitudinal striping, a characteristic sonographic sign for muscles. Ultrasound provides the best visualization of the insertion zones of the rectus muscles; the oblique muscles, however, cannot be differentiated due to their close relation to the adjacent rectus muscles.[28] The intraconal parts of the orbit are usually hard to investigate by ultrasonography; CT and MRI scans provide better visualization of the posterior orbital compartments.

Color-coded duplex sonography is suitable for measuring the blood circulation in the choroidea or central retinal and optic nerve vessels.[28] This technique is also sensitive for investigation a suspected cavernous sinus fistula.[34] Increased intracerebral pressure manifests in a swollen papilla (choked papilla), which is easily recognized.[35]

Sonographically the lacrimal glands are depicted as well-demarcated structures with homogeneous echogenicity in the lateral parts of the eyelids. Their axial extension is about 1 cm, and their echogenicity is quite similar to that of the thyroid gland or salivary glands (▶ Fig. 4.37c). Ultrasound has the highest sensitivity to recognize tumors or abscesses of the lacrimal glands, along with a subperiostal abscess condition in the area of medial canthus.[29]

The diagnostic evaluation of bony structures by ultrasound is challenging, since it is only sensitive for investigation of the bony orbital rims (▶ Fig. 4.37d, ▶ Fig. 4.37e). Fracture lines along with significant dislocations are visible. Nevertheless, estimation of the extension and severity of an orbital fracture is not possible by ultrasonography alone, and CT scans offer much better visualization of the entire orbit, midface and skull base (see Chapter 8).

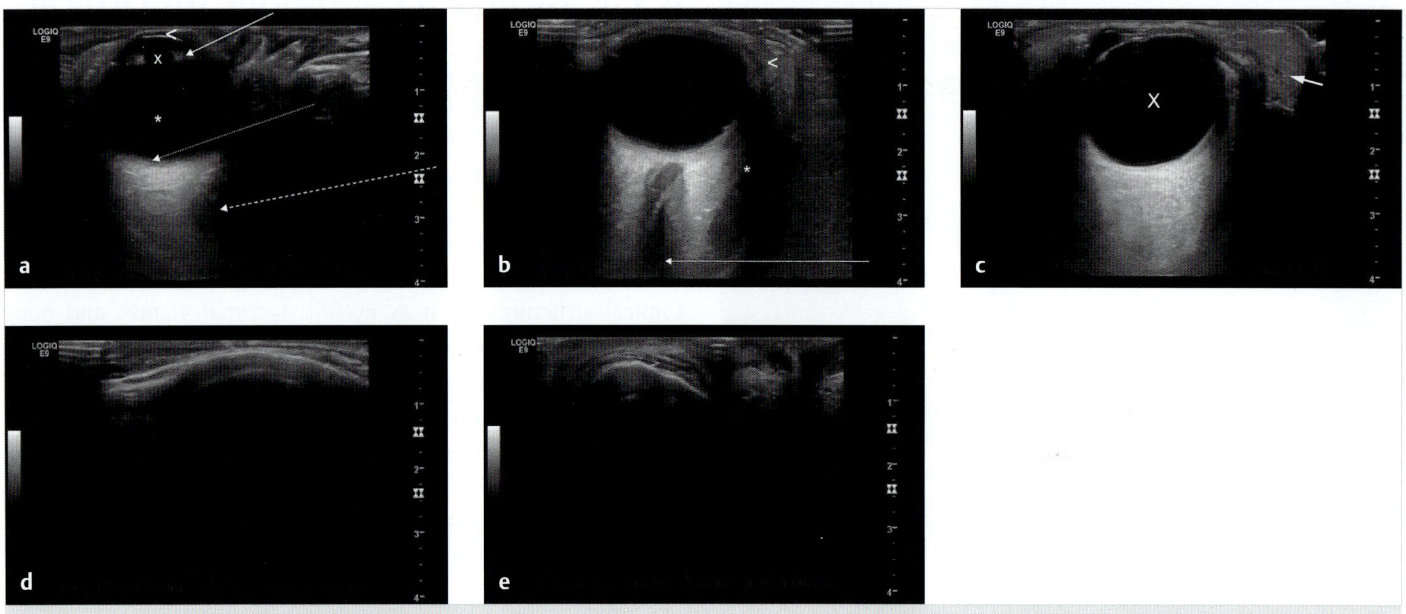

Fig. 4.37 Ultrasound examination of the orbit. **(a)** Normal ultrasound anatomy. The cornea (<), the lens (×), the iris (*arrow*), and the vitreous body (*) are clearly visible. The insertions of the extraocular muscles display as spindle-shaped hypoechoic structures (*dashed arrow*). The choroidea, retina and sclera cannot be differentiated in the dorsal parts of the eye bulb, due to their nearly similar echogenicity (*dotted arrow*). **(b)** Ultrasound of the eye bulb, axial section. The optic nerve (*arrow*), lateral rectus muscle (*), and the lacrimal gland (<) are clearly visible. **(c)** Axial section through the lacrimal gland (*arrow*). The gland parenchyma displays with homogenous echogenicity. ×, eyeball. **(d)** Ultrasound of the infraorbital bone rim. **(e)** Ultrasound of the lateral orbital bone rim with well-defined bony surfaces. However, the deeper parts of the bone cannot be assessed by ultrasonography.

4.7.3 Ultrasound Examination of Particular Orbital Diseases

Hereditary Malformations

Coloboma

Coloboma is regarded as a development-related schistasis of the eyeball. According to the severity, ectatic coloboma, with a bulging of the eyeball wall, or coloboma cysts can be differentiated. Sonography is highly sensitive in recognition of a coloboma, which is commonly accompanied by microphthalmus.[29,30]

Teratomas and Dermoids

Teratomas and dermoids are regarded as hereditary tumors and frequently occur clinically in the first years of life. Sonographically dermoids display as hypoechoic, sharply-bordered cystic masses with dorsal enhancement, located typically in the bony orbital rim.[29,30] Teratomas, on the other hand, contain hyperechoic as well as hypoechoic areas, with the hyperechoic structures commonly presenting with calcifications.[29,30]

Inflammatory Diseases

Acute inflammations and chronic inflammations can be differentiated within the inflammatory diseases of the orbit. The chronic category includes Grave's orbitopathy and idiopathic orbital inflammatory disease (orbital pseudotumor), the sonographic characteristics of which will be detailed in the next subsection, "Orbital Tumors."

Acute Inflammations

Either acute inflammatory diseases of the orbit originate directly in orbital structures themselves (dacryocystitis; lid phlegmon) or the orbit becomes secondarily involved by the spread of an acute inflammation of the paranasal sinuses (orbital complication). Sonography is sensitive and offers the possibility to differentiate between preseptal and postseptal extension of the disease.

Four stages can be differentiated in orbital complications (see Chapter 6): In stage I of the disease an inflammatory concomitant swelling of the upper and/or lower lid occurs. Sonographically the stage is characterized by a relaxation of the soft tissue of the eyelids. Due to the acute inflammatory process the tissue appears distinctly more hypoechoic. However, circumscribed hypoechoic or anechoic structures, indicating abscess formation, are not visible (▶ Fig. 4.38). Subperiostal abscess, which is regarded as stage II of the disease, displays as a circumscribed hypoechoic or anechoic structure with dorsal enhancement between the orbital lamina and the orbital soft tissue. The medial rectus muscle along with the eyeball are frequently laterally displaced.[29] Color-coded duplex sonography reveals only minor intralesional perfusion with areas of perfusion losses. Orbital phlegmon is characterized by a diffuse relaxation of the soft tissue in the entire orbit, as well preseptally and postseptally. The tissue appears partly hypoechoic and partly hyperechoic, but circumscribed abscess formations cannot usually be detected.

Acute inflammations of the eyelids can be caused by small injuries to the lid skin. The sonographic characteristics are similar to those of the inflammatory swelling concomitant with acute sinusitis. The findings are usually limited to the preseptal compartment. Abscess conditions are characterized by irregular structures with dorsal enhancement, which are located fairly superficially in most cases.

Acute dacryoadenitis is clinically characterized by swelling and reddening and paragraph-shape of the upper lid. The sonographic appearance is characteristic, with relaxation of the entire lacrimal gland tissue in the lateral lid and orbital area with some hypoechoic and some hyperechoic parts. The presence of some irregular structures might be an indication of microabscess formation.

Graves's Ophthalmopathy

Ultrasonography is can reveal the proliferation of adipose tissue occurring in the retrobulbar compartment and peribulbar in the area of the eyebrows.[36] The thickened extraocular muscles can also be identified (▶ Fig. 4.39). However, the retrobulbar area is hard to investigate by ultrasound alone and in such cases MRI is preferable. Ultrasound does not allow identification of the predominant pathology responsible for the exophthalmos with increase of intraorbital pressure, whether it is the proliferation of retrobulbar adipose tissue or thickening of extraocular muscles. However, ultrasound is suitable for monitoring of immunosuppressive therapy and for estimation of disease activity.[26,36]

Orbital Tumors

Benign Tumors and Pseudotumors

Idiopathic orbital inflammatory disease (orbital pseudotumor) is characterized by a hypoechoic mass that is poorly limited to the surrounding tissue and is adjacent to the extraocular muscles and cannot distinguished from them. Thus, differential diagnosis

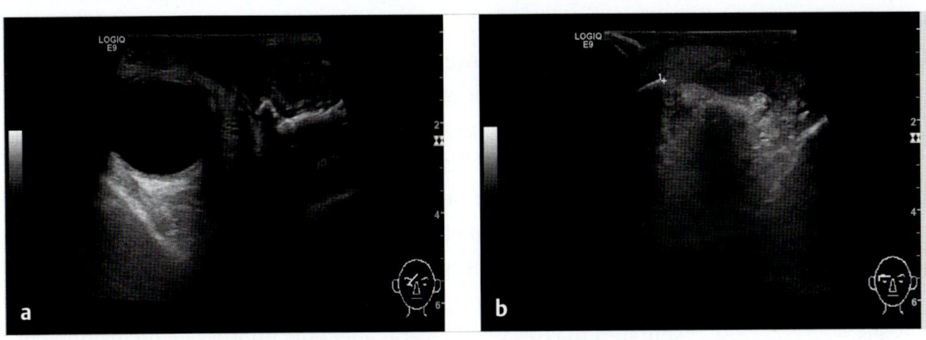

Fig. 4.38 Intraorbital complication due to an acute sinusitis. (a) Inflammatory upper lid swelling. The soft tissue shows as hypoechoic with no signs of abscess formation. (b) Acute dacryoadenitis of the lacrimal gland on the right side. The parenchyma shows as hypoechoic and loosened up.

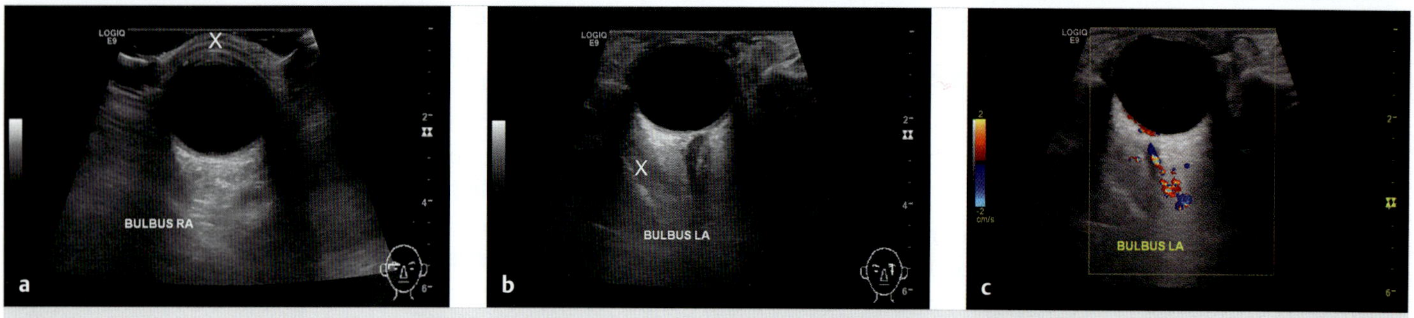

Fig. 4.39 Ultrasound of the left orbit affected by Graves's orbitopathy, axial section. **(a)** Thickening of the eye lids (×) along with a significant exophthalmos is visible. **(b)** The medial rectus muscle is thickened to a diameter of 2 cm (×). **(c)** Color-coded duplex sonography reveals a dilated arterial blood vessel, which perfuses the medial rectus muscle.

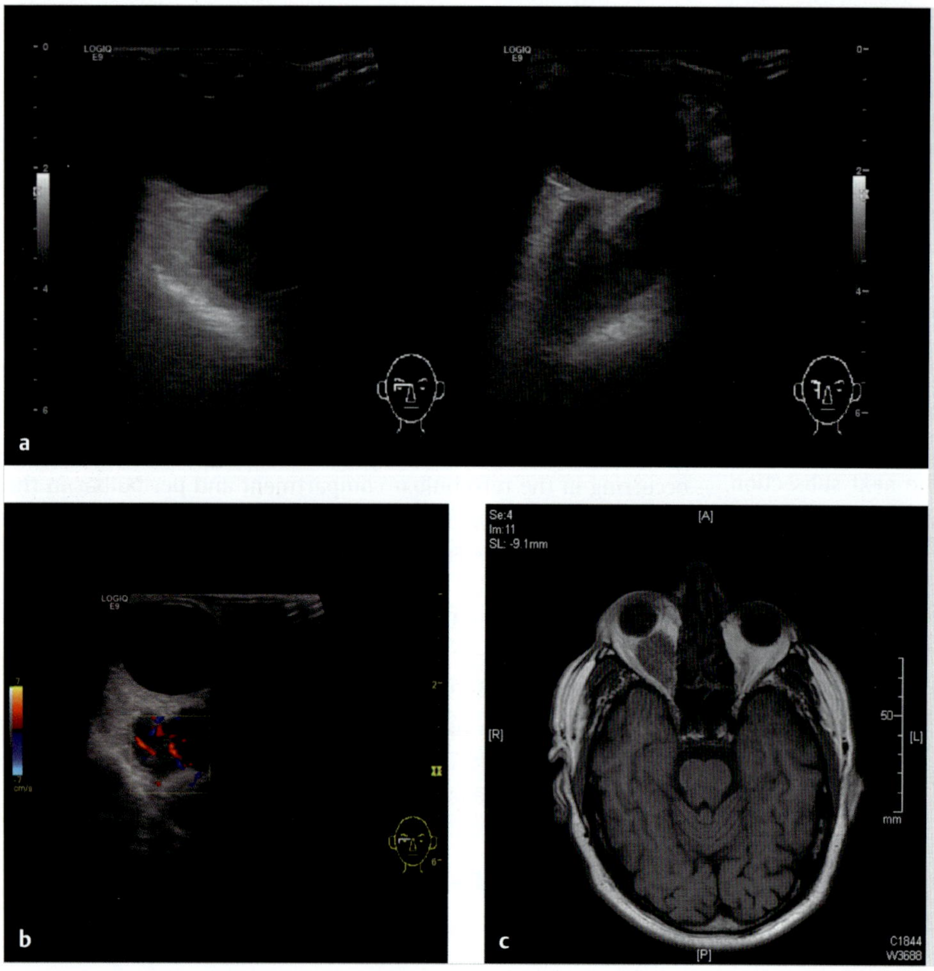

Fig. 4.40 Ultrasound examination of an orbital pseudotumor on the right eye. **(a)** Axial (left) and longitudinal (right) sections. The lesion displays as a hypoechoic, poorly demarcated retrobulbar located tumor. **(b)** Color-coded duplex sonography reveals numerous blood vessels and high perfusion of the lesion. **(c)** MRI of the same patient.

must exclude a muscle tumor. Some blood vessels are detectable by color-coded duplex sonography. However, no distinct perfusion pattern can be identified (▶ Fig. 4.40). The sonographic characteristics of this disease are essentially quite similar to those of a malignant lymphoma. Sonography can be used to obtain material for cytologic examinations by fine needle aspiration biopsy under direct view.[37]

Mucoceles infiltrating the orbit display as hypoechoic or anechoic masses with clear borders. In most cases there is an additional finely granular internal echo, which is due to protein molecules and cell debris in the mucocele content. Dehiscence of the bony walls, enabling the mucocele to grow into the orbit, can be detected in many cases (▶ Fig. 4.41). Color-coded duplex sonography does not reveal any intralesional vessels.

Cavernous hemangiomas are considered the most frequent benign orbital tumors; they have either retrobulbar or peribulbar location and can be identified by sonography. They usually display as hypoechoic masses with inhomogeneous echogenicity, and sometimes with worse demarcation toward the adjacent adipose tissue. Color-coded duplex sonography helps in identification of the afferent and draining blood vessels. The masses present with a dense and irregular blood vessel pattern that shows high blood flow velocity. Thrombosed hemangiomas have significantly worse perfusion. Sonography is suitable for interstitial laser therapy of hemangiomas, with the possibility of placing the laser transducer head into the lesion under direct visual control. The coagulation effect is visible real time.

Lymphangiomas represent hereditary lesions in most cases.[38] They appear sonographically as clearly separated, hypoechoic, septated masses with several anechoic impressive inclusions, corresponding to lymph cysts. Color-coded duplex sonography reveals perfusion patterns in the tumor capsule along with the

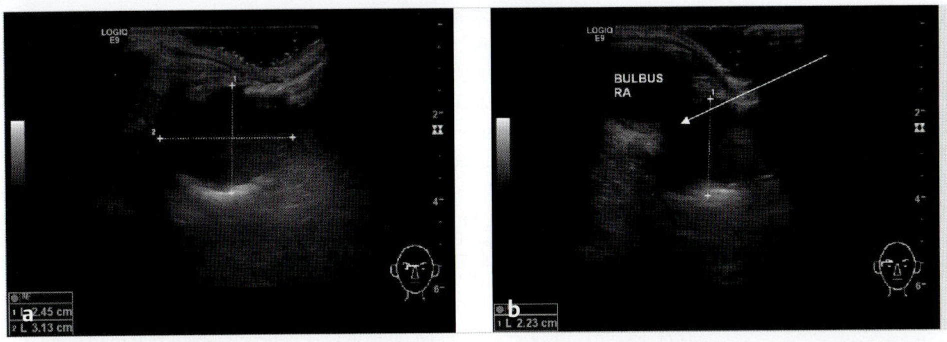

Fig. 4.41 Ultrasound examination of a mucocele of the right frontal sinus affecting the orbit. **(a)** Hypoechoic lesion with dorsal enhancement and lateral displacement of the eyeball. **(b)** A defect in the bony medial orbital wall is clearly visible (*arrow*).

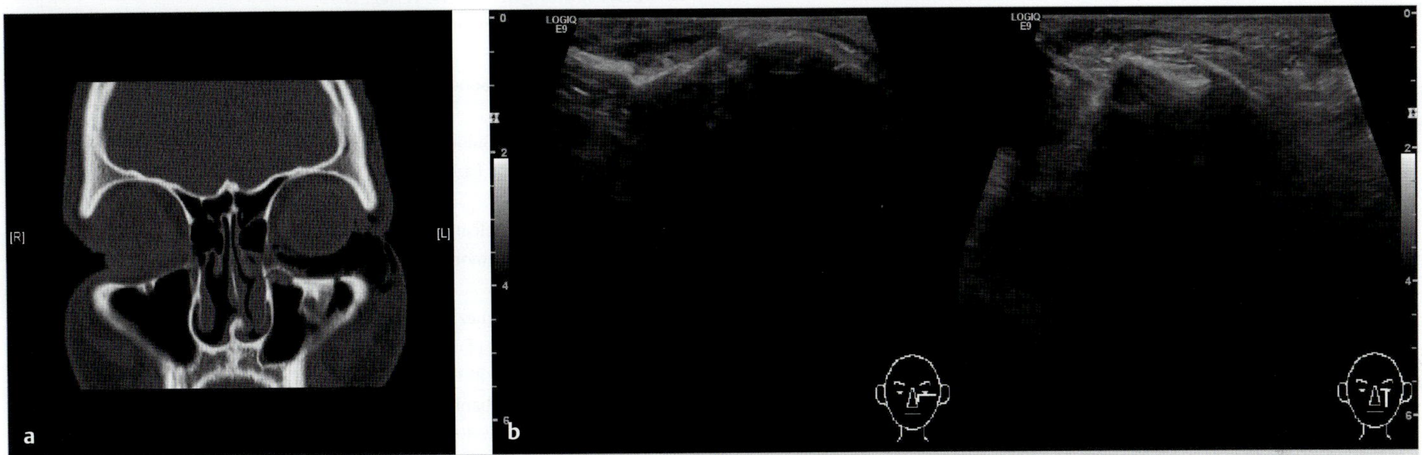

Fig. 4.42 Fracture of the bony infraorbital rim and zygoma bone fracture. The disruption of the bone with dislocation of bony fragments is clearly visible. **(a)** CT scan of a patient with zygoma bone fracture (coronal section). **(b)** Ultrasound examination of the same patient reveals disruption of the bone (left, axial section; right, longitudinal section).

septa. Intralesional bleeding can lead to fluid levels and sedimentation due to the blood constituents inside the lymph cysts.[29] Surgical excision is the therapy of choice. A minor invasive therapeutic procedure is sclerosing of the lesions, for which sclerosing agents are administered intralesionally under sonographic control.[38]

The most frequent benign tumors of the lacrimal glands are **pleomorphic adenomas**, which show sonographic conditions quite similar to those of pleomorphic adenoma of the salivary glands. The tumor displays as a hypoechoic, polycyclic limited intraglandularly located mass with clear borders and dorsal enhancement. Color-coded duplex sonography reveals only minor perfusion of these masses with detectable blood vessels in the tumor's capsule.

Malignant Tumors

Sonographically, **retinoblastoma** is characterized by a well-perfused hyperechoic mass that is directed toward the vitreous body. Calcifications occur frequently, which can be identified by intralesional hyperechoic irregular structures with dorsal sound mitigation or sound extinction.[39]

Rhabdomysarcomas originate in the extraocular muscles, impressing as hypoechoic masses that cannot be differentiated from the muscle. The tumor has a notably worse demarcation from the adjacent tissue and shows signs of infiltrative growth pattern. Color-coded duplex sonography reveals numerous blood vessels.[29]

Intraorbital metastases of malignant tumors of other provenance frequently originate in breast cancer, gastrointestinal cancer, kidney cancer, or thyroid cancer. Hence, they do not depict a uniform sonographic appearance. Hypoechoic or echo-complex masses with inhomogeneous echogenicity are common. A cytologic or histologic examination is required when metastasis is suspected.

Frequent malignant tumors of the **lacrimal glands** include adenocarcinoma, adenoid cystic carcinoma, and carcinoma ex pleomorphic adenoma. There are no specific sonographic characteristics but most of them display as hypoechoic lesions with unsharp borders, inhomogeneous echogenicity, and signs of infiltrative growth pattern.

Malignant lymphomas of the orbit appear sonographically as hypoechoic, roundish or oval masses in the lacrimal glands or peribulbar region with clear borders.[37] Color-coded duplex sonography reveals diffuse perfusion in most cases. Sonography is also suited for monitoring during chemotherapy or radiation therapy.[31,40,41]

Fractures

Sonography is appropriate for investigation of the soft tissue, eyelids, or peribulbar compartments in orbital injuries. However, only the superficially located bony walls—i.e., lateral and medial orbital walls, infra-orbital rim, and supra-orbital rim—can properly be evaluated; the extent and depth of the injury cannot be evaluated sonographically. Here, CT scan is more sensitive and a superior modality. Fractures display sonographically as a discontinuity of the affected bones and frequently a "stair," so that the degree of dislocation can be evaluated (▶ Fig. 4.42). In blow-out fractures adipose tissue and inferior rectus muscle prolapsed into the maxillary sinus can be visualized. A valuable indication for ultrasound is in patients for whom no exposure to ionizing radiation should occur (children; pregnant women). However, in cases of deep and extensive bony fractures, in patients with impaired eyeball motility or vision loss, a CT scan is mandatory.

Ultrasound can provide very valuable information for localizing intraorbital or intrabulbar foreign bodies.[42,43]

References

[1] Bücheler E, Lackner K-J, Thelen M. Einführung in die Radiologie. Diagnostik und Interventionen. 11th ed. Stuttgart: Thieme; 2005

[2] International Medical College. Wiki. Orbitafrakturen: Klassifikation und Diagnostik. http://www.med-college.de/de/wiki/artikel.php?id=381. Accessed November 1, 2016

[3] Reiser M, Kuhn F-P, Debus J. Radiologie. 3rd ed. Stuttgart: Thieme; 2011

[4] Hassler W, Unsöld R, Schick U. Raumforderungen der Orbita. Diagnostik und operative Behandlung. Dtsch Arztebl. 2007; 104(8):497,499, 500

[5] Jakobiec FA, Jones IS. Orbital Inflammations. In: Jones IS, Jakobiec FA, eds. Diseases of the Orbit. Hagerstown, MD: Harper and Row; 1979

[6] Som PM, Curtin HD. Head and Neck Imaging. 4th ed. St. Louis, MO: Mosby; 2003:578

[7] Rootman J, Ed. Diseases of the Orbit. Philadephia, PA: JP Lippincott; 1988

[8] Blodi FC, Gas JD. Inflammatory pseudotumour of the orbit. Br J Ophthalmol. 1968; 52(2):79–93

[9] Flanders AE, Mafee MF, Rao VM, Choi KH. CT characteristics of orbital pseudotumors and other orbital inflammatory processes. J Comput Assist Tomogr. 1989; 13(1):40–47

[10] Birch-Hirschfeld A. Zur Diagnostik und Pathologie der orbitalen Tumoren. Dtsch Ophthalmol Ges. 1905; 32:127–135

[11] Mombaerts I, Goldschmeding R, Schlingemann RO, Koornneef L. What is orbital pseudotumor? Surv Ophthalmol. 1996a; 41(1):66–78

[12] Mafee MF, Goodwin J, Dorodi S. Optic nerve sheath meningiomas. Role of MR imaging. Radiol Clin North Am. 1999; 37(1):37–58, ix

[13] Spagnolo F, Caltabiano G, Queirolo P. Uveal melanoma. Cancer Treat Rev. 2012; 38(5):549–553

[14] Mafee MF. Uveal melanoma, choroidal hemangioma, and simulating lesions. Role of MR imaging. Radiol Clin North Am. 1998; 36(6):1083–1099, x

[15] Avery RA, Fisher MJ, Liu GT. Optic pathway gliomas. J Neuroophthalmol. 2011; 31(3):269–278

[16] Yousem DM, Zimmermann RD, Grossmann RI. Neuroradiology: The Requisites. Philadelphia, PA: Mosby; 2010

[17] Demirci H, Shields CL, Karatza EC, Shields JA. Orbital lymphoproliferative tumors: analysis of clinical features and systemic involvement in 160 cases. Ophthalmology. 2008; 115(9):1626–1631, 1631.e1–1631.e3

[18] Henderson JW, Farrow GM. Orbital tumors. 2nd ed. New York, NY: Brian C. Decker; 1980

[19] Harris GJ, Jakobiec FA. Cavernous hemangioma of the orbit. J Neurosurg. 1979; 51(2):219–228

[20] Porterfield JF, Zimmermann LE. Rhabdomyosarcoma of the orbit; a clinicopathologic study of 55 cases. Virchows Arch Pathol Anat Physiol Klin Med Anat. 1962; 335:329–344

[21] Hintschich C, Stefani FH. Tumoren der Lider und der Orbita. In: Wollenberg B, Zimmermann F, eds. Manual Kopf-Hals-Karzinome. München: W. Zuckschwerdt; 2003:256

[22] Castellucci P, Zinzani P, Pourdehnad M, et al. 18F-FDG PET in malignant lymphoma: significance of positive findings. Eur J Nucl Med Mol Imaging. 2005; 32(7):749–756

[23] O'Doherty MJ, Macdonald EA, Barrington SF, Mikhaeel NG, Schey S. Positron emission tomography in the management of lymphomas. Clin Oncol (R Coll Radiol). 2002; 14(5):415–426

[24] Miyamoto J, Tatsuzawa K, Owada K, Kawabe T, Sasajima H, Mineura K. Usefulness and limitations of fluorine-18-fluorodeoxyglucose positron emission tomography for the detection of malignancy of orbital tumors. Neurol Med Chir (Tokyo). 2008; 48(11):495–499, discussion 499

[25] Hande PC, Talwar I. Multimodality imaging of the orbit. Indian J Radiol Imaging. 2012; 22(3):227–239

[26] Rose GE, Verity DH. Neuro-ophthalmology of orbital disease. Handb Clin Neurol. 2011; 102:467–491

[27] Jecker P. Ultraschalluntersuchung der Nasennebenhöhlen und der Orbita. In: Welkoborsky HJ, Jecker P, Maurer J, Mann WJ, eds. Ultraschall im Kopf-Hals-Bereich. Stuttgart: Thieme Verlag; 2013

[28] Dudea SM. Ultrasonography of the eye and orbit. Med Ultrason. 2011; 13(2): 171–174

[29] Gaßner I, Mair M. Sonographie von Bulbus oculi und Orbita. Kind & Radiologie. 2006; 3:34–39

[30] Gaßner I, Mair M. Bulbus oculi und Orbita. In: Hofmann V, Deeg KH, Hoyer PF, eds. Ultraschall in Pädiatrie und Kinderchirurgie. Stuttgart: Thieme Verlag; 2005: 191ff

[31] Ciocâlteu AM, Ardeleanu S, Checheriță IA. [The role of ultrasonography exam in orbital-ocular tumors]. Rev Med Chir Soc Med Nat Iasi. 2011; 115(4):1113–1118

[32] Fernández-Domínguez J, García-Rodríguez R, Mateos V. [Transorbital echography for assessment of optical nerve atrophy in demyelinating diseases: a pilot study]. Rev Neurol. 2012; 54(10):587–592

[33] Karami M, Janghorbani M, Dehghani A, Riahinejad M. Orbital Doppler evaluation of blood flow velocities in optic neuritis. Korean J Ophthalmol. 2012; 26 (2):116–122

[34] Shokoohi H, Taheri MR, Boniface KS, Abdulmohsen A, Janet L. Orbital ultrasound in the selective screening of a dural-cavernous sinus fistula. Eur J Emerg Med. 2013; 20(2):137–139

[35] Foster T, Tayal VS, Saunders T, Norton J. Emergency ultrasound optic nerve sheath measurement to detect increased intracranial pressure in head injury patients: preliminary study of interobserver variability in normal human subjects. Acad Emerg Med. 2003; 10:487–488 (Abstract)

[36] Chang SH, Papageorgiou KI, Ang M, King AJ, Goldberg RA. High-resolution ultrasound as an effective and practical tool to analyze eyebrow profile expansion in thyroid-associated periorbitopathy. Ophthal Plast Reconstr Surg. 2013; 29(5):382–385

[37] Orlandi D, Sconfienza LM, Lacelli F, et al. Ultrasound-guided core-needle biopsy of extra-ocular orbital lesions. Eur Radiol. 2013; 23(7):1919–1924

[38] Aslan A, Büyükkaya R, Tan S, Erdoğan C, Hakyemez B. Efficacy of ultrasonography in lymphatic malformations: diagnosis, treatment and follow-up: a case report. Med Ultrason. 2013; 15(3):244–246

[39] Chawla B, Hada M, Kashyap S, Bakhshi S. Orbital retinoblastoma in an adult. Orbit. 2013; 32(2):146–148

[40] Alkatan HM, Alaraj A, El-Khani A, Al-Sheikh O. Ocular adnexal lymphoproliferative disorders in an ophthalmic referral center in Saudi Arabia. Saudi J Ophthalmol. 2013; 27(3):227–230

[41] Rasmussen PK, Coupland SE, Finger PT, et al. Ocular adnexal follicular lymphoma: a multicenter international study. JAMA Ophthalmol. 2014; 132(7): 851–858

[42] Srirangam R, Gokhale SK, Kulkarni AU, Gadre KS. Unusual intraorbital foreign body. BMJ Case Rep. 2012; 2012

[43] Patel SN, Langer PD, Zarbin MA, Bhagat N. Diagnostic value of clinical examination and radiographic imaging in identification of intraocular foreign bodies in open globe injury. Eur J Ophthalmol. 2012; 22(2):259–268

Chapter 5

Diseases of the Eyelids and the Eye

5

5 Diseases of the Eyelids and the Eye

This chapter provides a brief overview of diseases of the eye and ocular adnexa that may involve or be part of orbital diseases or represent important differential diagnoses. Refer to standard textbooks for further detail.

5.1 Diseases of the Eyelids

B. Wiechens and M. A. Varde

5.1.1 Inflammatory Diseases

Hordeolum/Chalazion

A hordeolum is an acute bacterial infection of the sebaceous glands of the eyelid. If the sebaceous glands adjoining the ciliary follicles are infected, it is termed Hordeolum externum, which differentiates itself from Hordeolum internum, where the meibomian glands are infected. Clinically, acute onset, erythematous, painful swelling of the lid margin can be seen. Local application of antibiotics and warm compresses is the treatment of choice.

A chalazion represents a chronic noninfectious inflammation, mainly of the meibomian glands (▶ Fig. 5.1). It is often associated with meibomian gland dysfunction or blepharitis. A well-circumscribed indolent swelling of the tarsal plate can be seen, sometimes associated with a granuloma on the tarsal conjunctiva. Treatment involves local application of warmth and lid hygiene measures to address the underlying blockage of the meibomian gland orifices, along with topical application of steroids and antibiotics. Incision and curettage is required where conservative treatment is unsuccessful. A routine histologic examination of the specimens obtained is recommended to exclude sebaceous gland carcinoma, which may masquerade as a chalazion. Histology of a chalazion shows a typical granulomatous picture with abundant giant cells.

Lid Abscess

Abscesses in the periocular region can occur as in any other region of the body. The underlying cause is often a folliculitis involving the eyelids or eyebrow cilia. Clinically localized pain, redness, and swelling of the involved lid are seen. Incision and drainage of the abscess may often be needed as conservative treatment alone may not suffice. Daily wound toilette, local and systemic antibiotic administration similar to abscess treatment in general are recommended.

Preseptal Cellulitis

Preseptal cellulitis is an infection of the eyelids superficial to the orbital septum. It can be caused by local skin infections, but also by sinusitis or septic dental foci. Clinical signs are lid swelling and redness as well as mechanical ptosis. However, ocular motility is not affected, neither will there be signs of compressive optic neuropathy (e.g., afferent pupillary defect, vision loss) or exophthalmos. Treatment is targeted to the underlying disease as well as administration of antibiotics. Oral antibiotics would suffice in most cases, but in severe cases, especially in children, intravenous administration of antibiotics is required. A preseptal cellulitis can breach the septum and progress to orbital cellulitis (see Chapter 6).

5.1.2 Malignant Tumors of the Eyelids

Basal Cell Carcinoma

Basal cell carcinoma (BCC) is a malignant tumor arising from the basal cells of the epidermis. These tumors are the most common malignant tumors in humans and predominantly occur in aged, light-skinned individuals. The underlying cause is mainly DNA damage due to ultraviolet radiation. Thus, BCCs frequently occur in sun-exposed areas, particularly the face and can appear multilocularly, often involving the eyelids (▶ Fig. 5.2). BCCs account for

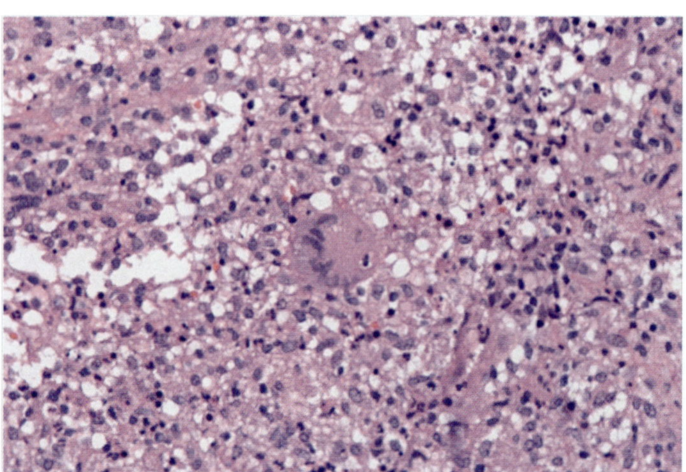

Fig. 5.1 Chalazion (hematoxylin & eosin staining). The lesion shows a significant lymphocytic infiltration and characteristic giant cells (center).

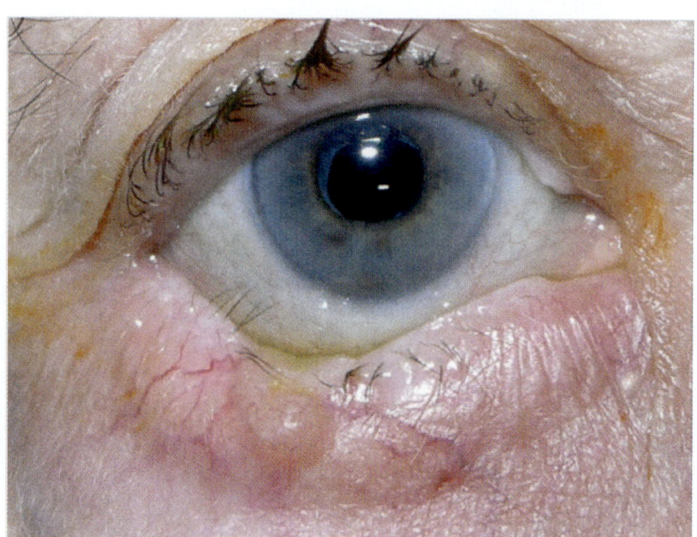

Fig. 5.2 Basal cell carcinoma of the lower lid. Nodular-configured lesion with irregular-shaped telangiectatic borders and loss of eyelashes.

nearly 90% of all malignant eyelid tumors amongst Caucasians, whereas they are rarely found amongst Asians and Africans. BCCs can also affect younger individuals, especially immunocompromised patients, patients with xeroderma pigmentosum or Gorlin–Goltz-syndrome.[1]

The tumors usually display an infiltrative growth pattern with a high recurrence rate in cases of incomplete tumor excision, though metastases occur rarely and late.

Common localizations for basal cell carcinoma are the lower lid as well as the medial and lateral canthus. Involvement of the medial canthus carries a poor prognosis, since orbital infiltration from here is more likely.

Clinically and histologically BCC can be divided into several subgroups, such as nodular (solid), pigmented, and sclerodermiform tumors. Sclerodermiform tumors show an occult growth pattern and often a lack of ulceration. Since the diagnosis is often delayed, there is a higher prevalence for deep infiltration of orbital structures. Accordingly, prognosis is worse in these cases.

Complete micrographically controlled surgical excision followed by reconstruction of the area is the treatment of choice. In rare cases, orbital exenteration may be required to achieve margin clearance, especially in cases with orbital infiltration. Local radiotherapy can be considered in patients with nonresectable tumors or as adjuvant therapy. Metastasizing BCCs have a very limited prognosis. Since 2013, the Hedgehog-signal pathway inhibitor vismodegib (Erivedge, Roche) is available for treatment of locally advanced tumors not amenable to surgery or radiotherapy and of metastasized BCC.

Squamous Cell Carcinoma

Squamous cell carcinomas (SCCs) arise from the skin or conjunctiva either de novo or from a precancerous lesion. About 10% of malignant eyelid tumors are SCCs. They also occur most commonly in elderly, light-skinned individuals; similarly to BCC, ultraviolet radiation exposure may be a risk factor for SCC. Other risk factors include mechanical and chemical irritants as well as infection with human papilloma virus (conjunctival SCC)[1] (▶ Fig. 5.3).

SCC usually demonstrates infiltrative growth and a tendency for lymphogenous and hematogenous metastasis.

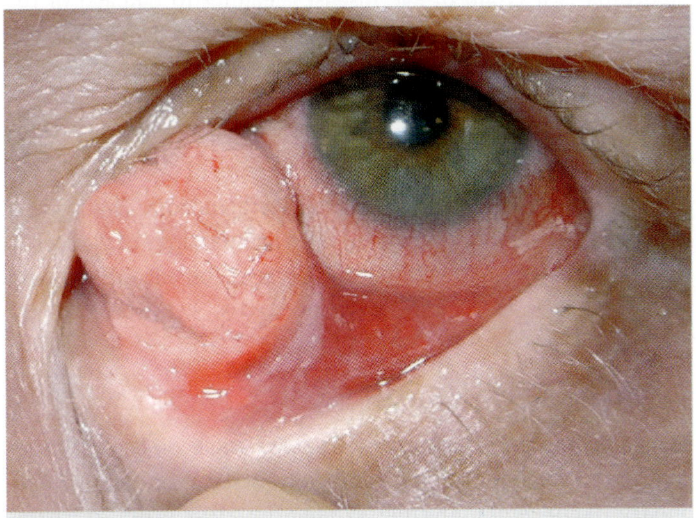

Fig. 5.3 Squamous cell carcinoma of the conjunctiva of the inferior fornix. The tumor's surface is partially keratinized with papillomatous blood vessels.

Treatment of choice is complete excision with histologically clear margins. In some cases of SCC, adjuvant or primary radiotherapy might be indicated. Conjunctival SCC often requires adjuvant chemotherapy with mitomycin C, interferon alfa, or 5-fluorouracil. When regional lymph node metastases occur, an additional neck dissection is indicated.

The prognosis of this tumor depends on the tumor stage, with a 5-year mortality of 0 to 40%.[2]

Sebaceous Gland Carcinoma

Sebaceous gland carcinomas (SGCs) arise from the epithelial cells of the meibomian, Zeiss, or other sebaceous glands located in the tarsus, caruncle, cilia, and eyebrows. Chalazion and unilateral chronic blepharitis should be considered important ophthalmologic differential diagnoses. SGC is mainly seen in middle-aged or elderly patients. While this tumor is very common in Asia, it only rarely occurs in whites. In contrast to BCC and SCC, sebaceous gland carcinoma is frequently localized in the upper lid (▶ Fig. 5.4).

Histologically, SGCs are characterized by a pagetoid growth pattern, with diffuse intraepithelial spread which is clinically not readily apparent. Thus, map biopsies are mandatory in excising SGCs.

SGCs can show lymphogenous as well as hematogenous metastasis. The local recurrence is approximately 30%[1] and depends on the clearance as well as adjuvant therapy. The prognosis depends largely on tumor stage, underlining the importance of an early diagnosis. Since SGC can mimic inflammatory diseases of the eyelids and ocular surface, the diagnosis is frequently delayed. This is one of the main reasons for a relatively high mortality of 5 to 40%.[2,3]

Recommended therapeutic options include complete surgical excision with histologically clear margins, sometimes needing orbital exenteration. Adjuvant cryotherapy or chemotherapy may also be indicated.

Malignant Melanoma of the Eyelids

Malignant melanoma of the eyelids may be cutaneous, conjunctival, or combined. The main risk factor for the development of malignant melanoma of the eyelid skin is UV light exposure, which does not seem to be of such impact in malignant melanoma of the conjunctiva. Melanomas of the eyelids can appear as

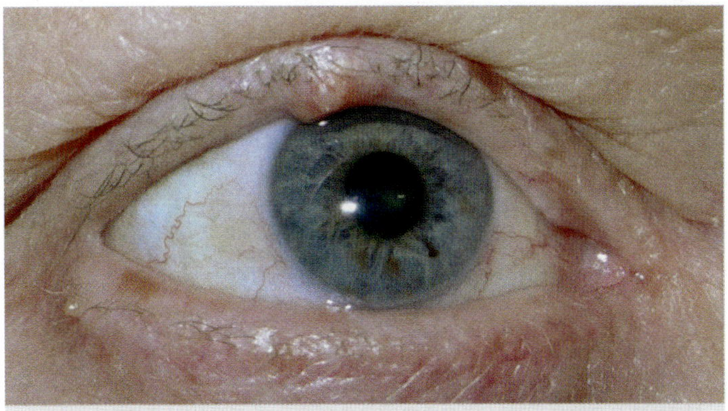

Fig. 5.4 Small carcinoma of the sebaceous glands in the upper lid, in this case a tumor recurrence following R0 resection of the same tumor 2 years before. Incorporation of lipids into the tumor leads to a yellowish color of the lesion.

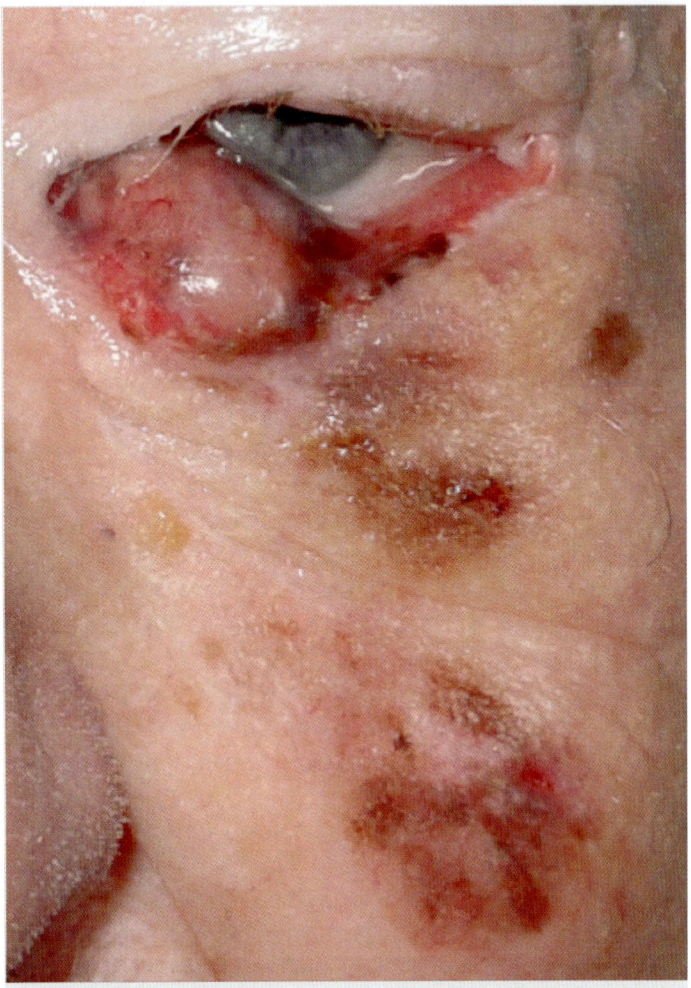

Fig. 5.5 Lentigo maligna melanoma with some amelanotic parts in the conjunctiva.

lentigo maligna melanoma (▶ Fig. 5.5), superficial spreading melanoma, or nodular melanoma. They can develop de novo or from precancerous lesions. The prognosis is worse when the tumor has infiltrated the lid margin and the conjunctiva. As well as advanced tumor stage, another negative prognostic factor is infiltration of the palpebral conjunctiva and caruncle.

Sentinel node biopsy (SNLB)[4] is required for accurate staging of cutaneous malignant melanoma of the eyelids; the diagnostic accuracy of this method in conjunctival melanoma is currently unclear.

Depending on tumor stage, mortality can be as high as 25%.[1] To improve the prognosis, early diagnosis and complete tumor excision is recommended.

Adjuvant treatment procedures, i.e. radiotherapy, brachytherapy, or local application of chemotherapeutics, are appropriate, particularly in conjunctival melanomas and their precancerous lesions. The latest agents for adjuvant systemic therapy are targeting specific genetic mutations in melanoma cells (e.g., vemurafenib) or have an immunomodulatory effect (e.g., ipilimumab). The prognosis in metastasizing melanomas is guarded.

Cutaneous Neuroendocrine Carcinoma (Merkel Cell Carcinoma)

Merkel cell carcinoma (MCC) originates from Merkel cells that represent stem cells of the epidermis associated with tactile sensitivity (▶ Fig. 5.6). It is a rare form of tumor, but often involves the eyelids (10% of all cases)[5,6] and commonly affects elderly light-skinned individuals. Virus infection with the so-called Merkel cell polyomavirus is discussed as an important etiology, comparable to squamous cell carcinoma due to HPV-infection.

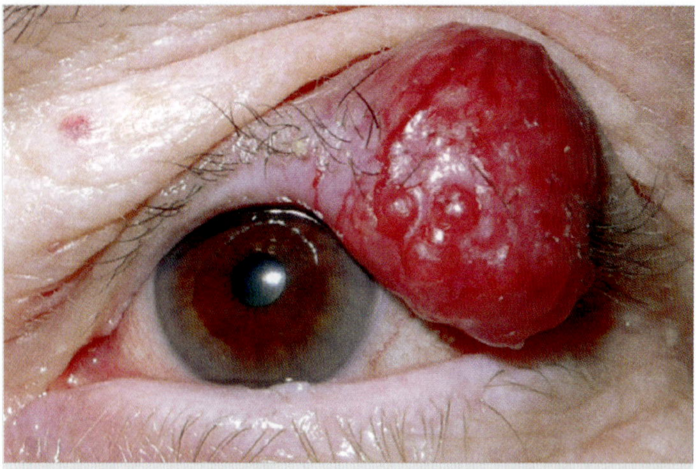

Fig. 5.6 Merkel cell carcinoma in the lateral upper lid on the left eye. The lesion shows significant vascularization along with a shiny surface.

Merkel cell carcinomas grow rapidly, with a tendency for local tumor recurrences as well as lymph node and distant metastasis. In a recently published study, a 5-year survival rate of 50% was found.[7] The prognosis depends significantly on the tumor stage.

Treatment of choice is a complete tumor excision with histologically clear margins, and combination with adjuvant radiotherapy. Other therapeutic strategies comprise immunomodulation with interferon alfa or tumor necrosis factor α.[8,9]

5.2 Diseases of the Eye

B. Wiechens

5.2.1 Glaucoma

Glaucoma is a group of eye diseases leading to damage of the optic nerve that results in irreversible visual field defects and can lead to blindness. The etiology is multifactorial. The main mechanisms involved are a reduction in optic nerve perfusion and increased intraocular pressure.

Orbital diseases may lead to a deterioration of underlying glaucoma or to a development of secondary glaucoma. This section will give only a brief overview on the systematology of glaucoma. For in-depth information about the disease, consult the standard text books.

Clinical Classification

Glaucoma can be differentiated as open-angle or angle-closure glaucoma. Depending on the pathogenesis, it can be primary, secondary, or congenital/juvenile. While primary glaucoma develops without any underlying ocular pathology, secondary glaucoma is usually related to an ocular condition or to a side effect of systemic medication.

Primary Glaucoma

Primary Open-angle Glaucoma (POAG)

Epidemiology

POAG represents nearly 90% of glaucoma in adults. The incidence of the disease increases significantly after the age of 40 years, reaching a peak between 60 and 70 years. Some studies suggest a genetic predisposition as POAG is frequently seen to accumulate in families.

Etiology and Pathogenesis

One of the main causes for the disease is an increased outflow resistance for the aqueous humor in the trabecular meshwork, the reason for which is yet unknown. The resulting increase of intraocular pressure leads to damage of the retinal ganglion cells and consequently of the optic nerve.

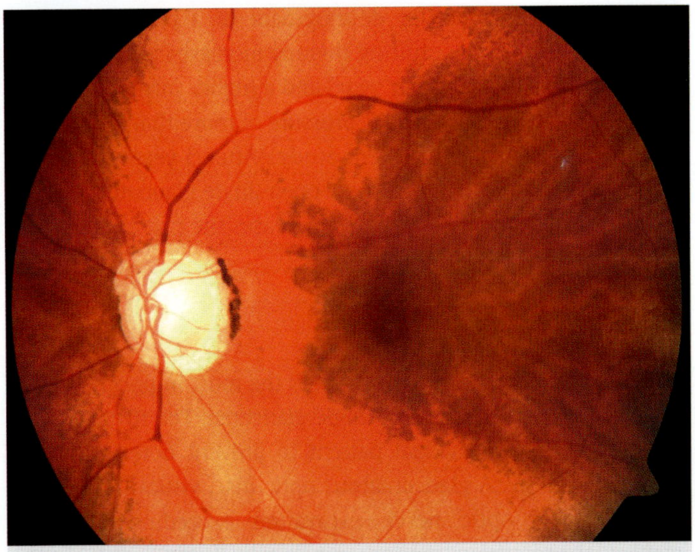

Fig. 5.7 Cupping of the optic disc.

Clinical Symptoms

POAG does not cause any symptoms until it is well advanced. General complaints of patients, such as burning sensation, feeling of pressure behind the eye, redness, or temporary blurred vision are not usually associated with chronic open-angle glaucoma. The damage to the optic nerve causes slow progressive visual field loss, which can become significant before patients go to see an ophthalmologist.

Gonioscopy reveals the iridocorneal angle to be open and without any pathologic findings. Depending on the stage of the disease, the optic nerve shows more or less pronounced cupping on ophthalmoscopy (▶ Fig. 5.7). It is important to detect asymmetry. In some cases viewing the fundus in red-free light will detect focal defects of the nerve fiber layer. Splinter-shaped hemorrhages at the optic disc margin can be indicative of glaucoma progression.

Diagnosis and Differential Diagnosis

For the diagnosis of glaucoma, measurement of the intraocular pressure (IOP), gonioscopy, ophthalmoscopy, perimetry (▶ Fig. 5.8), and results of a diurnal variation profile are important issues. Nowadays, photographs of the optic disc and tomography of the optic nerve and nerve fiber layer (i.e., optical coherence tomography, OCT/Heidelberg retinal tomography) are employed for clinical follow-up.

However, increased IOP is not always seen in glaucoma. Hence it is necessary to distinguish two other entities closely linked to glaucoma when contemplating differential diagnosis: normal-tension glaucoma and ocular hypertension.

Normal-tension Glaucoma

In this disease the typical findings for glaucoma— progressive optic nerve neuropathy and glaucomatous visual field defects— are present but the intraocular pressure is normal. These patients commonly are found to have low blood pressure (especially during the night) and vasospasms of peripheral blood vessels of the hands and feet. Hence, in addition to ophthalmologic diagnosis, systemic investigations to exclude rheologic risk factors and 24-hour blood pressure profile measurements are recommended.

Ocular Hypertension

In patients with this disease, increased intraocular pressure can be present for years without any pathologic findings of the optic disc or of the visual field. For this reason, periodic ophthalmologic examinations are recommended in patients with ocular

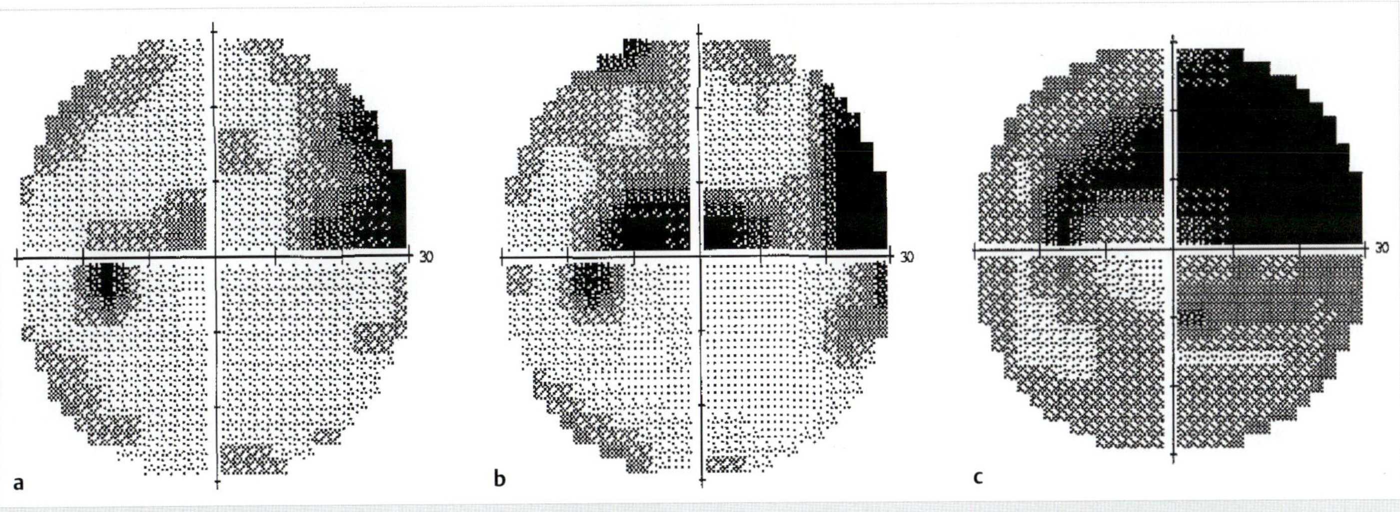

Fig. 5.8 **(a–c)** Perimetry showing a typical increase of a glaucomatous visual field defect over time (follow-up 2 years).

hypertension. The risk for development of a primary chronic open-angle glaucoma requiring therapy increases with lower age of the patient (about 2% per year) and a higher intraocular pressure (7% in cases of intraocular pressure of more than 26 mm Hg) (Ocular Hypertension Treatment Study). After 5 years the cumulative conversion rate into chronic open-angle glaucoma is about 9.5%.[10] Positive family history also increases the risk for glaucoma development.

Treatment

Decrease of the intraocular pressure is the most important aim of any therapy in primary open-angle glaucoma. The IOP has to be adjusted for any individual patient to prevent deterioration of optic neuropathy. A glaucomatous optic disc, visual field defect, asymmetry of optic nerve excavation exceeding 20%, and intraocular pressure of more than normal values (21 mm Hg) are considered indicators for the initiation of treatment. Basically an intraocular pressure of 30% below the initial values should be achieved, with pressures being within the normal range (10–21 mm Hg).

Decrease of intraocular pressure by medical treatment can be achieved through inhibition of aqueous humor production or enhancement of trabecular or uveoscleral drainage. Several drugs are available: parasympathomimetics, sympathomimetics, sympatholytics, prostaglandin analogues, carbonic anhydrase inhibitors, and—for acute cases—also osmotic agents such as mannitol 20% or Glycerosteril 10% (Fresenius). Treatment should be initiated with only one drug (e.g., beta blockers, if no contraindications) or prostaglandin analogues. When sufficient control of intraocular pressure is not achieved, a change of the substance class is indicated. If needed, combination therapy can be used. If progression of the glaucoma occurs despite reduction in IOP, the target IOP has to be further reduced (below 15 mm Hg or even below 12 mm Hg).

Surgical treatment is indicated if the intraocular pressure cannot be reduced to target levels despite multidrug treatment or if the patient cannot tolerate drug treatment due to allergic reaction or other side effects. The following surgical procedures are available:

- Laser-assisted trabeculoplasty.
- Trabeculectomy (filtration surgery).
- Deep sclerectomy.
- Canaloplasty.
- Cyclocryocoagulation/cyclophotocoagulation.
- Glaucoma drainage implants and shunts.

For further details, refer to textbooks of surgical procedures in ophthalmology.

Primary Angle-closure Glaucoma

Primary angle-closure glaucoma is less common than open-angle glaucoma, with a frequency of only about 5% of all glaucoma cases.[11]

Etiology and Pathogenesis

Angle-closure glaucoma is caused by a shallow anterior chamber with a narrow iridocorneal angle. Hyperopia, thickened lens (in cases with progressive cataract), and previous trauma with anterior displacement of the lens are risk factors. These mechanisms lead to an impairment of drainage of intraocular fluid from the anterior chamber. In addition, accumulation of aqueous humor in the posterior chamber can increase the anterior vaulting of the iris, causing additional angle-closure. As a result, there is an acute or intermittent increase of intraocular pressure (acute angle-closure glaucoma). In cases with anatomical disposition, acute angle-closure glaucoma can be triggered by pupillary dilatation leading to blockage of the iridocorneal angle with excessive increase of intraocular pressure.

Clinical Symptoms

The severity of clinical symptoms depends on the rate and level of rise in IOP. In severe cases, patients present with sudden redness and intense pain of the affected eye with radiation to the periorbital region. There can be additional symptoms such as upper abdominal pain with nausea and vomiting, headache, thoracic pain, and general feeling of illness. Acute visual loss might be masked by these general symptoms and lead to delayed diagnosis and treatment.

Ophthalmologic findings of acute glaucoma, which usually occurs unilaterally, are mixed conjunctival and ciliary injection, corneal edema, unreactive mid-dilated pupil (pressure-related damage of the sphincter pupillae muscle), and high intraocular pressure (palpation often showing a "rock-hard" globe) (▶ Fig. 5.9). Funduscopy is usually difficult due to corneal opacity.

Patients with chronic or intermittent angle-closure glaucoma commonly report transient blurred vision and perception of colored halos around light sources, which are due to the prismatic effect of the corneal epithelial edema.

Examination with a slit lamp reveals a shallow anterior chamber. In the acute setting gonioscopy is usually not possible because of the significant corneal epithelial edema. In cases of previous angle-closure, spot-shaped opacities in the anterior aspect of the lens might be seen.

Diagnosis

Diagnosis of angle-closure glaucoma is similar to that of open-angle glaucoma.

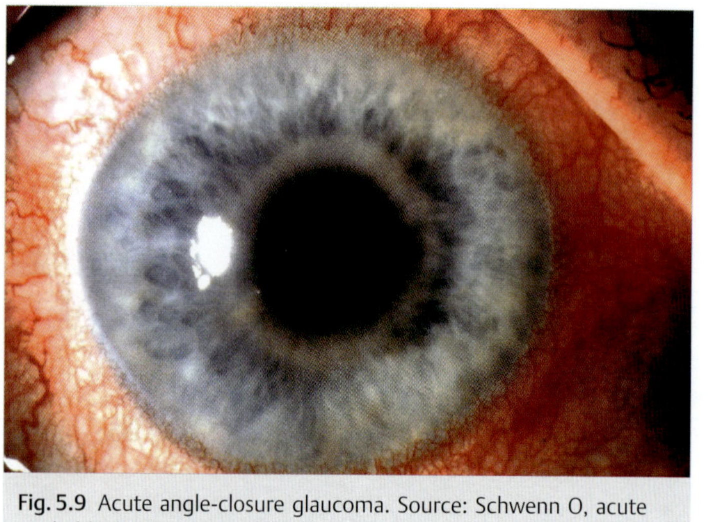

Fig. 5.9 Acute angle-closure glaucoma. Source: Schwenn O, acute angle block, chronic Angular block glaucoma and its differential diagnoses. Ophthalmology up2date 3: 2013, 299-309, Fig. 6.

Therapy

Acute angle-closure glaucoma is an emergency and requires immediate ophthalmologic attention, initiated by medical and followed by surgical treatment. The aim of immediate medical therapy is to decrease the intraocular pressure and open the iridocorneal angle. Contraction of the pupil by topical administration of pilocarpine 1 to 2% is a mainstay of treatment. Additional systemic administration of acetazolamide (10 mg/kg body weight, intravenously) reduces the production of aqueous humor. After cardiopulmonary risk factors have been excluded, an osmotic reduction of the vitreous can be achieved by additional systemic administration of hyperosmolar solutions (e.g. mannitol 1–1.5 g/kg body weight). With supplemental topical medication, that is, beta-blockers, alpha-2 agonists, and carbonic anhydrase inhibitors, a further decrease of intraocular pressure can be achieved. Severe pain during acute angle-closure is treated with analgesics.

Causative treatment of acute angle-closure glaucoma is surgical iridectomy (in cases with corneal edema) or YAG-laser iridotomy (in cases with clear media). As the nonaffected eye is often at risk for developing angle-closure glaucoma as well, prophylactic YAG-laser iridotomy should also be performed.

Further surgical therapeutic options depend on the factors underlying the disease. In cases, of anterior lens vaulting, a lens extraction should be performed, because medical glaucoma therapy alone is unsuccessful in the long term, and filtration surgery may lead to malignant glaucoma.[11] Additional medical treatment after control of the intraocular pressure is usually not necessary. However, in chronic cases, goniosynechiae can occur. In patients with suspected combination with primary open-angle glaucoma, further local glaucoma therapy is recommended.

Secondary Glaucoma

Secondary glaucoma encompasses glaucoma for which other eye conditions (e.g., pseudoexfoliation, pigment dispersion, intraocular inflammation, hemorrhage, and tumors), systemic diseases (e.g., diabetes mellitus, atherosclerosis), or side effects of systemic medication (especially steroids) are causative. Similarly to primary glaucoma, secondary open-angle glaucoma is distinguished from secondary angle-closure glaucoma.

Secondary Open-angle Glaucoma

Under normal anatomical conditions this type of glaucoma is caused by increase of ocular outflow resistance due to deposition of different substances in the trabecular meshwork. Pseudoexfoliation glaucoma belongs to this group of diseases. It is fairly common and is characterized by excessive production and deposition of extracellular matrix fibrils on the lens, zonular fibers, and trabecular meshwork. The origin of these proteins is still unclear, but it has been shown that these matrix proteins are deposited in other organs of the body too and that there is a genetic predisposition.

Pigment dispersion glaucoma, which is common in young myopic males, is characterized by release of iris pigment with subsequent deposition on the back surface of the cornea, on the iris, and the trabecular meshwork. In some patients a concave iris configuration can be recognized as the underlying pathomechanism.

Inflammatory glaucoma is characterized by sedimentation of proteins or by primary inflammation of cellular structures in the trabecular meshwork with consequent increase in intraocular pressure.

Phacolytic Glaucoma

Leaking of lens proteins through capsular defects in mature cataracts causes this rare condition. The proteins as well as macrophages lead to a blockage of the trabecular meshwork.

Steroid Response Glaucoma

Topical or systemic glucocorticoid therapy can induce deposition of mucopolysaccharides into the trabecular meshwork with consecutive increase of intraocular pressure. About 20 to 25% of the population are "steroid-responders." Usually, the IOP comes back to normal after discontinuation of treatment, but temporary medication may be required.

Secondary Angle-closure Glaucoma

Secondary angle-closure glaucoma is characterized by a closure due to scarring of the iridocorneal angle. **Neovascularization glaucoma** belongs to this group. Ischemic retinal diseases (e.g., advanced diabetic retinopathy or ischemic retinal vein occlusion) can lead to neovascularization of the iris through release of VEGF and other growth factors with consecutive scarring and blockage of the iridocorneal angle. Secondary angle-closure glaucoma can also occur in orbital diseases[12] (see the subsection "Glaucoma in Orbital Diseases" later).

Posttraumatic glaucoma

Direct injuries with resulting cicatrization of the iridocorneal angle or following sedimentation of blood or exudate can lead to an increase in intraocular pressure.

Tumor related glaucoma

Tumors located in the iris or ciliary body (e.g., melanoma or metastases) can lead to a blockage of the iridocorneal angle with development of secondary glaucoma.

Treatment

The underlying cause should be the mainstay of treatment of secondary glaucoma, but often, the treatment is similar to that of primary glaucoma. If sufficient control of intraocular pressure is not achieved, filtration or cyclodestructive surgery may be indicated.

Congenital Glaucoma

Primary and secondary congenital glaucoma can be distinguished. From data for Germany, the incidence of primary glaucoma is as high as 1:15,000 to 1:20,000 births per year. It most commonly (> 70% of cases) occurs bilaterally and manifests usually before the 6th to 12th months of life.

Secondary glaucoma can present as part of systemic diseases (metabolic diseases, neurofibromatosis, von Hippel-Lindau angiomatosis, and other phakomatoses). Secondary glaucomas can present and manifest during childhood.

Classic symptoms of congenital glaucoma are increased sensitivity to light and epiphora. Typical clinical signs are increased corneal diameter with large eye (buphthalmus), conjunctival redness, and corneal edema and breaks in Descemet's membrane (Haab's striae). Sometimes reversible optic disc cupping is also seen.

Diagnosis can be challenging. It includes measurement of intraocular pressure, gonioscopy, and examination of the anterior and posterior aspect of the eye as well as ultrasound.

Treatment is usually surgical (goniotomy, trabeculotomy). Lifelong ophthalmologic follow-up and possibly topical antiglaucomatous medications are required.

Glaucoma in Orbital Diseases

Changes of intraocular pressure can appear either as coincidentally with an orbital disease or as a side effect of it. This phenomenon was described fairly early in the ophthalmic literature.[13]

Intraocular pressure can be influenced by orbital entities through four primary pathophysiologic mechanisms[14]:

- Structural bony anomalies in congenital defects, posttraumatically and following surgery.
- Mass effects due to tumor growth or infiltrative disease.
- Vascular alterations leading to increased venous pressure in the orbit (e.g., certain arteriovenous malformations, carotid cavernous sinus fistulas).
- Inflammation and infection with alteration of vascular blood supply in orbital cellulitis or Graves's orbitopathy.

Although there is no direct correlation between disease severity, localization, and nature of orbital diseases with variations of the intraocular pressure, it is reasonable to conclude that orbital pathology can lead to a rise in IOP. Due to special anatomical conditions of the orbit (see Chapter 1 and Chapter 2) inflammatory diseases of the orbit or tumors may lead to increased hydrostatic pressure in the orbit. This leads to a disturbance of blood flow in the orbital veins and, since venous valves are not present in the orbit, an increase of the episcleral venous pressure. As a consequence, these conditions can bring about structural changes affecting Schlemm's canal and an increase of intraocular pressure.

Numerous orbital diseases can increase intraocular pressure (see ▸ Table 5.1). This list of orbital diseases underlines that a thorough ophthalmologic examination, including measurement of intraocular pressure, should be done in all patients with orbital diseases. It is important to note that the intraocular pressure is evaluated not only in the primary position of the eye but also in upgaze and downgaze. Compression of the globe in upgaze can lead to an increase of IOP in case of inferior rectus muscle fibrosis (common in Graves's orbitopathy). Regular perimetry should also be performed in all patients with orbital diseases, not only because of possible development of glaucoma but also to exclude visual field changes due to optic nerve compression.

Table 5.1 Overview of orbital diseases that can lead to changes in intraocular pressure (according to Nassr et al 2009[14])

Congenital anomalies	• Orbito-cranio-facial dysplasias • Clefts • Microphthalmos
Orbital and head trauma	• Orbital fractures • Carotid–cavernous sinus fistulas • Orbital compartment syndrome • Traumatic orbital hematoma and intramuscular hemorrhage • Posttraumatic subgaleal hematoma
Orbital inflammations	• Orbital pseudotumor • Graves's orbitopathy • Orbital cellulitis • Tolosa–Hunt syndrome • Allergic/infectious orbital inflammation • Foreign body granuloma • Posterior scleritis
Vascular malformations	• Intraorbital varix • Carotid–cavernous sinus fistula • Superior vena cava syndrome • Arteriovenous malformations • Cerebrovascular trauma • Antiphospholipid antibody syndrome
Orbital tumors and cysts	• Cavernous hemangioma • Lymphangioma • Lymphoid proliferation • Orbital osteoma • Lymphoproliferative disorders • Leukemia • Plasma cell tumors • Tumors of the lacrimal gland • Intraorbital malignant melanoma • Invasive uveal melanoma • Optic nerve meningioma • Glioma of the optic nerve • Neurofibromatosis • Juvenile xanthogranuloma • Invasive adenoma of the pituitary gland with orbital infiltration • Medulloepithelioma of the optic nerve • Intraorbital metastases • Orbital cysts
Other orbital diseases	• Orbital amyloidosis • Mucopolysaccharidosis • Phakomatoses • Collagen vascular diseases • Side effects of drugs or radiation therapy

5.2.2 Corneal Diseases

This section focuses on the description of corneal diseases that occur in conjunction with orbital diseases or that are of differential diagnostic importance. Essentially, infectious keratitis and exposure keratitis as well as neurotrophic keratopathy will be subjects of discussion.

Pathogenesis

The cornea together with the sclera is the envelope of the globe. Its water content is between 70 and 80% with a protein content of 18–20% and a polysaccharide content of about 4%. Due to its avascular, highly organized multilayered architecture (corneal epithelium, basement membrane, Bowman's layer, corneal stroma, Descemet's membrane, and corneal endothelium), the cornea is translucent for the passage and refraction of light (▸ Fig. 5.10). With a diameter of about 11.7 mm (range 10–13 mm)—the horizontal diameter being slightly larger than the vertical—and a radius of 7.7–7.8 mm, the cornea has a refractive power of about 43 diopters, accounting for 70% of the refractive power of the eye.[15] The tear film and the aqueous humor provide the nutrition of the avascular cornea. The limbal conjunctival vessels supply the stem cells that provide the epithelial surface. The

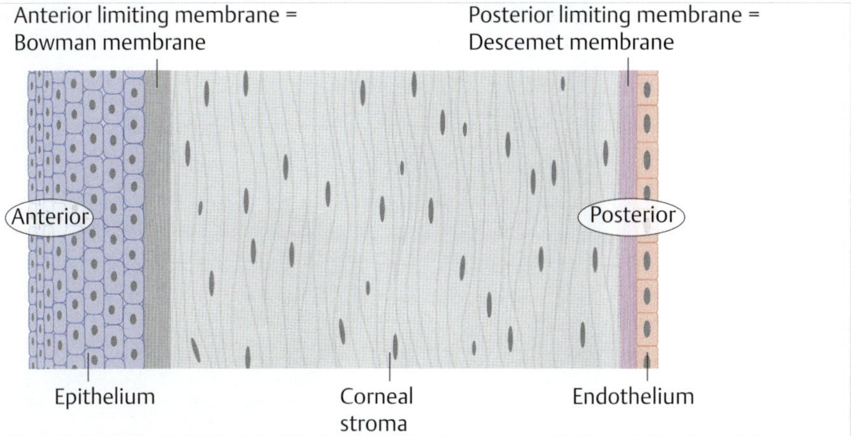

Fig. 5.10 Anatomy of the cornea.

tear film is important for wetting the corneal surface. Its components (lysozyme, lactoferrin, betalysin, and antibodies) also play an important role in the defense against environmental toxins and pathogenic organisms.

The transparency of the cornea is maintained by the regular pattern of collagen lamellae in the corneal stroma, and by keeping the stromal water content stable. Also crucial are the corneal epithelium as a barrier to the tear fluid, and active ion pumps of the corneal endothelium.

The cornea contains numerous nonmyelinated nerve fibers originating in the first branch of the trigeminal nerve. The sensitive innervation is crucial in the defense against environmental influences (reflex eyelid closure, pain, lacrimation).

Due to these properties and the potential for rapid regeneration of the corneal epithelium, the cornea shows a diversity of defense mechanisms to maintain its function. Corneal problems potentially leading to loss of vision can be caused by impairment of any of these mechanisms:

- Malposition of eyelids.
- Lack of eyelid closure due to exophthalmos or neurogenic diseases (lagophthalmos).
- Impaired lubrication of the cornea (dry eye syndrome).
- Corneal diseases.
- Blepharitis.
- Eyelid or lacrimal gland infections.
- Contact lenses.
- Neurogenic diseases.
- Immunosuppressive agents.
- Trauma.

The following issues can be causative for keratitis development:

- Genetics.
- Physical agents (e.g., ultraviolet radiation).
- Mechanical effects: following trauma, in cases with lid malpositions, trichiasis/dystichiasis, and by scar formation following inflammation.
- Infectious agents: bacterial, viral, mycotic or parasitic,
- Neurogenic causes: lagophthalmos, neurotrophic keratitis.

Many of these issues are seen in conjunction with orbital diseases and they are described in detail here.

Infectious Keratitis

Keratitis is defined as corneal inflammation and stromal defects (ulcers) of the cornea, which are caused either by pathogenic agents or immunologically. (General guideline No. 13: "Keratitis" of the German Ophthalmologic Society).[16]

Etiology and Pathogenesis

With the defense mechanisms described above, the cornea and conjunctiva can impede any pathogenic agents from penetrating into deeper tissue layers under normal conditions. Intact corneal epithelium is crucial to achieving this function. Impairment of surface integrity (defects of corneal epithelium) can lead to a penetration of pathogens into deeper corneal layers. This infection leads to a typical inflammatory reaction, with opacification of superficial or deep corneal layers (▶ Fig. 5.11). When an organism enters the stroma, liquefaction of the bradytrophic corneal tissue may occur, with inflammatory response in the anterior chamber (inflammatory corneal endothelial precipitates, inflammatory cells in the anterior chamber, hypopyon), spontaneous perforation of the cornea with leakage of intraocular fluid, and iris incarceration. This can lead to an infection of the posterior segment of the eye (endophthalmitis).

Diagnosis

Superficial swabbing or obtaining material from the base of the ulcer should be performed in every case of infectious keratitis to

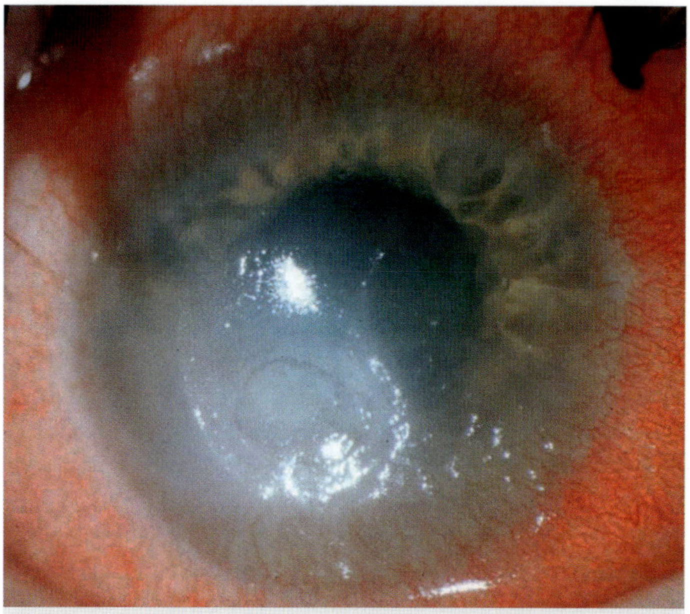

Fig. 5.11 Bacterial keratitis.

identify pathogenic organisms. Infectious keratitis is common in patients with contact lenses (about 30% in the United States). In these cases, contact lenses and their storage and rinsing solutions should be sent for microbiological analysis. Although microbiological culture and sensitivity testing takes some time (particularly for fungal growth), treatment should be initiated immediately. Change of the medication can be performed as needed after the antibiogram is available.

Apart from the patient's history, the ophthalmologic examination should include corneal sensitivity and syringing of the lacrimal pathway since its obstruction carries the risk of a potential reservoir for infectious organisms.

Bacterial Keratitis

The majority of infectious keratitis is of bacterial origin (about 90%). The most common organisms are staphylococci (*Staphylococcus epidermidis, S. aureus*), streptococci (*Streptococcus pneumoniae*), *Pseudomonas aeruginosa* and *Chlamydia* species.

Predisposing risk factors for bacterial keratitis are conjunctival diseases, eyelid disorders (lid malpositions, lagophthalmos, blepharitis), diseases of the lacrimal gland or lacrimal pathways (reservoir for pathogenic organisms), dry eye syndrome, injuries, and general illnesses (e.g. neurodermititis, immune-compromised patients, consumptive diseases).

Treatment

Depending on the severity of ocular involvement, topical administration of broad-spectrum antibiotics on an hourly basis is recommended. Cycloplegia is needed when the anterior chamber is involved. However, prompt oral or intravenous administration of antibiotics is required in cases with rapid progressive course or when deeper parts of the globe are involved.

In cases of deep corneal ulcerations, conjunctival or amnion membrane grafting may be indicated. A tectonic penetrating keratoplasty might be necessary in severe cases of spontaneous corneal perforation or abscess formation. However, risk factors (as mentioned above) should be treated in any case, either medically or surgically.

Viral Keratitis

The most common pathogen for viral keratitis is herpes simplex virus 1 (HSV-1). Herpes simplex virus 2 (HSV-2), varicella zoster virus, and adenoviruses (with the exception of epidemic keratoconjunctivitis) are found less frequently.

Herpes Simplex Virus Keratitis

About 90% of the general population is carrier for this neurotropic virus. Keratitis mostly occurs following reactivation of a herpes simplex infection, predisposing factors being physiological stress in patients with compromised immunity (i.e. upper respiratory tract infections) or following UV-radiation exposure. Clinical symptoms are characterized by visual loss, foreign body sensation, epiphora, and significant sensitivity to light.

Three forms of corneal herpes infection can be distinguished depending on the depth of corneal involvement:

- Dendritic keratitis with impairment or complete loss of corneal sensitivity (▶ Fig. 5.12).

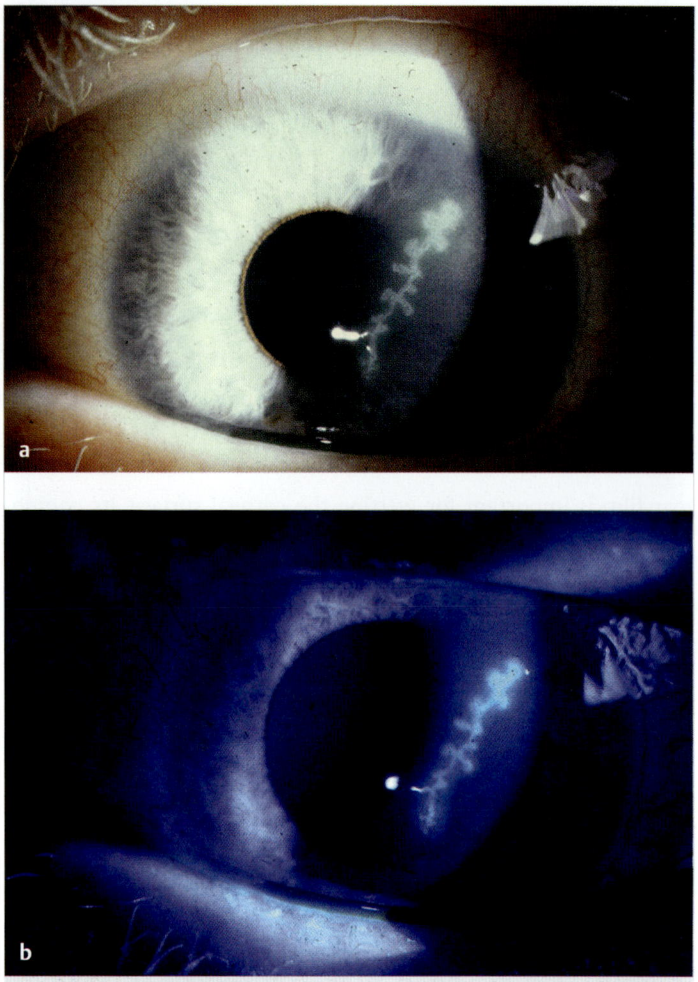

Fig. 5.12 Dendritic keratitis. **(a)** Epithelial linear branching corneal ulcer. **(b)** After staining with fluorescein dye.

- Disciform keratitis with disc-shaped infiltration and opacification of the stroma.
- Endothelial keratitis with concomitant anterior uveitis and secondary glaucoma due to swelling of the endothelial layer (endotheliitis) and the trabecular meshwork (trabeculitis).

Clinical Symptoms and Diagnosis

Usually the diagnosis of dendritic keratitis with linear, slightly branched and elevated epithelial swelling is clinically apparent. Epithelial defects can be demonstrated by slit-lamp examination after fluorescein staining.

Disciform keratitis is characterized by a typical disc-shaped opacification of the corneal stroma. As the stromal keratitis is known to develop recurrences quite often, this commonly results in corneal vascularization originating from the limbus with scar formation and recurrent epithelial defects (metaherpetic keratitis).

Signs of a herpesvirus-related anterior chamber involvement, which can also result in secondary glaucoma due to endothelial inflammation, are corneal condensations, loss of iris pigment epithelium (with transillumination of the iris), appearance of inflammatory cells in the anterior chamber, and flare.

The diagnosis of HSV-keratitis is often made clinically. In unclear cases, however, conjunctival scrapings, impression cytology, or aqueous humor specimens may be tested by cytology, culture, or polymerase chain reaction (PCR) to identify HSV.

Treatment

Topical administration of antiviral agents (e.g., acyclovir eye ointment) is the first-line treatment in cases with herpes simplex virus keratitis. An additional administration of topical or systemic steroids and systemic treatment with acyclovir (initially intravenously, followed by oral treatment with 5 × 400 mg over several weeks) is recommended in all cases with stromal or endothelial involvement.

Varicella Zoster Keratitis

Usually the initial infection with varicella zoster virus is seen as smallpox in childhood. The virus remains dormant in the sensitive cranial nerve, dorsal root, and autonomic ganglia. They can be reactivated just as the herpes simplex virus. An ophthalmic zoster infection occurs if the ophthalmic nerve (first branch of the trigeminal nerve) is involved.

Clinical Symptoms and Diagnosis

In most cases, patients present with severe pain and typical lesions of the skin in the area supplied by the nerve involved (▶ Fig. 5.13). Lesions involving the nose tip (Hutchinson's sign) are signs of an involvement of the nasociliary nerve, which provides sensitive innervation of the inner nose, the orbit, and the eye. The risk of development of an intraocular inflammation is increased in these cases due to common innervation. Other symptoms and clinical findings are quite similar to that of herpes simplex virus keratitis.

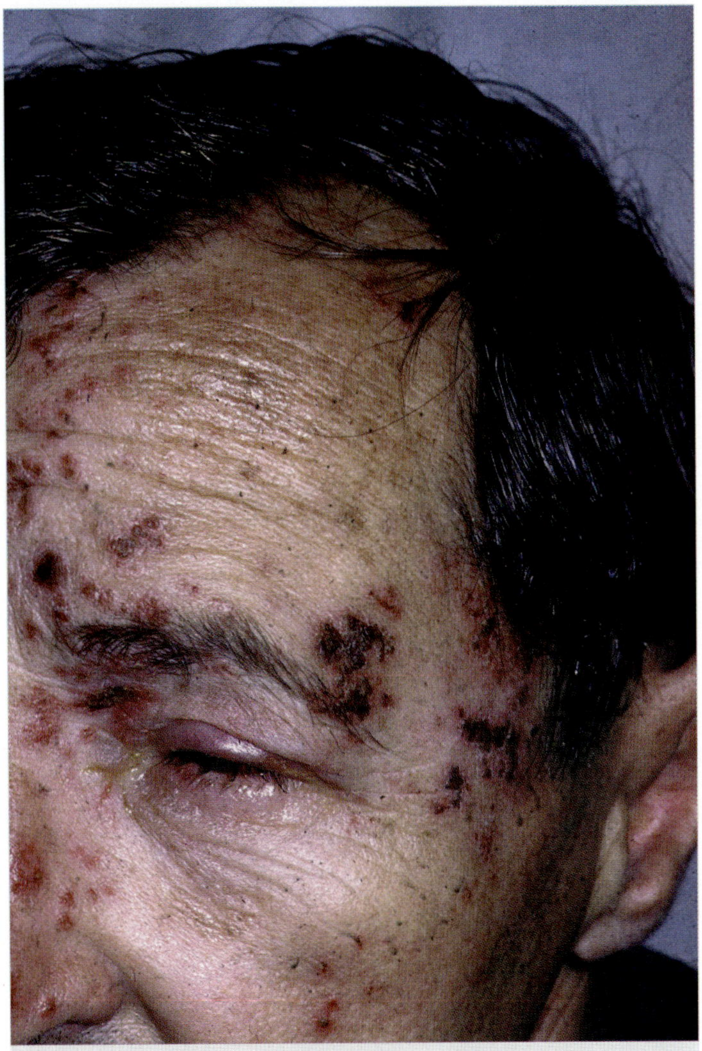

Fig. 5.13 Patient with ophthalmic varicella zoster infection.

Treatment

Therapy must follow an interdisciplinary approach involving ophthalmologists and dermatologists. Ophthalmologic therapy is similar to that of a herpes simplex virus keratitis. Skin lesions are usually treated with locally administered tinctures. As about 30% of patients suffer from paresthesia or neuralgia for several weeks or months, analgesic therapy might be recommended.

Epidemic Keratoconjunctivitis

This disease of the cornea and conjunctiva takes its name from its easy transmission and epidemic outbreaks. It is caused by adenovirus types 8, 19, and 37. The incubation period following smear infection is about 8–10 days. The partner eye is often affected up to 14 days after onset of the disease.

Clinical Symptoms and Diagnosis

In the beginning typically only one eye is involved. Characteristic symptoms are epiphora, sensitivity to light, foreign body sensation, and general feeling of illness. Painful swelling of regional preauricular lymph nodes is often associated. Slit-lamp examination reveals conjunctival swelling and injection along with swelling of the plica semilunaris in severe cases. Pseudomembranes of the conjunctiva can be seen. Sometimes bleeding is observed following therapeutic removal of these membranes. Nummular keratitis develops in 25–30% of all patients, often when conjunctival involvement is settling down. It is characterized by typical subepithelial round opacities of the cornea, which may lead to impairment of vision and increased glare for several weeks and may persist.

Treatment

The disease is self-limiting with a duration of about 14 days. Treatment is symptomatic and comprises mainly the use of artificial tears, since there is no specific antiviral agent available. Additional administration of topical antibiotics is appropriate to prevent bacterial superinfections. The use of topical steroids is a subject of ongoing discussion. Steroids can cause regression of bothersome nummuli, but application of steroids should be avoided because of a higher recurrence rate.

Secondary prophylaxis with adequate hygienic measures and avoidance of direct contact between patients and healthy persons is of particular importance to prevent the spread of disease.

Mycotic Keratitis

Risk factors for development of a mycotic keratitis are similar to those of other forms of keratitis. The multiplication of fungi occurs in the corneal stroma and leads to necrosis and inflammatory reactions in the tissue. If Descemet's membrane is breached, intraocular infection can occur. Mycotic keratitis accounts for about 6–10% of keratitis cases. Most common pathogenic organisms are *Aspergillus* species, followed by *Candida* and *Fusarium* species.

Clinical Symptoms and Diagnosis

As the disease usually begins slowly, patients may initially experience only minor symptoms. Slit-lamp examination reveals frequently raised, whitish corneal infiltrations with blurred edges.

Small satellites occurring in the periphery are typical findings of fungal keratitis. Involvement of the anterior chamber can lead to hypopyon, which has characteristically no distinct horizontal level but has blurred edges or is ascending toward the midline.

When taking specimens for microbiological analysis, it is important to obtain material from the depth of the lesion. In some cases, topical cyclosporine A (1 or 2%) or tacrolimus (0.03%) eyedrops may be helpful to reduce nummuli. Microbiological identification of fungi is often difficult and can be delayed. Therefore, if a fungal infection is suspected clinically, a direct smear can be done with special stains (e.g., PAS, Gomori, acridine orange).

Treatment

Immediate topical treatment should be initiated, also in cases of clinical suspicion without waiting for microbiology results. However, systemic therapy with amphotericin B, nystatin, or natamycin is often needed only in cases with intraocular involvement. Topical administration of fluconazole 0.2%, voriconazole, or amphotericin B eye drops 0.15–0.5% following corneal epithelial abrasion (as it does not penetrate the epithelium) is the line of treatment.[17] Therapeutic penetrating keratoplasty should be performed in therapy-refractive cases or in progressive keratitis with risk of endophthalmitis. The explanted cornea should be submitted for histopathology and microbiologic investigation.

Protozoic Keratitis

This form of keratitis is caused mainly by acanthamoebae, initially often unrecognized, frequently diagnosis is made only in advanced disease. The disease is almost exclusively seen in contact lens users. According to estimations by the German Ophthalmological Society, in Germany about 200 episodes per year occur in contact lens carriers.[20] Amebas exist in air-conditioning systems, soil, and tap water and can therefore be transferred to the eye.

Clinical Symptoms and Diagnosis

Patients usually see an ophthalmologist because of long-term keratitis, conjunctival redness, glare and ultimately severe pain. Slit-lamp examination reveals a ring infiltrate located intraepithelially or in the anterior stroma. It can therefore occasionally be confused with a herpes virus keratitis. In contrast to viral keratitis, patients with acanthamoeba keratitis commonly complain of severe pain.

Identification of the causative protozoa is difficult and only possible in appropriately equipped specialized laboratories. For analysis, corneal material can be taken by deep scraping or biopsy. Special stains (calcofluor white) and phase-contrast microscopy are used for identification of the single-celled organism.

Treatment

A triple combination of drugs is applied with polyhexamethylene biguanide 0.02% eye drops, propamidine isoethionate 0.1% eye drops, and a broad-spectrum antibiotic (as surface bacteria are the nutritional basis of the amebas). Cycloplegics should also be given. In many cases this treatment has to be given for a longer time.

Superficial Punctate Keratitis

Superficial punctate keratitis (SPK) is a frequently occurring unspecific keratitis. It can be acquired due to the following conditions or circumstances:

- Mechanical irritations (e.g., contact lenses, trichiasis, subtarsal foreign bodies),
- Dry eye (keratoconjunctivitis sicca).
- Allergic or infectious conjunctivitis.
- Following UV exposure or other physical or chemical irritants.
- In combination with other forms of keratitis.

Clinical Symptoms and Diagnosis

Typical symptoms include epiphora, foreign body sensation, severe pain, and only minor impairment of visual acuity.

The main finding is multiple small, punctate corneal lesions that can either involve the entire cornea, or—depending on the cause—affect only particular parts of the cornea. The diagnosis is verified by staining with fluorescein or Rose Bengal.

Treatment

Depending on the severity of the patient's symptoms, topical tear substitutes of variable viscosity are usually sufficient along with treatment of the underlying disease. Topical administration of antibiotics is necessary only in very rare cases. Depending on the cause of the disease, superficial punctate keratitis will usually heal in 24–36 hours because of the high regenerative potential of the cornea.

Corneal Epithelial Defect

Corneal erosion or epithelial defect of the cornea commonly occurs due to trauma. However, it can also arise spontaneously or in conjunction with other corneal disorders.

Clinical Symptoms and Diagnosis

Symptoms are mainly severe pain, epiphora and blepharospasm. Clinical examination frequently reveals conjunctival redness and corneal defects that can be stained by fluorescein (▶ Fig. 5.14).

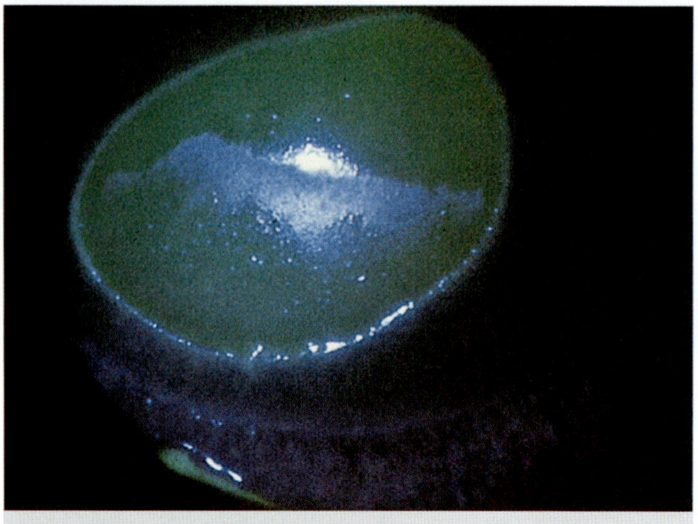

Fig. 5.14 Corneal epithelial defect stained with fluorescein. Source: Burk A, Burk R. Checklist Ophthalmology, 5th edition. Thieme: Stuttgart, 2014; Fig. 23.7.

Treatment

Depending on the size of the corneal defect, closure usually occurs within 24–48 hours with only local lubrication. The reason for this rapid healing is the high proliferation rate of basal cells and centripetal migration of peripheral corneal epithelial cells from the limbus. Treatment with an antibiotic ointment or therapeutic contact lens with antibiotic-containing eye drops might be necessary in cases with recurrent erosions or delayed wound healing.

Neurotrophic Keratitis

Neurotrophic keratitis is a degenerative inflammatory corneal disease, which is caused by a lesion of the first branch of the trigeminal nerve (ophthalmic nerve). Denervation, loss of corneal sensitivity is followed by neurotrophic changes. Underlying causes can be previous herpesvirus infections, tumors in the course of the nerve, or surgical procedures.

Clinical Symptoms and Diagnosis

Usually patients do not complain of any pain due to the loss of sensitivity. Most patients consult the ophthalmologist for conjunctival redness accompanied by slowly progressive visual loss. A corneal perforation may be present in very rare cases on first presentation. Clinical signs are dominated by a central corneal opacity with epithelial or stromal defects. Normally there is no corneal inflammatory reaction. In advanced stages of the disease a descemetocele or corneal perforation can occur. The clinical course might then be complicated by secondary infections.

Treatment

Early initiation of treatment with artificial tears, topical administration of antibiotics, and use of moisture goggles usually leads to a rapid improvement. Penetrating keratoplasty or amnion membrane transplantation should be performed in advanced cases with descemetoceles, perforations, or iris prolapse. However, prognosis of corneal transplants is limited due to the impaired healing and propensity for recurrence. Injection of botulinum toxin into the levator muscle for induction of a temporary protective ptosis or lateral tarsorrhaphy is recommended to achieve a temporary or long-term protection of the corneal surface.

Exposure Keratitis

Lagophthalmos is defined as incomplete eyelid closure mostly due facial nerve paresis, scar formation following injuries or surgery, or exophthalmos (e.g., Graves's ophthalmopathy) (▸ Fig. 5.15).

Clinical Symptoms and Diagnosis

The symptoms are quite similar to those of neurotrophic keratitis and punctate keratopathy. If a positive Bell phenomenon is present (outward and upward rotation of the eyeball during lid closure), findings usually occur in the lower third of the cornea because this part remains exposed due to lack of eyelid closure (exposition keratopathy). Diagnosis is similar to that of neurotrophic keratitis.

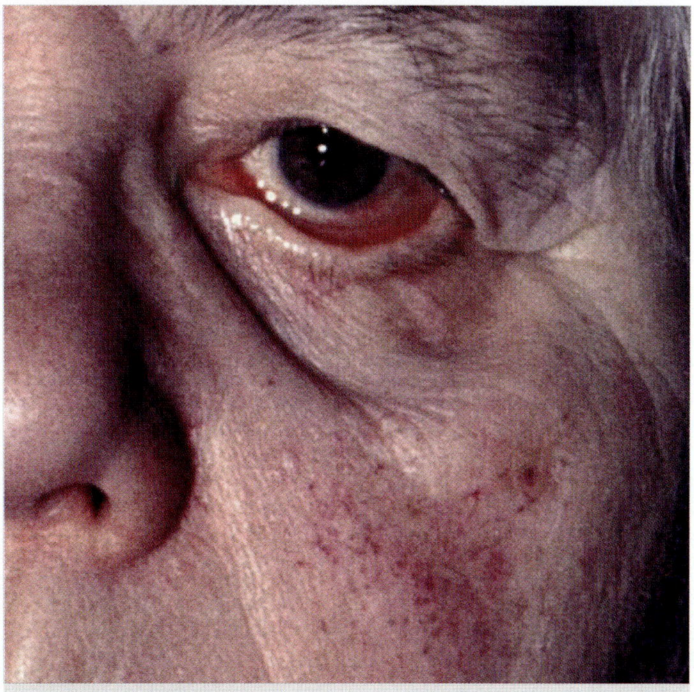

Fig. 5.15 Keratitis e lagophthalmo.

Treatment

Therapy is quite similar to that of neurotrophic and superficial punctate keratitis.

There is a vast variety of other corneal diseases that may lack association with orbital disorders. For further information, refer to textbooks and specialized literature in ophthalmology.

5.3 Occlusion of Intraocular and Intraorbital Vessels

B. Wiechens

Vascular disorders of the eye can occur on the basis of an underlying general disease or secondary to orbital diseases. This is due to the uniqueness of the orbital blood vessels and their close proximity to orbital structures and the eye. The microvessels of the orbit form a complex network whose density increases from orbital apex towards the globe.[21] The ophthalmic artery originates from the internal carotid artery and, on its course through the orbit, gives rise to many ocular and orbital vessels. Depending on the passage of the ophthalmic artery over or under the optic nerve, the central retinal artery and the ciliary arteries are its first branches (see Chapter 1). Both vessels are end arteries. The orbit is supplied by multiple anastomoses from the ophthalmic artery and branches of the external carotid artery via collaterals. For this reason ischemic events in the orbit (orbital infarction syndrome) are rare but are documented.[22,23]

The prognosis of ocular vessel occlusion secondary to orbital diseases depends largely on the localization and extent of the disease process affecting the vasculature of the eye. The variety of symptoms derives from the fact that the branching of the ophthalmic vessels shows a marked variation.[24]

5

5.3.1 Vascular Occlusions of the Retina and the Optic Nerve

Vascular occlusions of the retina and the optic nerve occur frequently. In most cases systemic diseases are causative. For this reason interdisciplinary collaboration between various disciplines is of great significance in order to investigate vascular risk factors.

Vascular occlusions of the retina or of the optic nerve secondary to orbital diseases are very rare. Among others they have been documented after orbital cellulitis,[25,26,27,28,29] systemic vasculitis,[30,31] and tumors (optic nerve sheath meningioma, optic nerve glioma, etc.)

Arterial, venous, and combined occlusions can be differentiated. As symptoms and prognosis of vascular occlusions vary, they will be discussed in more detail in the following sections.

5.3.2 Arterial Vascular Occlusions of the Retina/Choroid (Central Retinal Artery, Branch Retinal Artery, and Ophthalmic Artery Occlusion)

Central retinal artery occlusion (CRAO) can be differentiated from occlusions of its temporal or nasal branches (branch retinal artery occlusions, BRAO) (▶ Fig. 5.16, ▶ Fig. 5.17). CRAO is more frequent than BRAO.[32] Acute and chronic stages can be differentiated.[33]

Symptoms and Diagnosis

Patients complain of a sudden, painless impairment of visual acuity, a total visual field defect (due to central retinal artery occlusion), or a partial visual field defect (due to branch retinal artery occlusion). In approximately 15–20% of the population an additional artery is present, the cilioretinal artery, which supplies the retina between the optic nerve and the macula. If this artery is present, central vision may be preserved in cases of CRAO or BRAO.

Some patients may exhibit prodromes such as transient deterioration in visual acuity or blurred vision (amaurosis fugax). In retinal artery occlusions, patients experience a sudden loss of vision. However, complete blindness, as in ophthalmic artery occlusion, is rather rare. A relative afferent pupillary defect can be present. Funduscopically, edema of the nerve fiber layer with a loss of transparency of the retina is visible in the area that is supplied by the affected artery or arterial branch. The cherry red spot" of the macula (▶ Fig. 5.16) can be recognized as a pathognomonic sign of central artery occlusion. This feature is due to the fovea lacking the nerve fiber layer (Henle's nerve fiber layer), giving a direct view onto the retinal pigment epithelium and the choroid, which still is perfused. Occasionally, small yellow cholesterol embolic plaques can be visible at the occlusion site (Hollenhorst plaques).

Diagnosis of CRAO is usually not challenging. However, in most instances it is difficult to differentiate CRAO from ophthalmic artery occlusion (OAO, ~5% of patients). In contrast to CRAO patients, patients with OAO often complain of sudden blinding. A "cherry red spot" is often absent because the choroidal perfusion is compromised. In rare cases there may be exceptions because of circulatory anastomoses. Even complete occlusion of the ophthalmic artery may possibly leave the eye without symptoms.

An interdisciplinary examination with a focus on the cardiovascular system should be undertaken to determine vascular risk factors, such as hyperlipidemia, arterial hypertension, diabetes mellitus, or atherosclerosis (e.g., carotid artery stenosis).[34] In young patients care should be taken to identify platelet and factor abnormalities or collagen vascular/connective tissue diseases. Due to the different long-term treatment regimens, differentiation between nonarteritic and arteritic vascular occlusions has particular significance.

Treatment and Prognosis

Treatment consists of ocular massage, reduction of intraocular pressure to improve retinal perfusion, sublingual isosorbide dinitrate, intravenous acetazolamide. Intravenous mannitol, methylprednisolone, streptokinase, retrobulbar tolazoline, and various anticoagulants may be helpful in some cases.[34] Thrombolysis may

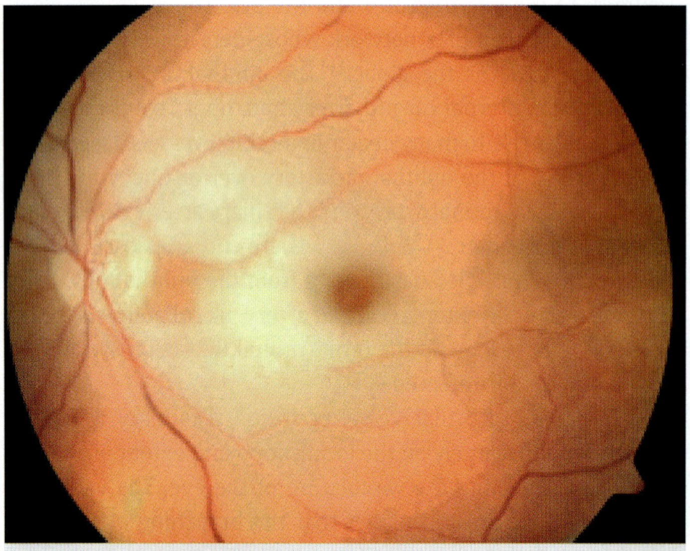

Fig. 5.16 Central retinal artery occlusion.

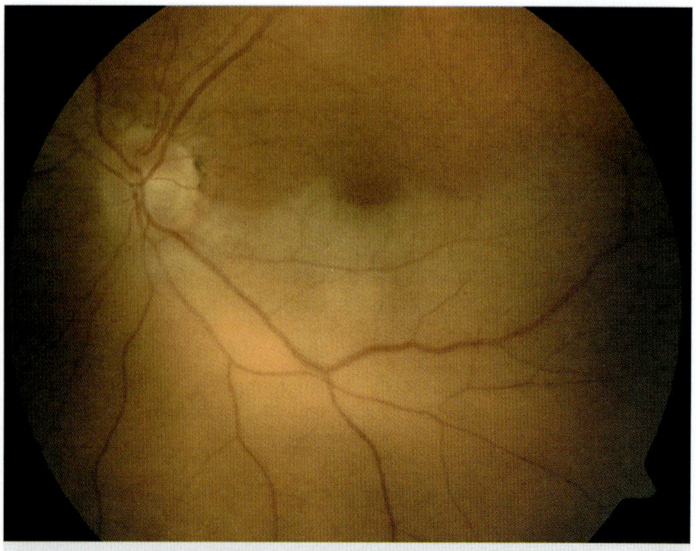

Fig. 5.17 Occlusion of the inferior retinal artery branch.

also be a therapeutic option. The European Assessment Group for Lysis in the Eye (EAGLE), however, did not find a statistically significant difference between lysis and standard therapy (60% vs. 57.1%). Thus thrombolysis is no longer recommended because of its high rate of side effects (37% vs. 4.3%).[35]

In conclusion, therapeutic options and prognosis are unsatisfactory. A final visual acuity of 0.1 or better can be achieved only in a small number of patients.[32] If the arterial vascular occlusion is of arteritic origin, long-term therapy with steroids (depending on the erythrocyte sedimentation rate), managed on an interdisciplinary basis, is indicated. Regular follow-up examinations are mandatory to minimize the risk of future vascular events.

In the long-term, optic nerve atrophy can develop. Due to regression of retinal edema, the retina becomes transparent again. Nevertheless, visual field defects and low vision often persist.

5.3.3 Venous Retinal Vascular Occlusions (Central Retinal Vein, Hemicentral Retinal Vein, and Branch Retinal Vein Occlusion)

Approximately two-thirds of all retinal vascular occlusions are of venous origin. Prevalence ranges from 0.7% (< 60 years of age) to 4.6% (> 80 years of age).[36,37] Three distinct types can be differentiated: central retinal vein occlusion (CRVO, ischemic, nonischemic, impending), hemicentral retinal vein occlusion, and branch retinal vein occlusion (BRVO) (▶ Fig. 5.18, ▶ Fig. 5.19). Branch retinal vein occlusion is more frequent than central vein occlusion.

Risk factors are age; systemic diseases, such as diabetes mellitus; arterial hypertension; coagulation disorders; ocular diseases, such as glaucoma; as well as oral contraceptives and smoking.

The pathogenesis is multifactorial in which local thrombogenesis plays a key role. Predilection sites for a local venous thrombosis are the common adventitial sheath at arteriovenous crossings posterior to the lamina cribrosa.[38] Atherosclerotic changes in the arterial wall may cause compression of the adjacent vein and alter local hemodynamic properties, favoring thrombogenesis and occlusion of the vein.[39]

Symptoms and Diagnostics

Patients present with sudden, painless unilateral blurred vision. Deterioration of visual acuity is reported in different degrees of severity by many patients. Sometimes patients notice prodromes over several days' duration such as transient episodes of blurring with improvement during the day. If the macula is not involved, branch retinal vein occlusion can be asymptomatic and may only be discovered incidentally.

In addition to a clinical ophthalmologic examination, perimetry, fluorescein angiography (Video 5.1), and optical coherence tomography represent the most important diagnostic procedures. Typical funduscopic changes in the affected area are disc hemorrhages, increased tortuosity and dilatation of the retinal veins, "dot/blot and flame-shaped" retinal hemorrhages, cotton wool spots, and retinal edema. Fluorescein angiography allows determination of the extent of capillary nonperfusion and the presence of neovascularization (in advanced stages) and of macular edema. Optical coherence tomography is a noninvasive procedure and useful in the assessment and monitoring of macular edema (▶ Fig. 5.20).

As with retinal arterial occlusion, physical examination and laboratory tests to determine vascular risk factors are recommended in all patients. The complex pathogenesis of the disease requires treatment of all risk factors.

Treatment and Prognosis

The treatment of the acute stage of retinal vein occlusion has to be separated from long-term management of the disease. In acute central vein occlusion (in symptomatic retinal branch vein occlusion currently not fully accepted), an isovolemic hemodilution may be advantageous along with strict blood pressure monitoring, with the aim of a temporary reduction of the hematocrit to a therapeutic target range of 35–38%[40,41] for up to 6 weeks after initial treatment.

The prognosis for visual recovery in acute stages of the disease can be positively influenced in some cases. The long-term course, however, is determined by the recurrence of macular edema and, in ischemic vein occlusions, by neovascularization and its complications.

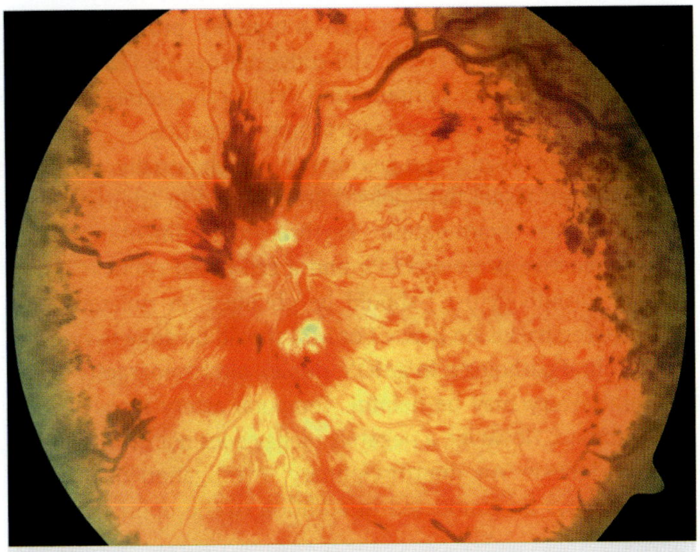

Fig. 5.18 Central retinal vein occlusion.

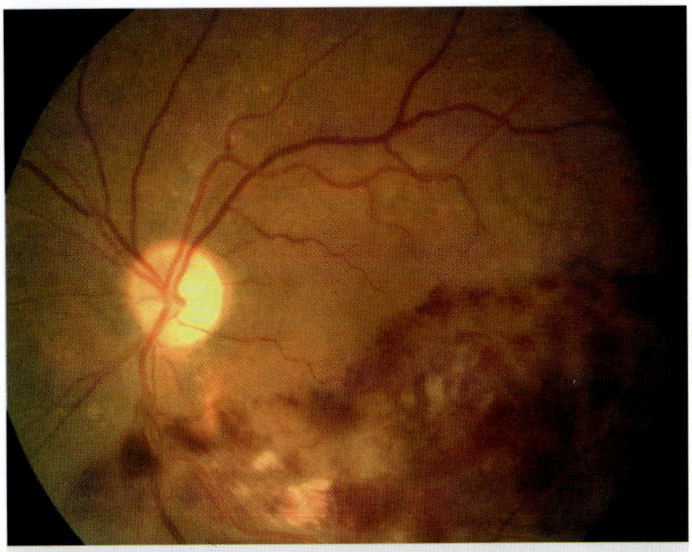

Fig. 5.19 Occlusion of the inferior branch retinal vein.

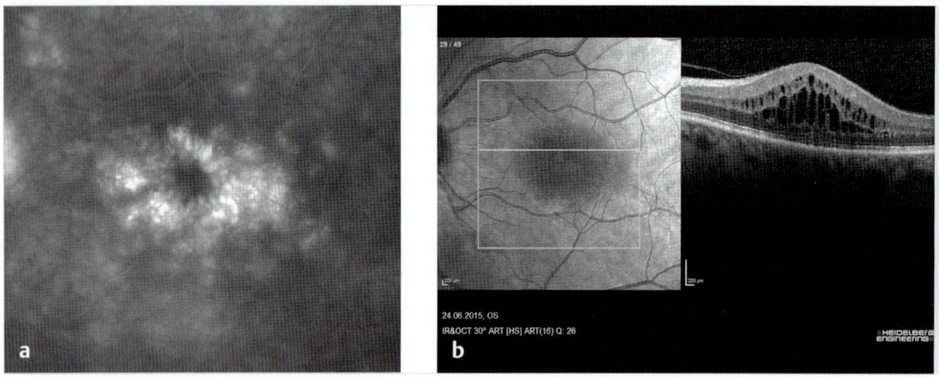

Fig. 5.20 Cystoid macular edema (Copyright: Heidelberg Engineering; reproduced with permission). **(a)** Fluorescence angiography. **(b)** Spectral domain OCT.

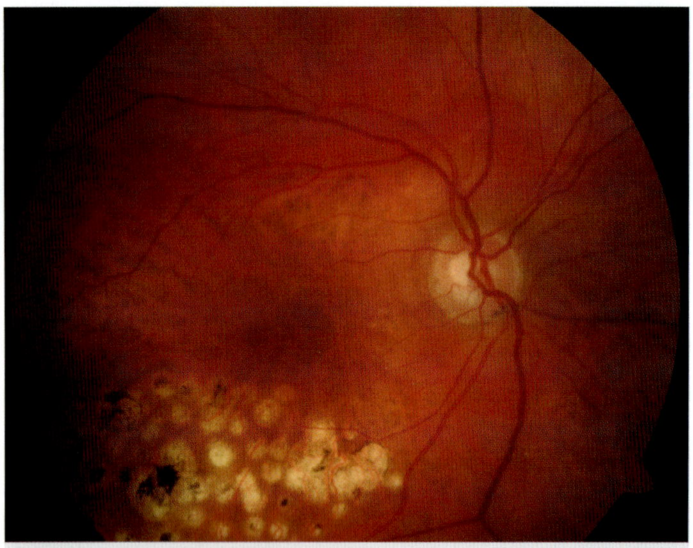

Fig. 5.21 Laser coagulation in a patient with a branch retinal vein occlusion.

Photocoagulation (scatter or sector) is the treatment of choice to improve vision and to prevent late-onset complications such as retinal neovascularization, vitreous hemorrhage, and neovascular glaucoma[42,43] (▶ Fig. 5.21). However, results after grid laser coagulation in cystoid macula edema are disappointing. Intravitreal injection of anti-VEGF-substances such as ranibizumab, aflibercept, pegaptanib, or bevacizumab as well as triamcinolone and dexamethasone implants has been shown to be successful and can be regarded to date as the gold standard.[44] Surgical interventions to increase venous flow, such as radial optic neurotomy (RON) or adventitial sheathotomy, have recently been advocated. Results of studies do not support therapeutic benefit. Hence operative interventions are not generally recommended at the time being.[45]

The prognosis of retinal vein occlusion is more favorable than that of retinal artery occlusion. Natural course and results after treatment are expectedly better in BRVO than in CRVO. Vision recovers over time in about one-third of patients. In another third of patients, predominantly those with central venous occlusion, late-onset complications such as retinal neovascularization, vitreous hemorrhage, neovascular glaucoma with long-term visual disturbances can occur, so that recurrent treatment is needed.

5.3.4 Anterior Ischemic Optic Neuropathy (Nonarteritic/Arteritic)

Depending on the etiology, anterior ischemic optic neuropathy is divided into

- **Nonarteritic** anterior ischemic optic neuropathy (naAION) caused by atherosclerosis.
- **Arteritic** anterior ischemic optic neuropathy (aAION) associated with temporal arteritis (giant cell arteritis).

naAION occurs in patients of middle and higher age. Risk factors are diabetes mellitus, arterial hypertension, and hyperlipidemia, as well as sleep-apnea syndrome, sildenafil, and optic disc drusen. In addition, nocturnal hypotension seems to play a significant role in the development of the disease.[46]

The incidence of naAION is higher than that of aAION, which predominantly occurs in patients of higher age associated with temporal arteritis. Approximately 15–20% of patients with arteritis temporal are afflicted with aAION, with a female predisposition.

Symptoms and Diagnosis

Patients usually notice a sudden, unilateral, severe visual loss. In patients with naAION this visual impairment is predominantly noted in the morning after awakening. In aAION frequent accompanying symptoms are headache, jaw claudication, unintentional weight loss, and myalgias, sometimes followed—within days—by similar symptoms and sudden visual loss in the second eye.

Ophthalmoscopically, there are a typically prominent optic disc, radial disc hemorrhages, and congested vessels (▶ Fig. 5.22). Nodular, tender, and nonpulsating temporal arteries are frequently observed in patients with temporal arteritis.

Color vision testing and perimetry (which usually reveals a wedge-shaped visual field defect) are required in addition to an ophthalmologic examination. Erythrocyte sedimentation rate (ESR), C-reactive protein (CRP), and a cell blood count (CBC; to identify thrombocytosis) should be obtained. In isolated cases with progressive vision loss, CT or MRI should be done to rule out intracerebral pathology. In aAION, duplex ultrasonography of the temporal artery may be helpful. Temporal artery biopsy is the gold standard. However, a negative biopsy does not confirm a negative diagnosis. An interdisciplinary investigation of patients should always be conducted in addition to the ophthalmologic work-up.

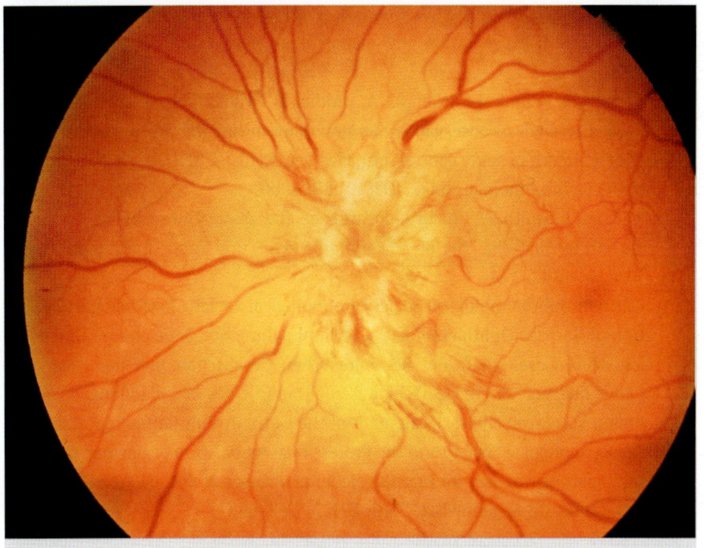

Fig. 5.22 Anterior ischemic optic neuropathy.

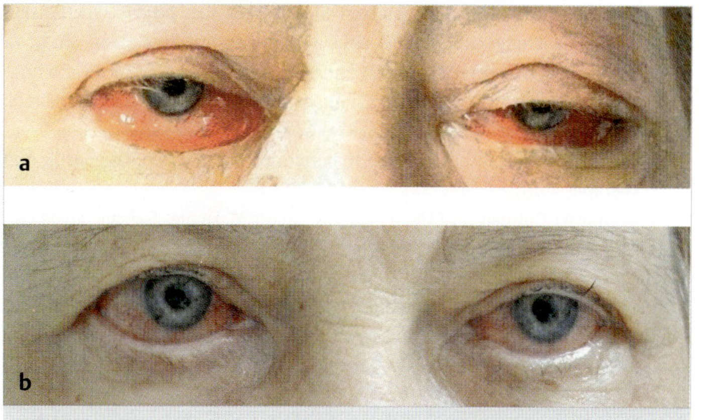

Fig. 5.23 Chemosis of the conjunctiva due to an internal carotid artery–cavernous sinus fistula. (a) Before therapy. (b) Following neuroradiologic intervention.

The differential diagnosis includes:

- Papilledema.
- Papillitis/optic nerve neuritis.
- Optic disc drusen.
- Disc malformations.
- Inflammatory or infiltrative changes of the optic disc.
- High hyperopia.

Treatment and Prognosis

Systemic steroids may be helpful in aAION and also in naAION.[47]

Administration of high-dose steroids is recommended in patients with aAION, initially 1000 mg/day for 5 days. To minimize the high risk of involvement of the second eye, long-term treatment with steroids and monitoring of clinical symptoms, ESR, and CRP is recommended for at least 6 months. Steroids are slowly tapered off.

In naAION short-term administration of steroids at 1–1.5 mg/kg body weight is sufficient. Some trials have investigated the effectiveness of isovolemic hemodilution. The significance of this treatment currently cannot be determined. However, treatment of the underlying systemic disease is crucial.

Even after immediate treatment prognosis in both forms is poor. Visual recovery has been reported; unfortunately, it is not the rule.

5.3.5 Occlusion of Intraorbital Vessels

Acute occlusion of intraorbital vessels is a rare event and is usually a sequela of other diseases in which the orbit becomes involved:

- Periorbital diseases with orbital infiltration (sinusitis, tumors).
- Trauma with direct injury of the vascular structures.
- Orbital hematoma.
- Congenital or acquired malformations.
- Previous surgery.
- Adverse effects of drug treatment (e.g., oral contraceptives).

Periorbital infections that have spread to the orbit (e.g., upper lid abscess; frontal, maxillary, or ethmoidal sinusitis) can lead to orbital cellulitis. Acute and chronic inflammatory reaction in orbital tissues and an increase in intraorbital pressure can be complicated by an alteration of orbital and retinal vascular circulation. Vascular occlusion may occur in orbital and retinal arteries and veins.[24,25,26,27,28,31]

Similarly, traumatic, iatrogenic or spontaneous orbital hematomas can cause an interruption in the orbital and ocular blood supply.[22,18]

Orbital arteriovenous malformations, carotid cavernous sinus fistulas (▶ Fig. 5.23, ▶ Fig. 3.5), ophthalmic artery aneurysms, and orbital varix (characterized by intermittent protrusion of the eye when the Valsalva maneuver is performed) entail a considerable risk of an orbital hematoma or an alteration in intraorbital hemodynamics.[19]

An exact patient history, the ophthalmologic examination, and further diagnostic imaging procedures (MRT, CT, angiography, ultrasound) usually lead to the correct diagnosis. Treatment is conducted on an interdisciplinary basis depending on the pathological findings, the extent of the symptoms, the age of the patient and the prognosis.

References

[1] Rohrbach JML, Lieb WE, Küper K, et al. Tumoren des Auges und seiner Adnexe. Stuttgart: Schattauer; 1998

[2] Donaldson MJ, Sullivan TJ, Whitehead KJ, Williamson RM. Squamous cell carcinoma of the eyelids. Br J Ophthalmol. 2002; 86(10):1161–1165

[3] Wali UK, Al-Mujaini A. Sebaceous gland carcinoma of the eyelid. Oman J Ophthalmol. 2010; 3(3):117–121

[4] Pflugfelder A, Kochs C, Blum A, et al. German Society of Dermatology. S3-guideline "diagnosis, therapy and follow-up of melanoma" – short version. J Dtsch Dermatol Ges. 2013; 11(6):563–602

[5] Albores-Saavedra J, Batich K, Chable-Montero F, Sagy N, Schwartz AM, Henson DE. Merkel cell carcinoma demographics, morphology, and survival based on 3870 cases: a population based study. J Cutan Pathol. 2010; 37(1):20–27

[6] Rice RD, Jr, Chonkich GD, Thompson KS, Chase DR. Merkel cell tumor of the head and neck. Five new cases with literature review. Arch Otolaryngol Head Neck Surg. 1993; 119(7):782–786

[7] Lemos BD, Storer BE, Iyer JG, et al. Pathologic nodal evaluation improves prognostic accuracy in Merkel cell carcinoma: analysis of 5823 cases as the basis of the first consensus staging system. J Am Acad Dermatol. 2010; 63(5):751–761

[8] Durand JM, Weiller C, Richard MA, Portal I, Mongin M. Treatment of Merkel cell tumor with interferon-alpha-2b. Br J Dermatol. 1991; 124(5):509

[9] Ito Y, Kawamura K, Miura T, et al. Merkel cell carcinoma. A successful treatment with tumor necrosis factor. Arch Dermatol. 1989; 125(8):1093–1095

[10] Kass MA, Heuer DK, Higginbotham EJ, et al. for the, Ocular Hypertension Treatment Study Group. The Ocular Hypertension Treatment Study: a randomized trial determines that topical ocular hypotensive medication delays or prevents the onset of primary open-angle glaucoma. Arch Ophthalmol. 2002; 120(6):701–713, discussion 829–830

[11] Pfeiffer N. Glaukom und okuläre Hypertension. Grundlagen, Diagnostik und Therapie. Stuttgart, New York: Thieme; 2005:13

[12] Zborowski-Gutman L, Gutman I, Chen V, Sharir M, Findler G. Acute angle closure glaucoma precipitated by orbital pseudotumour. Br J Ophthalmol. 1988; 72(2):142–144

[13] Guist G, II. Entzündliche Orbitalprozesse und Glaukom. [Inflammatory orbital processes and glaucoma]. Z Augenheilkd. 1925; 55:308–317

[14] Nassr MA, Morris CL, Netland PA, Karcioglu ZA. Intraocular pressure change in orbital disease. Surv Ophthalmol. 2009; 54(5):519–544

[15] Lang GK. Hornhaut (Kornea). In: Lang GK, ed. Lehrbuch der Augenheilkunde. 4th ed. Stuttgart, New York: Thieme; 2008:105–142

[16] Leitlinie Nr. 13 Keratitis [Guideline no. 13: Keratitis] Stand 17.08.2011. Deutschen Ophthalmologischen Gesellschaft e.V. (DOG) and Berufsverbandes der Augenärzte e.V. (BVA); 2011

[17] Behrens-Baumann W, Finis D, MacKenzie C, Roth M, Geerling G. [Keratomycosis - Therapy Standards and New Developments]. [in German]. Klin Monbl Augenheilkd. 2015 Jun;232(6):754764. doi: 10.1055/s-0035-1546032. Epub 2015 Jun 17.

[18] Mitteilung aus der Vorab-Pressekonferenz anlässlich des 111th Kongresses der Deutschen Ophthalmologischen Gesellschaft (DOG) [Opening announcement]; September 12, 2013; Berlin

[19] Bron AJ, Tripathi RC, Tripathi BJ. Wolff's Anatomy of the Eye and Orbit. 8th ed. London: Chapman & Hall Medical; 1997

[20] Maier P1, Feltgen N, Lagrèze WA. Bilateral orbital infarction syndrome after bifrontal craniotomy. Arch Ophthalmol 2007;125(3):422423.

[21] Wiroteurairueng T, Poungvarin N. Orbital infarction syndrome in nephrotic syndrome patient with extensive carotid arteries occlusion. J Med Assoc Thai. 2007; 90(11):2499–2505

[22] Luo QL, Orcutt JC, Seifter LS. Orbital mucormycosis with retinal and ciliary artery occlusions. Br J Ophthalmol. 1989; 73(8):680–683

[23] Bhola RM, Dhingra S, McCormick AG, Chan TK. Central retinal artery occlusion following staphylococcal orbital cellulitis. Eye (Lond). 2003; 17(1):109–111

[24] Komolafe OO, Ashaye AO. Combined central retinal artery and vein occlusion complicating orbital cellulitis. Niger J Clin Pract. 2008; 11(1):74–76

[25] Coşkun M, Ilhan Ö, Keskin U, et al. Central retinal artery occlusion secondary to orbital cellulitis and abscess following dacryocystitis. Eur J Ophthalmol. 2011; 21(5):649–652

[26] Das JK, Choudhury BD, Medhi J. Orbital abscess and hemi-occlusion of the central retinal vein in a child. Orbit. 2007; 26(4):295–297

[27] Proctor CM, Magrath GN, de Castro LE, Johnson JH, Teed RG. Orbital cellulitis complicated by central retinal artery occlusion. Ophthal Plast Reconstr Surg. 2013; 29(2):e59–e61

[28] Menezo V, Lightman S. The eye in systemic vasculitis. Clin Med (Lond). 2004; 4(3):250–254

[29] Sudhakar P, Shah GV, Saponara F, Fullen DR, Trobe JD. Central retinal artery occlusion secondary to orbital inflammation in lupus erythomatosus profundus. J Neuroophthalmol. 2012; 52:93–94

[30] Mirshahi A, Feltgen N, Hansen LL, Hattenbach L-O. Retinal vascular occlusions: an interdisciplinary challenge. Dtsch Arztebl Int. 2008; 105(26):474–479

[31] Lang GE. Netzhaut: Retinale Arterienverschlüsse. In Lang GK, ed. Augenheilkunde. 4th ed. Stuttgart, New York: Thieme; 2008:321ff

[32] Varma DD, Cugati S, Lee AW, Chen CS. A review of central retinal artery occlusion: clinical presentation and management. Eye (Lond). 2013; 27(6):688–697

[33] Feltgen N, Reinhard T, Kampik A, Jurklies B, Brückmann H, Schumacher M. [Lysis therapy vs. conservative therapy: randomised and prospective study on the treatment of acute central retinal artery occlusion (EAGLE study)]. [in German]. Ophthalmologe. 2006; 103(10):898–900

[34] Mitchell P, Smith W, Chang A. Prevalence and associations of retinal vein occlusion in Australia. The Blue Mountains Eye Study. Arch Ophthalmol. 1996; 114(10):1243–1247

[35] German Ophthalmological Society, Retinological Society, Professional Association of German Ophthalmologists. Stellungnahme der Deutschen Ophthalmologischen Gesellschaft, der Retinologischen Gesellschaft und des Berufsverbands der Augenärzte Deutschlands zur Therapie des Makulaödems beim retinalen Venenverschluss. [Statement of the German Ophthalmological Society, the Retinological Society and the Professional Association of German Ophthalmologists on Therapy for Macular Oedema in Cases of Retinal Vein Occlusion]. Klin Monatsbl Augenheilkd. 2010; 227(7):542–556

[36] Hayreh SS. Structure of the optic nerve. In: Ischemic Optic Neuropathies. Berlin, Heidelberg, New York: Springer; 2011:7–34

[37] Hansen LL. Central retinal vein occlusion. In: Joussen AM, Gardner TW, Kirchhof B, Ryan SJ, eds. Retinal Vascular Disease. Berlin, Heidelberg, New York: Springer; 2007:443–466

[38] Glacet-Bernard A, Zourdani A, Milhoub M, Maraqua N, Coscas G, Soubrane G. Effect of isovolemic hemodilution in central retinal vein occlusion. Graefes Arch Clin Exp Ophthalmol. 2001; 239(12):909–914

[39] Wolf S, Arend O, Bertram B, et al. Hemodilution therapy in central retinal vein occlusion. One-year results of a prospective randomized study. Graefes Arch Clin Exp Ophthalmol. 1994; 232(1):33–39

[40] The Central Vein Occlusion Study Group. Natural history and clinical management of central retinal vein occlusion. Arch Ophthalmol. 1997; 115(4):486–491

[41] Hayreh SS, Zimmerman MB, Podhajsky P. Incidence of various types of retinal vein occlusion and their recurrence and demographic characteristics. Am J Ophthalmol. 1994; 117(4):429–441

[42] Feltgen N, Pielen A, Hansen L, et al. [Intravitreal drug therapy for retinal vein occlusion–pathophysiological mechanisms and routinely used drugs]. [in German]. Klin Monatsbl Augenheilkd. 2010; 227(9):681–693

[43] Hasselbach HC, Ruefer F, Feltgen N, et al. Treatment of central retinal vein occlusion by radial optic neurotomy in 107 cases. Graefes Arch Clin Exp Ophthalmol. 2007; 245(8):1145–1156

[44] Hayreh SS. Ischemic optic neuropathy. Prog Retin Eye Res. 2009; 28(1):34–62

[45] Hayreh SS, Zimmerman MB. Non-arteritic anterior ischemic optic neuropathy: role of systemic corticosteroid therapy. Graefes Arch Clin Exp Ophthalmol. 2008; 246(7):1029–1046

[46] Rose GE, Verity DH. Acute presentation of vascular disease within the orbit-a descriptive synopsis of mechanisms. Eye (Lond). 2013; 27(3):299–307

[47] Smoker WR, Gentry LR, Yee NK, Reede DL, Nerad JA. Vascular lesions of the orbit: more than meets the eye. Radiographics. 2008; 28(1):185–204, quiz 325

Suggested Further Reading

Krachmer JH, Mannis MJ, Holland EJ. Cornea. 2nd ed. Vol. 1, 2. Philadelphia, PA: Elsevier Mosby; 2005

Chapter 6

Orbital Complications

6

6 Orbital Complications

S. Graß and H.-J. Welkoborsky

6.1 Introduction

A disease or symptom of a disease spreading from the outside to the internal structures of the orbit is referred to as an "orbital complication." Orbital complications can have traumatic causes (fractures, hemorrhages), inflammatory causes (acute sinusitis, dacryoadenitis), allergic causes, or autoimmune causes (Graves's orbitopathy).

6.2 Intraorbital Hemorrhages

6

6.2.1 Iatrogenic Hemorrhage due to Endonasal Surgery of the Sinuses

Intraoperative or postoperative bleeding into the orbit can be caused by sinus surgery. This can result in an orbital compartment syndrome, which, in the worst case, may be associated with a loss of vision (cf. Chapter 2). Immediate treatment of this complication is always indicated.

According to literature, orbital complications following paranasal sinus surgery (functional endoscopic sinus surgery [FESS]) occur in 0.07% of cases.[1,2] The use of image-guided navigation systems seems to reduce the risk of complications.[3]

Pathogenesis

Intraconal and Retrobulbar Hemorrhage

Intraconal or retrobulbar hemorrhage is usually caused by trauma to the anterior ethmoid artery, rarely also by trauma to the posterior ethmoid artery. The anterior ethmoid artery is particularly at risk in endonasal sinus surgery due to its close position to the ethmoid sinuses.[4,5] An injury to the artery results in its retraction into the orbit, with subsequent acute intraorbital hemorrhage. This increase of intraorbital pressure leads to an orbital compartment syndrome with the risk of blindness due to ischemia of the optic nerve (cf. Chapter 2.4).[6]

Peribulbar Hemorrhage

Peribulbar hemorrhage is usually caused by trauma of the periorbita in the front portion of the orbit. This type of complication is less severe than intraconal or retrobulbar hemorrhage. However, the displacement of the eyeball leads to a secondary increase in pressure, which, in severe cases, is accompanied by traction or pressure to the optic nerve. Clinically, this leads to proptosis and a decrease in visual acuity.

Therapy

Treatment depends on the location of the hemorrhage. In lighter peribulbar bleedings without a disturbance of eye motility and without visual loss, conservative measures (cooling) can be sufficient. In peribulbar bleeding leading to proptosis, eyeball displacement, or even loss of vision, immediate endonasal orbital decompression is the treatment of choice. Targeted hemostasis by location of the retracted artery is not advisable, since it is rather difficult to find and the manipulation in the orbit leads to a further increase in pressure. Therefore, first a resection of the **orbital lamina of the ethmoid bone** and then the **slitting of the periorbita** should be performed in surgery. Necessary pressure relief can be achieved in this way. Lateral **canthotomy** and **cantholysis** are emergency procedures for additional pressure relief.[7] In retrobulbar or intraconal bleeding associated with a loss of visual acuity, the measures described are often not sufficient, indicating an additional decompression of the optic nerve.

Orbital Decompression

Resection of the Orbital Lamina of the Ethmoid Bone

First a resection of the ethmoidal cell system and exposure of the skull base is performed via an endonasal, transethmoidal approach. Then the orbital lamina of the ethmoid bone (lamina papyracea) is located in its entire anterior and posterior extension and resected.[8]

Slitting of the Periorbita

To achieve further decompression, the periorbita is slit from anterior, leading to a prolapse of orbital adipose tissue. This procedure ensures the endonasal drainage of the hematoma.

Lateral Canthotomy

If sufficient pressure relief cannot be achieved by the measures described above, a lateral canthotomy (widening of the canthus) is indicated. Some authors describe this as an emergency measure (▶ Fig. 6.1a).[2,9,10] Here, the soft tissue of the eye angle is transconjunctivally cut down to the bony orbital rim. According to the literature, an intraocular pressure reduction of about 14.2 mm Hg can be achieved with this measure.[11]

Cantholysis

During the subsequent inferior cantholysis the lateral palpebral ligament and the infra-orbital septum are transected to achieve a prolapse of orbital fat. This results in the retraction of the eye, leading to a further pressure reduction of about 30.4 mm Hg. A complementary method in which the upper, stronger proportion of the canthal tendon is cut ("superior cantholysis"; ▶ Fig. 6.1b) to achieve even further pressure relief has been described more recently. Pressure can be decreased by additional 19.2 mm Hg[11,12] using this method.

Decompression of the Optic Nerve

Endonasal decompression of the optic nerve can be performed with the aid of a microscope or an endoscope. After ethmoid and sphenoid sinus surgery, the bone shell of the optic nerve is located in the lateral sphenoid sinus wall and resected round a circumference of 180°. Afterwards, the nerve sheath is slit in order to relieve pressure. During sphenoid sinus surgery, attention should be paid to the internal carotid artery in the area of the lateral sphenoid sinus wall. The optic canal is located craniolateral to the internal carotid artery. Both structures are characterized by

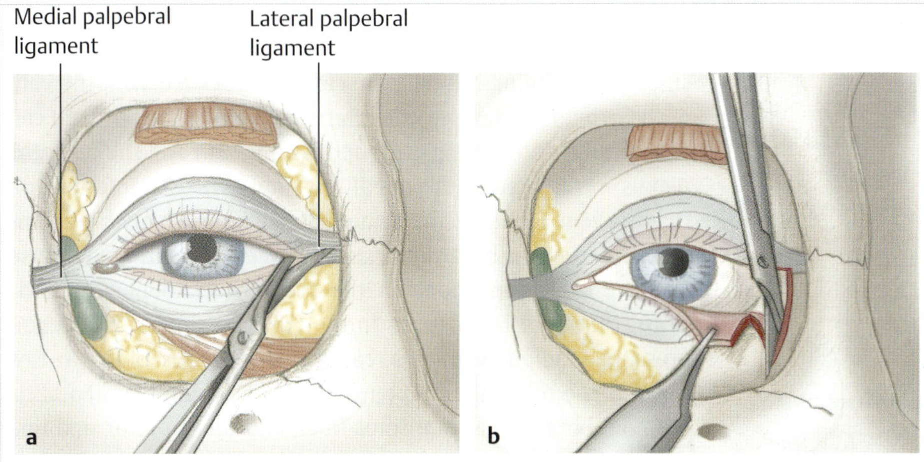

Fig. 6.1 Emergency procedures to relieve orbital pressure. (Reproduced from Strutz J, Mann W, eds. Praxis der HNO-Heilkunde, Kopf- und Halschirurgie. 2nd ed. Stuttgart: Thieme; 2010:459. Fig. 10:22.) **(a)** Lateral canthotomy. **(b)** Inferior cantholysis.

protrusions in the lateral sphenoid sinus wall. A triangular depression, usually found between the optic nerve channel and the internal carotid artery, can provide guidance (see Chapter 1). If possible, the decompression of the optic nerve should be performed using a computer-assisted navigation system.

Prognosis

If intraocular pressure is increased, relief within 24 hours is recommended. Due to a correlation between the duration of nerve injury and postoperative increase of visual acuity, pressure relieve within 8 hours is even better. The more quickly decompression occurs, the better the expected postoperative visual results.[8] With consistently combined conservative and surgical treatment, visual recovery is expected to range between 68% and 80%.[13,14]

> **Memorize** M!
>
> With a rate of 0.07%, iatrogenic hemorrhage in the course of sinus surgery is rare. Due to the anatomical location, bleeding of the anterior ethmoid artery occur more frequently than bleeding of the posterior ethmoid artery. This may result in an intraconal/retrobulbar or a peribulbar hematoma, while the first is considered to be the more serious complication. Prompt initiation of therapy possibly with surgical procedures (resection of the orbital lamina of the ethmoid bone, slitting of the periorbita, lateral canthotomy, cantholysis, or decompression of the optic nerve) is essential to counteract a permanent loss of vision and blindness.

6.2.2 Bleeding into the Orbit as a Result of Trauma

A cranial or craniocerebral trauma combined with fractures of the bony orbital walls that are associated with an additional injury of arteries can result in severe bleeding into the orbit.

Pathogenesis

In pathogenic terms there are basically two ways of posttraumatic hemorrhage into the orbit:

- The ruptured blood vessels (e.g., anterior/posterior ethmoid artery) retract into the eye socket and quickly cause an increase in intraorbital pressure due to acute bleeding.
- Fracture lines crossing arteries that run in bone canaliculi (e.g., the infra-orbital artery) can cause direct bleeding from the bone fragment into the orbit.

The compression of the optic nerve leads to nerve damage, which may be associated with loss of vision or even blindness (= orbital compartment syndrome) (see Chapter 2.3).

Bleedings from the **supra-orbital artery** can result from a fracture of the orbital roof. It arises from the ophthalmic artery, runs through the orbit, and exits through the supra-orbital rim via the supra-orbital foramen.

As part of a zygomatic fracture, the **infra-orbital artery**, a branch of the maxillary artery, can be injured in its course. The artery runs from the pterygopalatine fossa through the maxillary foramen and infra-orbital canal, to exit via the infra-orbital foramen. Le Fort II and III fractures as well as skull base fractures can also damage the infra-orbital artery, especially in the superior and inferior orbital fissures.

The **ophthalmic artery** may be injured in skull base fractures that run through the optic canal.

Escher III and IV fractures (skull base fractures) can result in injury of the **anterior** or **posterior ethmoid artery**. The anterior ethmoid artery arises from the ophthalmic artery and passes through the anterior ethmoidal foramen from the orbit into the cranial cavity. The posterior ethmoid artery is also a branch of the ophthalmic artery and runs through the posterior ethmoidal foramen from the orbit into the cranial cavity.

Clinical Symptoms

Clinically, the acute condition presents a rapidly progressing, hard swelling (on palpation) of the upper and/or lower eyelid with progressive exophthalmos. Ocular motility is initially unimpeded, but then quickly limited. The lid seems to be retracted due to the exophthalmos. After a while, a reddish-bluish tissue discoloration can be observed (monocular hematoma) (▶ Fig. 6.2). Visual acuity may decrease rapidly in acute hemorrhage.

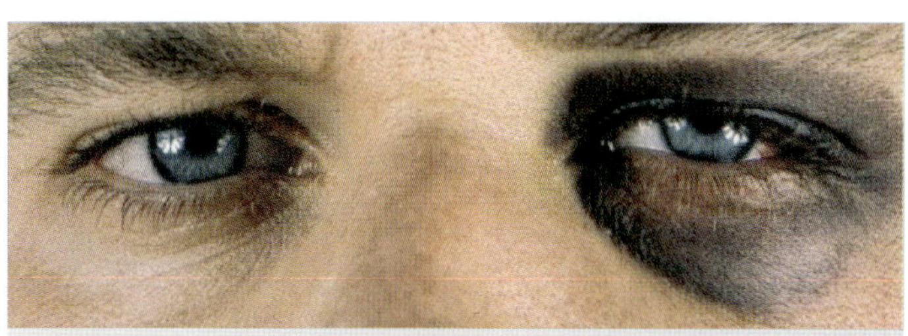

Fig. 6.2 Monocular hematoma (left).

Therapy

Like iatrogenic bleedings, traumatic bleeding into the orbit requires immediate endonasal orbital decompression, possibly also a decompression of the optic nerve by resection of the orbital lamina of the ethmoid bone, slotting of the periorbita, and where necessary also lateral canthotomy and cantholysis as well as decompression of the optic nerve (see "Therapy" in Chapter 6.2.1).

M!

Memorize:

- Supra-orbital artery: fracture of the orbital roof.
- Infra-orbital artery: zygomatic fracture, skull base fracture.
- Ophthalmic artery: skull base fracture through the optic canal.
- Anterior or posterior ethmoid artery: skull base fracture.

6

6.3 Orbital Complications of Acute Sinusitis

6.3.1 Pathogenesis

Orbital and intracranial complications can occur alongside acute sinusitis. Due to the close anatomical proximity, orbital complications are usually caused by an ethmoidal or frontal sinusitis (75%). Maxillary or sphenoid sinusitis is comparatively rare as a cause.[6] As the pathogenesis of sinogenic orbital complications is different in children, this topic will be discussed separately in Chapter 6.6.

A bacterial sinusitis episode is usually precipitated by an upper respiratory tract infection/rhinitis accompanied by sinusitis. Viral sinusitis are mostly caused by rhinoviruses (30–40%), less often also by coronaviruses, human parainfluenza viruses, human respiratory syncytial viruses, influenza viruses, adenoviruses, coxsackieviruses/echo viruses, and other viruses.[6] Bacterial sinusitis is usually a superinfection of a viral infection. The most common causative pathogens are *Streptococcus pneumoniae* (31%) and *Haemophilus influenzae* (21%). Anaerobes, *Staphylococcus aureus, Streptococcus pyogenes, Moraxella catarrhalis*, and gram-negative bacteria are found less frequently (▶ Table 6.1).[6,15]

Acute sinusitis has a multifactorial etiology but in most cases it is based on a ventilation disturbance of the sinuses due to a narrowing around the osteomeatal unit of the middle nasal meatus. Viral rhinitis leads to an edematous swelling of the mucosa around the sinus ostium with resultant secretion. It results in a local inflammatory response of the nasal sinuses and consecutive shift of the ostia.[6]

Table 6.1 Pathogens of acute bacterial sinusitis[6]

Pathogen	Frequency (%)
Streptococcus pneumoniae	31
Haemophilus influenzae	21
Anaerobes (e.g., Bacteroides, Peptostreptococcus, Fusobacterium)	6
Staphylococcus aureus	4
Streptococcus pyogenes	2
Moraxella catarrhalis	2
Gram-negative bacteria (e.g., *Pseudomonas aeruginosa, Klebsiella pneumoniae, Escherichia coli*)	9

The inflammation can be transferred to the orbit via bone gaps and blood vessels, especially through veins. Veins of the paranasal sinuses and the nasal cavity are closely associated with the veins of the orbit. For example, the ethmoidal vein of the ethmoid cells anastomose with the superior ophthalmic vein and the pterygoid plexus in the area of the maxillary sinus with the inferior ophthalmic vein. Orbital veins do not contain venous valves, enabling blood to flow in both directions between the ethmoid sinuses and the orbit dependent on the pressure gradient within the veins. During inflammations in the ethmoid sinuses, the venous pressure gradient increases, causing the venous blood to flow towards the orbit (see chapter 1.5.2).[16] The orbital lamina of the ethmoid bone, the frontal sinus floor, and the superior, and inferior orbital fissure are bony areas of predilection for inflammatory progression (▶ Fig. 6.3). The activation of an inflammatory cascade causes pressure to increase within the retrobulbar compartment, which might quickly be accompanied by optic nerve damage and amaurosis. On the other hand, bacterial toxins lead to direct nerve or dural sheath damage (optic neuritis) requiring immediate surgical source control (see Chapter 2).

6.3.2 Phases of Orbital Complications

The transfer of a sinogenic inflammation onto the orbit can result in various stages of orbital complications, while these stages can gradually evolve into each other or skip certain phases. Any orbital complication indicates an ophthalmological examination.

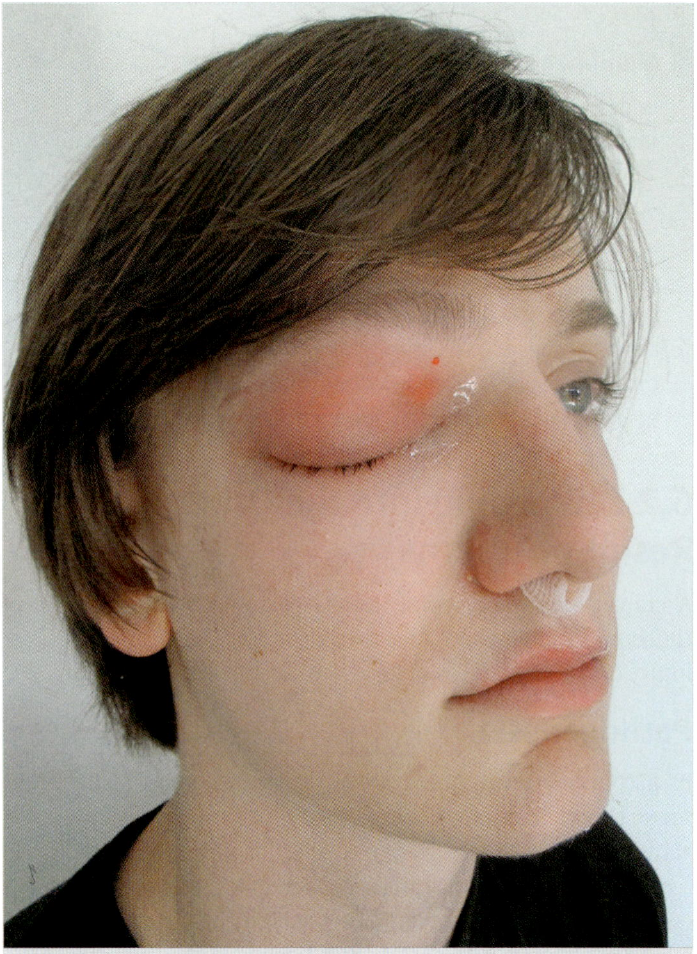

Fig. 6.3 Sinogenic genesis of orbital complication with swelling and redness of the upper lid.

Table 6.2 Overview of different classifications of orbital complications

Stage	Chandler (1970)[17]	Kastenbauer (1992)[18]	Stammberger (1993)[19]
I	Preseptal cellulitis	Orbital edema	Inflammatory eyelid edema
II	Orbital cellulitis	Orbital periostitis	Periorbital osteitis/ edema
III	Subperiostal abscess	Subperiosteal abscess	Subperiosteal abscess
IV	Orbital abscess	Orbital apex syndrome	Intraorbital infiltration/ abscess
V	Cavernosus sinus thrombosis	Orbital cellulitis	Cavernosus sinus thombosis

A number of different phase classifications for orbital complications can be found in the literature. ▶ Table 6.2 outlines three different classifications that are commonly used.

From the author's own experience, the following classification of orbital complications has proved to be useful.[6,8]

Stage I: Orbital edema

An orbital edema manifests clinically as an inflammatory, usually unilateral, upper and/or lower lid swelling during frontal or ethmoidal sinusitis. Soft tissue inflammation is limited to the anterior orbit ("preseptal cellulitis"). Ocular motility is unimpaired and visual acuity is not reduced. The eye can usually be actively opened.

Stage II: Periostitis of the orbit

Periostitis is characterized by a transfer of the inflammation to the periosteum of the orbit, resulting in a soft tissue edema behind the orbital septum (postseptal cellulitis; synonym, orbital cellulitis), which may lead to proptosis. Ocular motility may be painful yet not restricted. At this stage, visual impairment is not yet present. The eye can usually only be opened passively.

Stage III: Subperiosteal abscess

A subperiosteal abscess is defined as a withdrawal of the periorbita from the orbital lamina of the ethmoid bone due to an inflammatory infiltration. Displacement of the periorbita accompanies the abscess. The resulting motility disorder leads to double vision. Periostitis and a subperiosteal abscess are often clinically indistinguishable. Usually, the abscess becomes visible through computed tomography or magnetic resonance imaging (▶ Fig. 6.4).

Stage IV: Orbital abscess

Should a subperiosteal abscess spread to the periorbita it causes an orbital abscess, including motility disorders, diplopia, and visual loss. An orbital abscess can occur at multiple sites, both preseptal and postseptal (medial orbital wall, cranial to the eyelids, in the upper and/or lower eyelid, and in the lacrimal gland). The diagnosis of an orbital abscess requires a CT or MRI scan.

Stage V: Orbital cellulitis with orbital apex syndrome

An orbital abscess can transform into orbital cellulitis, leading to ophthalmoplegia due to paralysis of the cranial nerves II, III, IV, and VI, and can cause amaurosis. In pathogenic terms, this stage presents a breakthrough of the pus through the periorbita as a result of the subperiosteal orbital abscess. The inflammation then spreads very quickly to the orbital adipose tissue, muscles, and nervous structures (▶ Fig. 6.5).

M!

Memorize:

Orbital complications
- Stage I: Orbital edema
- Stage II: Periostitis of the orbit
- Stage III: Subperiosteal abscess
- Stage IV: Orbital abscess
- Stage V: Orbital cellulitis with orbital apex syndrome

(= ophthalmoplegia, amaurosis)

6.3.3 Therapy

Initiation of inpatient treatment is necessary as soon as any sinusitis causes orbital complications. Depending on the clinical symptoms, a conservative approach might be sufficient; otherwise, surgical procedures are indicated.

Conservative Treatment Measures

Conservative treatment includes mainly the treatment of the sinusitis itself with decongestant agents and intravenous antibiotic therapy.

Decongestion of nasal mucous membranes is achieved by inhalation with saline (3 times daily), 0.1% xylometazoline-containing nasal spray or gel (3 times daily), or the insertion of decongestant strips into the middle nasal meatus (2 times daily). Mucolytics such as acetylcysteine can be added for dissolution of mucus.

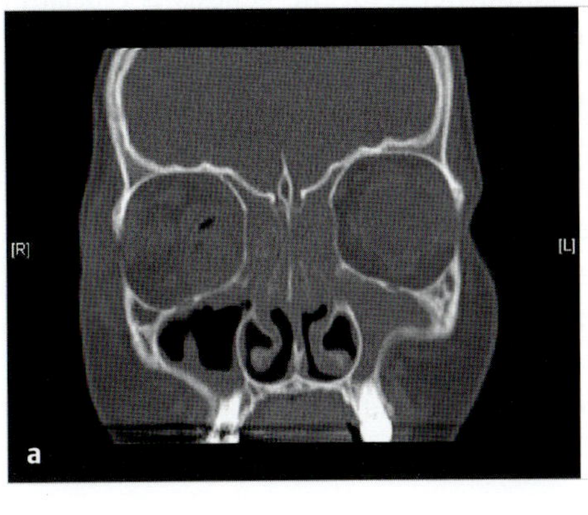

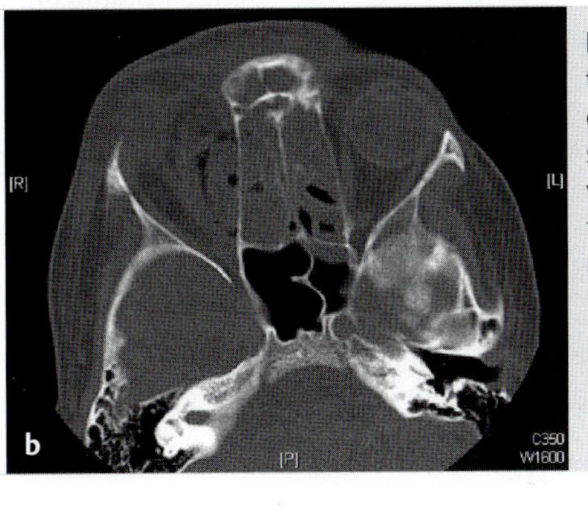

Fig. 6.4 CT scans of a subperiosteal abscess at the medial orbital wall on the right side, based on an adjacent ethmoid sinusitis. Air inclusions suggest gas-forming bacteria. **(a)** The coronal view presents the medial rectus muscle and the trochlear displaced laterally. A fine tissue lamella between the abscess and orbital content might indicate an intact periorbita. **(b)** The axial view presents the exophthalmos.

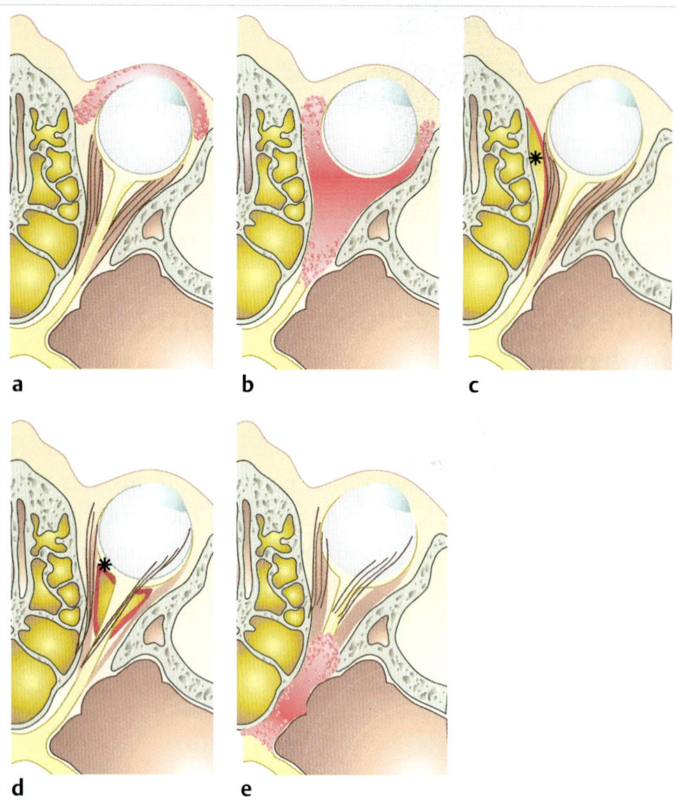

Fig. 6.5 Phases of orbital complication. (Reproduced from Strutz J, Mann W, eds. Praxis der HNO-Heilkunde, Kopf- und Halschirurgie. 2nd ed. Stuttgart: Thieme: 2010:439. Fig.10:14.)

Table 6.3 Therapeutic management of orbital complications due to an acute sinusitis according to stage of the disease

Stage	Conservative therapy	Surgical procedures
I	Decongestant agents	Progression at 24 hours despite conservative therapy: surgical source control
	Intravenous antibiotic therapy	
II	Decongestant agents	Progression at 24 hours despite conservative therapy: surgical source control
	Intravenous antibiotic therapy	
III	Intravenous antibiotic therapy	Indication of immediate surgical procedure: surgical source control
	Heparin	
	Intravenous corticoid therapy	
IV	Intravenous antibiotic therapy	Indication of immediate surgical procedure: endonasal orbital relief, eventually with additional transfacial access depending on abscess localization
	Heparin	
	Intravenous corticoid therapy	
V	Intravenous antibiotic therapy	Indication of immediate surgical procedure: endonasal orbital relief, eventually with additional transfacial access depending on abscess localization
	Heparin	
	Intravenous corticoid therapy	

Intravenous antibiotic therapy uses broad-spectrum penicillin (i.e., ampicillin + sulbactam) or—in patients with allergy to penicillin—with clindamycin as it reacts well with soft tissue and bony structures. (*Caution*: cross-reactivity between penicillins and cephalosporins is possible).

In stages I and II of orbital complications, conservative therapy can be sufficient at first. Since most of the stage I and II complications improve within 24 hours of consistent therapy, conservative management is justified. However, if progression of clinical symptoms including visual and/or motility loss and increased exophthalmos is observed after 24 hours, CT scanning of the paranasal sinus system and the optic nerve canal (axial and coronal planes) should be performed and surgical intervention is mandatory.[6]

In addition, intravenous cortisone therapy for additional detumescence and inflammatory reduction and application of heparin to prevent venous sinus thrombosis are recommended in stages III to V.

Surgical Treatment

The following clinical symptoms are an indication for surgical intervention:

- Deterioration of clinical findings within 24 hours.
- Visual loss.
- Impairment of eye motility.

Surgical procedures include sinus surgery as source control; abscess relief in cases of subperiostal or orbital abscess; and orbital decompression in cases of orbital cellulitis (▶ Table 6.3).

Prognosis

The prognosis in terms of postoperative visual improvement seems to be dependent on the following factors: initial blindness (complete loss of vision) indicates a negative prognosis; also a long interval before surgical intervention (> 48 hours) is associated with significant deterioration of visual recovery, a fact that is explained by the pathophysiological processes that take place during an inflammatory response of the optic nerve (see Chapter 2). With timely diagnosis and consistent treatment (intravenous antibiotic therapy and possibly surgical measures) the prognosis of visual loss in the context of an orbital abscess or orbital cellulitis is as high as a 68 to 100% recovery rate.[20,21,22,23,24]

6.4 Orbital Complications of Other Cause

Orbital complication can have other causes than traumatic, iatrogenic, or sinogenic ones. Knowledge of the genesis is crucial in order to be able to initiate appropriate therapeutic strategies.

6.4.1 Orbital Emphysema

Orbital emphysema describes an abnormal intraorbital accumulation of air. Due to the relatively loose tissue texture and numerous fascial spaces, air can spread throughout the entire orbit. The extent of emphysema, particularly retrobulbar and intraconal, is only visible via CT scan or MRI scan of the orbit.

Pathogenesis

A precondition for the emergence of orbital emphysema is a physical connection between intraorbital soft tissues and the air-filled spaces. The most common cause is a fracture of the bony medial and cranial orbital wall or of the orbital floor with subsequent opening to the sinus system.[25] Forceful nose blowing increases pressure into the sinuses, pushing air into orbital soft tissue. Hence, about 33% of skull base and craniocerebral trauma are accompanied by soft tissue emphysema.[26] Sporting activity is the second most common cause for the development of orbital emphysema. Weight training considerably tightens abdominal muscles[27]: this leads to pressure in the sinus system. Energy exceeding 2.08 J exerted on the orbital lamina of the ethmoid bone during this pressure increase cause to a fracture that allows air to enter into the orbit.[28] A similar mechanism is the cause for orbital emphysema resulting from heavy nose blowing or diving with hyperbaric breathing gas bottles, which can also trigger a fracture of the lamina papyracea.[29,30,31,32] Finally, accidents can also facilitate air entering into the orbit through the conjunctiva, for example, when working with machines that produce a strong air pressure (such as high-pressure air jets).[28] In those cases, however, lesions of the conjunctiva and the eyeball usually predominate.

Clinical Symptoms

Clinically, a soft and resilient swelling of the upper and lower lid is usually present. Palpation is mostly accompanied by typical tissue crepitation. Eyelid motility may be limited in cases with significant accumulations of air in the soft tissue of the eyelids, while ocular motility is generally neither obstructed nor painful. Invading air can have space-occupying effects, but the pressure generated in this way is often not sufficient to decrease visual acuity. In the context of emphysema this has been described only in case reports.[30,33,34] Key et al report three cases of orbital emphysema triggered by trauma that led to rapidly progressive visual loss and required immediate surgical decompression. Nonetheless, patients presenting with orbital emphysema should receive thorough clinical ophthalmologic examination.

Therapy

Orbital emphysema usually requires conservative therapy. Since there is a very high probability that fractures are followed by bacterial dissemination from intranasal sites via the sinuses into the orbit, treatment is recommended to include broad-spectrum antibiotics (e.g., aminopenicillins, cephalosporins, clindamycin) for 5 to 7 days, accompanied by cooling measures and the administration of a nonsteroidal, anti-inflammatory drugs such as ibuprofen (4 × 600 mg/day).[25,27,35] Orbital decompression is indicated only in exceptional circumstances, namely in the course of a rapid deterioration of vision.[32,34] The procedure corresponds to that described under "Therapy" in Chapter 6.2.1.

As an emergency procedure for immediate relief, some authors suggest the transpalpebral insertion of a large-caliber needle through which excess air can escape.[31]

The overall prognosis is positive. In most cases the resorption of excessive air takes up to a week. Loss of vision that initially necessitated surgical decompression is usually completely regressed with a full recovery of visual acuity.[34]

6.4.2 Dysthyroid Optic Neuropathy

A special form of orbital complication is dysthyroid optic neuropathy (DON), which can occur in course of active thyroid orbitopathy and may lead to a rapid loss of vision requiring immediate surgical treatment. The loss of vision often represents the most serious symptom for patients.[36]

Pathogenesis

Endocrine orbitopathy is an autoimmune disease characterized by the proliferation of retrobulbar adipose tissue and a thickening of the extraocular muscles due to myositis. A detailed discussion of the disease's pathogenesis is given in Chapter 7, so it is only briefly mentioned here. The consequence of these mechanisms is a massive increase in intrabulbar and intraocular pressure. At the same time, the venous pressure in the superior ophthalmic vein increases, which may contribute to a further elevation of intraocular pressure.[37] All the elevated pressure gradients act on the optic nerve and this results in proptosis-induced stress on the nerve.[38] In about 5% of cases, this leads to the development of dysthyroid optic neuropathy characterized by a rapid loss of vision, among other things.[38] From a pathogenetic view, the two factors—pressure increase and autoimmunologically triggered inflammatory response—act on the optic nerve during the deterioration of visual acuity.

Clinical Symptoms

The prominent clinical symptoms of active Graves's ophthalmopathy include chemosis, upper lid retraction, proptosis, and ocular motility disorders. The intraocular pressure is increased. Within only a few days, deterioration of visual acuity or even blindness may also occur.

Therapy

High-dose corticosteroids are administered over a period of 3 to 4 days.[39] Additionally, orbital decompression is indicated for improvement or recovery of visual acuity if no significant improvement is achieved by corticosteroid treatment within 1 to 2 weeks.[38] This reduces pressure on the nerve and leads to almost normal blood flow in the superior ophthalmic vein.[37] Despite these therapeutic procedures, the prognosis regarding visual recovery is uncertain. If there has been a loss of vision during DON prior to the initiation of therapy, the rate of complete remission is about 40%.[39]

6.4.3 Dentogenic Abscesses

Pathogenesis

After sinogenic causes, dentogenic processes are the second most common cause of orbital complications. Most of these abscesses are triggered by the following[40]:

- Mouth–antrum connection after dental procedures.
- Periapical periodontitis (acute apical inflammation).
- Deep marginal periodontitis (chronic apical inflammation).
- Alveolitis (inflammation of bony tooth socket) after tooth extraction in the upper jaw.
- Submucosal abscess.

- Infected implants.
- Over pressed filling material after a dental root canal treatment.
- Iatrogenic origin from excessive pushing of instruments in dental root canal treatment.
- Traumatic damage to the front teeth of the upper jaw.
- Dentogenic maxillary sinusitis.
- Infected odontogenic maxillary cysts that have grown in the maxillary sinus (radicular, follicular, or occlusion cysts).
- Odontogenic tumors.

Often the third molar of the mandible or maxilla (37.5%), the first molar of the maxilla (12.5%), or the second molar of the lower jaw (12.5%) is the origin of infection.[41] The root tip of the maxillary canine extends almost up to the orbit (which is why it is also called the "eye tooth") and is often the focus of an orbital complication.[41]

6

The infection is usually a secondary infection that is transferred to the orbit either hematogenously, lymphogenously, or by continuity through bone gaps on the maxillary sinus and the orbital floor (see Chapter 6.2.1).[41]

The polymicrobial bacterial spectrum of odontogenic inflammation usually differs from the spectrum of sinogenic orbital abscesses. It comprises aerobic bacteria such as streptococci and staphylococci and anaerobic bacteria, predominantly oral pathogenic anaerobes such as *Peptostreptococcus, Fusobacterium*, and *Prevotella* species.[40,42]

Clinical Symptoms

Typical symptoms are toothache and headache as well as increased body temperature. Clinically, usually swelling and reddening of the cheek and/or the lower lid is observed with the possibility of upper lid edema. Affected teeth are touch-sensitive and cause headaches. Depending on the inflammatory stage, the development of chemosis, proptosis, dysmotility or even amaurosis and ophthalmoplegia is possible.

Therapy

Axial and coronal CT scans of the paranasal sinus system are essential for assessing the anatomy and the extent of the complication,. Intravenous antibiotic therapy should be initiated using aminopenicillin with a β-lactamase inhibitor, possibly combined with metronidazole. Lincosamides (e.g., clindamycin) can be used as an alternative.[40,41,42] Surgical therapy includes elimination of the focus of infection with tooth extraction or root resection and abscess drainage performed by a dental surgeon or an oral and maxillofacial surgeon.[40,41] In cases where the inflammation leads to the formation of an abscess in the orbit or to orbital cellulitis, procedures referred to under "Surgical treatment" in Chapter 6.3.3 are to be carried out as well.

6.4.4 Infection of the Cheek Skin

Pathogenesis

An infection in the facial area (skin injury, furuncle, atheroma, etc.) can act as an access point for the transmission of an inflammation to the internal structure of the orbit and cause swelling around the eye. Bacteria such as staphylococci and streptococci are usually detectable. The inflammation is transmitted through the bloodstream, usually venous, to the internal structures of the orbit, where it can cause orbital complications. It should be noted that the transition of inflammations through the angular vein can cause venous sinus thrombosis and thrombophlebitic sepsis.[43]

Clinical Symptoms

The clinical picture shows classical signs of inflammation, such as pain, swelling, redness, and warmth in the access area as well as swelling of the affected eyelids, which can be associated with chemosis. In advanced stages, the inflammation can manifest itself in erysipelas or abscess formation.[43]

Therapy

The focus of therapeutic procedures is on intravenous antibiotic therapy with a broad-spectrum penicillin (e.g., ampicillin + sulbactam) or alternatively with clindamycin. Incision for pus drainage is necessary in treating abscesses.

6.4.5 Dacryoadenitis

Pathogenesis

Dacryoadenitis is an inflammation of the lacrimal gland. Two different types are distinguished [44]:

- Acute dacryoadenitis: acute, infectious, usually unilateral (exception: infection with mumps).
- Chronic dacryoadenitis: chronic, noninfectious, usually bilateral.

Acute dacryoadenitis is often associated with a common cold or flu, but it might also be predisposed by a preexisting immune deficiency. Acute inflammation is usually of bacterial origin. Typical bacteria are staphylococci, streptococci, and pneumococci. Viruses, such as mumps and measles virus, influenza virus, herpes simplex/zoster, and the Epstein–Barr virus are less common.[44]

Systemic diseases (e.g., sarcoidosis, Wegener's granulomatosis, Sjögren's syndrome, amyloidosis) in the course of tuberculosis or leukemia or triggered by an orbital pseudotumor are examples of causes of **chronic dacryoadenitis**.[44]

Clinical Symptoms

The main symptoms of dacryoadenitis are epiphora and often conjunctivitis. Pressure-sensitivity and redness and swelling of the upper eyelid are common, the latter presenting the typical paragraph form (▶ Fig. 6.6). Motility disorders and proptosis are also possible. A fulminant course may lead to orbital cellulitis. Differential diagnosis should also consider a phlegmon of the upper lid, for example, after superficial skin injuries.[44,45]

Therapy

The form of treatment depends on the underlying disease. For an infectious origin, local treatment with antibiotic drops (e.g., gentamycin, neomycin, or ofloxacin) and disinfectant envelopes might be sufficient, or, depending on the progression of the disease, systemic antibiotic treatment with a broad-spectrum penicillin (e.g., ampicillin + sulbactam), a cephalosporin, or clindamycin is indicated.[44,45] Colliquation with abscess formation, both well visualized sonographically, requires surgical abscess incision.

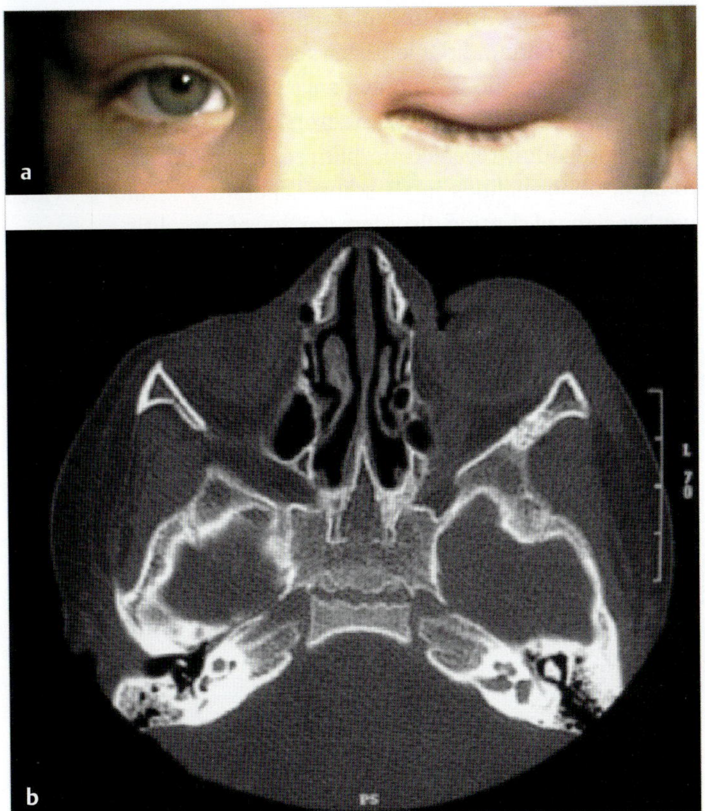

Fig. 6.6 Dacryoadenitis on the left eye. **(a)** Paragraph form of the upper lid due to a dacryoadenitis. **(b)** CT scan of paranasal sinuses in axial plane with visible swelling in the left lacrimal gland.

6.4.6 Insect Bites

Pathogenesis

Insect bites can be primary or secondary causes of a local inflammatory response and a resulting orbital complication:

- **Primary inflammation:** direct effect of a pollutant (e.g., insect toxin) on the tissue.
- **Secondary inflammation:** indirect effect of bacterial superinfection on the tissue.

Clinical Symptoms

Depending on the localization of insect bites, orbital structures can be involved, including painfully restricted lid opening as well as abscess formation or even periocular necrotizing fasciitis.[46]

Primary Inflammation

A **slight local reaction** shows a reddened, painful swelling in the area of the bite, which is usually less than 10 cm in diameter and declines within 24 hours.[47]

Severe local reactions present swellings of more than 10 cm that can persist for days and are accompanied by lymphadenitis and a deteriorating general condition. These reactions are likely of allergic nature, but not IgE-mediated. They occur in up to 25% of the population.[47]

It is only on very rare occasions that insect bites cause illnesses that might be fatal (rhabdomyolysis, hemolysis, cerebral disorders, hepatic and renal damage).[47]

Secondary Inflammation

If a secondary infection of an insect bite develops, overheating accompanied by a phlegmonous or suppurative soft tissue inflammation can follow in addition to the clinical picture described above.

Therapy

Primary Inflammation

Local treatment of an insect bite includes topical corticosteroid cream or gel. Oral administration of an antihistamine (H_1-blocker) may be added. A severe organ disease requires systemic and symptomatic therapy.[47]

Secondary Inflammation

If an insect bite developed into a bacterial superinfection, intravenous antibiotic therapy with broad-spectrum penicillin (e.g., ampicillin + sulbactam), a cephalosporin, or clindamycin should be induced. Surgical intervention is necessary in case of abscess formation (see Chapter 6.4.4).

6.4.7 Allergic Diseases

Pathogenesis

Allergic blepharitis (= contact dermatitis) is caused by a cell-mediated antigen–antibody reaction that is usually a late-phase response. Preservatives in cosmetics, eye drops, or ointments are the most common triggering allergens.[48]

A special form of allergic reaction is **angioedema** (Quincke's edema), an acute-response type. It presents acute swelling of the subcutaneous tissue and submucosal layer due to the activation of the bradykinin leading to vasodilation. An ACE inhibitor can be a triggering agent. Hereditary angioedema is based on a deficiency of C1-esterase inhibitors.[49]

Clinical Symptoms

Blepharitis presents edematous red swelling that usually affects the upper and lower lids. The skin appears to be crinkled like parchment. In course of the disease it changes in a flaky manner. These symptoms are accompanied by painful tension and itching of the skin.[48]

Angioedema, on the other hand, leads to an elastic, painless, nonitching swelling. It can occur on any part of the body but often affects the face and mucous membranes of the respiratory tract.[43] A life-threatening airway obstruction with suffocation should always be considered.

Therapy

The treatment of choice for **allergic blepharitis** includes the reduction of allergic reactions by avoidance of allergens as well as administration of corticoid ointments.[48]

Very strong allergic reactions and **angioedema** might indicate an additional application of intravenous corticosteroids, antihistamines and, if necessary, substitution of a C1 esterase inhibitor. If the edema is suspected to be ACE inhibitor-induced, use should be discontinued permanently.[43]

6.4.8 Conjunctivitis

Pathogenesis

Conjunctivitis is an inflammation of the conjunctiva of the eye of *infectious* or *noninfectious* causes. It can be classified into different categories, the following being the most common types[49,50]:

- **Bacterial conjunctivitis**: usually caused by staphylococci, streptococci, and pneumococci or by chlamydiae.
- **Viral conjunctivitis (= epidemic keratoconjunctivitis)**: frequent in infections with adenovirus type 8 or 19.
- **Mycotic and parasitic conjunctivitis**: caused, inter alia, by *Candida albicans*, *Aspergillus*, *Acanthamoeba*, *Microsporidium* and *Leishmania*. These organisms play a minor role and are rather rare in civilized countries.
- **Mechanically induced conjunctivitis**: external stimuli as well as dry conjunctiva are triggers for this kind of conjunctivitis.
- **Allergic conjunctivitis**: of special importance for patients with atopy in reaction to seasonal pollen allergies with rhinoconjunctivitis. Animal hair, cosmetics, and drugs can also be causative allergens.

Clinical symptoms

Typical symptoms of conjunctivitis are[49,50]:

- Pain, foreign-body sensation and itching.
- Hyperemia (redness of the conjunctiva).
- Purulent secretion.
- Chemosis (conjunctival swelling).
- Epiphora (excessive lacrimation).
- Pseudoptosis (narrowing of the palpebral fissure).
- Photophobia (aversion to light).
- Blepharospasm (eyelid squint).
- Possible formation of membranous and pseudomembranous deposits and blisters.

Therapy

Treatment depends on the inflammatory cause. Cooling packs and artificial lacrimal fluid can support all kinds of symptom relief.

In uncomplicated progressions of **bacterial conjunctivitis**, local antibiotic therapy (ointments, drops; e.g., using gentamicin, neomycin, or ofloxacin) leads to rapid improvement. Cortisone-containing combination drugs (e.g. dexamethasone) can be added.[49] Chlamydial conjunctivitis is treated locally and systemically with tetracyclines. If the disease takes a therapy-resistant, progressive course, systemic treatment with a broad-spectrum antibiotic (e.g., ampicillin + sulbactam) should be induced. **Viral conjunctivitis**, however, usually heals without any specific treatment.[49]

6.4.9 An Unusual Cause for an Orbital Complication

Lourdes Del Rosso and colleagues report an unusual case of orbital complication.[51] A 63-year-old man with multiple nonsurgical medical conditions took, among other things, 1 × 325 mg aspirin and 1 × 75 mg clopidogrel for 2 years on a daily basis. For the last two months of observation he supplemented his diet with a daily dosage of 1 × 1000 IU vitamin E and fish oil. Also suffering from obstructive sleep apnea syndrome (OSAS), he used a CPAP (continuous positive airway pressure) mask at night for 5 years without any problems. Then unexplained periorbital skin hematoma occurred, first around the left later also around the right eye. The patient's history showed no evidence suggesting problems with the CPAP mask, trauma, physical exertion, pain, or other discomfort. Examination revealed no blurred vision, no further hematoma or abnormalities in CT scans. Laboratory results provided neither signs of clotting disorders nor any of vasculitis.

Pathogenesis

The authors assume that a combination of various factors was responsible for the hematoma. Since both vitamin E and fish oil (omega-3 fatty acids) have anticoagulant properties, the intake combined with the antiplatelet drugs aspirin and clopidogrel may have led to an additionally increased risk of bleeding. Due to the CPAP mask, the hydrostatic pressure in the central ophthalmic vein could have been increased, leading to periorbital capillary damage. After the intake of vitamin E and fish oil was discontinued, the hematoma regressed and no further bleeding occurred.

Therapy

Patients presenting facial hematomas associated with a CPAP mask should be checked for increased bleeding tendency. A combined intake of anticoagulants with vitamin E and fish oil should be indicated only cautiously. Even at low pressure, CPAP masks can cause facial hematoma in patients taking anticoagulant drugs or anticoagulant nutritional supplements.

6.5 Summary

A summary of the main orbital complications is given in ▶ Table 6.4.

6.6 Special Features of Orbital Complications in Children

With an incidence of 3%, orbital complications are more likely to appear in children than in adults.[52,53] In children, these often accompany acute sinusitis.[54,55] However, sinogenic causes are not always the trigger, so that a precise patient history as well as the correct diagnosis is of crucial importance.[55,56,57] Differential diagnosis in children should also consider dacryocystitis, odontogenic causes, insect bites, allergic reactions, trauma or an orbital tumor.[58,59] Chronic rhinitis, frequently in children, can be mistaken for sinogenic causes.[58]

The cause of the orbital complication has to be uncovered as part of an interdisciplinary study (i.e., pediatrician, otolaryngologist, ophthalmologist, dentist). ENT analysis should always include an endoscopic examination of the nose, in this case especially of the middle nasal meatus. If the endoscopy shows pus in the middle nasal meatus, the child has a fever, and laboratory inflammation parameters are also elevated (CRP, leukocytes), it most likely indicates a focus in the sinuses.[60] Children usually present an ethmoid sinusitis, due to specifics characteristic of the development of the sinus system. Ethmoid sinuses are already developed at birth, but the maxillary and frontal sinuses are only fully developed by the age of 10 to 12 years.[55,61,62] The most common organisms of pediatric rhinosinusitis are *Streptococcus*

Table 6.4 Summary of significant orbital complications

Complication	Cause	Pathogenesis	Symptoms	Therapy
Hematoma	Hemorrhage	• Accidental • Iatrogenic (FESS) • Spontaneous	• Pressure increase • Orbital compartment syndrome • Exophthalmos • Blindness	• Lateral canthotomy • Cantholysis • Endonasal orbital decompression
Inflammation	Transmission of an inflammation	Spread of a bacterial infection (sinogenic, odontogenic)	• Stage I (orbital edema) • Stage II (periostitis) • Stage III (subperiosteal abscess) • Stage IV (orbital abscess) • Stage V (orbital cellulitis; apex orbit syndrome)	• Intravenous antibiotic therapy • CT scans of paranasal sinuses • Operative elimination of the cause of inflammation
Emphysema	Entrance of air into the orbit	• Traumatic (fractures) • Iatrogenic	Soft tissue emphysema, rarely with space-occupying effects and visual disturbance	Cooling; rarely operative procedures necessary for relief
Dysthyroid optic neuropathy (DON)	Autoimmune disease (hyperthyroidism)	• Auto-immunologically induced inflammation of the extraocular muscles (myositis) • Proliferation of retrobulbar adipose tissue • Pressure increase	• Ocular motility disorder • Rapid visual loss • Chemosis • Exophthalmos	• Corticosteroids • Orbital decompression
Conjunctivitis	Inflammation of the conjunctiva	• Bacterial • Viral • Mycotic, parasitic • Allergic • Mechanical	• Itching • Hyperemia • Epiphora • Blepharospasm • Purulent secretion	• Antibiotic eye drops • Systemic antibiotic therapy • If necessary, operative abscess drainage
Dacryoadenitis	Inflammation of the lacrimal gland	• Acute: infectious (bacterial/ viral) • Chronic: noninfectious (systemic disease, tubercu-losis, leukemia, orbital pseudotumor)	• Epiphora • Signs of inflammation and paragraph form of the upper lid • Caution: upper lid abscess, or • -phlegmon	• Antibiotic eye drops • Systemic antibiotic therapy • If necessary, operative abscess drainage
Allergic reaction	1. Allergic eyelid eczema (allergens) 2. Angioedema (ACE-inhibitors, C1-esterase-inhibitor deficiency)	Allergic reaction: 1. Acute response - type I 2. Late phase response - type IV	1. Painfully itchy eyelid eczema 2. Painless nonitching facial edema	• Allergen avoidance • Corticosteroids • Antihistamines • C1-esterase-inhibitors

pneumoniae (36%) and *Haemophilus influenzae* (23%). *Moraxella catarrhalis* is more common in children (19%) than in adults (2%). If the focus is odontogenic, mostly anaerobic bacteria such as bacteroides, fusobacteria, and peptostreptococci are detectable.[6]

All children clinically presenting an orbital complication should be hospitalized and receive intravenous antibiotic therapy; see Chapter 6.3.3. A progression of the disease despite 24 hours of conservative therapy, restricted eye motility, and loss of vision or abscess formation visible on MRI or CT scans is an indication for immediate surgery.[54,58,62,63,64,65,66,67,68,69] If not already done, preoperative imaging (MRI or CT) is required.

CT scanning in children is a matter of critical discussion because of considerations of radiation exposure. CT, in contrast to magnetic resonance imaging allows for an exact evaluation of osseous structures. However, radiation exposure can induce cataract formation, brain tumors, or leukemia, especially in small children. The cumulative dose of two or three CT head examinations (~60 mGy) can triple the risk of developing a brain tumor; that of 5 to 10 CT examinations can triple the risk of leukemia.[70,71] Radiation dosage should therefore be reduced to a minimum. Beside the MRI and low-dose CT programs, digital volume tomography (DVT) is an imaging alternative that has an effective dosage of ~0.3 mSv.[72,73]

In a study by Welkoborsky and colleagues, 49 children were hospitalized and treated for eye swelling.[61] Of these children, 18 (36.7%) developed an orbital complication due to acute sinusitis. 21 children (61%) showed orbital swelling of nonsinogenic inflammatory origin (infected sebaceous cyst, infected insect bites, herpes simplex infection with bacterial superinfection, conjunctivitis, or odontogenic focus) that also required a comprehensive diagnostic evaluation and therapy; 4 children (8.2%) presented a facial trauma; 3 children (6.1%) suffered from an orbital tumor (hemangioma, undifferentiated sarcoma, glioma). In 2 other children (4.1%), allergic rhinosinusitis caused the orbital swelling, and in 1 child (2.0%) an intraorbital foreign body (a piece of wood) was responsible for the orbital complication.

Thus, orbital complications in children are challenging since they can be caused by many diseases. Careful clinical evaluation and anamnesis with the collaboration of parents is mandatory in uncovering the exact cause, which is crucial for consequent therapy.

References

[1] Ramakrishnan VR, Kingdom TT, Nayak JV, Hwang PH, Orlandi RR. Nationwide incidence of major complications in endoscopic sinus surgery. Int Forum Allergy Rhinol. 2012; 2(1):34–39

[2] Maharshak I, Hoang JK, Bhatti MT. Complications of vision loss and ophthalmoplegia during endoscopic sinus surgery. Clin Ophthalmol. 2013; 7:573–580

[3] Dalgorf DM, Sacks R, Wormald PJ, et al. Image-guided surgery influences perioperative morbidity from endoscopic sinus surgery: a systematic review and meta-analysis. Otolaryngol Head Neck Surg. 2013; 149(1):17–29

[4] Keerl R, Weber R, Drees G, Draf W. [Individual learning curves with reference to endonasal micro-endoscopic pan-sinus operation]. Laryngorhinootologie. 1996; 75(6):338–343

[5] Lisbona Alquezar MP, Fernández Liesa R, Lorente Muñoz A, et al. [Anterior ethmoidal artery at ethmoidal labyrinth: Bibliographical review of anatomical variants and references for endoscopic surgery]. Acta Otorrinolaringol Esp. 2010; 61(3):202–208

[6] Kühnel T. Nase und Nasennebenhöhlen. In: Strutz J, Mann W, eds. Praxis der HNO-Heilkunde, Kopf- und Halschirurgie. 2nd ed. Stuttgart: Thieme; 2010:395–469

[7] Oester AE, Jr, Fowler BT, Fleming JC. Inferior orbital septum release compared with lateral canthotomy and cantholysis in the management of orbital compartment syndrome. Ophthal Plast Reconstr Surg. 2012; 28(1):40–43

[8] Strutz J, Welkoborsky H-J. Chirurgische Therapie der Orbita. In: Strutz J, Mann W, eds. Praxis der HNO-Heilkunde, Kopf- und Halschirurgie. 2nd ed. Stuttgart: Thieme; 2010:778–789

[9] Lima V, Burt B, Leibovitch I, Prabhakaran V, Goldberg RA, Selva D. Orbital compartment syndrome: the ophthalmic surgical emergency. Surv Ophthalmol. 2009; 54(4):441–449

[10] Saussez S, Choufani G, Brutus JP, Cordonnier M, Hassid S. Lateral canthotomy: a simple and safe procedure for orbital haemorrhage secondary to endoscopic sinus surgery. Rhinology. 1998; 36(1):37–39

[11] Yung CW, Moorthy RS, Lindley D, Ringle M, Nunery WR. Efficacy of lateral canthotomy and cantholysis in orbital hemorrhage. Ophthal Plast Reconstr Surg. 1994; 10(2):137–141

[12] Anderson RL. Medial canthal tendon branches out. Arch Ophthalmol. 1977; 95(11):2051–2052

[13] Chen YA, Singhal D, Chen YR, Chen CT. Management of acute traumatic retrobulbar haematomas: a 10-year retrospective review. J Plast Reconstr Aesthet Surg. 2012; 65(10):1325–1330

[14] Han JK, Caughey RJ, Gross CW, Newman S. Management of retrobulbar hematoma. Am J Rhinol. 2008; 22(5):522–524

[15] Aring AM, Chan MM. Acute rhinosinusitis in adults. Am Fam Physician. 2011; 83(9):1057–1063

[16] Gonsch G. Einflussfaktoren auf den Verlauf und die Therapie orbitaler Komplikationen bei Sinusitis [Dissertation]. Würzburg: Bayerischen Julius-Maximilians-Universität Würzburg; 2007:10

[17] Chandler JR, Langenbrunner DJ, Stevens ER. The pathogenesis of orbital complications in acute sinusitis. Laryngoscope. 1970; 80(9):1414–1428

[18] Kastenbauer E. Komplikationen der Entzündungen der Nasennebenhöhlen und des Oberkiefers. In: Naumann HH, Helms J, Herberhold C, Kastenbauer E, eds, Oto-Rhino-Laryngologie in Klinik und Praxis. Vol 2. Stuttgart: Thieme; 1992:234–246

[19] Stammberger H. Komplikationen entzündlicher Nasennebenhöhlenerkrankungen einschließlich iatrogen bedingter Komplikationen. Eur Arch Otorhinolaryngol. 1993 Suppl I:4–15

[20] Balogun BG, Balogun MM, Adekoya BJ. Orbital cellulitis: clinical course and management challenges. the Lagos State University Teaching Hospital experience. Nig Q J Hosp Med. 2012; 22(4):231–235

[21] Ben Amor M, Khalifa Z, Romdhane N, et al. [Orbital complications of sinusitis]. J Fr Ophtalmol. 2013; 36(6):488–493

[22] De Melo WM, Sonoda CK, Hochuli-Vieira E, Gabrielli MA, Gabrielli MF. Paranasal sinus infection causing orbital subperiosteal abscess: surgical management of this devastating entity. Oral Maxillofac Surg. 2013; 17(2):131–135

[23] Serra EC, Sverzut CE, Trivellato AE. Orbital abscess after facial trauma. Braz Dent J. 2009; 20(4):341–346

[24] Khalifa BC. Extent of resection of the lamina papyracea in medial subperiosteal abscess. Otolaryngol Head Neck Surg. 2011; 145(1):161–164

[25] Ababneh OH. Orbital, subconjunctival, and subcutaneous emphysema after an orbital floor fracture. Clin Ophthalmol. 2013; 7:1077–1079

[26] Karabekir HS, Gocmen-Mas N, Emel E, et al. Ocular and periocular injuries associated with an isolated orbital fracture depending on a blunt cranial trauma: anatomical and surgical aspects. J Craniomaxillofac Surg. 2012; 40(7): e189–e193

[27] Ozdemir O. Orbital emphysema occurring during weight lifting. Semin Ophthalmol. 2015; 30(5–6):426–428

[28] Hwang K, Kim DH, Lee HS. Orbital fracture due to high-pressure air injection. J Craniofac Surg. 2011; 22(4):1506–1507

[29] Bolognini A, Delehaye E, Cau M, Cosso L. Barotraumatic orbital emphysema of rhinogenic origin in a breath-hold diver: a case report. Undersea Hyperb Med. 2008; 35(3):163–167

[30] Furlani BdeA, Diniz B, Bitelli LG, Martins EN. [Sight-threatening orbital emphysema after nose blowing: case report]. Arq Bras Oftalmol. 2009; 72(2): 251–253

[31] Singh M, Phua VM, Sundar G. Sight-threatening orbital emphysema treated with needle decompression. Clin Experiment Ophthalmol. 2007; 35(4):386–387

[32] Al-Shammari L, Majithia A, Adams A, Chatrath P. Tension pneumo-orbit treated by endoscopic, endonasal decompression: case report and literature review. J Laryngol Otol. 2008; 122(3):e8

[33] Key SJ, Ryba F, Holmes S, Manisali M. Orbital emphysema - the need for surgical intervention. J Craniomaxillofac Surg. 2008; 36(8):473–476

[34] Chaudhry IA, Al-Amri A, Shamsi FA, Al-Rashed W. Visual recovery after evacuation of orbital emphysema. Orbit. 2007; 26(4):283–285

[35] Hiraoka T, Ogami T, Okamoto F, Oshika T. Compressed air blast injury with palpebral, orbital, facial, cervical, and mediastinal emphysema through an eyelid laceration: a case report and review of literature. BMC Ophthalmol. 2013; 13:68

[36] Du Y, Ye H, Li K, et al. Vision-related quality of life tends to be more severely impaired in patients with dysthyroid optic neuropathy. Curr Eye Res. 2014; 39(5):532–536

[37] Onaran Z, Konuk O, Oktar SO, Yücel C, Unal M. Intraocular pressure lowering effect of orbital decompression is related to increased venous outflow in Graves orbitopathy. Curr Eye Res. 2014; 39(7):666–672

[38] Cascone P, Rinna C, Reale G, Calvani F, Iannetti G. Compression and stretching in Graves orbitopathy: emergency orbital decompression techniques. J Craniofac Surg. 2012; 23(5):1430–1433

[39] Currò N, Covelli D, Vannucchi G, et al. Therapeutic outcomes of high-dose intravenous steroids in the treatment of dysthyroid optic neuropathy. Thyroid. 2014; 24(5):897–905

[40] Wandasiewicz IT. Die funktionelle Behandlung bei der dentogenen Sinusitis maxillaris [Dissertation]. Graz: Medizinische Universität Graz; 2008:46–80

[41] Schmelzle R, Heiland M. Weichteilinfektionen. In: Schwenzer N, Ehrenfeld M, eds. Zahnärztliche Chirurgie—Zahn-Mund-Kiefer-Heilkunde. 4th ed. Stuttgart: Thieme; 2009:119–121

[42] AWMF online. Leitlinien Nr. 007/086: Odontogene Sinusitis maxillaris. Available at: http://www.awmf.org/uploads/tx_szleitlinien/007-086_S2_Sinusitis_maxillaris_abgelaufen.pdf. Accessed August 10, 2016

[43] Hintschich C. Lidschwellungen. In: Kampik A, Grehn F, eds. Augenärztliche Differentialdiagnose. 2nd ed. Stuttgart: Thieme; 2008:97–121

[44] Wagner P, Lang GK. Tränenorgane. In: Lang GK, eds. Augenheilkunde. 5th ed. Stuttgart: Thieme; 2010:62

[45] Fechner UP, Teichmann KD, eds. Medikamentöse Augentherapie. 4th ed. Stuttgart: Thieme; 2000:267–268

[46] Poitelea C, Wearne MJ. Periocular necrotising fasciitis–a case report. Orbit. 2005; 24(3):215–217

[47] Przybilla B, Ruëff F. Insektenstiche: Klinisches Bild und Management. Dtsch Arztebl Int. 2012; 109(13):238–248

[48] Wagner P, Lang GK. Lider (Palpebrae). In: Lang GK, ed. Augenheilkunde. 5th ed. Stuttgart: Thieme; 2010:40

[49] Lang GK, Lang GE. Bindehaut (Konjunktiva). In: Lang GK, ed. Augenheilkunde. 5th ed. Stuttgart: Thieme; 2010:70–81

[50] Heiligenhaus A, Rösel M. Konjunktivitis. In: Kampik A, Grehn F, eds. Augenärztliche Differentialdiagnose. 2nd ed. Stuttgart: Thieme; 2008:74–88

[51] DelRosso L, McCarty DE, Hoque R. "Why did my CPAP beat me up?" Bilateral periorbital ecchymosis associated with continuous positive airway pressure therapy. J Clin Sleep Med. 2012; 8(6):730–732

[52] Hicks CW, Weber JG, Reid JR, Moodley M. Identifying and managing intracranial complications of sinusitis in children: a retrospective series. Pediatr Infect Dis J. 2011; 30(3):222–226

[53] Giusan AO, Kubanova AA, Uzdenova RKh. [Rhinosinusogenic orbital complications: the prevalence and principles of treatment]. Vestn Otorinolaringol. 2010; 4(4):64–67

[54] Yu LG, Li N, Jiang Y, Han M. [Clinical analysis of orbital complications of acute pediatric sinusitis]. Zhonghua Er Bi Yan Hou Tou Jing Wai Ke Za Zhi. 2012; 47 (4):314–316

[55] Bagheri A, Tavakoli M, Aletaha M, Salour H, Ghaderpanah M. Orbital and preseptal cellulitis: a 10-year survey of hospitalized patients in a tertiary eye hospital in Iran. Int Ophthalmol. 2012; 32(4):361–367

[56] Shinder R, Nasser QJ, Gutman J, Brejt S, Williams MD, Esmaeli B. Idiopathic inflammation of the orbit and contiguous structures. Ophthal Plast Reconstr Surg. 2012; 28(4):e82–e85

[57] Meara DJ. Sinonasal disease and orbital cellulitis in children. Oral Maxillofac Surg Clin North Am.. 2012; 24(3):487–496

[58] Chaudhry IA, Al-Rashed W, Arat YO. The hot orbit: orbital cellulitis. Middle East Afr J Ophthalmol. 2012; 19(1):34–42

[59] Moubayed SP, Vu TT, Quach C, Daniel SJ. Periorbital cellulitis in the pediatric population: clinical features and management of 117 cases. J Otolaryngol Head Neck Surg. 2011; 40(3):266–270

[60] Welkoborsky H-J, Graß S, Deichmüller C, Bertram O, Hinni ML. Orbital complications in children: differential diagnosis of a challenging disease. Eur Arch Otorhinolaryngol. 2015; 272(5):1157–1163

[61] Lehnerdt G, Peraud A, Berghaus A, et al. Orbitale und intrakranielle Komplikationen akuter Sinusitiden. Diagnostik und Therapie bei Kindern und Jugendlichen. HNO. 2011; 59(1):75–86, quiz 87–88

[62] Cavaliere M, Volino F, Parente G, Troisi S, Iemma M. [Endoscopic treatment of orbital cellulitis in pediatric patients: transethmoidal approach]. Arch Soc Esp Oftalmol. 2013; 88(7):271–275

[63] Bedwell J, Bauman NM. Management of pediatric orbital cellulitis and abscess. Curr Opin Otolaryngol Head Neck Surg. 2011; 19(6):467–473

[64] Ketenci I, Unlü Y, Vural A, Doğan H, Sahin MI, Tuncer E. Approaches to subperiosteal orbital abscesses. Eur Arch Otorhinolaryngol. 2013; 270(4): 1317–1327

[65] Upile NS, Munir N, Leong SC, Swift AC. Who should manage acute periorbital cellulitis in children? Int J Pediatr Otorhinolaryngol. 2012; 76(8):1073–1077

[66] Brugha RE, Abrahamson E. Ambulatory intravenous antibiotic therapy for children with preseptal cellulitis. Pediatr Emerg Care. 2012; 28(3):226–228

[67] Gavriel H, Yeheskeli E, Aviram E, Yehoshua L, Eviatar E. Dimension of subperiosteal orbital abscess as an indication for surgical management in children. Otolaryngol Head Neck Surg. 2011; 145(5):823–827

[68] Dewan MA, Meyer DR, Wladis EJ. Orbital cellulitis with subperiosteal abscess: demographics and management outcomes. Ophthal Plast Reconstr Surg. 2011; 27(5):330–332

[69] Wald ER, Applegate KE, Bordley C, et al. American Academy of Pediatrics. Clinical practice guideline for the diagnosis and management of acute bacterial sinusitis in children aged 1 to 18 years. Pediatrics. 2013; 132(1):e262–e280

[70] Pearce MS, Salotti JA, Little MP, et al. Radiation exposure from CT scans in childhood and subsequent risk of leukaemia and brain tumours: a retrospective cohort study. Lancet. 2012; 380(9840):499–505

[71] Bernier M-O, Rehel J-L, Brisse HJ, et al. Radiation exposure from CT in early childhood: a French large-scale multicentre study. Br J Radiol. 2012; 85 (1009):53–60

[72] Pindrik J, Huisman TA, Mahesh M, Tekes A, Ahn ES. Analysis of limited-sequence head computed tomography for children with shunted hydrocephalus: potential to reduce diagnostic radiation exposure. J Neurosurg Pediatr. 2013; 12(5):491–500

[73] Morton RP, Reynolds RM, Ramakrishna R, et al. Low-dose head computed tomography in children: a single institutional experience in pediatric radiation risk reduction: clinical article. J Neurosurg Pediatr. 2013; 12(4):406–410

Chapter 7

Endocrine Orbitopathy

7

7 Endocrine Orbitopathy

7.1 Etiology and Pathogenesis

George J. Kahaly

7.1.1 Etiology

Endocrine orbitopathy (EO) is the most common extrathyroidal manifestation of Graves's disease and/or autoimmune thyroid disease. The EO can occur before, during, or after the onset of the thyroid disease.[1] The eyes are usually affected asymmetrically. Although women are affected more frequently by EO, men are often confronted with a particularly difficult progression of the disease.[2] The general manifestation age lies between 40 and 50 years. The EO typically occurs combined with Graves's disease and positive TSH (thyroid stimulating hormone) receptor antibodies. It occurs only rarely with Hashimoto's thyroiditis with antibodies against thyroperoxidase or thyroglobulin instead, or (even less commonly) with no autoimmune thyroid disease present. Of the 250 EO patients who were studied prospectively at the Johannes Gutenberg University orbital center in Mainz, Germany, 231 (92.4%) had Graves' disease, 12 (4.8%) had Hashimoto's thyroiditis, and 7 (2.8%) had no autoimmune thyroid disease.[3] The prevalence of EO in the general population is estimated to be 16 women and 3 men per 100,000 per year.[4] A clinically relevant progression of the EO can be observed in about one-fourth of all patients with Graves's disease. If one includes palpebral changes as well, the number increases to 40%. Using computer tomography or magnetic resonance imaging, or by measuring the intraocular pressure, subclinical abnormalities were revealed in most patients with Graves's disease. Nevertheless, severe forms of EO are observed in only 3 to 5% of all cases.[5,6]

> **Memorize**
>
> EO is usually associated with autoimmune thyroid disease. Approximately 25% of all patients with Graves's disease suffer from orbital symptoms. Severe progressions of the EO occur in only 3 to 5% of all patients.

7.1.2 Pathogenesis

Immune Pathogenesis of Orbital Changes

The immune process in the orbital space is composed of inflammatory reactions, the proliferation of connective and adipose tissue (both around the outer eye muscles as well as within the perimysium and endomysium), and finally an excessive production of glycosaminoglycans from orbital fibroblasts. The inflammatory reaction is mainly characterized by an infiltration of T lymphocytes ($CD4^+$, $CD8^+$, $CD45RO^+$, $CD45RB^+$) in particular, whereby plasma cells and macrophages are increased.[7] The proliferation of lymphocytes, plasma cells, and macrophages leads to a stimulation of the orbital fibroblasts, and to a massive production of collagen and mucopolysaccharides. The orbital fibroblasts are uniquely sensitive to certain cytokines, which explains the anatomical localization of the immune response. The fibroblasts release proinflammatory cytokines (especially interleukins IL-6 and IL-8) and thus stimulate the nuclear factor κB.[8]

The volume of the eye muscles can increase up to 2 to 3 times its usual size. Most commonly affected are the inferior and medial rectus muscles. It has been shown in animal models that a secondary effect is the obstruction of orbital veins, depending on the respective anatomical circumstances. This results in additional edema formation and amplification of the inflammatory response.[9] A part of the orbital fibroblasts are so-called preadipocytes that can be converted into fat cells, as observed in vitro.[10] During this conversion, the preadipocytes increasingly express the TSH receptor, supporting the theory that this receptor is an important autoantigen in the orbital immune response.

There are hints that T lymphocytes with similar molecular T-cell receptor repertoires can migrate into both the thyroid tissue and the orbital tissue, which suggests antigen similarities of both tissue types.[11,12] Both the TSH receptor as well as a TSH receptor variant have been detected in orbital connective and adipose tissue at RNA and protein levels. Since the cloning of the TSH receptor, there are numerous indications for its extrathyroidal and orbital presence.[13,14,15,16,17,18] The extracellular portions of the TSH receptor thus come into consideration as cross-reacting antigenic determinants for T lymphocytes and as a target structure for EO patients. This perception is supported by the fact that in animal experiments the injection of TSH receptors triggers both Graves's disease and characteristics of EO. However, a functional TSH receptor or other thyroid antigens have not yet been detected in orbital tissue.[19,20] Investigations revealed that there is in fact a link between the activity and severity of the EO and the height of the measured TSH receptor antibody titers.[21] On the other hand, there are also indications regarding other orbital proteins with which the immune system reacts.[22] Orbital T cells react with the patient's own orbital protein fragments, although lymphocytes should be tolerant against autologous tissues.[23] Hence, the characterization of these antigenic structures is likely to bring further enlightenment regarding the pathogenetic backgrounds of the EO.

After the acute process including lymphocytic infiltration of the orbital tissue and the activation of fibroblasts, there follows a chronic stage. The histopathological correlate is an increasing fibrosis. Consequently, the transformation and proliferation of the tissue within the—anatomically rather narrow—orbital space leads to a pressure increase, which causes the characteristic symptoms of the EO (▶ Fig. 7.1).

> **Memorize**
>
> As part of the EO, the volume of the eye muscles (usually the inferior and medial rectus muscles) will increase by up to 2 to 3 times its usual size. There is a relationship between the activity and severity of the EO and the amplitude of the measured TSH receptor antibody titers. (See also ▶ Fig. 7.1.)

Pretibial Myxedema and Acropachy

The EO is not only closely related to autoimmune-determined thyroid disorders; it is part of a complex disease pattern that can

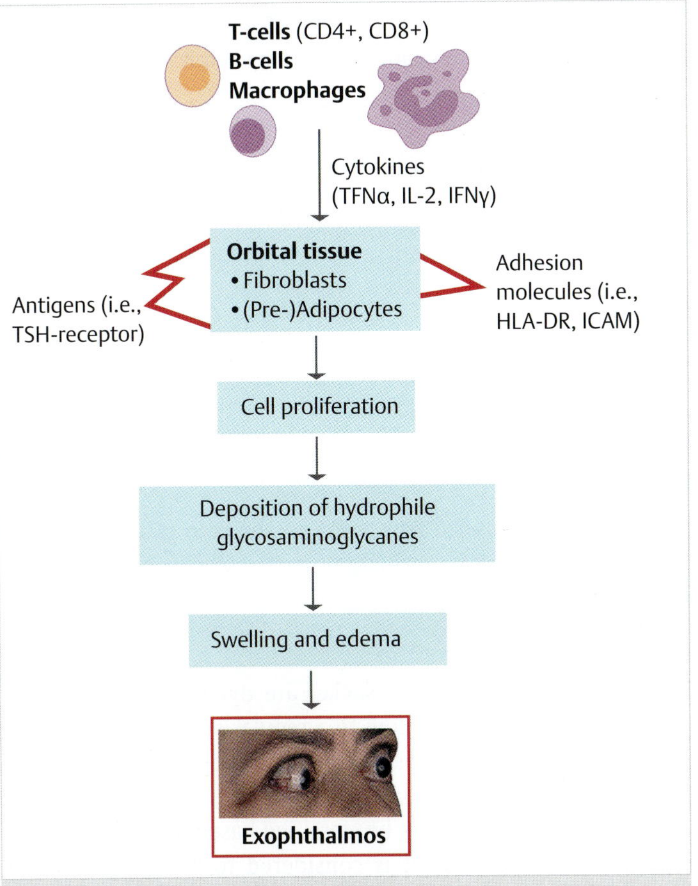

Fig. 7.1 Pathogenesis of endocrine orbitopathy (EO).

affect several organs. Besides the thyroid and eye manifestations in the progression of autoimmune hyperthyroidism, it may, for example, come to changes in the morphology and functioning of the heart.[24] About 5% of patients suffering from Graves's disease and EO also show a peculiar gelatinous inflammatory swelling in the area of the lower leg and forefoot (pretibial myxedema), as well as alterations in their fingers and toes (acropachy). Patients with an endocrine dermopathy regularly show EO and high titers of TSH receptor antibodies. As in the thyroid and orbital tissue of patients suffering from Graves's disease, specialized T lymphocytes can also be detected in the actively inflamed pretibial myxedema tissue. The accumulation of glycosaminoglycans and other dermal connective tissue components in the dermal subcutis due to the cytokine-based stimulation of pretibial fibroblasts is the morphological correlate of nodular or diffuse pachyderma related to the pretibial myxedema (▶ Fig. 7.2).

Risk Factors

Patients should refrain from smoking and avoid psychological stress, as, according to the evidence, both are modifiable risk factors that amplify the autoimmune process.[25] Studies have shown that patients suffering from Graves's disease developed EO significantly more often when smoking.[26] It was also revealed that nicotine negatively affects therapeutic success regarding radioactive iodine therapy,[27] steroid therapy, and retrobulbar radiotherapy.[28] The phenotype and function of peripheral T lymphocytes are also affected by smoking, and the production of acute-phase proteins, complement factors, and interleukin-1 is enhanced.[29] It is also known that emotionally stressful incidents favor the occurrence of autoimmune hyperthyroidism,[30] and that chronic psychological stress as well as genetic predisposition influence antithyroid therapy negatively.[31,32]

> **Memorize**
>
> Smoking and psychological stress are risk factors that amplify the autoimmune process.

7.2 Clinical and Laboratory Investigations

George J. Kahaly

7.2.1 Clinical Investigations

Patients suffering from EO usually report slowly increasing local discomfort that is more pronounced in the morning than in the

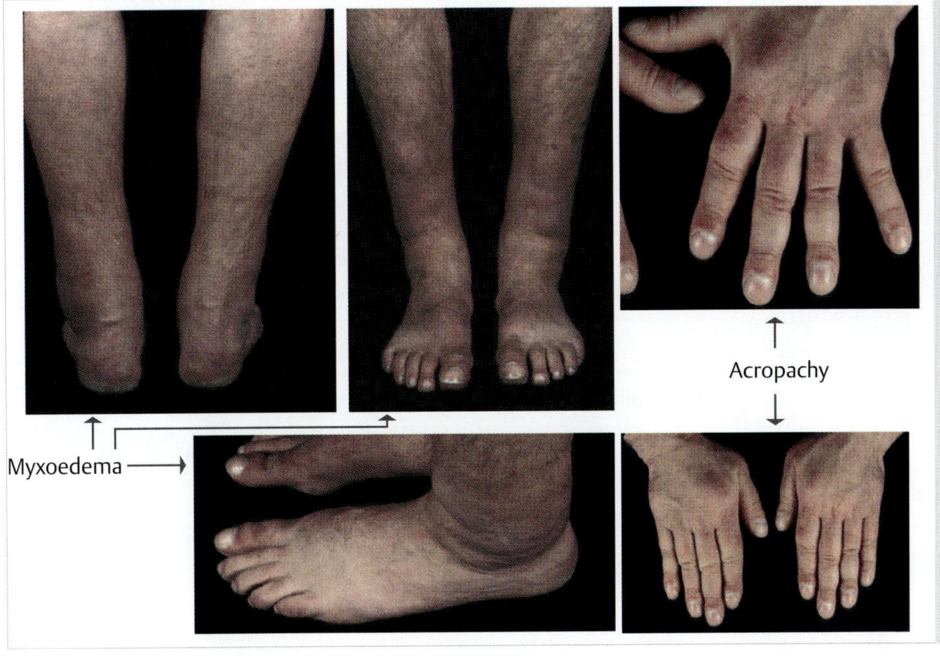

Fig. 7.2 Pretibial myxedema and acropachy.

7

Table 7.1 Symptoms and signs of an EO by frequency

Symptom	Frequency
Lid retraction	90%
Inflammatory soft tissue symptoms (eyelid swelling, lid reddening, caruncle swelling, conjunctiva reddening, chemosis)	80%
Exophthalmos	50–60%
Corneal moistening defect	> 50%
Eye bulb motility disorders	40%
Impairment of visual acuity	3–5%

Table 7.2 Diagnostic measures on suspicion of optic neuropathy

Pupillary reactions (relative afferent pupillary deficit, RAPD)
Visual field examinations
Color vision
Visual evoked potentials (VEP)
Determination of visual acuity (→ rather late)

evening.[33] Usually, the focus is on eyelid reactions; other symptoms such as periorbital edema, pain and pressure behind the eyes, photosensitivity, foreign body sensation, lacrimation, and exophthalmos come in varying degrees of severity and frequency (▶ Table 7.1). Severe conjunctivitis, local infections, and corneal defects are possible results of an incomplete eyelid closure. The eye muscle changes result in motility disorders of the eye, with consequent diplopia. A severe complication is pinching of the optic nerve, which may result in the loss of visual acuity and visual field failures or even complete blindness.[2,6]

In a study on the natural disease progression in 59 patients with EO, the symptomatology improved in 65% spontaneously; in 22% it remained unchanged; and only 13% of patients showed deterioration.[34] Activations are described in connection with a recurrence of the underlying thyroid disease or after surgical orbital decompression operations.[35] In about half of the patients, the measurement of TSH receptor antibody titers allowed an estimation of the severity and course of the EO.[36]

In principle, all eye sections should be examined ophthalmologically. The degree of the exophthalmos is determined and quantified by measuring the sagittal distance between the corneal apex and the lateral osseous orbital rim (Hertel exophthalmometer). Examination of the motility of the extraocular muscles and the resulting diplopia is important for potential surgery later. Pathological pupillary responses, visual field defects, and disturbed color vision are early signs of optic nerve compression that may be detected by an ophthalmologist even before a reduction of central vision acuity occurs (▶ Table 7.2). From visual evoked potentials, early stages of optic nerve dysfunction may also be revealed before the decrease of visual acuity.[37]

Table 7.3 Clinical Activity Score, CAS. One point is given for each feature

• Retrobulbar pain (in primary gaze)
• Retrobulbar pain on attempted up-, side-, or downgaze
• Redness of the eyelids
• Inflammatory eyelid swelling
• Redness of the conjunctiva
• Chemosis
• Inflammation of caruncle or plica
• Increase of 2 mm or more in proptosis in the last 1–3 months
• Decrease in visual acuity in the last 1–3 months
• Decrease in eye movements of 8° or more in the last 1–3 months

Memorize

Clinical symptoms and signs of EO are shown in ▶ Table 7.1. Diagnostic measures regarding suspected optic neuropathy are shown in ▶ Table 7.2.

The changes within the eye socket are dynamic processes that cannot be described according to a regular scheme. For an accurate assessment of the disease's progression, the activity and severity of the EO are evaluated using established scores.

The activity of the EO can be classified based on a 7-point scale (▶ Fig. 7.3; ▶ Table 7.3). It is considered to be clinically active when inflammatory processes with edematous swelling, disruption of the venous outflow, and thickening of the affected muscles dominate (▶ Fig. 7.4). Patients complain about bulging eyes, burning, foreign body sensation, and peribulbar pressure pain. These symptoms can be intensified when moving. Eyelids, conjunctiva, and lacrimal caruncle may be swollen and/or red.

The severity of the EO is classified based on a 6-class scheme[38] (▶ Fig. 7.5; ▶ Table 7.4). Principally, the disease is considered to be severe if a corneal injury or optic nerve compression is present. To date, the evidence-based recommendations of the European interdisciplinary working group (European Group on Graves's orbitopathy = EUGOGO) for the management of EO[39,40] distinguish the following severity classifications.

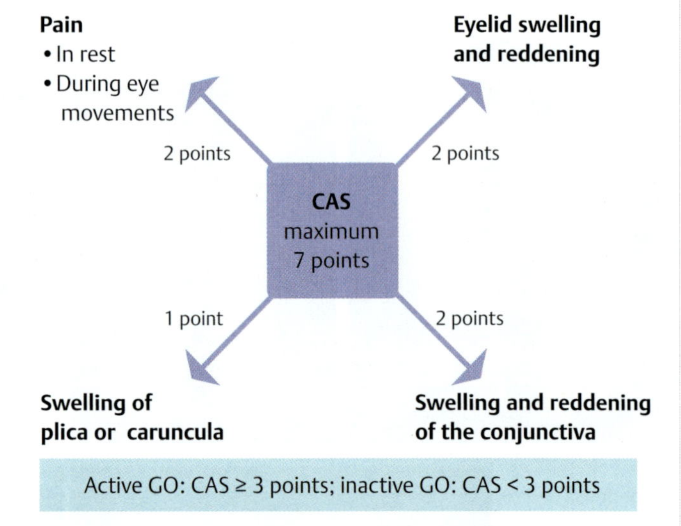

Fig. 7.3 Activity of endocrine orbitopathy according to the Clinical Activity Score (CAS).

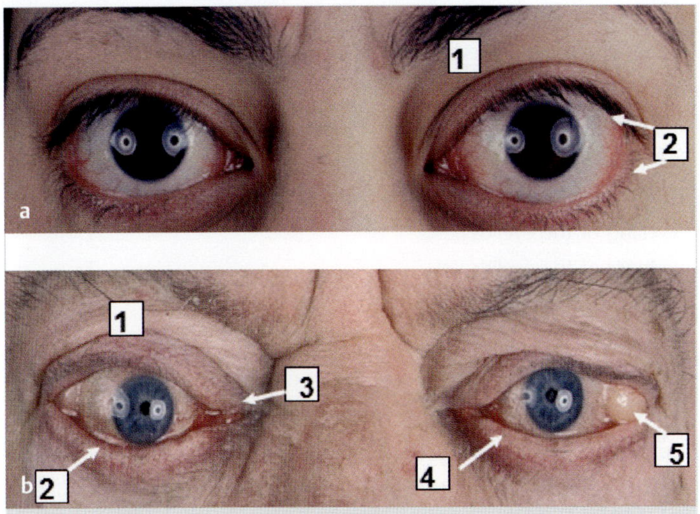

Fig. 7.4 **(a)** Inactive endocrine orbitopathy. Discrete eyelid swelling (1), upper- and lower-lid retraction (2), more severe on the left eye (CAS = 1). **(b)** Active endocrine orbitopathy. Eyelid swelling and reddening (1), chemosis (2), plica and caruncle swelling (3), conjunctival reddening (4). According to the pathologic findings visible in this photograph, a CAS of 6 points is justified. A prolapse of orbital fat tissue also occurs (5).

Fig. 7.4 Clinical EO activity.

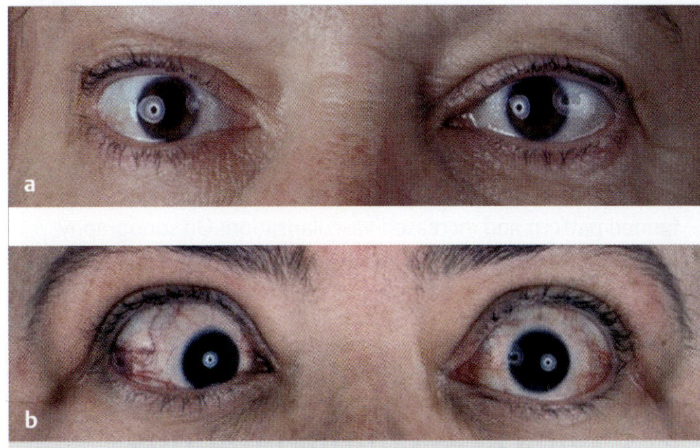

Fig. 7.5 **(a)** Mild endocrine orbitopathy. Eyelid swelling, slight upper lid retraction on the right eye, only mild exophthalmos. According to the light reflex nearly physiological eye bulb position (at least in the primary position). **(b)** Severe endocrine orbitopathy. The significant eyelid symptoms along with the strabismus indicate a serious disease. An optic nerve compression occurred additionally in this case which is not visible in this photograph.

- **Mild EO**: in patients whose daily lives are only insignificantly affected by the signs and symptoms of the EO, so that neither immunosuppressive nor surgical therapy is appropriate. These patients usually show one or several of the following symptoms: minor eyelid retraction (≤ 2 mm), mild soft tissue involvement, exophthalmos ≤ 3 mm above the standard value according to age and race, temporary or missing diplopia, corneal inflammation, which responds to a local treatment with a tear replacement solution.
- **Moderate to severe EO**: in patients without impairment of eyesight, yet whose daily lives are affected by the symptoms of the disease, justifying immunosuppressive (with active EO) or surgical (with inactive EO) therapy. Patients of this category usually suffer from one or more of the following symptoms: eyelid retraction ≥ 2 mm; moderate to severe soft tissue involvement; exophthalmos ≥ 3 mm above the standard value according to age and race; inconstant or constant diplopia.
- **Eyesight endangering EO**: patients with optic neuropathy and/or corneal decompensation. This category requires immediate intervention.

Table 7.4 EO severity classification

Class	Criterion	Elaboration
1	Clinical signs of EO	For example: eye lid reactions
2	Degree of inflammation/soft tissue involvement	For example: corneal reddening and swelling
3	Exophthalmos	Using the Hertel exophthalmometer
4	Eye bulb motility disorders	For example: diplopia/strabismus
5	Corneal involvement	For example: superficial punctate keratopathy or corneal ulceration
6	Optic nerve involvement	Loss of visual acuity/neuropathy

Memorize

The activity of the EO is assessed using a clinical activity score (CAS, 7-point score). Based on clinical symptoms, the disease is categorized as mild, moderate to severe, or eyesight endangering EO.

7.2.2 Laboratory Examinations and Medical Imaging

The EO usually manifests in close temporal relation (6–12 months) to hyperthyroidism.[25] The procedure along a standardized diagnostic staging system has been proven effective[41] and also allows for evaluation of the progression of the disease. The primary task is clinical and laboratory control of the thyroid function including the determination of basal serum values for TSH, free T_4 and free T_3.[42] The presence of thyroidal antibodies (specific TSH receptor, thyroid peroxidase, and thyroglobulin antibodies) facilitates the attribution of the thyroid dysfunction to Graves's disease in the case of clinically inconclusive findings. The thyroid examination is completed by ultrasonography of the thyroid gland and possibly scintigraphy. The quite typical ultrasound image of Graves' disease shows a diffuse goiter with hypoechoic, fanned pattern, as well as a significantly increased vascularization of the enlarged organ. A scintigram usually depicts the thyroid as diffusely retentive. In patients suffering from Hashimoto's thyroiditis the thyroid is depicted as an extensive or circumscribed hypoechoic region.

Medical imaging techniques regarding the orbit (CT and/or MRI) are only applicable preoperatively and are used in unclear or unilateral cases.[43,44,45] In this regard, ocular myositis or idiopathic orbital inflammation is the most common differential diagnosis of EO.[46]

> **Memorize**
>
> As part of the diagnostic process, clinical and laboratory tests (of thyroid function and thyroid antibodies) are supplemented by ultrasonography. The sonographic image of Graves's disease is fairly typical: diffuse enlarged goiter showing a hypoechoic, fanned pattern and increased vascularization. On sonography Hashimoto's thyroiditis shows an extensive or circumscribed hypoechoic texture.

7.2.3 Clinical Recommendations for Practical Use

Patients suffering from EO in an acute stage should be monitored closely and in an interdisciplinary fashion in order to detect possible impairment of visual acuity, vision field defects, or corneal lesions at an early stage. Semiannual control examinations are recommended, even after reaching a stable euthyroid condition.[47] In analogy to the relapse predictions regarding hyperthyroidism during Graves's disease, TSH receptor antibody determination can also predict aggravation of EO in patients with high antibody levels. This information may influence treatment decisions, though these should be taken only by experienced specialists. The therapy can only be considered optimal if carried out as an **interdisciplinary collaboration**, involving experts working together in coordination. With the establishment of specialized orbital centers and a correspondingly consistent exploration of influencing factors and pathophysiological relations as well as of genetic factors, a better targeted therapy of the EO will be available, including, for example, improvement of the quality of life, which is significantly negatively affected.[48] Ideally, this objective will be reached by the founding of specialized orbital centers.[49] The Department of Medicine of the Johannes Gutenberg University Medical Center in Mainz, Germany, for example, offers a weekly multidisciplinary consultation period conducted by endocrinologists and relevant experts from the eye, ENT, radiotherapy, and psychosomatic clinics as an inherent part of its patient care.

> **Memorize**
>
> Patients with EO in the acute stage must be monitored closely and interdisciplinary. Using TSH receptor antibody determination, an aggravation of the EO can be predicted in patients with high antibody levels.

7.3 Ophthalmological Findings and Complications

M. A. Varde and B. Wiechens

EO is an autoimmune disorder affecting the orbital tissues and leading to characteristic changes observable in clinical examination. Complications can lead to irreversible visual loss in case of corneal or optic nerve involvement. Changes in the appearance can cause psychological problems for patients and lead to depression.

Table 7.5 Clinical Activity Score based on.[51] Points 1–7 are accumulated in a first evaluation; in all following examinations points 1–10 are scored

Symptom/sign	Score
Spontaneous periorbital pain	1
Periorbital pain associated with ocular movement	1
Swelling of the eyelids	1
Redness of the eyelids	1
Conjunctival injection	1
Chemosis	1
Swelling and redness of the caruncle or plica semilunaris	1
Increase in exophthalmos by ≥ 2 mm	1
Limitation of monocular excursion by ≥ 8°	1
Visual impairment of more than 1 Snellen's line	1

7.3.1 Classification of Findings

Signs of periocular inflammation characterize the active stage of EO. The **Clinical Activity Score (CAS)** is used to assess the **activity of the disease**. The CAS is regarded the best predictive factor for the progression of EO and is therefore important for the planning of anti-inflammatory treatment strategies such as steroid therapy, immunosuppressive therapy, or radiotherapy.[50] The CAS is based on clinical signs and does not require imaging (▸ Table 7.5). It is important to ensure that the findings are actually caused by active inflammation. Symptoms of dry eye, a common condition in EO, may also cause pain, variations in visual acuity, and conjunctival redness, while chemosis in relation to itching can be caused by an allergic reaction.

The **severity of the disease** is evaluated using the **NOSPECS Score** (▸ Table 7.6). This score is also elicited in each consultation in order to assess the progression of EO and to decide on potential interventions. A disadvantage of the score is the fact that it implies a chronological progression from Stage 0 to Stage VI that does not necessarily occur in each individual case. For example, a compressive optic neuropathy is often associated with only slight exophthalmos and no corneal involvement.

A more recent classification is the LEMO, which takes into account the independence of signs and symptoms that occur as well as their severity.

Important clinical signs, symptoms, and complications of EO will subsequently be discussed in more detail.

Table 7.6 NOSPECS Score based on[51] to evaluate the severity of EO. Individual stages are divided into subgroups depending on severity. If multiple areas are involved the highest stage is the NOSPECS score

Symptom/sign	Stage
No symptoms or signs	0
Only signs no symptoms (lid retraction, lid lag)	I
Soft tissue involvement (periorbital swelling)	II
Exophthalmos	III
Involvement of extraocular muscles	IV
Corneal involvement (exposure keratopathy)	V
Compressive optic neuropathy with loss of visual acuity	VI

7.3.2 Dry Eye Syndrome

Dry eyes are not only a very common problem in otherwise healthy people but are also frequently found in EO and other autoimmune diseases. In general, two main causes of dry eyes can be differentiated: increased evaporation and hyposecretion. The components of the tear film are discussed in more detail in Chapter 15.1. Hyposecretion of tears is caused by direct lymphocytic infiltration of the lacrimal gland as well as being due to the effect of TSH receptor autoantibodies. Lid retraction, lagophthalmos and a decreased blink rate (as discussed below) result in increased evaporation of tears. The meibomian gland function is also affected by thyroid hormones. Even therapeutic measures for EO can lead to dry eyes: Hypothyroidism (e.g., after thyroablative treatment), irradiation of the orbit, and various surgical interventions in the lid area (ptosis surgery, blepharoplasty) are associated with dry eye syndrome.[52]

Patients complain of dryness and foreign-body sensation as well as pain and variations in visual acuity due to the resulting irregularity of the corneal surface. Symptoms are often disproportionate to the clinical findings and can be localized to the retrobulbar area; hence they have to be distinguished from pain associated with EO activity. In rare cases, extreme dryness can lead to corneal ulcers and blindness.

Clinical examination shows a diffuse conjunctival injection (to be clinically distinguished from the local injection close to the muscle insertions in active myositis) and conjunctival wrinkling (to be distinguished from chemosis related to inflammation) as well as superficial punctate keratopathy (punctate defects of the corneal epithelium visible with fluorescein stain). Visual acuity can be significantly reduced and simulate a decrease in vision due to optic nerve compression.

Application of artificial tears is the treatment of choice. In severe cases, a temporary closure of the lacrimal drainage system with punctal plugs or a tarsorrhaphy (described below) can be contemplated.

Dry eye can also occur as an initial symptom of EO, so the differential diagnoses should already include EO.[53]

7.3.3 Lid Retraction

Upper lid retraction with lateral flare is pathognomonic for EO (▶ Fig. 7.6). The resulting staring gaze is described as Kocher's sign, the visibility of the sclera above the limbus as Dalrymple's sign.

Lid retraction (enlargement of the palpebral fissure due to retraction of the upper or lower lid margin from the central cornea) in EO is caused by static and dynamic mechanisms. They can affect both the upper and the lower eyelid.

In the course of the disease, the direct involvement of the levator palpebrae superioris muscle leads to fibrosis and static retraction of the upper eyelid. The lower eyelids are accordingly affected on the lower lid retractors (see ▶ Fig. 16.2, ▶ Fig. 16.3).

One of the *dynamic* mechanisms of a true lid retraction is *hyperinnervation* of Müller's muscle in the upper lid (sympathetic part of the *capsulopalpebral fascia* in the lower lid) due to an increased sympathetic activity in hyperthyroidism.

A true lid retraction is generally visible in primary position, but particularly in downgaze (von Graefe's sign). This sign can be helpful in distinguishing a pseudo lid retraction.

Infiltration with subsequent **fibrosis of the inferior rectus muscle** is often part of the muscle involvement in EO. It results in a restrictive vertical strabismus and relative hyperinnervation of the main antagonist, the superior rectus muscle with the co-innervated levator palpebrae superioris muscle (LPS). This leads to an ipsilateral **pseudo lid retraction**. According to **Hering's law** this is followed by hyperinnervation of the contralateral LPS and therefore a contralateral pseudo lid retraction.

Another mechanism causing a pseudo lid retraction is a **contralateral** ptosis. Here, hyperinnervation of the ipsilateral LPS results in a contralateral upper lid retraction according to Hering's law. Manual lifting the ptotic eyelid corrects contralateral upper lid retraction. Pseudo lid retraction can also be caused by exophthalmos. Here, the protrusion of the eyeball causes a mechanical enlargement of the palpebral fissure.

For the correction of lid retraction, all these mechanisms have to be considered before lid surgery is planned (Chapter 7.4.4).

7.3.4 Indicators for Clinical Activity

In the active stage of EO, patients often present with bilateral swelling and redness of the eyelids. Conjunctival injection (hyperemia of the conjunctiva), chemosis (swelling of the conjunctiva), as well as swelling of the caruncle and plica semilunaris often occur in active disease (▶ Fig. 7.7). As mentioned before, this has to be distinguished from viral and allergic conjunctivitis as well as from irritation associated with dry eye.

7.3.5 Exophthalmos

The protrusion of the eye from the orbit is defined as **exophthalmos** (proptosis). EO presents axial proptosis, wherein the globe is displaced anteriorly without any horizontal or vertical displacement. The amount of exophthalmos is usually determined with the **Hertel exophthalmometer**, in which the position of the corneal apex is measured in relation to the lateral orbital rim in primary gaze (primary position). Hence, absolute values can vary significantly between individuals, depending on facial configuration, and are mainly used for follow-up examination.

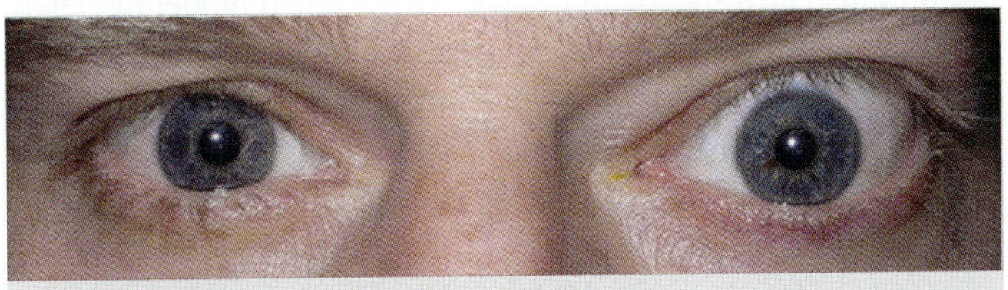

Fig. 7.6 Left upper lid retraction with characteristic lateral flare.

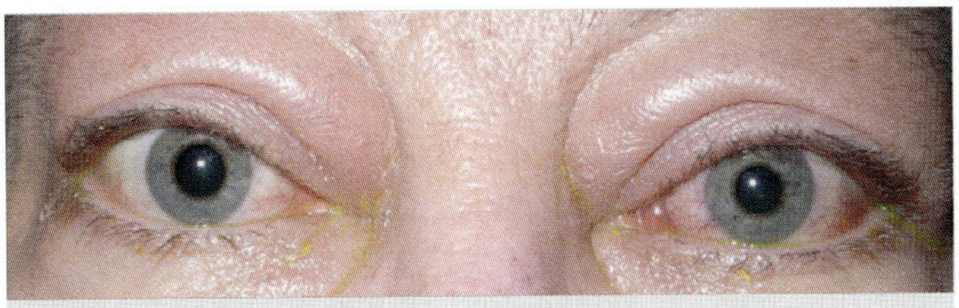

Fig. 7.7 Clinically active EO. Bilateral swelling and redness of the lids, conjunctival injection and swelling of the plica semilunaris in the left eye.

A nonaxial protrusion should always raise suspicion regarding the possibility of an extraconal mass in the orbit.

Exophthalmos associated with EO is caused by a proliferation of orbital adipose tissue, swelling of the extraocular muscles, and orbital edema due to increased expression of glycosaminoglycans.

Apart from considerable cosmetic impairment, exophthalmos is the main risk factor for severe exposure keratopathy with corneal ulceration.

7.3.6 Lagophthalmos

Lagophthalmos is mainly caused by lid retraction and proptosis. Incomplete involuntary blinking with complete arbitrary lid closure is described as blink lagophthalmos. The rare blinking, frequently observed in EO, is known as Stellwag's sign. A history of nocturnal lagophthalmos may be sought from carers and attendants. In assessing lagophthalmos, it is not only its degree that is important but, especially, whether corneal exposure exists. Bell's phenomenon is an important protective mechanism for the cornea. When closing the lids, the eyeball rotates upward, protecting the cornea under the upper lid. This reflex is suppressed by restriction due to fibrosis of the inferior rectus muscle, as is often the case in EO. In case of corneal exposure, surgical correction of the lagophthalmos is urgently required.

7.3.7 Ptosis

Ptosis can have an aponeurotic cause due to a chronic swelling of the periorbital tissue and stretching of the levator aponeurosis associated with an exophthalmos. However, it can also be a sign of myasthenia gravis that sometimes accompanies EO. According to the literature, 5 to 10% of myasthenia patients present autoimmune thyroiditis, but only 0.2% of patients with autoimmune thyroiditis present myasthenia.[54] However, diagnosis is important since the disease can be a vital threat.

Myasthenia should always be suspected in strabismus atypical for EO (exodeviation = outward squinting), and in cases presenting with variability in eyelid position along with strabismus.

7.3.8 Exposure Keratopathy

Exposure keratopathy refers to the severe dryness of the cornea due to incomplete eyelid closure (lagophthalmos). The tear film lubricates the corneal surface and is evenly distributed by blinking. It preserves the optical properties of the cornea, which are the basis for good visual acuity, and protects the integrity of the epithelium against microorganisms. Exposure keratopathy develops when the closure of the eyelid is impaired. In EO it is caused by any combination of **lid retraction, proptosis**, and **reduced Bell's phenomenon** due to restrictive strabismus. Ophthalmic examination includes staining of the cornea with fluorescein sodium. The yellow dye stains exposed basement membrane in case of deepithelialization and is clearly visible in the blue light of a slit lamp. In the early stages of exposure keratopathy, the inferior part of the cornea is often stained in a punctate pattern (superficial punctate keratopathy). Further progression can lead to corneal abrasions with extensive epithelial defects. Infection with bacteria or fungi can lead to corneal ulcers. If stromal melt is severe, an ulcer can lead to a perforation of the cornea with prolapse of intraocular tissue (▶ Fig. 7.8). An intraocular extension presents itself as hypopyon and can subsequently result in endophthalmitis (infiltration of the vitreous chamber and possibly the retina), panophthalmitis (inflammation of all ocular structures), and orbital cellulitis.

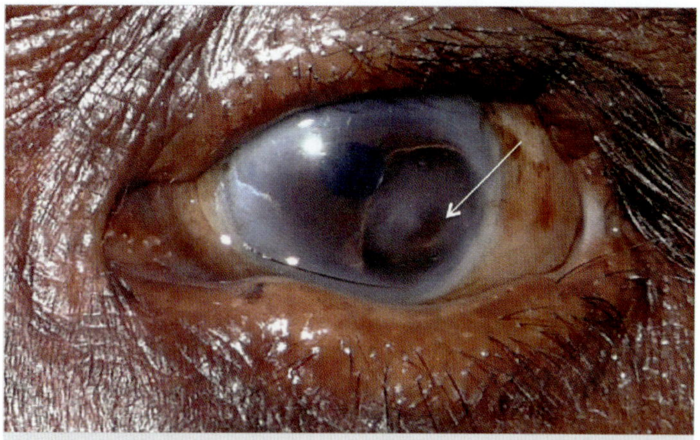

Fig. 7.8 Exposure keratopathy (in this case due to traumatic lagophthalmos). In the inferotemporal quadrant thinning of the corneal stroma without infiltrate. Centrally within the lesion lighter area indicating a descemetocele with chance of spontaneous perforation (*arrow*). With kind permission from Dr. B. Mukherjee, Sankara Nethralaya Eye Hospital, Chennai, India.

Exposure keratopathy is thus a serious complication of thyroid ophthalmopathy that necessitates urgent treatment (Chapter 7.4.4).

7.3.9 Strabismus

Involvement of the extraocular muscles leads to swelling and later fibrosis of affected muscles, with resulting restrictive strabismus. The medial rectus muscle and the inferior rectus muscle are most commonly affected. The restriction becomes most obvious in the opposite direction of gaze, hence in abduction and elevation. Patients initially notice diplopia only in extreme gazes. Later they may present with manifest strabismus and sometimes extreme angle deviation. Other muscles—including the oblique muscles—may also be affected. Cover testing and squint assessment as well as traction testing are performed to diagnose restrictive strabismus. Internal strabismus (esotropia) due to fibrosis of the medial rectus muscle and vertical deviation due to fibrosis of the inferior rectus muscle are most commonly observed (▶ Fig. 7.9). Less common is exotropia (diverging strabismus; an exception is myasthenia as shown above). Restrictive eye motility may subsequently lead to an increase in intraocular pressure (IOP) when looking in the opposite direction, which also represents a clinical sign. IOP usually increases in an upward gaze.

Progressive strabismus may be an indicator for disease activity but may also be a sign of an increase in fibrotic remodeling. There are therapeutic approaches to treating involved muscles with botulinum toxin in order to prevent contracture.[55] Strabismus surgery is the ultimate corrective treatment choice, but it should only be performed after reaching clinical inactivity, a euthyroid state, and stable squint angles. Since a variation in orbital volume may result in an altered globe position, surgical correction of strabismus in EO should only be carried out after orbital

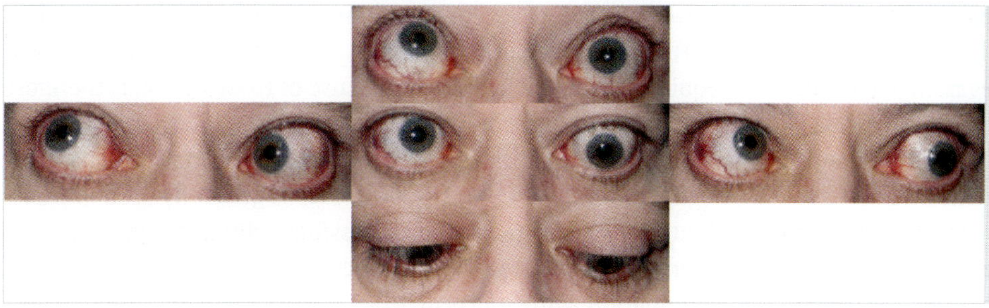

Fig. 7.9 Strabismus in inactive EO. In primary position esotropia and hypotropia of the left eye, limitation of upgaze, abduction limitation in the right eye.

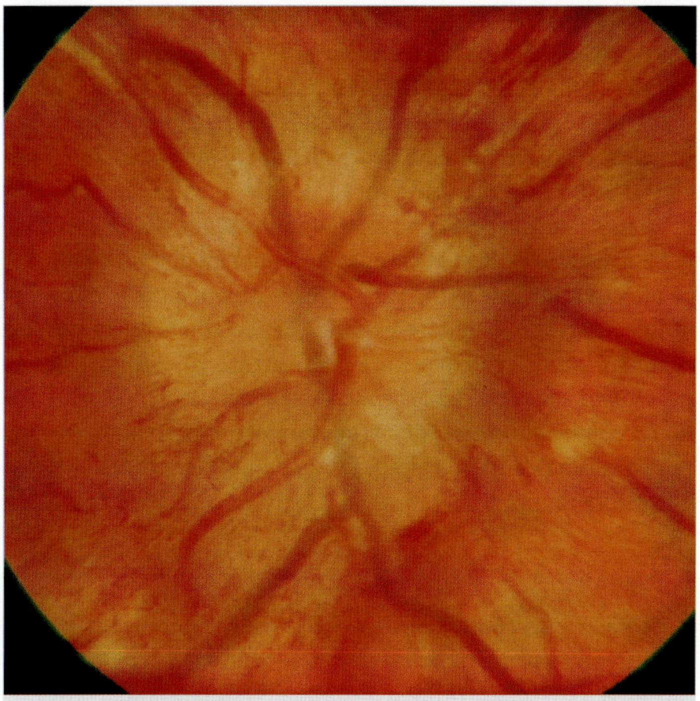

Fig. 7.10 Disc edema in compressive optic neuropathy. Blurring of the optic disc margins, hyperemia, and hemorrhages can be seen.

decompression. Strabismus surgery aims at increasing the area of binocular single vision and shifting it into the main field of view (straight and downgaze). Full functionality of the muscle cannot be restored, however.

7.3.10 Compressive Optic Neuropathy

Compressive optic neuropathy is the most serious of all EO complications apart from exposure keratopathy. It occurs only in the active stage of EO and may be an indication for emergency orbital decompression.

Clinical signs are loss of vision, relative afferent pupillary defect (RAPD), visual field loss, and impaired color vision. Funduscopy may show a hyperemic and swollen optic disc, possibly with disc hemorrhages (▶ Fig. 7.10). These patients often do not present with pronounced exophthalmos.

7.3.11 Glaucoma

Most studies have not shown increased incidence of glaucoma in patients with thyroid eye disease. However, elevated intraocular pressure is frequently observed and described. The main reason for increased IOP is the elevated venous pressure accompanying EO. The involvement of extraocular muscles and restriction of ocular movement leads to gaze-dependent increase in IOP, which might be overlooked in primary position measurements.[56] Regular ophthalmological examination is important to determine the timing for treatment.

Compressive optic atrophy may morphologically resemble glaucomatous optic atrophy.

7.4 Therapy

7.4.1 Immunosuppressive Therapy

George J. Kahaly

Introduction

First to be treated is generally the thyroid dysfunction as this alone often leads to an improvement of the symptoms.[57] It should be mentioned at this point that not only does the euthyroidism improve the course of the disease but some thyroid depressants themselves have a positive effect on the immunological reaction of the orbit as well. Methimazole effectively inhibits the formation of free radicals from monocytes.[58] Furthermore, a severe EO is often associated not only with thyroid dysfunction but also with the coexistence of a goiter.[59] In addition to the drug treatment of the hyperthyroidism, radioactive iodine therapy or a thyroidectomy can be considered. Studies show that radioactive iodine therapy is frequently associated with a deterioration of eye involvement.[60,61] Without question, a euthyroid state has to be reached and a hypothyroid metabolic condition must be avoided.

Considering that explanations of the development of the EO are largely based on assumptions, so far no causal therapy regimen is available. Hence, treatment objectives focus on relieving local discomfort, inhibiting autoimmune phenomena within the obit, and preventing possible complications. Local eye conditions, for example, dryness or conjunctivitis, can be treated with ophthalmic solutions or ointment.

> **Memorize**
>
> Generally, in patients suffering from EO, the thyroid dysfunction has to be treated at first, which means achieving euthyroidism and avoiding a hypothyroid metabolic condition. Also, patients have to give up smoking.

Glucocorticoids

It is recommended to use glucocorticoids in the acute phase of the disease. Comparative studies show that 70 to 75% of patients benefit from this kind of treatment. The systemic administration of glucocorticoids can be intravenous or oral, with a significant superiority of the intravenous application regarding the reduction of diplopia and the control of inflammatory processes. The increased effectiveness is accompanied by improved tolerance of treatment. Also, the intravenous bolus treatment involves a considerably lower weight gain and patients perceive the treatment as far less stressful. If the glucocorticoid treatment is continued for more than 3 months, vitamin D replacement therapy (5600 IU weekly) has to be administered. Accompanying bisphosphonate therapy should also be administered in patients who are at risk of osteoporosis.

An active principle of glucocorticoids is the inhibition of the nuclear factor κB (Chapter 7.1.2), which explains the anti-inflammatory effect of this therapy.[62] Randomized studies have shown the superiority of intravenous massive-dose steroid therapy (starting with 0.5 g weekly) for about 12 weeks compared to the oral glucocorticoid therapy (starting with 1 mg/kg bw/day).[63] Injections are superior to oral administration, especially with regard to the treatment of diplopia resulting from motility disorders and the fight against inflammatory processes. The increased effectiveness is accompanied by an improved tolerance of the steroid. This is partly true due to the comparatively rare occurrence of stomach pains and skin problems as well as a significantly lower weight gain during intravenous bolus therapy, which is why patients find the treatment to be far less stressful. In optic nerve involvement with impending visual loss, an initially high-dose intravenous therapy with 500 mg methylprednisolone is recommended for 3 days under close ophthalmic observation. If there is improvement of the symptoms of compression, conservative therapy may follow according to the dosage recommendations given earlier; in the event of another optic neuropathy, surgical intervention is unavoidable.

7

Retrobulbar steroid injection does not offer any advantages compared to systemic application and rather increases the local complication rate. During intravenous administration it has to be considered that cumulative steroid dosages of > 10 g of methylprednisolone are associated with increased liver toxicity: several cases of severe and partly fatal liver failure have been described in this dosage range. A predisposing factor could be preliminary liver damage as part of previous viral hepatitis.[64,65,66,67] Also, acute left heart failure has been observed under intravenous steroid therapy in previously clinically unremarkable cardiac patients.[68]

> **Memorize** M!
>
> Of patients with thyroid eye disease or EO, 70 to 75% obtain benefit from the use of glucocorticoids, with intravenous application being superior to oral treatment.

Nonsteroidal Immunosuppressive Agents

When there is insufficient response to the glucocorticoid medication and/or persistent inflammatory activity, the administration of nonsteroidal immunosuppressive agents is indicated.[69] These show successful results particularly regarding the soft tissue involvement; their major disadvantage—apart from the higher cost—is the risk of severe infections, which cannot be excluded. it is true also that such therapy is not yet fully established and requires further clinical trials. The use of these agents is therefore restricted to experienced medical centers.

During the treatment any possible side effects must be thoroughly monitored. Cyclosporine, which is generally used in transplantation medicine, can be successfully administered in cases of severe active EO. Treatment with cyclosporine (3–4 mg/kg bw) in combination with glucocorticoid is successful in serious cases and is superior to glucocorticoid monotherapy with regard to efficacy and relapse prophylaxis.[70] Cyclosporine inhibits the transcription of the IL-2 gene and suppresses the TSH receptor antibody production. In the treatment of EO, a low dosage of cyclosporine (3 mg/kg bw) is administered. The aim is to slow down the orbital inflammatory process and to prevent relapses after the glucocorticoid therapy. Liver values, kidney retention parameters, and blood pressure need to be monitored regularly. Patients should avoid alcohol consumption while under therapy.

Treatment with high dosages of immunoglobulin has proven to be effective, but due to the very high treatment costs and the risk of infections it is only rarely used.[71] Expectations of the success of somatostatin analogues were not realized.[72,73,74] As in diagnostics, advantage is taken of the increased expression of somatostatin receptors within the orbit. The response to octreotide therapy can be estimated with reference to previously performed octreotide scintigraphy.

> **Memorize** M!
>
> The administration of nonsteroidal immunosuppressive agents (e.g., cyclosporine) is indicated in case of an insufficient response to the glucocorticoid medication and/or persistent inflammatory activity.[69] Their use should be restricted to experienced medical centers only.

Antioxidants

Free radicals and oxidative processes stimulate the immune process in the thyroid and in the eye sockets and are responsible for a substantial part of the orbital damage. Experiments on cell cultures and in animal models as well as clinical studies have already provided specific indications regarding this concept. The most important antioxidant substances include vitamins (C, E, beta-carotene), omega-3 fatty acids (salmon, fish oils), alpha-lipoic acid, nicotinamide, and selenium in particular. Modulation of the inflammatory activity and the autoaggressive mechanisms by the essential trace element selenium have been observed. A randomized trial has demonstrated the protective effect of selenium regarding the inflammatory changes in autoimmune thyroiditis and thyroid eye disease.[75,76] This specific effect of selenium was expected from observations that suggested such immunomodulatory influence.[77,78] A significant clinical improvement was also achieved during a double-blind, randomized trial investigating rheumatoid arthritis.[79] Nonetheless, reliable proof in the form of controlled clinical studies on the effectiveness of antioxidants is still pending. Given the limited treatment alternatives, the low probability of side effects, and the high tolerance rate, supportive antioxidant therapy is likely to be a useful treatment approach in patients with EO.

Table 7.7 Conservative therapeutic procedures in active EO

Clinical signs	Therapy
Mild EO	Symptomatic
Remote subjective complaints	Lacrimal substitute, tanned lenses
Slight inflammatory signs	+ Selenium 300 µg/day for 6 months
Severe EO	Immunosuppressive
High inflammatory activity	Intravenous glucocorticoid administration 0.5 g/day; once/week for 10 weeks
Motility disorders and/or diplopia	0.75 g/day; once/week for 10 weeks
Alternative Treatment	Cyclosporine + steroids (experienced medical centers)
Optic nerve neuropathy	IV methylprednisolone 0.75–1 g/day; twice/week for 2 weeks
Preconditions: euthyroidism + nicotine abstinence	

Memorize

Free radicals and oxidative processes stoke the immune process in the thyroid and in the eye sockets. Antioxidant therapy (e.g., using selenium) is a useful supportive therapy measure in patients with EO.

Controls and Follow-up

Patients with thyroid eye disease in the active stage should be monitored closely and in interdisciplinary collaboration for early detection of possible deterioration of vision, visual field restriction, or corneal lesions. Using a functional TSH receptor antibody test based on a cell-based bioassay, a deterioration of the EO can be predicted in patients with high levels of simulating TSH receptor antibodies. This information can affect treatment decisions, which should be made only by specialists. The recommended conservative therapy regimen for patients with active EO is shown and explained in ▶ Table 7.7.

Memorize

The recommended conservative therapeutic procedure regarding patients with active EO is shown and explained in ▶ Table 7.7.

7.4.2 Radiotherapy of Endocrine Orbitopathy

H. Christiansen and R. M. Hermann

Its potential for regulating inflammation makes radiation therapy an important component in the treatment of EO. This treatment option is especially interesting as it shows similar effectiveness to the use of glucocorticoids but without their typical side effects.

Nonetheless, radiotherapy can act only in the active stage of the disease (CAS ≥ 3/7). Retrobulbar irradiation has no value in the treatment of an inactive, already fibrotic ("burnt out") phase of the disease[51] or in the treatment of a vision-threatening dysthyroid optic neuropathy.[40]

In assessing available studies, it must be kept in mind that both the inclusion criteria and the end points vary between the individual studies. For some groups, eye motility rates are more important,[80] while others focus on determining the exact volumes of intraorbital adipose tissue and eye muscles.[81]

Effectiveness of Radiation

Two prospectively randomized studies demonstrate the significance of radiotherapy (▶ Table 7.8). Mourits et al randomized 60 euthyroid patients without diabetes suffering from moderate-to-severe EO (defined as moderate motility disorders and consecutive diplopia or proptosis of ≥ 23 mm, or moderate to severe eyelid swelling) between 10 × 2 Gy irradiation per working day and 10 × 0 Gy placebo irradiation.[80] After 6 months, eye motility improved in 60% of patients in the 20 Gy group compared to 30% in the 0 Gy group ($p = 0.04$). This was mainly due to a

Table 7.8 Randomized studies of retrobulbar irradiation comparing different dose and fractionation schedules

Author	*n*	Retrobulbar irradiation	Results
Mourits et al[80]	60	10 × 2 Gy	6 months at 10 × 2 Gy: Motility and diplopia enhanced, quicker decrease of disease activity
		10 × 0 Gy	
Prummel et al[82]	88	10 × 2 Gy	6 months: no difference between therapy paths
		10 × 0 Gy	12 months at 10 × 2 Gy: eye bulb motility and diplopia enhanced, decreased need for alt. therapies
Gorman et al[81]	42	1 orbit 10 × 2 Gy	3 months: no difference between both orbits
		Contralaterally 10 × 0 Gy (actually ~10 × 0.2 Gy)	6 months: no difference between both orbits
Gerling et al[85]	86	8 × 0.3 Gy	6 months: no difference between therapy paths
		8 × 2 Gy	
Kahaly et al[86]	65	A: 20 × 1 Gy (weekly)	6 months: clinical response A 67% vs. B 55% and C 57% Conjunctivitis A 0%, B 18%, and C 36%
		B: 10 × 1 Gy (per work day)	
		C: 10 × 2 Gy (per work day)	
Where not otherwise specified, irradiation was carried out on working-day basis (that is 5 times/week).			
Only significant differences in the examined end points are included (or equal effectiveness, where no differences were found).			

reconstitution of the elevation. In the 20 Gy group the diplopia subsequently significantly improved. Patients also showed an earlier decrease in the clinical activity index of the EO. However, differences in exophthalmos, eyelid swelling, and disease activity were not found upon conclusion of the study.

In a second study, Prummel et al randomized 88 euthyroid patients with mild EO (defined as low motility impairment, low eyelid swelling, proptosis of < 24 mm) also between 20 Gy and 0 Gy placebo irradiation.[82] After 6 months, no significant differences between the different treatment measures was found; after 12 months, however, 52% of the 20 Gy group showed significant improvements (particularly regarding motility and diplopia) compared to 27% in the 0 Gy group ($p = 0.02$). Furthermore, the need for alternative treatments was significantly lower after the 20 Gy therapy (66% vs. 84%, $p = 0.049$). Yet there were no notable differences between the groups regarding quality of life and prognosis of EO symptomatology in clinical progression (14% vs. 16%).

7

In a meta-analysis of all available data, a Cochrane review identified an odds ratio of 1.92 (1:27–2.91) regarding the therapy success of orbital radiation compared to placebo irradiation.[83]

> **Memorize**
>
> Compared to the placebo irradiation, 6 to 12 months after treatment, percutaneous irradiation of the retrobulbar region with 10 × 2 Gy leads to a significant improvement of patient's eye motility, to a more rapid remission of the disease, and to a lesser need for alternative therapies in patients suffering from moderate-to-severe active EO.

Dose and Fractionation of Retrobulbar Irradiation

A randomized study that observed the treatment of 42 euthyroid, nondiabetic patients with moderate-to-severe EO appeared to question the previously described results.[81]

One orbit of each patient was normofractionally irradiated with 20 Gy; the other orbit received a placebo irradiation and could thus be regarded as an "internal control" group. After 6 months, each initially nonirradiated orbit was treated. This approach was made possible by a special irradiation technique: Each orbit was individually covered by angled fields (e.g., on the left side with gantry angles of 45° and 135°). Such a technique may only be used in studies, as a significantly higher tissue volume beyond the targeted structures is exposed to irradiation compared to the traditional technique with laterally opposing fields (see "Technique" below at the end of Chapter 7.4.2).

At 3 and at 6 months after treatment there was no difference between the 20 Gy and the placebo-irradiated orbit group in clinical or imaging end points. Although only one orbit was actually treated, the symptoms improved equally in both. This can be explained in various ways: radiogenically altered lymphocytes could have entered the contralateral orbit and triggered biological effects.[83] Furthermore, a higher proportion of patients in the inactive, chronic phase of the disease seem to have been recruited compared to the studies cited before.[84] Another important approach to explaining these findings was provided by the authors themselves after conducting phantom measurements: despite the special irradiation technique, the contralateral orbit treated with placebo irradiation actually received about 2 Gy. The intended 0 Gy dose in this area was not achieved. The low dosage received contralaterally might have triggered similar effects as the originally prescribed 10-fold higher dosage ipsilaterally.

This interpretation of the results is supported by another randomized trial,[85] in which 86 euthyroid patients with EO received a retrobulbar irradiation with 8 × 0.3 Gy per working day (total dose of 2.4 Gy) or 8 × 2 Gy. Although the clinical and imaging end points improved within 6 months after irradiation, no difference between the two treatment schedules was observed. Irradiation with 2.4 Gy was therefore as effective as irradiation with 16 Gy.

A protracted fractionated irradiation with low single doses may even be more effective than the standard dose of 10 × 2 Gy.[86] Kahaly et al. randomized 65 euthyroid patients with mild-to-moderate EO between 20 × 1 Gy weekly (treatment duration corresponding to 20 weeks: path A), 10 × 1 Gy per working day for 2 weeks (path B), or 10 × 2 Gy per working day for 2 weeks as the standard treatment (path C). The authors defined a distinct improvement in at least three objectifiable symptoms of the disease within 6 months as a significant therapy response. The response to treatment was significantly higher in path A at 67% than in path C (55%, $p = 0.007$) and in path B (59%). Radiation-induced conjunctivitis as an acute reaction did not occur in path A, but did occur in 18% of the patients in path B and in 36% of the patients in path C. Ultimately, the protracted 20-week low-dose concept proved to be more effective and better tolerated than the standard path.

In a pilot study with 18 patients, this concept was modified to 10 × 1 Gy administered once a week.[87] After 6 months, all patients showed significant improvements in all symptoms. However, there is still a need for prospective, randomized studies examining this fractionation scheme as well as the required total dosage.

Given these results, medical findings that see no clinical advantage in applying any kind of "dose escalation" up to 30 Gy (15 × 2 Gy) in therapy series compared to 10 × 2 Gy[88] can be considered reasonable.

In summary, the research just outlined shows the following:

1. The effectiveness of orbital irradiation especially in the treatment of an active moderate-to-severe EO[40] with a particular improvement of eye motility. Furthermore, the reduction of disease activity is accelerated, so that, if necessary, rehabilitation surgery of the eye muscles can be performed at an earlier stage.[84]
2. The effectiveness of low dosages of radiation: both 8 × 0.3 Gy per working day and 20 × 1 Gy once a week are effective. So far though, the two schemes have not been prospectively tested against each other. A total dosage of 2.4 Gy should not be accompanied by any side effects, and should be particularly suitable for patients with borderline blood glucose levels. On the other hand, a 20-week immunomodulatory therapy course has conceptual advantages compared to the 2-week treatment. Prior to any change of current treatment concepts, however, it should be noted that all studies covering the combination of steroid and irradiation therapy have used the 10 × 2 Gy standard fractionation.

> **Memorize**
>
> The total dose and fractionation required are not yet determined. An irradiation of 8 × 0.3 Gy per working day seems equally as effective as 8 × 2 Gy per working day. In one study, 20 × 1 Gy per week has proven to be more effective than 10 × 2 Gy per working day. In fact, radiobiological considerations of the modulation of molecular biological milieus support low total dosages and extended application periods.

Possible Molecular Biological Explanations

Very low doses of irradiation can exert notable anti-inflammatory and immunomodulatory effects. Various mechanisms have been described *in vitro*, of which only a selection can be mentioned:

- The endothelial adhesion of lymphocytes is reduced even at 0.3 to 0.7 Gy levels.[89]
- Low doses of radiation can already induce apoptosis in lymphocytes, which, in turn, on direct contact convert fixed macrophages into an anti-inflammatory phenotype.[90]
- The expression of proinflammatory cytokines such as IL-10 and TNF-α is decreased, whereas the expression of anti-inflammatory enzymes (TGF-β1) increases.[91]
- Low doses of radiation cause a differentiation of fibroblasts into fibrocytes, which play a crucial role regarding the progression of EO.[92,93]

These mechanisms can only reduce symptoms in the early, inflammatory stages of EO. Hence, retrobulbar irradiation is only suitable in active phases of the disease and should therefore be part of therapeutic considerations at an early stage;[94] it has no effect on already fibrotic tissues.

> **Memorize**
>
> Ionizing radiation shows anti-inflammatory and immunomodulatory effects, even at low dosages. Hence, radiation therapy in EO treatment can only be effective as long as the inflammation is still active and the fibrotic stage has not yet been reached.

Irradiation and Steroids

A randomized study demonstrated the equal effectiveness of oral prednisone and retrobulbar irradiation with 10 × 2 Gy per working day.[95] Prummel et al. randomized 56 patients with moderate-to-severe EO between oral prednisone (60 mg/day for 2 weeks, 40 mg/day for 2 week, 30 mg/day for 4 weeks, 20 mg/day for 4 weeks, for 3 months in total) + placebo irradiation, and retrobulbar irradiation at 20 Gy + placebo capsules. After 6 months, 50% of patients in the prednisone group showed a significant improvement of symptoms compared to 46% of irradiated patients. Steroid-treated patients showed significantly more side effects.

The **combination of irradiation and steroids** has several advantages. First, it combines the fast-acting steroid treatment with the radiation treatment that exerts its full effect only in the medium term (6–12 months). This prevents relapses after the discontinuation of steroids.[96] At the same time, steroids can deal with an initial increase of eyelid swelling at the beginning of the radiation treatment. Secondly, the combination of these two mechanisms of action is more effective than any individual treatment option alone.[40,97]

The highest effectiveness so far was observed when combining intravenous steroids and irradiation. Marcocci et al randomized 82 patients with moderate-to-severe EO between retrobulbar irradiation in combination with IV methylprednisolone (4 cycles of 15 mg/kg, 4 cycles of 7.5 mg/kg, where 1 cycle = 2 days bi-weekly) or in combination with oral prednisone (100 mg/day, tapering off over 5 months). During follow-up examinations within 12 months, 87.8% of the IV group showed a significant improvement in comparison with 63.4% in the oral group ($p < 0.02$).[98] Moreover, side effects were significantly less common in the IV treatment compared to the oral therapy (▶ Table 7.9).

> **Memorize**
>
> Retrobulbar irradiation and steroid administration complement each other perfectly in terms of impact and effectiveness.

Side Effects and Risks of Retrobulbar Irradiation

Retrobulbar irradiation in normofractionated standard dosage up to 20 Gy is usually well tolerated. About 35% of patients develop an acute reaction in the form of a reversible radiogenic conjunctivitis.[86]

However, an initial intensification of the inflammatory reaction might occur, triggering a transient exacerbation of the ocular symptoms of the EO. This is prevented by simultaneous treatment with steroids (see above).

The development of a **radiogenic retinopathy** is highly improbable as the threshold dose is approximately 30 to 35 Gy (see Chapter 14.5.7). However, with preexisting microangiopathies due to diabetes or arterial hypertension, an increase of such changes was observed even after low doses of radiation.[40] In 2 out of 42 patients in a prospective study,[81] microvascular changes

Table 7.9 Randomized studies on the significance of retrobulbar irradiation and treatment with corticosteroids

Author	*n*	Therapy	Results
Prummel et al[95]	56	10 × 2 Gy irradiation vs. orally administered prednisone	6 months: no difference between therapy paths
Marcocci et al[98]	82	A: 10 × 2 Gy + oral prednisone B: 10 × 2 Gy + IV prednisone	12 months: clinical response A 88%, B 64% Side effects due to steroids: B < A

7

were present before irradiation. Within 3 years after treatment, the changes increased in 1 patient, whereas in 2 others new changes occurred, while all 3 patients suffered from further risk factors (uveitis, poorly adjusted hypertension, elevated blood glucose levels).[99] Thus, diabetic or hypertensive retinal changes are considered absolute contraindications for retrobulbar irradiation. Also, diabetes *without* existing retinopathy is at least a relative contraindication. However, in these cases as well low-dose irradiation with up to 2.4 Gy total dosage can be safely administered.

The risk of accelerated **cataract** development is generally elevated by ionizing radiation. However, this does not influence the therapeutic decision because of exceptionally good treatment options (see Chapter 14.5.6). In various extensive examination series with long follow-up periods, the risk of a clinically significant cataract development was calculated to be about 10% within 10 years after 20 Gy retrobulbar irradiation,[100,101] with the dosage around the lenses adding up to about 10% of the prescribed overall radiation dose (see "Technique" below).

So far, no studies with long-term observation periods have been published describing **malignancy induced by retrobulbar irradiation.**[100,101] On the basis of long-term epidemiologic observations of atomic bomb victims and of patient populations after radiation treatment, mathematical models have been developed for estimating the stochastic lifetime risk for the occurrence of radiogenically induced tumors (ICRP).[102] To do this, specific tissue weighting factors are postulated for each organ individually, which are multiplied with the absorbed dosage to produce a so-called effective dose.

At a field size of 5 × 5 cm using 5 MV photons and taking into account the weighting factors, a cumulative effective dose of about 64 mGy can be estimated.[103] Based on this estimation and according to epidemiological data, a lifetime risk of 14/1,000 patients is postulated for the occurrence of radiogenically induced tumors.[104]

However, this mathematical model was developed for radiation protection and relates to the exposure of complete organ systems to ~1 Gy. Accordingly, other groups argue that a significantly lower risk of radiogenic cancer induction should be adopted, about 3/1,000.[105,106] A comparison of tumor induction rates calculated on the basis of the effective dosage and the actual occurrence of secondary tumors in patient populations irradiated for other benign diseases revealed an overestimation of risk of only 30 to 50% in the mathematical model.[107]

Through the use of smaller fields with individual avoidance of the brain (see "Technique" below) and by using 12 MV photon radiation at a dosage of 10 × 1.6 Gy, the cumulative dose—and therefore all risks—can be halved to about 34 mGy.[104]

This risk (up to 14/1,000, probably much lower) must be seen in relation to the tumor risk of the population who are not additionally radiogenically exposed. In 2008, the lifetime risk of a man in Germany to suffer from malignancy was 50.7% and to die from a malignancy 25.9%; in women the corresponding figures were 42.8% and 20.2% respectively.[108]

Another risk factor for radiogenically induced cancer is the patient's age by the time the radiation exposure occurs. The risk is reduced by the third decade of the patient's life; it starts to decrease steadily from the age of 40 years.[104] By limiting the application of radiation treatment to patients > 30 years of age, exposure of the high-risk juvenile patient population is avoided.

> M!
>
> **Memorize**
>
> In patients with pre-existing diabetic or hypertensive retinopathy, retrobulbar irradiation with 20 Gy is contraindicated. However, irradiation with lower overall dosages (8 × 0.3 Gy) should not be associated with any increased risk.
>
> The risk of developing a clinically relevant cataract amounts to approximately 10% within 10 years after 20 Gy retrobulbar irradiation, but is negligible regarding the indication for radiotherapy, due to there being exceptionally good treatment options.
>
> So far, no publication is available that describes a malignancy induced by retrobulbar irradiation of an EO. Radiation protection calculations defined a theoretical maximum risk of 1.4%, which in reality is most likely to be much lower, especially when using small collimated fields with high photon energies. Radiation exposure should be avoided in patients < 30 years of age.

Technique

The clinical target volume for irradiation is the "retrobulbar space." With techniques usually available, co-irradiation of the posterior eye segment is inevitable.

In the classical, therapy simulator–based approach, the patient is immobilized with an individually adjusted head mask. The position of the lenses can be determined accurately by metal plates that are placed and temporarily fixed on the eyelids. The use of contact lenses in which X-ray markers are embedded would be even more accurate. Using fluoroscopy, asymmetric lateral opposing fields—gantry positions 90° and 270°—are afterward determined. To avoid any kind of radiation divergence into the lenses, the isocenter is placed behind the eyelids and the anterior field segment is closed up to the center of the field (half-field technique). A table rotation provides the possibility to compensate differences in exophthalmos between the eyes. A typical field size is 4 × 4 cm. Using this procedure, the dosage at the lens can be reduced to about 10% of the therapeutic dose.[109] For reasons of radiation protection, it is necessary that the brain be dorsally blocked, cranial and caudal to the bony orbit, by multileaf collimators or individually created blocks (▶ Fig. 7.11b).

The dosage of radiation is at median level, so that a similar dose distribution is ensured in both orbits.

The use of higher photon energies (e.g., 12 MV) leads to a lower radiogenic exposure of at-risk structures, which reduces the radiocarcinogenic risk in particular.[104]

This approach is increasingly being replaced primarily by 3D-planned irradiation on the basis of computed tomography (▶ Fig. 7.11, ▶ Fig. 7.12). This usually leads the same field configuration but eliminates the lens markings (which especially in cases of pronounced eyelid swelling are imprecise) as these are directly defined in the imaging (▶ Fig. 7.11a). Furthermore, the field size can be chosen individually, so that dorsally only the orbital apex is exposed to the 95% isodose (▶ Fig. 7.12). Due to the mask support, only a limited security margin for positional variabilities (planning target volume) of a maximum of 5 mm need be covered.

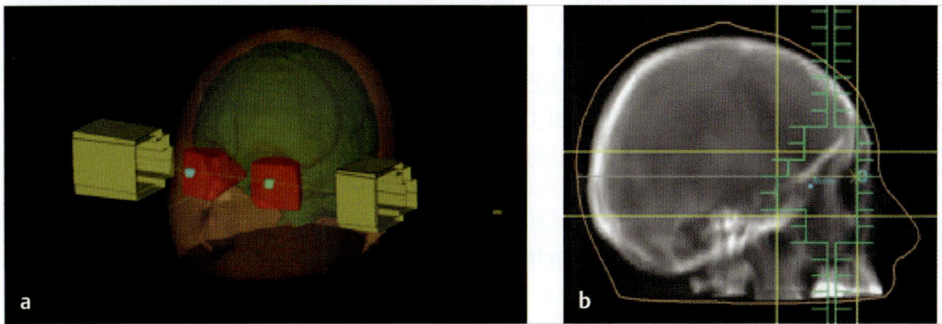

Fig. 7.11 **(a)** Beam paths of radiotherapy in a 3D reconstruction. Red highlights the target volume (retrobulbar space with safety margin); the lenses are marked in green. The individual formation of the irradiation fields due to the multileaf collimators is clearly visible. **(b)** "Beam's eye view": view from the direction of the beam source to a radiograph generated by the planning system. The yellow lines indicate the position of the field aperture, the green dashes the position of the leaves of the collimator (see "Operating Principle and Use of the Linear (Particle) Accelerator" in Chapter 14.2 (p. 230)). Due to the individually controllable positioning of those leaves, the radiogenic burden for the cerebrum can be significantly reduced. Only the area of the orbit within the yellow and green lines is irradiated. The central beam line has been placed directly behind the lenses (blue), to block the lenses and prevent radiation divergence.

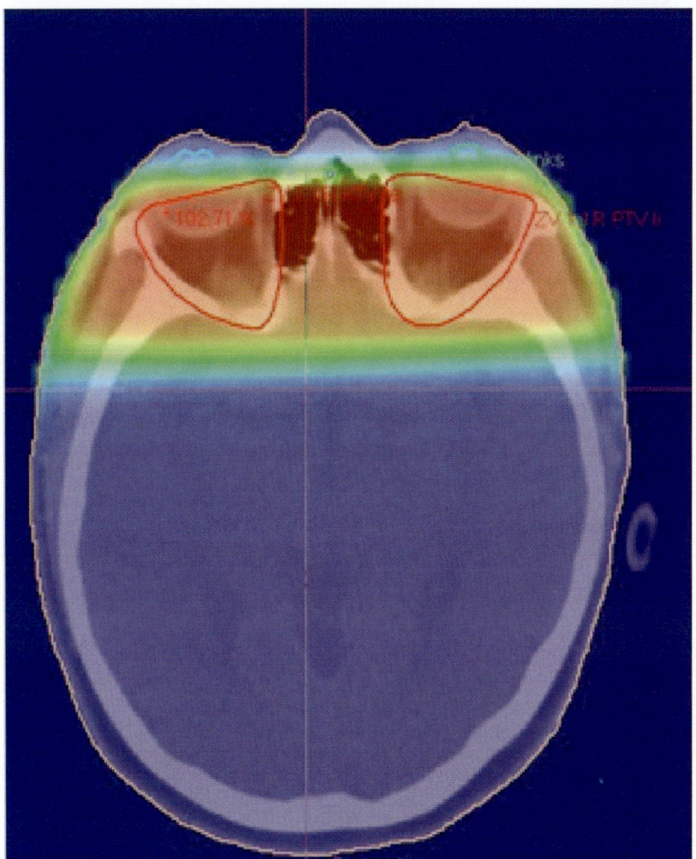

Fig. 7.12 Dose distribution obtained with the previously described technique. Red color represents the 100% isodose, yellow the 95% isodose. Toward the lenses, a steep drop of dosage is visible, which is due to avoidance of beam divergence in this direction.

7.4.3 Orbital Decompression

H.-J. Welkoborsky

According to recommendations of the European Group on Graves's Orbitopathy (EUGOGO) conservative therapy measures should be focused on the treatment of EO.[39,40,41] Intravenous corticosteroid therapy, combined with retrobulbar irradiation where necessary, is considered the therapy of choice. New therapeutic strategies such as immunomodulators or monoclonal antibodies engage the autoimmune mechanism of the disease, but their effectiveness cannot yet be finally assessed.[110,111]

The preceding sections have covered immunosuppressive therapy and retrobulbar irradiation as therapeutic measures. Surgical procedures, in contrast, are considered to be second-line treatment. They are recommended in cases of active thyroid eye disease with impending visual loss when conservative therapy is not successful after about 2 weeks and/or rapid vision loss occurs due to the high increase in pressure in the orbit (acute optic neuropathy due to thyroid dysfunction). These severe forms are present in some 5% of patients with thyroid eye disease.[112] Surgical measures in cases of inactive disease patterns primarily meet the purpose of rehabilitative surgery for an improvement of cosmesis. In the following, the possibilities of surgical orbital decompression are considered.

Definition

Orbital decompression can be defined as surgical intervention to reduce intraorbital pressure. Three different forms are distinguished:

- Bony decompression, in which one or more of the osseous orbital walls is removed.
- Transpalpebral (or transconjunctival) adipose tissue decompression, in which peribulbar and retrobulbar adipose tissue is resected via a transpalpebral approach.
- Surgical procedures using a combination of the two previously described techniques.

According to the number and position of the resected osseous walls, **orbital bony decompression** is differentiated as one-wall, two-wall, and three-wall decompression or as medial, inferior and lateral decompression. **"Balanced" decompression** is defined as the simultaneous removal of the medial and lateral orbital walls.[113] This simultaneous, balanced, removal of the osseous walls has the objective of providing sufficient space, medially and laterally, for the thickened and prolonged outer eye muscles and the increased adipose tissue, which significantly reduces the rate of postoperative diplopia.[113,114]

Epidemiologic studies show that the rate of orbital decompression in patients with EO in England rose from 0.06/100,000 in 1991 to 0.62/100,000 in 2008. In 2011 it was 0.56/100,000, while large regional differences were found.[115] The increase is attributed to the introduction of increasingly improved microsurgical operation techniques, while the drop in surgery rates since 2008 is mainly due to the improved knowledge of the pathophysiology of the disease, with evidence of the effectiveness of conservative treatment measures.

Indications

Depending on the activity degree of the disease there are three substantial indications for orbital decompression:

- In mild to severe EO after exhausting all conservative treatment options.
- In dysthyroid optic nerve neuropathy (DON) cases with no improvement after about 2 weeks, as an emergency intervention with intravenous administration of glucocorticoids. Emergency indicators [116] besides the rapid loss of vision caused by an intraorbital pressure increase are a massive motility disorder or even “frozen globe,” corneal ulcer, and massive proptosis with traction of the optic nerve.[112]
- In inactive or stable mild to severe EO as a cosmetically rehabilitative intervention, treating residual proptosis, double vision, and eye lid retraction. Treatment can be combined with simultaneous eyelid surgery.

Although in emergency situations a rapidly progressive visual loss forces surgery, cosmesis is usually the reason for elective surgery in the inactive or stable state of the disease.[117]

The objectives of orbital decompression are:

- Reduction of intraorbital pressure.
- Reduction of proptosis.
- Reduction of upper eyelid retraction with improved moistening of the cornea, which can facilitate the healing of a corneal ulcer.
- Improvement of eye motility.
- Cosmetic improvement.

In any case, preoperative investigations should include a clinical assessment of the disease activity degree as well as a diagnostic clarification of thyroid hormones. Furthermore, **ophthalmologic examination** must include the determination of visual acuity, visual field, intraocular pressure, and proptosis as well as an assessment of the ocular fundus and anterior eye including the cornea and palpebral fissure. If a decompression of the medial orbital wall is planned, an ENT examination with endoscopic assessment of the nasal cavity is necessary.

Imaging techniques are of decisive importance in the preparation of surgery. Magnetic resonance imaging (MRI) is used for the evaluation of soft tissue structures—that is, the determination of the degree of hypertrophy of the intraorbital muscles and adipose tissue. Computed tomography (CT) visualizes bony rims of the orbit. In many cases, both methods are applied preoperatively. Where possible, the operation should be carried out with the aid of a computerized navigation system. Navigation can rely on MRI and CT data individually, or on a combination of the two data sets by image fusion.

Regardless of the chosen surgical procedure, a surgical microscope or endoscope should always be used in an orbital decompression.[114]

Surgical Procedure of Orbital Decompression

The literature describes numerous surgical procedures. However, a meta-analysis conducted by the Cochrane Institute in 2011 showed that only very few evidence-based studies can be found, complicating a concluding assessment of individual surgical methods.[118] In principle, orbital relief can be reached by two different methods that in recent years have frequently been combined: simple removal of adipose tissue on the one hand (transpalpebral decompression by intraorbital fat removal),[119] and resection of one or more osseous orbital walls on the other (orbital bony decompression) with and without slitting of the periorbita.

Transpalpebral decompression is performed via an access point in the upper eyelid furrow (upper eyelid blepharoplasty) and subciliarly at the lower lid (▶ Fig. 7.13). Alternatively, a

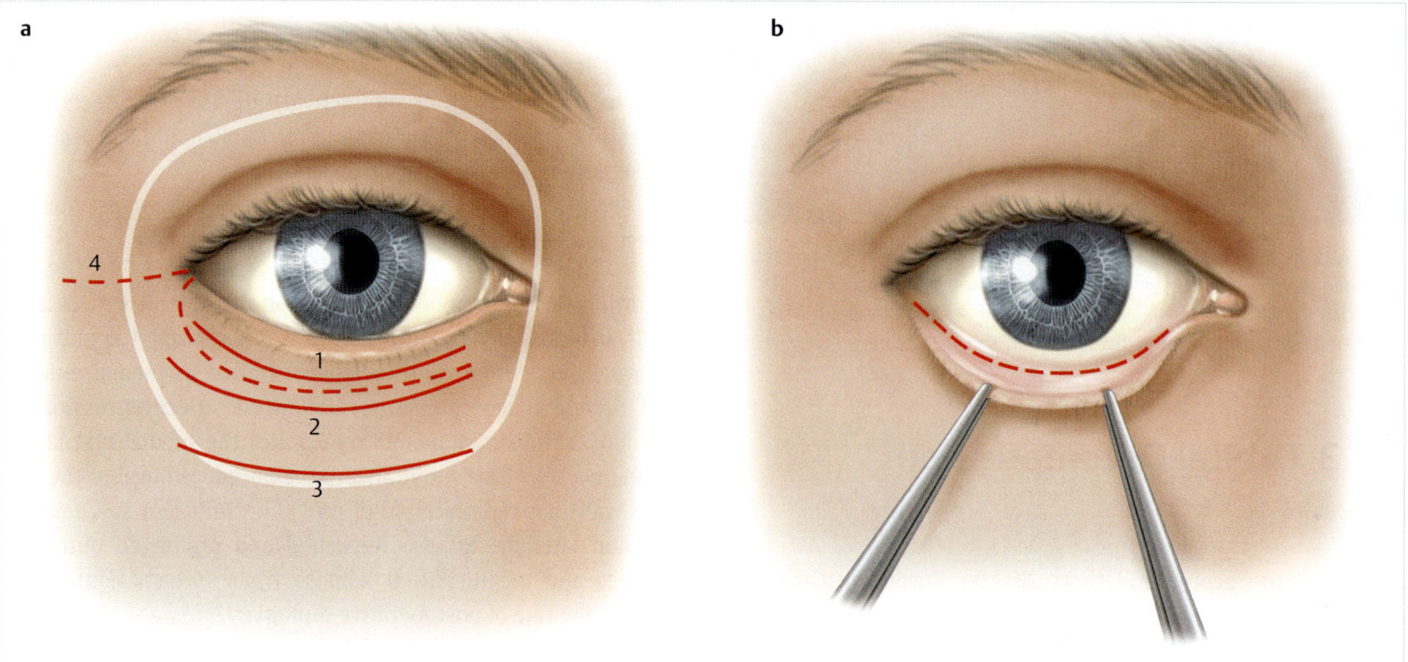

Fig. 7.13 Schematic illustration of incisions for transpalpebral orbital fat tissue resection. **(a)** Subciliary incision or incision in the lid furrow. **(b)** Transconjunctival incision.

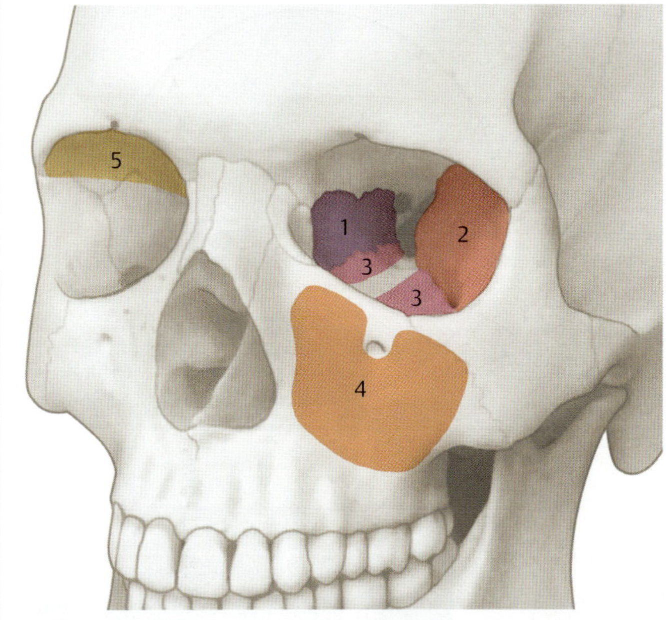

Fig. 7.14 Schematic illustration of the bony orbital walls which are partially resected for bony orbital decompression. (1) The medial orbital wall is resected up to the orbital apex, the resection of the lateral orbital wall (2) extends to the superior orbital fissure. For inferior decompression (3) the remainder of an inferomedial bone strut in the orbital floor, containing the infraorbital nerve is important. (4) Anterior wall of the maxillary sinus. (5) Orbital roof.

transconjunctival access can be chosen with the advantage of leaving no visible scar and having a significantly lower risk of postoperative development of ectropion. In upper eyelid blepharoplasty the orbicularis oculi muscle is transversely split, presenting the space above the aponeurosis of the levator palpebrae muscle. Afterwards, the orbital septum is cut medially, resulting in a prolapse of adipose tissue and enabling the dissection of excrescent fat from the periosteum and the medial rectus muscle.[119]

Orbital bony decompression is performed via a partial resection of the osseous orbital rims. Depending on the number of resected walls, the procedure is called one-wall, two-wall, or three-wall decompression. Resected walls are usually the medial, inferior (floor of the orbit), and lateral walls: resection of the orbital roof is usually not done (▶ Fig. 7.14).

Partial removal of the medial orbital wall (orbital lamina of the ethmoid bone) is performed via endoscopic or microscopic endonasal access. Initially, the ethmoidal cell system is resected from posterior to the transition into the supra-orbital recess in order to create sufficient space for the subsequent prolapse of orbital tissue. Then, the orbital lamina is localized and resected in its entire length. At this point, a protrusion of orbital matter with a still intact periorbita is already visible. This measure alone has a decompressing effect,[116] but this is considerably accentuated by the slitting of the periorbita in its entire length.[116,120] This is followed by a prolapse of adipose tissue as well as an expansion of the hypertrophied muscles (especially the medial rectus muscle) in the ethmoidal cell system (▶ Fig. 7.15). Since the pressure increase especially in the area of the orbital apex has a negative effect on the optic nerve, the resection of the medial wall has to be expanded up to the sphenoid sinus, that is, the orbital apex in the region of the anular tendon (anulus of Zinn).

Some authors recommend a retrocaruncular transconjunctival cut as an alternative to the endonasal access. The advantages are considered to be an increased overview over the surgical area in the resection of the medial orbital wall and the maxilloethmoidal bone pillar, the absence of externally visible scarring, and the possibility of expansion of the resection to the orbital floor.[116]

If necessary, decompression of the optic nerve can be performed simultaneously with the endonasal transethmoidal orbital decompression.[121] For this, the sphenoid sinus is opened and the sphenoid sinus sidewall is displayed. The optic nerve runs in its bone channel laterocranially in the side wall. After identification, the bone shell on the nerve is resected over a circumference of 180° and the nerve sheath is slit where necessary. Endonasal surgery procedures require a full understanding of the anatomical landmarks in order to avoid injury to the carotid artery, which usually runs in the lateral sphenoid sinus wall caudally to the optic nerve, and to the nerve itself.[122,123]

Decompression of the inferior orbital wall (floor of the orbit) can be achieved by an endonasal approach, a transantral approach via the maxillary sinus, or a transconjunctival approach (▶ Fig. 7.16). The remainder of an inferomedial bone strut in the area of the orbital floor is significant as it contains the infraorbital nerve. A resection of this bone strut results in both a caudal displacement of the bulbus and hypoesthesia in the supply area of the nerve.[124] Where required, the resection of the inferior orbital wall can be extended to the sections lateral to the infraorbital canal. Here, the in situ remainder of an inferomedial bone strut containing the nerve canal is important as well, to prevent a postoperative caudal displacement of the eye bulb on the one hand and hypoesthesia on the other hand.[116]

The resection of the lateral orbital wall requires a lateral orbitotomy. Incision can either run at or close behind the lateral orbital rim (*caution*: frontal branch and orbital branch of the facial nerve) or close to the hair border (▶ Fig. 7.17). Some authors also describe a transcanthal transconjunctival access route via the lateral canthus.[125] After exposure of the lateral orbital rim the temporal muscle is separated from the lateral orbital wall and shifted caudally. This is followed by the resection of the lateral orbital wall including parts of the zygomatic bone up to the greater wing of the sphenoid bone in the region of the inferior orbital fissure.[126,127]

Postoperative Findings

Orbital decompression surgery reduces hydrostatic pressure on the optic nerve and consequently decreases intraorbital pressure. In addition to the reduction of proptosis, this also results in an improvement of arterial blood flow and venous drainage of the nerve, which improves the axonal flow within the nerve, increasing visual acuity.[116,128,129] Additionally, it has been observed that one-sided decompression led to a decrease of the disease's clinical activity score (CAS) on both the operated and nonoperated sides, equally associated with improved venous drainage, lower intraorbital pressure, and a reduction of inflammatory cytokine expression.[130]

The **evaluation of the decompression effect** depends on the chosen surgical technique and is difficult insofar as few evidence-based studies have been published.[118,131] Thus, no general recommendations regarding specific surgical techniques can be derived.[118,131] In addition to the CAS, the following clinical

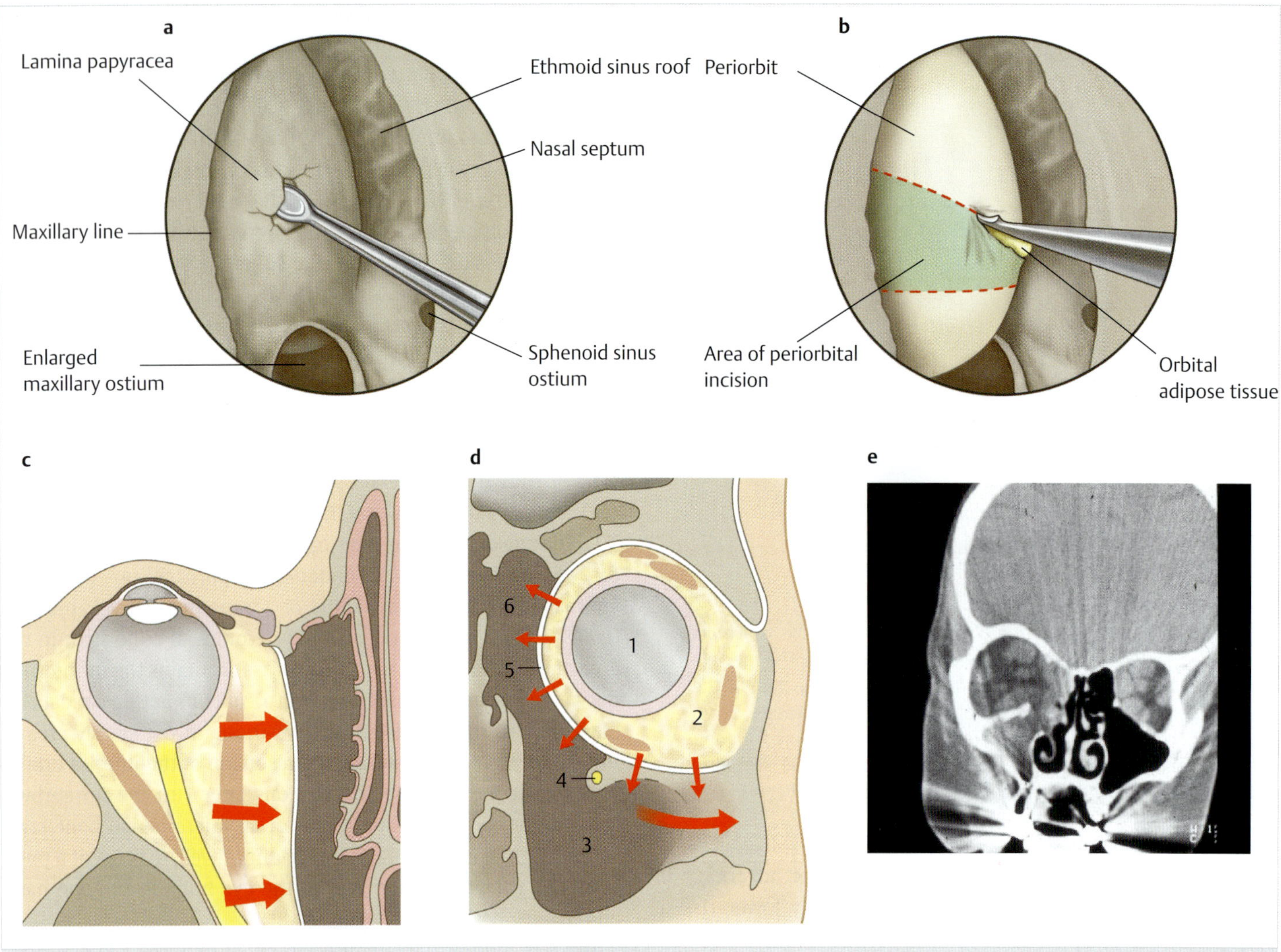

Fig. 7.15 Schematic illustration of a medial and medio-inferior orbital decompression using an endonasal endoscopic approach. **(a)** The lamina payracea is exposed and resected in its entire length. **(b)** At this point the periorbita remains still intact and is slit in its entire length after resection of the lamina papyracea. **(c)** This is followed by a prolapse of adipose tissue and an expansion of the hypertrophied medial rectus muscle in the ethmoidal cell system. **(d)** The decompression can be expanded laterally for resection of the medial parts of the orbital floor. The resection of the orbital floor is limited by the infra-orbital canal which remains intact. 1, eye bulb; 2, orbital adipose tissue; 3, maxillary sinus; 4, infra-orbital nerve; 5, periorbita; 6, ethmoid sinus. **(e)** CT scan some days after a medio-inferior orbital decompression on the right side. The prolapsed orbital tissue is clearly visible.

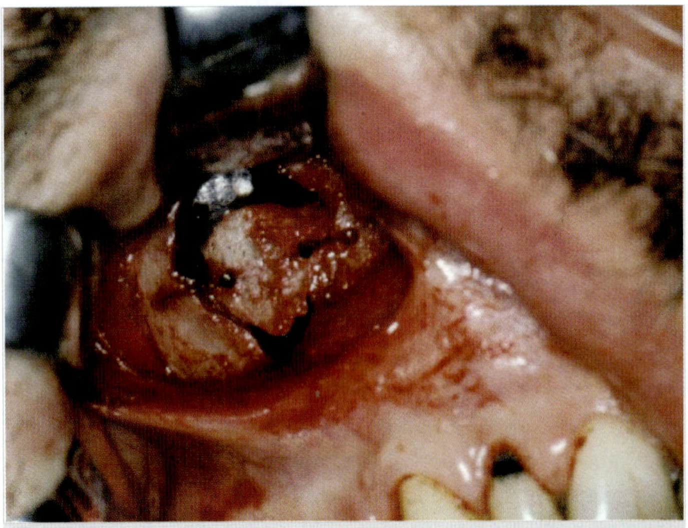

Fig. 7.16 Inferior decompression using a transantral approach. The soft tissue of the cheek are pushed away with a hook. Parts of the orbital floor are resected following the opening of the sinus via the anterior maxillary wall. The inferior decompression can alternatively also be performed via a transconjunctival or subciliary approach.

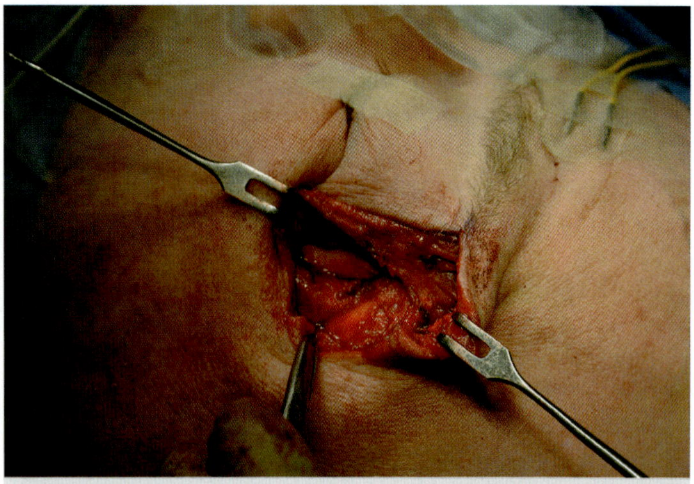

Fig. 7.17 Lateral orbital decompression. The bony lateral orbital wall has been resected, but the periorbita is still not slit.

parameters can be used postoperatively to assess the decompression effect: **visual acuity, proptosis**, and the postoperative occurrence or improvement of preoperatively existing **diplopia**.

Postoperative Visual Acuity

In the literature, indications regarding postoperative improvement of **visual acuity** vary between 25 and 100%. This seems to be independent of whether in addition to a two-wall decompression adipose tissue was resected or not. It should be noted that very different specifications are made regarding preoperative visual loss and postoperative visual improvements. In some cases, no data is provided (▶ Table 7.10). Nor do many studies include information on whether patients presented with active or inactive thyroid eye disease. Clauser et al report on a normalization of visual evoked potentials as a result of decompression surgery.[132] Similar observations were reported by other working groups, who stated that, in patients with traumatic optic neuropathy and profound visual loss, effects of optic nerve decompression can already be observed intraoperatively as a recovery of potentials immediately after opening the nerve-sheath.[133] Information on visual deterioration is found only sporadically, mostly indicating complications during surgery. Ultimately, however, it should be noted that in many cases recovery of visual acuity is achieved by orbital decompression surgery, a fact that is easily reconciled with pathophysiological processes that lead to vision loss and are interrupted by surgery.

Proptosis

There are various reports in the literature regarding the reduction of proptosis, ranging from 2.53 mm in the study by Alsuhaibani et al[134] to 8.1 mm in the study by Wang et al.[125] (cf. ▶ Table 7.10). An evaluation of these studies suggests the following.

1. The combination of bony decompression and fat resection leads to a stronger decrease in proptosis than fat resection alone.[118,135] Olivari's publication is an exception to this conclusion, describing an average 6 mm decrease of proptosis solely from performing adipose tissue resection.[119] Again, it must be taken into account that studies are usually based on retrospective analysis, and describe very different methods of bony decompression and fat resection. Thus, these studies have a valuable descriptive character but do not allow the derivation of generally valid, evidence-based conclusions and recommendations.[118] Hence, it is important to know whether the adipose

7

Table 7.10 Results of orbital decompression in relation to the reduction of the exophthalmos, to the improvement of visual acuity, and to diplopia depending on the surgical method used (ns = not specified)

Author	Year	Number of orbits (Number of Patients)	Decrease of Hertel value	Surgical technique	Improvement of visual acuity	Postoperative diplopia
Shepard et al[113]	1998	18	4.6 mm	Medial and lateral	100%	ns
Kacker et al[141]	2003	22	5.9 mm	Medial and lateral	100%	30.7% (4/13 patients)
Unal et al[138]	2003	13	6.9 mm	3-walls: medial, inferior and lateral	ns	57.1%
Graham et al[144]	2003	63	4.1 mm	Medial and lateral	ns	10% (4/40 patients)
Sellari-Francheschini et al[127]	2005	276	5.3 mm	Medial and lateral	ns	20%
Kahaly et al[117]	2007	264 (142)	3 mm	2-walls: medial, inferior additional adipose tissue reduction	ns	100 patients preoperative diplopia 4 patients additional postoperative diplopia
Olivari[119]	2010	1000 (511)	6.0 mm	Transpalpebral adipose tissue reduction	Preoperative 10.7% Postoperative 1.7%	Preoperative 72% patients diplopia Postoperative 18% patients diplopia
Alsuhaibani et al[134]	2011	38	2.53 mm	Medial and lateral	ns	ns
Rocchi et al[136]	2012	247	5.7 mm	Medial and lateral	ns	17.8%
			4.0 mm	Lateral		0%
Lal et al[146]	2013	24	3.7 mm	Medial and inferior	50%	0%
Fichter et al[137]	2013	30	3.0 mm	Lateral and adipose tissue reduction	ns	ns
Wang et al[125]	2013	66	8.1 mm	3-walls: lateral, medial, and orbital floor	25%	10.6% (7/66)
Roncevic et al[139]	2013	130	7.2 mm	3-walls: lateral, medial, and orbital floor as well as adipose tissue reduction	68%	4.6% (6/130 patients)
Onaran et al[128]	2014	72	6.2 mm	2-wall decompression and adipose tissue reduction	ns	ns
Lee et al[140]	2014	90	5.1 mm	2-wall-decompression and adipose tissue reduction	100%	14.5% (8/55 patients)

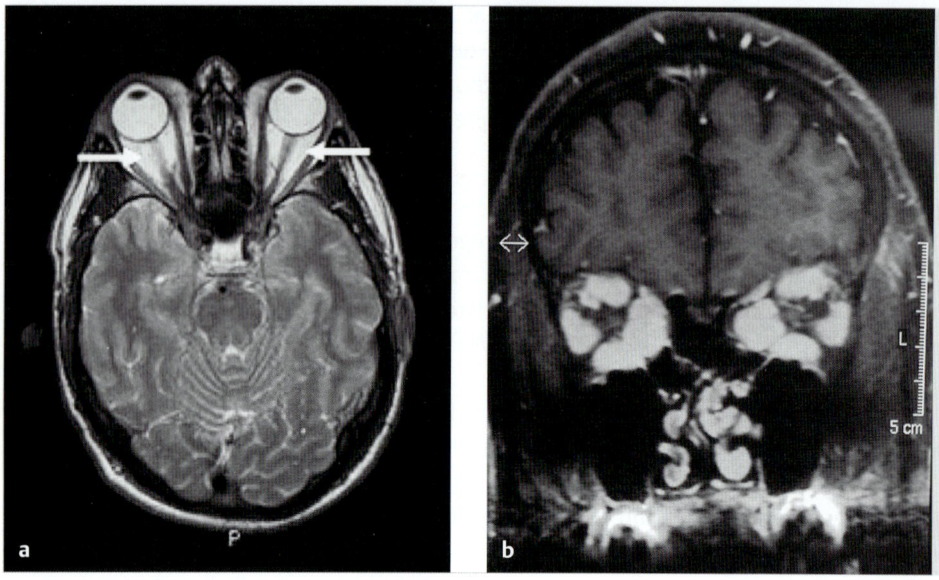

Fig. 7.18 Preoperative MRI scans. (a) In a patient with considerable proliferation of adipose tissue and slim extraocular muscles (adipose tissue type). (b) In a patient where excessive hypertrophy of the extraocular muscles is predominant (mucular type).

tissue resection, as described by Olivari, was conducted up to the orbital apex or limited to the peribulbar and retrobulbar area.

2. A purely lateral decompression seems to be less effective than a medial-inferior two-wall decompression in terms of reduction of proptosis.[114,136,137] However, specific features of the surgical technique have to be considered here as well, as it is of significance whether the resection of the medial orbital wall was performed transethmoidally or transconjunctivally.
3. Studies in which a three-wall decompression was performed (i.e., both the medial and the lateral and inferior orbital wall were resected) report the highest reduction of exophthalmos, which is unsurprising.[125,138,139]
4. An explanation for the huge differences found between the studies evaluated might also be pathology as the basis for surgical indications. Preoperative MRI of the orbit is used for determination. Where excessive adipose tissue in the orbit dominates the disease, thorough adipose tissue resection seems to be indicated and should lead to satisfactory results (adipose tissue type). In cases with predominant hypertrophy of intraorbital muscles (muscular type), a pure resection of adipose tissue is not likely to be sufficient and a bony decompression should be performed. Mostly, however, a combination of the two findings is observed (▶ Fig. 7.18). In these cases a combined bony decompression and resection of adipose tissue is indicated. This case-based, individualized surgical indication is referred to as "graded decompression".[140]

In summary and based on the author's experience:

1. In cases in which hypertrophy of intraorbital muscles or a combination of muscle hypertrophy and adipose tissue dominates the clinical picture, bony decompression is superior to just adipose tissue resection in terms of postoperative visual improvement and decrease of proptosis.
2. Decompression should always proceed to the orbital apex, as the highest hydrostatic pressure on the optic nerve is found here. To achieving this, exclusively lateral decompression surgery is less suitable than medial or combined medial–inferior decompression because the orbital apex cannot be reached laterally.[126] This is particularly important in cases where decompression of the optic nerve has to be performed simultaneously. There is some evidence in the literature supporting the assumption that a balanced decompression with or without fat resection is the most effective method and delivers relatively few complications.[118,141]
3. A simultaneous resection of adipose tissue leads to both decompression effects and a decline of the upper eyelid retraction and thus to a significant improvement of cosmesis (▶ Fig. 7.19) when performed retrobulbarly as well as peribulbarly.

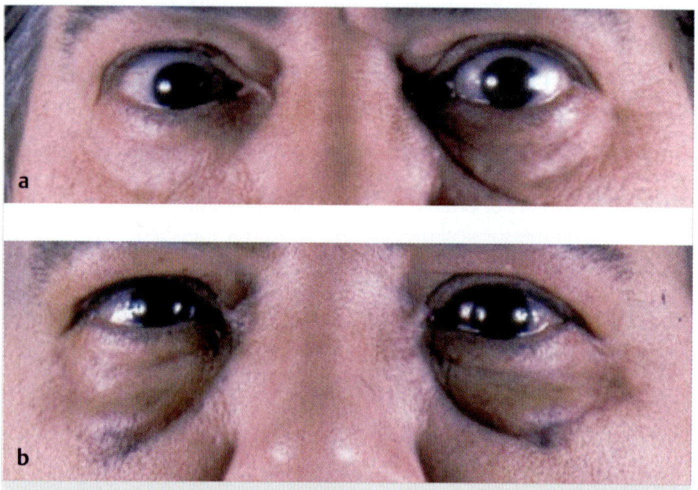

Fig. 7.19 Female patient with Graves's orbitopathy. (a) Preoperative view. (b) Postoperatively following combined endonasal transethmoid medial and inferomedial decompression along with resection of orbital adipose tissue via a transpalpebral approach.

This approach seems pragmatic and is based on clinical considerations. But as long as there are no existing evidence-based and particularly prospective and randomized studies comparing different surgical procedures on a large number of patients, a general recommendation cannot be made.[114,118,131]

Diplopia

Because the literature offers conflicting data, reduction of double vision is also difficult. Some studies do not mention rates of preoperative diplopia, others mention rates of preoperative diplopia only, and yet others mention only rates of postoperative diplopia. Also, it is often unclear how double vision is measured.[142] General standards cannot be derived from the reviewed literature. The rate of double vision ranges from 4.6% [139] through 34%[142] to 57%.[138] It seems to be dependent on the chosen surgical process among other things:

1. An adipose tissue reduction alone leads to a low rate of postoperative diplopia.[119]
2. In bony decompression the rate of postoperative diplopia in medial and inferior two-wall decompression is higher than in a solely lateral decompression.[116,136,143] This is understandable since medial and inferior decompression results in a prolapse of the hypertrophied and (due to proptosis) extended medial and inferior rectus muscles, which are then "too long" and are stretched, resulting in double images.
3. The rate of diplopia increases in cases of medial decompression that include the slitting of the periorbita.[120] If no inferomedial bone pillar is left during inferior decompression, the risk of double vision is also increased[124] (▶ Fig. 7.19).
4. Balanced decompression—a simultaneous resection of the medial and lateral orbital wall—reduces the rate of postoperative double vision compared to a three-wall decompression with additional resection of the orbital floor. It is reported with less than 10% to 20% of cases.[113,123,127,138,141,143,144,145]
5. Existing preoperative diplopia improves only partially after bony decompression regardless of the selected approach. In many cases, new double vision occurs [120,131,136,142].
6. The prognosis for postoperative diplopia is considered to be rather positive. It usually responds well to conservative measures of therapy (prisms, covers, orthoptics).[139,142,146,147,148,149]
7. If secondary strabismus surgery is necessary for the correction of diplopia, previous decompression has no negative influence on the outcome of the surgery.[120,150]

Thus, it can be concluded that orbital decompression surgery eliminates or improves preoperatively existing diplopia only in a subset of patients. Some patients postoperatively present new cases of diplopia. The highest rate of postoperative diplopia seems to be triggered by a combination of medial–inferior two-wall decompression with periorbita slitting. The lowest rate is observed after lateral decompression or simple adipose tissue reduction. The prognosis of diplopia is considered positive.

Complications

The literature covers only relatively few studies regarding complications after orbital decompression. In their meta-analysis, Leong et al report a complication rate of 9.3%.[131] The occurrence of complications depends on the surgical procedure chosen. Complication rates seem to be lower following the endonasal transethmoidal approach than with the endoscopic transantral method, which is explained by a better overview of the operating field and anatomically important structures.[118] The most common complication is postoperative double vision.

Complications can essentially be classified as ocular complications, sinogenic complications, and intracerebral complications.

Ocular Complications

In addition to postoperative diplopia **deterioration in vision** may occur. The cause is usually found in an injury of the optic

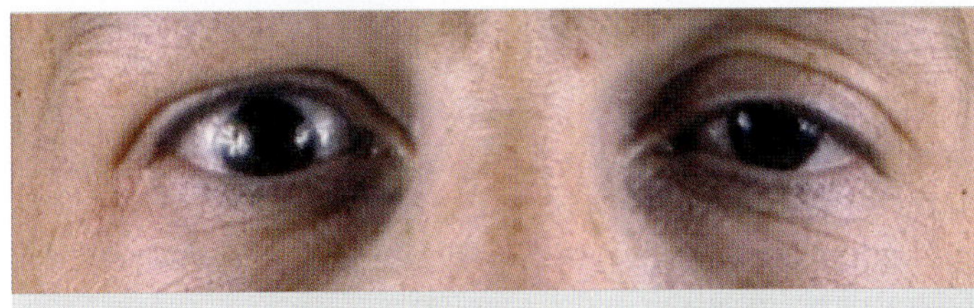

Fig. 7.20 Patient with a significant caudal displacement of the left eye bulb and severe double vision following resection of the entire orbital floor.

nerve or in pressure damage due to hemorrhage following injury to blood vessels. This complication occurs in less than 1% of cases, while the risk of optic nerve injury is lower in endonasal surgical procedures as the nerve and its channel can be observed under direct vision. Kahaly et al describe **eyeball motility disorders** in 22 out of 142 patients, however, these are usually only temporary.[117] In addition to a significant sensory disturbance in the distribution of the infraorbital nerve, a resection of the entire orbital floor in course of inferior decompression leads to caudal displacement of the eyeball (▶ Fig. 7.20).[124] **Oscillopsia** is reported as a complication after lateral decompression occurring in about 35% of cases and usually regressing spontaneously within months.[151] A **medial deviation** of the eyeball can occur after medial and lateral two-wall decompression and is usually relieved by exercise.[134] Ultimately, lateral orbitotomy can lead to a **depression of the temporal region**. This is due to the fact that the temporal muscle is separated from the lateral orbital wall and partially displaced caudally and was only partially relocated.[137]

Sinogenic Complications

Sinogenic complications occur in about 3.5% of cases. They are more common in connection with endonasal transethmoidal surgical procedures than after endoscopic transantral or transconjunctival access.[152] Complications include the following:

- **Bleeding**. Bleeding occurs following an injury of the anterior or posterior ethmoid artery. Less common are injuries to intraorbital vessels. Hemorrhage into the orbit may lead to renewed pressure increase despite decompression.
- **Sinusitis**. The most common sinogenic complication is postoperative sinusitis usually affecting the frontal sinus, less commonly the maxillary or sphenoid sinus. Pathogenically, sinusitis develops due to the relocation of the canals of the affected sinus with subsequent congestion of blood, wound exudate, and mucus followed by secondary infection. It is well treatable with antibiotics. However, cases have been described in which postoperative sinusitis led to blindness as a result of spread to the optic nerve.[153]
- **Adhesions and synechiae**. Adhesions to the lateral nose wall of orbital contents prolapsed into the ethmoidal cell system may lead to a blocking of the sinus ostium with a subsequent development of *chronic sinusitis*. This usually affects the frontal sinus. In many cases, follow-up surgery with re-opening of the sinus is necessary. To prevent the development of synechiae it is important to broadly open the frontal sinus and to drain it toward the nose during decompression surgery. A consistent endonasal treatment in the first postoperative week can also prevent synechiae.

Intracerebral Complications

Intracerebral complications are usually rare. Violation of the skull base may cause **rhinoliquorrhea**, which requires the covering of the defect. Injuries of the skull base may sometimes also result in **meningitis. Intracerebral hemorrhages** occur only with injuries of dural or brain vessels and are very rare.

7.4.4 Eyelid Surgery in Endocrine Orbitopathy

M. A. Varde and B. Wiechens

Introduction

7

Correction of eyelid malpositions in the context of EO is performed, wherever possible, in the **inactive stage** of the disease. Its aim is the restoration of eyelid function, rehabilitation, and the correction of the esthetic consequences of the disease. In rare cases, lid surgery becomes necessary in the active stage of the disease, for example, in patients with **exposure keratopathy**.

The most common malpositions of the eyelid in EO are **lagophthalmos, lid retraction**, and **ptosis**. Swelling of the soft tissues and an increase in the orbital adipose tissue causes **dermatochalasis** (excess skin) and orbital fat prolapse (▶ Fig. 7.21) (Chapter 7.3).

Generally, surgical procedures are avoided in the active stages of EO. Exceptions are exposure keratopathy not sufficiently treatable with conservative measures, and optic nerve compression. The technique of optic nerve decompression has been described in detail in earlier chapters. Before rehabilitative surgery of the periocular area can be considered, stable euthyroid state, clinical inactivity, and stable clinical findings (proptosis, strabismus, lid position) have to be ensured.

Correction of Lagophthalmos

In the acute stage of exposure keratopathy, a **tarsorrhaphy** may be necessary in rare cases. The surgical technique, as well as the technique of **chemotarsorrhaphy** with botulinum toxin, is described in Chapter 16.4 in the context of treatment for facial nerve palsy. The surgery is often challenging due to the swollen periorbital structures and frequent exophthalmos. Conservative measures for the protection of the ocular surface such as artificial tears and the creation of a moist chamber are analogous to those in facial nerve palsy.

Because of the exophthalmos it is often not possible to apply a moist chamber as the cornea comes into contact with the bandage. In these cases immediate orbital decompression (Chapter 7.4.3) can be considered.

Correction of Eyelid Retraction

Prior to eyelid surgery, orbital decompression—if indicated—and strabismus surgery have to be completed.[154] In cases of persistent significant exophthalmos, the cosmetic result anticipated from lid surgery is limited. A pseudo lid retraction is treated by correcting the relevant mechanisms (as discussed next).

Correction of Pseudo Lid Retraction

Differentiation between pseudo lid retraction and true lid retraction is crucial as the former has other causes (restrictive strabismus and exophthalmos) that have to be corrected *before* lid surgery is considered. Possible treatment options are recession of the frequently fibrosed inferior rectus muscle in the former scenario and orbital decompression in case of the latter.

Restrictive strabismus due to a fibrosed inferior rectus muscle can be diagnosed through the **cover test** and the **forced duction test (FDT)**. The FDT is carried out while the patient lies supine. The patient is instructed to desist from any voluntary eye movements as much as possible. A topical anesthetic (Proparacaine eyedrops) is used to adequately anesthetize the ocular surface. Using two fine-toothed surgical forceps, the globe is grasped at the limbus (for testing the vertical recti muscles at the 3 and 9 o'clock positions, and for testing the horizontal recti muscles at the 12 and 6 o'clock positions). Care is taken to not depress the globe into the orbit as this may lead to slackening of the recti muscles and a false negative test result. The globe is passively elevated and depressed to test the vertical recti, and adducted and abducted to test the horizontal recti. The resistance felt by the examiner to these passive movements is accessed. An increased resistance in one direction (for example, for elevation) gives a positive test for inferior rectus muscle indicating that the muscle is taut and fibrosed and hence restricts elevation of that globe.

Surgical correction of restrictive strabismus is mainly **recession of the fibrosed muscle**. Resection or plication surgeries are avoided as much as possible in EO. Surgery in these cases is frequently difficult due to advanced fibrosis. In case of an inferior rectus recession, a standard inferior conjunctival peritomy and dissection and exposure of the muscle are performed. It is paramount to meticulously dissect the muscle from its attachment to the lower-lid retractors and to the ligaments of the lower fornix. After securing the muscle with 6–0 absorbable sutures, it is disinserted from its original insertion, recessed and sutured back to the sclera. Unfortunately, the standard tables and the general rules which determine the amount of recession in regular cases are not suitable in EO. The tautness of the muscle on FDT, the tightness of the muscle on table during dissection, and the experience of the surgeon in such cases help in determining the amount of recession and there may still be surprises. Hence, recession with adjustable suture technique is a preferable variation, wherein the muscle is recessed with or without a "Hang-back" technique (the author prefers the former) and the sutures

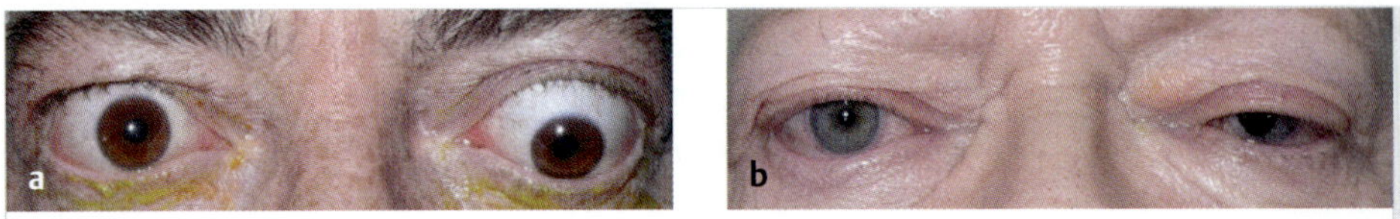

Fig. 7.21 Lid position abnormalities in Graves's orbitopathy. **(a)** Bilateral upper lid retraction with lateral flare. **(b)** Aponeurotic ptosis, dermatochalasis, orbital fat prolapse. The left pupil is dilated due to unrelated traumatic mydriasis.

are tied in a "bow-tie" knot. This allows final adjustments to be carried out once the anesthesia has worn off and the patient can cooperate for a cover test.

With the recession of the inferior rectus, a pseudo upper-lid retraction often corrects itself. An increase in the lower-lid retraction after a inferior rectus recession is caused by failure to adequately severe the attachments of the inferior rectus to the lower-lid retractors. These check-ligaments are attachments of the muscle to the inferior fornix. Nevertheless, with large recessions of the inferior rectus, a lower-lid retraction often occurs.

An alternative to strabismus surgery, mainly in the active stage of the EO, is the selective paralysis of the muscle by injecting botulinum toxin into the muscle belly. This can either be done under direct view or transconjunctivally monitored by electromyography.[155]

Correction of True Lid Retraction

The severity of upper lid retraction is classified as mild, moderate, and severe. Surgical correction of true lid retraction of the upper lid can be achieved by **Müllerectomy, levator disinsertion, levator recession**, or **blepharotomy** depending on severity. The correction of lower eyelid retraction can be achieved through **retractor recession** with a spacer graft.

One treatment option as a minimally invasive therapy approach or with clinical activity of the EO, is an **injection of botulinum toxin A**[156] or **triamcinolone**[157] **into the levator palpebrae superioris (LPS) muscle**. The upper lid is everted and approximately 10 units of Botox A or 20 mg of triamcinolone are injected subconjunctivally at the upper edge of the tarsus (▶ Fig. 7.22). The injections may be repeated where necessary.

A **Müller muscle excision (Müllerectomy)** is a treatment option in cases with mild lid retraction. This procedure is preferably carried out transconjunctivally. After administering a suitable local anesthetic-epinephrine mixture, a traction suture is applied to the upper lid and the lid is everted over a **Desmarres retractor**. Some local anesthetic is injected under the Müller muscle at the upper tarsal border. The conjunctiva with Müller muscle is incised

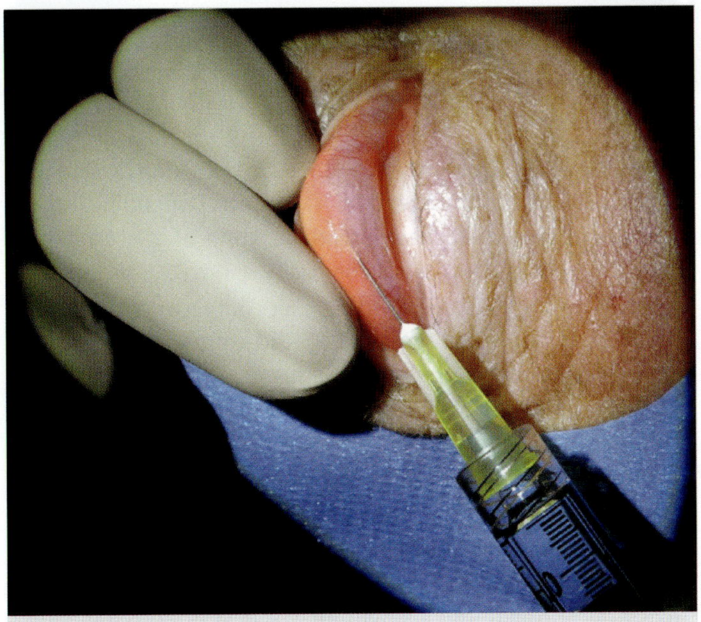

Fig. 7.22 Transconjunctival injection of botulinum toxin to the superior tarsal border for treatment of pronounced retraction and entropion of the upper lid in a patient with active GO.

and separated from the LPS. The Müller muscle is carefully dissected and excised completely. Since the surgery is done under local anesthesia, the lid height and contour can be checked intraoperatively.

In case of residual retraction, a Müllerectomy can be supplemented with a graduated disinsertion or recession of the LPS. The levator is disinserted in stages. Here it is important to separate the lateral attachments of the LPS, since "lateral flare" is cosmetically annoying.[158]

A **levator recession and Müllerectomy via a transcutaneous approach** is another surgical option and can be achieved with a hangback recession of the levator (▶ Fig. 7.23) or with a spacer graft taken from sclera or bovine pericardium. The advantage of the anterior approach is the possibility of combination with a blepharoplasty as well as the easier exposure of the anatomical structures.

The graded **blepharotomy**[159] is mainly done in moderate-to-severe upper lid retraction. Here, a lid crease incision on the upper lid is deepened in layers separating almost the entire lid, until the desired effect is obtained, oftentimes separation is carried out until the conjunctiva is reached. Then the skin is closed superficially.

Lower lid retraction often requires a spacer graft for its correction; this is sutured in between the lower edge of the tarsal plate and the lid retractors. Donor sclera or bovine pericardium are particularly suitable graft tissues. Where necessary, a horizontal lid shortening procedure can be done. However, the possibility of retraction of a tightened lower lid in a protruding globe has to be taken into account.

Correction of Ptosis

Aponeurotic ptosis in EO does not significantly differ from those observed in age-related changes, trauma or associated with contact lens wear. However, in EO, there is often significant increase and prolapse of the orbital fat as well as cicatricial changes of the levator palpebrae superioris muscle due to the chronic inflammation.

Aponeurotic ptosis can be corrected by transcutaneous or transconjunctival levator reinsertion. It can be combined with an upper lid blepharoplasty. If the surgery is done under local anesthesia, the surgeon has the option of assessing lid height and contour during the surgery.

With transcutaneous (anterior approach) **levator reinsertion**, a lid crease incision is done and the dissection plane deepened onto the tarsal plate. Dissection is continued superiorly underneath the orbicularis muscle until the orbital septum is visible. This is incised horizontally and the preaponeurotic fat pad is retracted so that the aponeurosis of the LPS becomes visible as a white layer. The aponeurosis is often found to be disinserted, can be attenuated, or shows fatty infiltration. A 5–0 polypropylene suture is placed in the intact part of the aponeurosis and secured to the tarsal plate, making sure there is no full thickness bites through the tarsus. The first suture is placed at the level of the lid apex, mostly in the medial third of the lid. The lid height is checked and modified if needed. A second suture is placed laterally to the first one and the eyelid contour is re-checked. Before the wound is closed, where necessary, a resection of orbital fat from the medial and middle fat pad is carried out and the eyelid contour and shape are checked once more[160] (▶ Fig. 7.24).

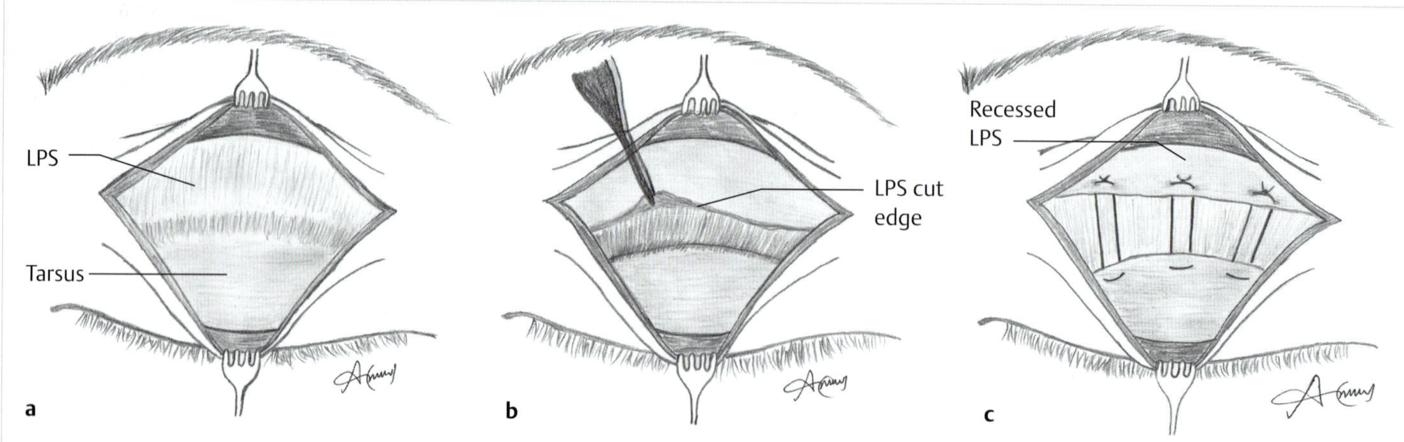

Fig. 7.23 Levator recession with hangback sutures. **(a)** Dissection of LPS via an anterior approach. **(b)** Excision of the underlying Müller's muscle. **(c)** Disinsertion of the medial and lateral horn of the LPS and re-suturing to the tarsal plate with 6-0 hangback sutures.

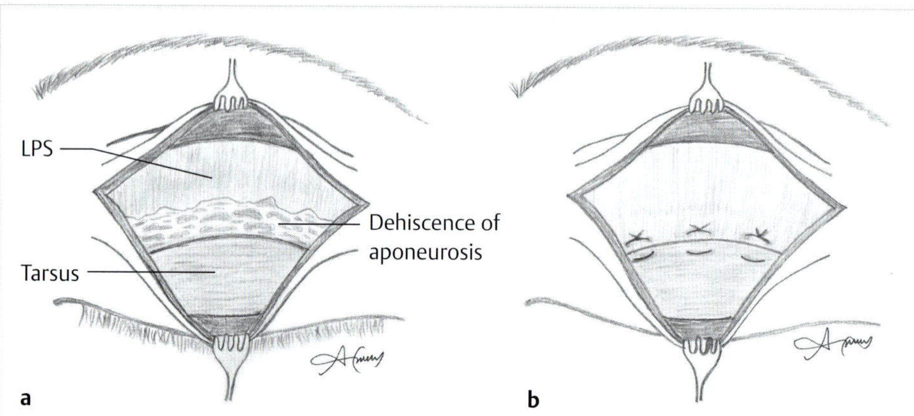

Fig. 7.24 Anterior approach levator reinsertion. **(a)** Lid crease incision, dissection onto the tarsal plate and the septum. Incision of the septum to display the levator muscle. **(b)** Reattachment of the intact aponeurosis to the tarsal plate with 5-0 polypropylene sutures.

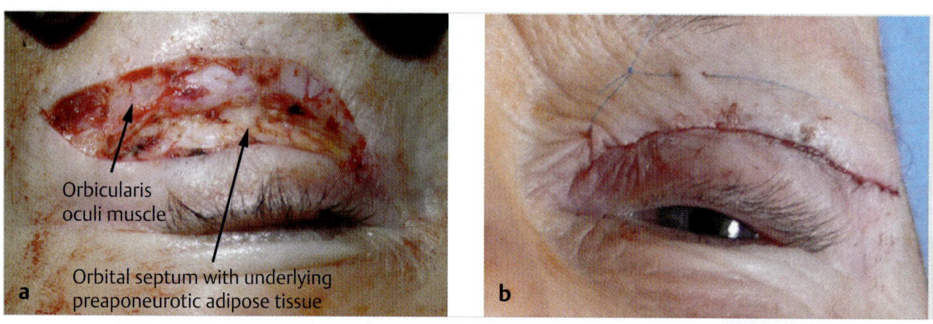

Fig. 7.25 Upper lid blepharoplasty. **(a)** Excision of skin and underlying orbicularis. **(b)** Intracutaneous wound closure.

Levator surgery can also be combined with an **upper lid blepharoplasty** (described below).

A further option for correcting ptosis is **transconjunctival levator tuck** ("white line advancement"), in which the levator aponeurosis is displayed via a conjunctival incision analogous to the Müllerectomy and sutured to the upper edge of the tarsal plate with absorbable sutures.[161,162]

Correction of Dermatochalasis and Orbital Fat Prolapse

Upper lid blepharoplasty is generally carried out transcutaneously. The incision is drawn before infiltration and at least 20 mm of skin should remain between the lower edge of the eyebrow and eyelashes so that lagophthalmos due to excessive skin removal is avoided. The lower part of the incision is in the lid crease, the upper part depends on the extent and location of the excess skin. After administration of local anesthetic, the skin incision is performed and the skin is excised. Depending on the nature of the dermatochalasis and the tone of the orbicularis muscle, the orbicularis can also be partly removed. The septum is opened over the medial and middle fat compartment and, after cauterization, fat is excised until the lid contour is satisfactory before the wound is closed (▶ Fig. 7.25). Care has to be taken not to remove too much orbital fat, since this might lead to superior sulcus deformity and a sunken appearance.

Adjuvant procedures with an upper eyelid blepharoplasty are, for example, ptosis correction by **levator reinsertion** (as above) and **repositioning of the lacrimal gland** into the lacrimal gland fossa with a 5–0 absorbable suture. Dissection is carried out superiorly through the blepharoplasty access and the lateral superior orbital edge is displayed. The lacrimal gland, which often prolapses with its capsule, is sutured to the periosteum of the lacrimal gland fossa.

For **lower lid blepharoplasty** the *transcutaneous approach* in case of a dermatochalasis, or the *transconjunctival approach* for only fat excision, are suitable.

For a **transcutaneous lower lid blepharoplasty** a subciliary incision is used with a lateral extension. The skin to be excised is best assessed using nontoothed forceps with the patient looking up or with the mouth open so as to avoid postoperative ectropion due to overcorrection. A **lateral canthopexy** (placing a suture from the lateral palpebral ligament into the periosteum of the lateral orbital rim without opening the lateral canthus) should be done in case of lid laxity. With evident lid laxity, a simultaneous **lateral tarsal strip procedure** or horizontal lid shortening should be performed. A skin–muscle flap is elevated and the orbital septum is exposed. The septum is incised over the lateral, middle, and medial fat compartment and fat is excised after cauterization until the lid contour is satisfactory.

For **transconjunctival lower lid blepharoplasty**, after eversion of the lower lid an incision is made in the fornix through which the orbital fat can directly be viewed. Careful dissection and excision of orbital fat can be done in the three compartments. One should note that the inferior oblique muscle separates the medial from the middle fat pad and is thus prone to injury. The conjunctival incision is sutured with an absorbable 8–0 suture.

In summary, eyelid surgery is the last stage in the functional and cosmetic rehabilitation of patients with Graves's disease. It is done in the inactive and stable stage of the disease after orbital and strabismus surgery and consists mainly of blepharoplasty, as well as the correction of lid retraction and ptosis.

References

[1] Bartley GB, Fatourechi V, Kadrmas EF, et al. Chronology of Graves' ophthalmopathy in an incidence cohort. Am J Ophthalmol. 1996; 121(4):426–434

[2] Kendler DL, Lippa J, Rootman J. The initial clinical characteristics of Graves' orbitopathy vary with age and sex. Arch Ophthalmol. 1993; 111(2):197–201

[3] Ponto KA, Pitz S, Pfeiffer N, Hommel G, Weber MM, Kahaly GJ. Endokrine Orbitopathie. Lebensqualität und berufliche Belastung. [Quality of life and occupational disability in endocrine orbitopathy]. Dtsch Arztebl Int. 2009; 106 (17):283–289

[4] Bartley GB, Fatourechi V, Kadrmas EF, et al. The incidence of Graves' ophthalmopathy in Olmsted County, Minnesota. Am J Ophthalmol. 1995; 120(4): 511–517

[5] Orgiazzi J. Pathogenesis. In: Wiersinga WM, Kahaly GJ, eds. Graves' Orbitopathy: A Multidisciplinary Approach. Basel: Karger; 2007:41–56

[6] Kahaly G, Förster G, Pitz S, Rösler HP, Mann W. Aktuelle interdisziplinäre Diagnostik und Therapie der endokrinen Orbitopathie. [Recent interdisciplinary diagnosis and therapy of endocrine orbitopathy]. Dtsch Med Wochenschr. 1997; 122(1–2):27–32

[7] Saber E, McDonnell J, Zimmermann KM, Yugar JE, Feldon SE. Extraocular muscle changes in experimental orbital venous stasis: some similarities to Graves' orbitopathy. Graefes Arch Clin Exp Ophthalmol. 1996; 234(5):331–336

[8] Sorisky A, Pardasani D, Gagnon A, Smith TJ. Evidence of adipocyte differentiation in human orbital fibroblasts in primary culture. J Clin Endocrinol Metab. 1996; 81(9):3428–3431

[9] Heufelder AE, Herterich S, Ernst G, Bahn RS, Scriba PC. Analysis of retroorbital T cell antigen receptor variable region gene usage in patients with Graves' ophthalmopathy. Eur J Endocrinol. 1995; 132(3):266–277

[10] Heufelder AE, Wenzel BE, Scriba PC. Antigen receptor variable region repertoires expressed by T cells infiltrating thyroid, retroorbital, and pretibial tissue in Graves' disease. J Clin Endocrinol Metab. 1996; 81(10): 3733–3739

[11] Feliciello A, Porcellini A, Ciullo I, Bonavolontà G, Avvedimento EV, Fenzi G. Expression of thyrotropin-receptor mRNA in healthy and Graves' disease retro-orbital tissue. Lancet. 1993; 342(8867):337–338

[12] Paschke R, Vassart G, Ludgate M. Current evidence for and against the TSH receptor being the common antigen in Graves' disease and thyroid associated ophthalmopathy. Clin Endocrinol (Oxf). 1995; 42(6):565–569

[13] Otto E, Förster G, Kuhlemann K, Hansen C, Kahaly GJ. TSH receptor in endocrine autoimmunity. Clin Exp Rheumatol. 1996; 14 Suppl 15:S77–S84

[14] Hiromatsu Y, Sato M, Inoue Y, et al. Localization and clinical significance of thyrotropin receptor mRNA expression in orbital fat and eye muscle tissues from patients with thyroid-associated ophthalmopathy. Thyroid. 1996; 6(6): 553–562

[15] Crisp MS, Lane C, Halliwell M, Wynford-Thomas D, Ludgate M. Thyrotropin receptor transcripts in human adipose tissue. J Clin Endocrinol Metab. 1997; 82(6):2003–2005

[16] Major BJ, Cures A, Frauman AG. The full length and splice variant thyrotropin receptor is expressed exclusively in skeletal muscle of extraocular origin: a link to the pathogenesis of Graves' ophthalmopathy. Biochem Biophys Res Commun. 1997; 230(3):493–496

[17] Burch HB, Sellitti D, Barnes SG, Nagy EV, Bahn RS, Burman KD. Thyrotropin receptor antisera for the detection of immunoreactive protein species in retroocular fibroblasts obtained from patients with Graves' ophthalmopathy. J Clin Endocrinol Metab. 1994; 78(6):1384–1391

[18] Kahaly G, Otto E, Förster G, et al. T cells and orbital connective tissue in endocrine orbitopathy. Exp Clin Endocrinol Diabetes. 1996; 104 Suppl 4:79–83

[19] Gerding MN, van der Meer JW, Broenink M, Bakker O, Wiersinga WM, Prummel MF. Association of thyrotrophin receptor antibodies with the clinical features of Graves' ophthalmopathy. Clin Endocrinol (Oxf). 2000; 52(3):267–271

[20] Wall JR, Hayes M, Scalise D, et al. Native gel electrophoresis and isoelectric focusing of a 64-kilodalton eye muscle protein shows that it is an important target for serum autoantibodies in patients with thyroid-associated ophthalmopathy and not expressed in other skeletal muscle. J Clin Endocrinol Metab. 1995; 80(4):1226–1232

[21] Otto EA, Ochs K, Hansen C, Wall JR, Kahaly GJ. Orbital tissue-derived T lymphocytes from patients with Graves' ophthalmopathy recognize autologous orbital antigens. J Clin Endocrinol Metab. 1996; 81(8):3045–3050

[22] Perros P, Crombie AL, Kendall-Taylor P. Natural history of thyroid associated ophthalmopathy. Clin Endocrinol (Oxf). 1995; 42(1):45–50

[23] Prummel MF, Wiersinga WM, Mourits MP, Koornneef L, Berghout A, van der Gaag R. Effect of abnormal thyroid function on the severity of Graves' ophthalmopathy. Arch Intern Med. 1990; 150(5):1098–1101

[24] Kahaly GJ, Dillmann WH. Thyroid hormone action in the heart. Endocr Rev. 2005; 26(5):704–728

[25] Lazarus JH, Marino M. Orbit–thyroid relationship. In: Wiersinga WM, Kahaly GJ, eds. Graves' Orbitopathy: A Multidisciplinary Approach. Basel: Karger; 2007:27–33

[26] Pfeilschifter J, Ziegler R. Aktuelle interdisziplinäre Diagnostik und Therapie der endokrinen Orbitopathie. Rauchen und endokrine Orbitopathie. [Current interdisciplinary diagnosis and therapy of endocrine orbitopathy. Smoking and endocrine orbitopathy]. Dtsch Med Wochenschr. 1997; 122(34–35): 1060–1061

[27] Bartalena L, Martino E, Marcocci C, et al. More on smoking habits and Graves' ophthalmopathy. J Endocrinol Invest. 1989; 12(10):733–737

[28] Bartalena L, Marcocci C, Tanda ML, et al. Cigarette smoking and treatment outcomes in Graves ophthalmopathy. Ann Intern Med. 1998; 129(8):632–635

[29] Eckstein A, Quadbeck B, Mueller G, et al. Impact of smoking on the response to treatment of thyroid associated ophthalmopathy. Br J Ophthalmol. 2003; 87(6):773–776

[30] Holt PG. Immune and inflammatory function in cigarette smokers. Thorax. 1987; 42(4):241–249

[31] Winsa B, Adami HO, Bergström R, et al. Stressful life events and Graves' disease. Lancet. 1991; 338(8781):1475–1479

[32] Yoshiuchi K, Kumano H, Nomura S, et al. Psychosocial factors influencing the short-term outcome of antithyroid drug therapy in Graves' disease. Psychosom Med. 1998; 60(5):592–596

[33] Wiersinga WM, Kahaly GJ. Graves' Orbitopathy. A Multidisciplinary Approach: Questions and Answers. Basel: Karger; 2010

[34] Pearce S, Kendall-Taylor P. Natural history. In Wiersinga WM, Kahaly GJ, eds. Graves' Orbitopathy: A multidisciplinary Approach: Questions and Answers. Basel: Karger Publishers; 2010:77–87

[35] Kalmann R, Mourits MP. Late recurrence of unilateral graves orbitopathy on the contralateral side. Am J Ophthalmol. 2002; 133(5):727–729

[36] Eckstein AK, Plicht M, Lax H, et al. Thyrotropin receptor autoantibodies are independent risk factors for Graves' ophthalmopathy and help to predict severity and outcome of the disease. J Clin Endocrinol Metab. 2006; 91(9): 3464–3470

[37] Salvi M, Spaggiari E, Neri F, et al. The study of visual evoked potentials in patients with thyroid-associated ophthalmopathy identifies asymptomatic optic nerve involvement. J Clin Endocrinol Metab. 1997; 82(4): 1027–1030

[38] Dickinson AJ. Clinical manifestations. In: Wiersinga WM, Kahaly GJ, eds. Graves' Orbitopathy: A Multidisciplinary Approach: Questions and Answers. Basel: Karger; 2010:1–25

[39] Bartalena L, Baldeschi L, Dickinson AJ, et al. Consensus statement of the European group on Graves' orbitopathy (EUGOGO) on management of Graves' orbitopathy. Thyroid. 2008; 18(3):333–346

[40] Bartalena L, Baldeschi L, Dickinson A, et al. European Group on Graves' Orbitopathy (EUGOGO). Consensus statement of the European Group on Graves' orbitopathy (EUGOGO) on management of GO. Eur J Endocrinol. 2008; 158 (3):273–285

[41] Ponto KA, Pitz S, Mann WJ, Weber MM, Pfeiffer N, Kahaly GJ. [Management of Graves' orbitopathy: evidence-based recommendations]. Dtsch Med Wochenschr. 2009; 134(49):2521–2524

[42] Marcocci C, Pinchera A. Thyroid treatment. In: Wiersinga WM, Kahaly GJ, eds. Graves' Orbitopathy: A Multidisciplinary Approach: Questions and Answers. Basel: Karger; 2010:100–110

[43] Kahaly GJ. Imaging in thyroid-associated orbitopathy. Eur J Endocrinol. 2001; 145(2):107–118

[44] Müller-Forell W, Kahaly GJ. Neuroimaging of Graves' orbitopathy. Best Pract Res Clin Endocrinol Metab. 2012; 26(3):259–271

[45] Pitz S. Orbital imaging. In: Wiersinga WM, Kahaly GJ, eds. Graves' Orbitopathy: A Multidisciplinary Approach: Questions and Answers. Basel: Karger; 2010:57–65

[46] Mourits MP. Diagnosis and differential diagnosis of Graves' orbitopathy. In: Wiersinga WM, Kahaly GJ, eds. Graves' Orbitopathy: A Multidisciplinary Approach: Questions and Answers. Basel: Karger; 2010:66–76

[47] Boborides K, Perros P. General management plan. In: Wiersinga WM, Kahaly GJ, eds. Graves' Orbitopathy. A Multidisciplinary Approach: Questions and Answers. Basel: Karger; 2010:88–95.

[48] Wiersinga WM. Quality of life. In: Wiersinga WM, Kahaly GJ, eds. Graves' Orbitopathy: A Multidisciplinary Approach: Questions and Answers. Basel: Karger Publishers; 2010:211–220

[49] Wiersinga WM. Combined thyroid-eye clinics. In: Wiersinga WM, Kahaly GJ, eds. Graves' Orbitopathy: A multidisciplinary Approach: Questions and Answers. Basel: Karger; 2010:96–99

[50] Terwee CB, Prummel MF, Gerding MN, Kahaly GJ, Dekker FW, Wiersinga WM. Measuring disease activity to predict therapeutic outcome in Graves' ophthalmopathy. Clin Endocrinol (Oxf). 2005; 62(2):145–155

[51] Mourits MP, Prummel MF, Wiersinga WM, Koornneef L. Clinical activity score as a guide in the management of patients with Graves' ophthalmopathy. Clin Endocrinol (Oxf). 1997; 47(1):9–14

[52] Rocha EM, Mantelli F, Nominato LF, Bonini S. Hormones and dry eye syndrome: an update on what we do and don't know. Curr Opin Ophthalmol. 2013; 24(4):348–355

[53] Gupta A, Sadeghi PB, Akpek EK. Occult thyroid eye disease in patients presenting with dry eye symptoms. Am J Ophthalmol. 2009; 147(5):919–923

[54] Yaman A, Yaman H. Ocular myasthenia gravis coincident with thyroid ophthalmopathy. Neurol India. 2003; 51(1):100–101

[55] Krzizok T. Botulinumtoxin-Injektionen zur Behandlung von Strabismus. Welche Indikationen haben sich bewährt? [Botulinum toxin injections for the treatment of strabismus. Which indications are still useful today?]. Ophthalmologe. 2007; 104(9):759–762

[56] Haefliger IO, von Arx G, Pimentel AR. Pathophysiology of intraocular pressure increase and glaucoma prevalence in thyroid eye disease: a mini-review. Klin Monatsbl Augenheilkd. 2010; 227(4):292–293

[57] Benker G, Kahaly GJ, Reinwein D. What can the European Multicenter Trial on the treatment of Graves' disease with antithyroid drugs teach us about the course of thyroid-associated orbitopathy (TAO)? European Multicenter Trial Group. Exp Clin Endocrinol Diabetes. 1999; 107 Suppl 5:S186–S189

[58] Weetman AP, Holt ME, Campbell AK, Hall R, McGregor AM. Methimazole and generation of oxygen radicals by monocytes: potential role in immunosuppression. Br Med J (Clin Res Ed). 1984; 288(6416):518–520

[59] Eckstein A, Esser J. Endokrine Orbitopathie. Pathogenese, klinisches Bild und Untersuchung, stadienabhängige Therapie. [Endocrine orbit disorders. Pathogenesis, clinical presentation and examination, stage-dependent therapy]. Ophthalmologe. 2003; 100(10):857–880

[60] Tallstedt L, Lundell G. Radioiodine treatment, ablation, and ophthalmopathy: a balanced perspective. Thyroid. 1997; 7(2):241–245

[61] Ponto KA, Zang S, Kahaly GJ. The tale of radioiodine and Graves' orbitopathy. Thyroid. 2010; 20(7):785–793

[62] Kazim M, Goldberg RA, Smith TJ. Insights into the pathogenesis of thyroid-associated orbitopathy: evolving rationale for therapy. Arch Ophthalmol. 2002; 120(3):380–386

[63] Kahaly GJ, Pitz S, Hommel G, Dittmar M. Randomized, single blind trial of intravenous versus oral steroid monotherapy in Graves' orbitopathy. J Clin Endocrinol Metab. 2005; 90(9):5234–5240

[64] Weissel M, Hauff W. Fatal liver failure after high-dose glucocorticoid pulse therapy in a patient with severe thyroid eye disease. Thyroid. 2000; 10(6): 521

[65] Marinó M, Morabito E, Brunetto MR, Bartalena L, Pinchera A, Marocci C. Acute and severe liver damage associated with intravenous glucocorticoid pulse therapy in patients with Graves' ophthalmopathy. Thyroid. 2004; 14 (5):403–406

[66] Salvi M, Vannucchi G, Sbrozzi F, et al. Onset of autoimmune hepatitis during intravenous steroid therapy for thyroid-associated ophthalmopathy in a patient with Hashimoto's thyroiditis: case report. Thyroid. 2004; 14(8):631–634

[67] Le Moli R, Baldeschi L, Saeed P, Regensburg N, Mourits MP, Wiersinga WM. Determinants of liver damage associated with intravenous methylprednisolone pulse therapy in Graves' ophthalmopathy. Thyroid. 2007; 17(4):357–362

[68] Gursoy A, Cesur M, Erdogan MF, Corapcioglu D, Kamel N. New-onset acute heart failure after intravenous glucocorticoid pulse therapy in a patient with Graves' ophthalmopathy. Endocrine. 2006; 29(3):513–516

[69] Kahaly GJ. Management of moderately severe Graves´ orbitopathy. In: Wiersinga WM, Kahaly GJ, eds. Graves' Orbitopathy: A Multidisciplinary Approach. Basel: Karger; 2007:120–152

[70] Kahaly G, Schrezenmeir J, Krause U, et al. Ciclosporin and prednisone v. prednisone in treatment of Graves' ophthalmopathy: a controlled, randomized and prospective study. Eur J Clin Invest. 1986; 16(5):415–422

[71] Kahaly G, Pitz S, Müller-Forell W, Hommel G. Randomized trial of intravenous immunoglobulins versus prednisolone in Graves' ophthalmopathy. Clin Exp Immunol. 1996; 106(2):197–202

[72] Krassas GE, Kaltsas T, Dumas A, Pontikides N, Tolis G. Lanreotide in the treatment of patients with thyroid eye disease. Eur J Endocrinol. 1997; 136(4):416–422

[73] Kung AW, Michon J, Tai KS, Chan FL. The effect of somatostatin versus corticosteroid in the treatment of Graves' ophthalmopathy. Thyroid. 1996; 6(5): 381–384

[74] Krassas GE, Kahaly GJ. The role of octreoscan in thyroid eye disease. Eur J Endocrinol. 1999; 140(5):373–375

[75] Spallholz JE, Boylan LM, Larsen HS. Advances in understanding selenium's role in the immune system. Ann N Y Acad Sci. 1990; 587:123–139

[76] Marcocci C, Kahaly GJ, Krassas GE, et al. European Group on Graves' Orbitopathy. Selenium and the course of mild Graves' orbitopathy. N Engl J Med. 2011; 364(20):1920–1931

[77] Gärtner R, Gasnier BC, Dietrich JW, Krebs B, Angstwurm MW. Selenium supplementation in patients with autoimmune thyroiditis decreases thyroid peroxidase antibodies concentrations. J Clin Endocrinol Metab. 2002; 87(4): 1687–1691

[78] Gärtner R, Gasnier BC. Selenium in the treatment of autoimmune thyroiditis. Biofactors. 2003; 19(3–4):165–170

[79] Peretz A, Neve J, Duchateau J, Famaey JP. Adjuvant treatment of recent onset rheumatoid arthritis by selenium supplementation: preliminary observations. Br J Rheumatol. 1992; 31(4):281–282

[80] Mourits MP, van Kempen-Harteveld ML, García MB, Koppeschaar HP, Tick L, Terwee CB. Radiotherapy for Graves' orbitopathy: randomised placebo-controlled study. Lancet. 2000; 355(9214):1505–1509

[81] Gorman CA, Garrity JA, Fatourechi V, et al. A prospective, randomized, double-blind, placebo-controlled study of orbital radiotherapy for Graves' ophthalmopathy. Ophthalmology. 2001; 108(9):1523–1534

[82] Prummel MF, Terwee CB, Gerding MN, et al. A randomized controlled trial of orbital radiotherapy versus sham irradiation in patients with mild Graves' ophthalmopathy. J Clin Endocrinol Metab. 2004; 89(1):15–20

[83] Rajendram R, Bunce C, Lee RWJ, Morley AM. Orbital radiotherapy for adult thyroid eye disease. Cochrane Database Syst Rev. 2012(7):CD007114

[84] Perros P, Krassas GE. Orbital irradiation for thyroid-associated orbitopathy: conventional dose, low dose or no dose? Clin Endocrinol (Oxf). 2002; 56(6): 689–691

[85] Gerling J, Kommerell G, Henne K, Laubenberger J, Schulte-Mönting J, Fells P. Retrobulbar irradiation for thyroid-associated orbitopathy: double-blind comparison between 2.4 and 16 Gy. Int J Radiat Oncol Biol Phys. 2003; 55(1): 182–189

[86] Kahaly GJ, Rösler HP, Pitz S, Hommel G. Low- versus high-dose radiotherapy for Graves' ophthalmopathy: a randomized, single blind trial. J Clin Endocrinol Metab. 2000; 85(1):102–108

[87] Cardoso CC, Giordani AJ, Wolosker AMB, et al. Protracted hypofractionated radiotherapy for Graves' ophthalmopathy: a pilot study of clinical and radiologic response. Int J Radiat Oncol Biol Phys. 2012; 82(3):1285–1291

[88] Petersen IA, Kriss JP, McDougall IR, Donaldson SS. Prognostic factors in the radiotherapy of Graves' ophthalmopathy. Int J Radiat Oncol Biol Phys. 1990; 19(2):259–264

[89] Kern PM, Keilholz L, Forster C, Hallmann R, Herrmann M, Seegenschmiedt MH. Low-dose radiotherapy selectively reduces adhesion of peripheral blood mononuclear cells to endothelium in vitro. Radiother Oncol. 2000; 54(3): 273–282

[90] Voll RE, Herrmann M, Roth EA, Stach C, Kalden JR, Girkontaite I. Immunosuppressive effects of apoptotic cells. Nature. 1997; 390(6658):350–351

[91] Rödel F, Keilholz L, Herrmann M, Sauer R, Hildebrandt G. Radiobiological mechanisms in inflammatory diseases of low-dose radiation therapy. Int J Radiat Biol. 2007; 83(6):357–366

[92] Bahn RS. Graves' ophthalmopathy. N Engl J Med. 2010; 362(8):726–738

[93] Hermann RM, Fest J, Christiansen H, et al. Radiosensitization dependent on p53 function in bronchial carcinoma cells by the isoflavone genistein and estradiol in vitro. Strahlenther Onkol. 2007; 183(4):195–202

[94] Alpert TE, Alpert SG, Bersani TA, Hahn SS, Bogart JA, Chung CT. Radiotherapy for moderate-to-severe Graves' ophthalmopathy: improved outcomes with early treatment. Cancer J. 2003; 9(6):472–475

[95] Prummel MF, Mourits MP, Blank L, Berghout A, Koornneef L, Wiersinga WM. Randomized double-blind trial of prednisone versus radiotherapy in Graves' ophthalmopathy. Lancet. 1993; 342(8877):949–954

[96] Wiersinga WM, Prummel MF. Graves' ophthalmopathy: a rational approach to treatment. Trends Endocrinol Metab. 2002; 13(7):280–287

[97] Bartalena L, Marcocci C, Chiovato L, et al. Orbital cobalt irradiation combined with systemic corticosteroids for Graves' ophthalmopathy: comparison with systemic corticosteroids alone. J Clin Endocrinol Metab. 1983; 56(6):1139–1144

[98] Marcocci C, Bartalena L, Tanda ML, et al. Comparison of the effectiveness and tolerability of intravenous or oral glucocorticoids associated with orbital radiotherapy in the management of severe Graves' ophthalmopathy: results of a prospective, single-blind, randomized study. J Clin Endocrinol Metab. 2001; 86(8):3562–3567

[99] Robertson DM, Buettner H, Gorman CA, et al. Retinal microvascular abnormalities in patients treated with external radiation for graves ophthalmopathy. Arch Ophthalmol. 2003; 121(5):652–657

[100] Marcocci C, Bartalena L, Rocchi R, et al. Long-term safety of orbital radiotherapy for Graves' ophthalmopathy. J Clin Endocrinol Metab. 2003; 88(8):3561–3566

[101] Marquez SD, Lum BL, McDougall IR, et al. Long-term results of irradiation for patients with progressive Graves' ophthalmopathy. Int J Radiat Oncol Biol Phys. 2001; 51(3):766–774

[102] International Commission on Radiological Protection (ICRP) 1990 Recommendations of the International Commission on Radiological Protection. ICRP Publication 60. Ann ICRP. 1991; 21:1–3

[103] Snijders-Keilholz A, De Keizer RJW, Goslings BM, Van Dam EW, Jansen JT, Broerse JJ. Probable risk of tumour induction after retro-orbital irradiation for Graves' ophthalmopathy. Radiother Oncol. 1996; 38(1):69–71

[104] Broerse JJ, Snijders-Keilholz A, Jansen JT, Zoetelief J, Klein C, Seegenschmiedt MH. Assessment of a carcinogenic risk for treatment of Graves' ophthalmopathy in dependence on age and irradiation geometry. Radiother Oncol. 1999; 53(3):205–208

[105] Blank LE, Barendsen GW, Prummel MF, Stalpers L, Wiersinga W, Koornneel L. Probable risk of tumor induction after retro-orbital irradiation for Graves' ophthalmopathy. [letter]. Radiother Oncol. 1996; 40(2):187–189

[106] Trott KR, Kamprad F. Estimation of cancer risks from radiotherapy of benign diseases. Strahlenther Onkol. 2006; 182(8):431–436

[107] Jansen JT, Broerse JJ, Zoetelief J, Klein C, Seegenschmiedt HM. Estimation of the carcinogenic risk of radiotherapy of benign diseases from shoulder to heel. Radiother Oncol. 2005; 76(3):270–277

[108] Krebs in Deutschland. 2007/2008. 8th ed. Berlin: Robert Koch-Institut und die Gesellschaft der epidemiologischen Krebsregister in Deutschland e.V.; 2012

[109] Wiersinga WM. Perspective–Part III: retrobulbar irradiation in Graves orbitopathy: the Dutch experience. Ophthal Plast Reconstr Surg. 2002; 18(3): 175–176

[110] Chen TS, Figueira E, Lau OC, et al. Successful "medical" orbital decompression with adjunctive rituximab for severe visual loss in IgG4-related orbital inflammatory disease with orbital myositis. Ophthal Plast Reconstr Surg. 2014; 30(5):e122–e125

[111] Eckstein A, Berchner-Pfannschmidt U, Führer D, Esser J. [Update on endocrine orbitopathy]. Ophthalmologe. 2013; 110(11):1079–1096

[112] Cascone P, Rinna C, Reale G, Calvani F, Iannetti G. Compression and stretching in Graves orbitopathy: emergency orbital decompression techniques. J Craniofac Surg. 2012; 23(5):1430–1433

[113] Shepard KG, Levin PS, Terris DJ. Balanced orbital decompression for Graves' ophthalmopathy. Laryngoscope. 1998; 108(11 Pt 1):1648–1653

[114] Siracuse-Lee DE, Kazim M. Orbital decompression: current concepts. Curr Opin Ophthalmol. 2002; 13(5):310–316

[115] Dharmasena A, Keenan TD, Goldacre MJ. Orbital decompression for thyroid-associated orbitopathy in England: trends over time and geographical variation. Orbit. 2014; 33(2):109–114

[116] Verity DH, Rose GE. Acute thyroid eye disease (TED): principles of medical and surgical management. Eye (Lond). 2013; 27(3):308–319

[117] Kahaly GJ, Bumb P, Pitz S, et al. [Decompression surgery for endocrine orbitopathy]. Med Klin (Munich). 2007; 102(9):714–719

[118] Boboridis KG, Bunce C. Surgical orbital decompression for thyroid eye disease. Cochrane Database Syst Rev. 2011(12):CD007630

[119] Olivari N. Endokrine ophthalmopathie – chirurgische therapie. In: Praktische Plastische Chirurgie. Heidelberg: Kaden Verlag; 2004:239–254

[120] Mainville NP, Jordan DR. Effect of orbital decompression on diplopia in thyroid-related orbitopathy. Ophthal Plast Reconstr Surg. 2014; 30(2):137–140

[121] Metson R, Pletcher SD. Endoscopic orbital and optic nerve decompression. Otolaryngol Clin North Am. 2006; 39(3):551–561, ix

[122] Song Y, Song J, Liu Q, Li Y, Yao D. Study on measurements for margin of safety in lateral operation of a transnasoethmoid-sphenoid approach to decompress the optic canal. J Craniofac Surg. 2014; 25(1):243–246

[123] Takahashi Y, Miyazaki H, Ichinose A, Nakano T, Asamoto K, Kakizaki H. Anatomy of deep lateral and medial orbital walls: implications in orbital decompression surgery. Orbit. 2013; 32(6):409–412

[124] Bleier BS, Lefebvre DR, Freitag SK. Endoscopic orbital floor decompression with preservation of the inferomedial strut. Int Forum Allergy Rhinol. 2014; 4(1):82–84

[125] Wang Y, Xiao LH, Yang ZK, Li YY. [Modified orbital decompression for severe thyroid associated ophthalmopathy]. Zhonghua Yan Ke Za Zhi. 2013; 49(3): 242–249

[126] Fichter N, Schittkowski MP, Vick HP, Guthoff RF. [Lateral orbital decompression for Graves' orbitopathy. Indication, surgical technique, and treatment success]. Ophthalmologe. 2004; 101(4):339–349

[127] Sellari-Franceschini S, Berrettini S, Santoro A, et al. Orbital decompression in graves' ophthalmopathy by medial and lateral wall removal. Otolaryngol Head Neck Surg. 2005; 133(2):185–189

[128] Onaran Z, Konuk O, Oktar SO, Yücel C, Unal M. Intraocular pressure lowering effect of orbital decompression is related to increased venous outflow in Graves orbitopathy. Curr Eye Res. 2014; 39(7):666–672

[129] Takahashi Y, Nakamura Y, Ichinose A, Kakizaki H. Intraocular pressure change with eye positions before and after orbital decompression for thyroid eye disease. Ophthal Plast Reconstr Surg. 2014; 30(1):47–50

[130] Oh SR, Tung JD, Priel A, et al. Reduction of orbital inflammation following decompression for thyroid-related orbitopathy. BioMed Res Int. 2013; 2013 (13):794984

[131] Leong SC, Karkos PD, Macewen CJ, White PS. A systematic review of outcomes following surgical decompression for dysthyroid orbitopathy. Laryngoscope. 2009; 119(6):1106–1115
[132] Clauser LC, Tieghi R, Galie' M, Franco F, Carinci F. Surgical decompression in endocrine orbitopathy. Visual evoked potential evaluation and effect on the optic nerve. J Craniomaxillofac Surg. 2012; 40(7):621–625
[133] Welkoborsky HJ, Möbius H, Bauer L, Wiechens B. Traumatische Optikusneuropathie. Langzeitergebnisse nach endonasaler mikrochirurgischer Dekompression des N. opticus. [Traumatic optic nerve neuropathy. Longterm results following microsurgical optic nerve decompression]. HNO. 2011; 59(10): 997–1004
[134] Alsuhaibani AH, Carter KD, Policeni B, Nerad JA. Orbital volume and eye position changes after balanced orbital decompression. Ophthal Plast Reconstr Surg. 2011; 27(3):158–163
[135] Chang M, Baek S, Lee TS. Long-term outcomes of unilateral orbital fat decompression for thyroid eye disease. Graefes Arch Clin Exp Ophthalmol. 2013; 251(3):935–939
[136] Rocchi R, Lenzi R, Marinò M, et al. Rehabilitative orbital decompression for Graves' orbitopathy: risk factors influencing the new onset of diplopia in primary gaze, outcome, and patients' satisfaction. Thyroid. 2012; 22(11):1170–1175
[137] Fichter N, Krentz H, Guthoff RF. Functional and esthetic outcome after bony lateral wall decompression with orbital rim removal and additional fat resection in graves' orbitopathy with regard to the configuration of the lateral canthal region. Orbit. 2013; 32(4):239–246
[138] Unal M, Leri F, Konuk O, Hasanreisoğlu B. Balanced orbital decompression combined with fat removal in Graves ophthalmopathy: do we really need to remove the third wall? Ophthal Plast Reconstr Surg. 2003; 19(2):112–118
[139] Roncevic R, Savkovic Z, Roncevic D. Results of diplopia and strabismus in patients with severe thyroid ophthalmopathy after orbital decompression. Indian J Ophthalmol. 2014; 62(3):268–273
[140] Lee KH, Jang SY, Lee SY, Yoon JS. Graded decompression of orbital fat and wall in patients with graves' orbitopathy. Korean J Ophthalmol. 2014; 28:1–11
[141] Kacker A, Kazim M, Murphy M, Trokel S, Close LG. "Balanced" orbital decompression for severe Graves' orbitopathy: technique with treatment algorithm. Otolaryngol Head Neck Surg. 2003; 128(2):228–235
[142] Souchier M, Adenis JP, Sabatier A, Robert PY. [Management of induced diplopia after orbital decompression: study of 87 interventions in 51 patients]. J Fr Ophtalmol. 2013; 36(2):103–111
[143] Goldberg RA, Perry JD, Hortaleza V, Tong JT. Strabismus after balanced medial plus lateral wall versus lateral wall only orbital decompression for dysthyroid orbitopathy. Ophthal Plast Reconstr Surg. 2000; 16(4):271–277
[144] Graham SM, Brown CL, Carter KD, Song A, Nerad JA. Medial and lateral orbital wall surgery for balanced decompression in thyroid eye disease. Laryngoscope. 2003; 113(7):1206–1209
[145] van der Wal KG, de Visscher JG, Boukes RJ, Smeding B. Surgical treatment of Graves orbitopathy: a modified balanced technique. Int J Oral Maxillofac Surg. 2001; 30(4):254–258
[146] Lal P, Thakar A, Tandon N. Endoscopic orbital decompression for Graves' orbitopathy. Indian J Endocrinol Metab. 2013; 17(2):265–270
[147] Jackson JL. Nonsurgical management of diplopia after orbital decompression surgery. Am Orthopt J. 2012; 62:29–33
[148] Silbert DI, Matta NS, Singman EL. Diplopia secondary to orbital surgery. Am Orthopt J. 2012; 62:22–28
[149] Fraine L. Nonsurgical management of diplopia. Am Orthopt J. 2012; 62:13–18
[150] Kim MH, Park KA, Oh SY. The effect of previous orbital decompression on results of strabismus surgery in patients with Graves' ophthalmopathy. J AAPOS. 2013; 17(2):188–191
[151] Fayers T, Barker LE, Verity DH, Rose GE. Oscillopsia after lateral wall orbital decompression. Ophthalmology. 2013; 120(9):1920–1923
[152] Antisdel JL, Gumber D, Holmes J, Sindwani R. Management of sinonasal complications after endoscopic orbital decompression for Graves' orbitopathy. Laryngoscope. 2013; 123(9):2094–2098
[153] Haller D, Gosepath J, Mann WJ. The management of acute visual loss after sinus surgery–two cases of rhinogenic optic neuropathy. Rhinology. 2006; 44 (3):216–218
[154] Rootman J. Diseases of the orbit: A multidisciplinary approach. Philadelphia: Lippincott; 2003: 628
[155] Dawson E, Ali N, Lee JP. Botulinum toxin injection into the superior rectus for treatment of strabismus. Strabismus 2012; 20: 24–25
[156] Shih MJ, Liao SL, Lu HY. A single transcutaneous injection with Botox for dysthyroid lid retraction. Eye 2004; 18: 466–469
[157] Lee JM, Lee H, Park M, et al. Subconjunctival injection of triamcinolone for the treatment of upper lid retraction associated with thyroid eye disease. J Cran Surg 2012; 23: 1755–1758
[158] Ben Simon GJ, Mansury AM, Schwarcz RM, et al. Transconjunctival Muller muscle recession with levator disinsertion for correction of eyelid retraction associated with thyroid-related orbitopathy. Am J Ophth 2005; 140: 94–99
[159] Hintschich C, Haritoglou C. Full thickness eyelid transsection (blepharotomy) for upper eyelid lengthening in lid retraction associated with GravesÅL disease. Br J Ophth 2005; 89: 413–416
[160] Tyers AG, Collin JRO. Colour atlas of ophthalmic plastic surgery. Edinburgh: Churchill Livingstone; 1995: 338
[161] Patel V, Malhotra R. Transconjunctival blepharoptosis surgery: a review of posterior approach ptosis surgery and posterior approach white-line advancement. Open Ophth J 2010; 4: 81–84
[162] Patel V, Salam A, Malhotra R. Posterior approach white line advancement ptosis repair: the evolving posterior approach to ptosis surgery. Br J Ophth 2010; 94: 1513–1518

Chapter 8

Traumatology and Traumatic Optic Neuropathy

8

8 Traumatology and Traumatic Optic Neuropathy

C. Deichmueller and H.-J. Welkoborsky

8.1 Introduction

Etiologically, both bony and soft tissue injuries of the orbit are a result of accidents, falls, or physical altercations (▶ Table 8.1). Two groups can be distinguished here: in elderly patients (> 60 years) these injuries are often caused by falls;[1] in young (mostly male) patients, assaults and sporting accidents are the leading causes. In terms of frequency, traffic and workplace accidents follow.

Injury mechanisms are highly dependent on locoregional features. While in Innsbruck (Austria) and Grenoble (France) (winter) sports accidents are the primary cause,[5,7] assault dominate in the United States and in Germany.[2,3,9] In Brazil, India, and the United Arab Emirates, traffic accidents are predominant (in UAE 5.5%, with camel participation), with falls and assault following in frequency in India and in Brazil, respectively. With a rate of 4%, assault is only rarely observed in the United Arab Emirates.[4,6,8] Since the 1980s, mid-facial injuries in car accidents have significantly declined in industrialized countries due to the statutory use of seat belts. This trend was reinforced by the introduction of airbags, explaining the shift of injury frequencies, with assault becoming the primary cause for trauma.[10,11,12] Seasonal influences are also reported.[13] Furthermore, with a ratio of 4:1 men are significantly more often affected than women. The median age is approximately 38 years.[14,15,16]

8

In many cases, associated injuries of the skull base can be observed, necessitating a thorough medical history and physical examination. Since patients presenting orbital fractures have often suffered multiple traumas, it can be complicated to obtain an accurate history.[17,18]

8.2 Patient History

Depending on the patient's vigilance, a direct or an indirect patient history should be sought. In either case, the following facts need to be collected:

- Type of accident (fall, sports, work accident, assault).
- Time and course of the accident.
- Retrograde amnesia, loss of consciousness, and possibly duration.
- Preexisting conditions and social history.
- Principal complaints and impairment (e.g., loss of vision, diplopia).
- Limitations of daily routine due to symptoms.

Table 8.1 Frequencies of orbital wall fracture causes[2,3,4,5,6,7,8,9]

Cause	Frequency
Falls	10–38%
Sports accidents	5–31%
Assaults	4–41%
Traffic accidents	12–59%
Work accidents	0.8–5%
Others	0.8–3%

8.3 Clinical Examination

First, a complete endoscopic ENT and ophthalmic examination is necessary (see Chapter 3). In comatose patients, a determination of visual evoked potentials can provide information on the functioning of the visual system.[19]

8.4 Instrumental Diagnostics

If clinical examination does not reveal evidence suggesting a bone injury of the facial skeleton, occipitomental radiography of the sinuses is sufficient for a preliminary assessment. The suspicion of a nasal bone fracture indicates an additional lateral radiograph of the nose. Besides possible fracture lines, the occipitomental sinus radiograph reveals a blow-out fracture showing the typical image of a hanging drop (see ▶ Fig. 4.1).

If radiation exposure is contraindicated (e.g., in children or during pregnancy), sonography can supply valuable information, for example, on fracture lines in the osseous nasal framework or the infraorbital rim (see ▶ Fig. 4.42).[20]

If the clinical examination or the subsequent occipitomental sinus radiograph suggests a fracture, a CT scan of the orbit as well as the paranasal sinuses should be performed. This provides information on the presence of fractures and accompanying bone injuries. Also, the extent of the fracture and the path of its fracture lines can only be determined using CT.[21]

8.5 Symptoms

Fracture signs in the orbit and the midface, as in other bone injuries, can be classified as certain and uncertain signs (▶ Table 8.2). Certain fracture signs include crepitation of bone fragments, malposition (elevation), abnormal mobility, and presence of fracture lines in diagnostic imaging. Characteristics of uncertain fracture signs are swelling, soft tissue emphysema, diplopia, impairment such as a trismus, dysesthesia, and pain. Many patients report an initial epistaxis that usually stops without treatment. A black eye or periorbital hematoma is one of the major symptoms occurring shortly after trauma (▶ Fig. 8.1; see also ▶ Fig. 6.2). Trauma to the orbital floor causes a descent of the eyeball, resulting in consecutive enophthalmos. Double images stem from eye motility disorders that might be caused by swelling or by an incarceration of extraocular muscles in the fracture gap; for example, of the

Table 8.2 Certain and uncertain fracture signs in orbital and midfacial fractures

Certain fracture signs	Uncertain fracture signs
Crepitation of bone fragments	Swelling
Deformation (step formation)	Emphysema
Motility disorder	Diplopia
Diagnostic imaging	Functional disorders (e.g. trismus)
	Sensory disturbance
	Dental percussion attenuation
	Pain

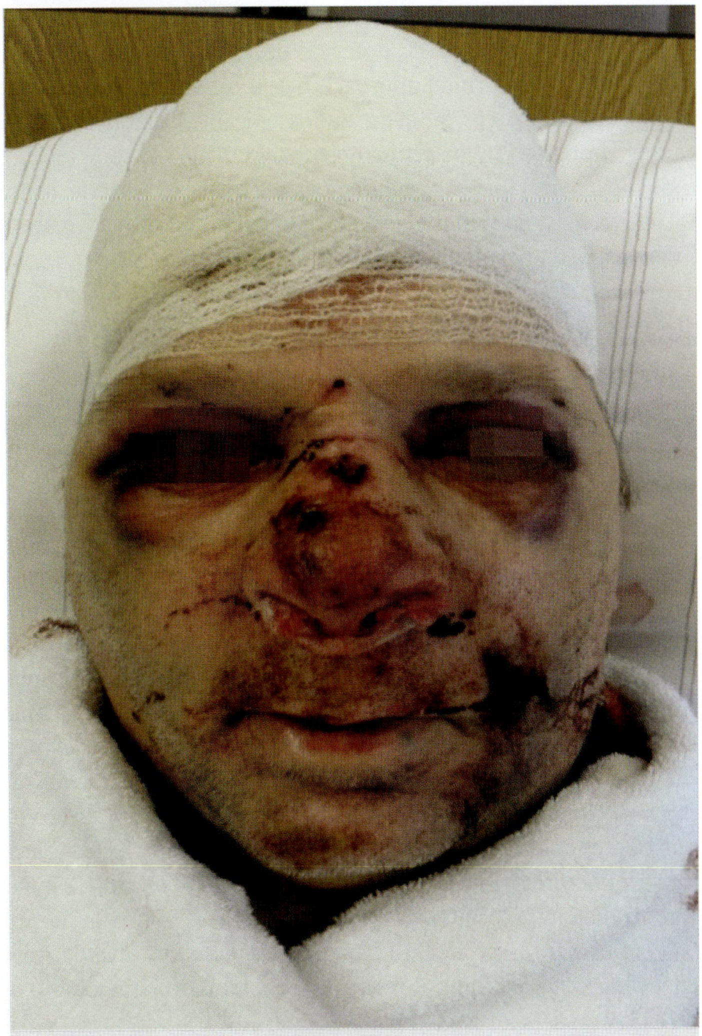

Fig. 8.1 Patient with monocular hematoma in LeFort III fracture (bilateral) and Escher IV fracture (right).

inferior rectus muscle. Depending on the affected muscle, diplopia is reinforced when gazing up or laterally. Additionally, a traction test in this case is pathologic.

Trauma often leads to shearing injuries around the infraorbital nerve canal but only rarely to ruptures. A result is sensory loss in the supply area of the infraorbital nerve (terminal branch of the maxillary division of the trigeminal nerve, V_2). Traumatic optic neuropathy (TON), which occurs in up to 5% of all craniocerebral injuries and facial trauma, leads to a loss of vision. In unconscious patients, this can be diagnosed by a missing pupillary response (afferent pupillary defect).[22] With endonasal pressure increase (e.g., on nose blowing or pressing) the size of hairline cracks is sufficient to allow air to enter the surrounding tissue of the paranasal sinuses. Emphysema in the area of the upper and lower lid with corresponding crackle is the first indication, but it might also spread over the entire affected side of the face (▶ Fig. 8.2). Other symptoms mentioned in ▶ Table 8.3 depend on associated injuries.

8.6 Orbital Soft Tissue Injuries

Soft tissue injuries of the orbit may occur in isolation or in combination with bone injuries. These especially include eyelid and bulbar injuries.

Due to the possibility of contamination, tetanus protection must always be secured. In inconclusive cases or those that are

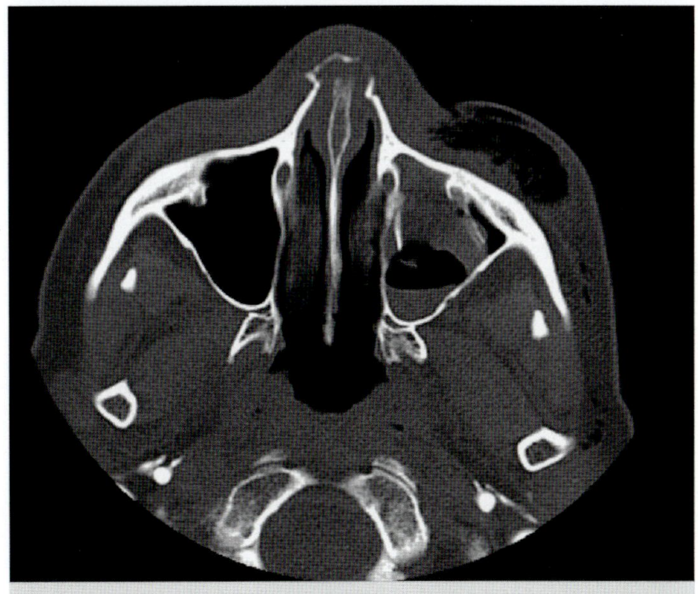

Fig. 8.2 Patient presenting pronounced air emphysema of cheek soft tissue in an orbital floor fracture on the left and nasal bone fracture (axial CT scan).

not in line with general vaccination recommendations (currently every 10 years for adults), simultaneous vaccination with tetanus immunoglobulin and active vaccine must be applied.[23] For animal bites, postexposure immunoprophylaxis against rabies might be indicated.

8.6.1 Lacerations

Various injury patterns can be distinguished. Accidents mostly produce tear crush wounds with lacerated edges and occasional tissue defects. Abrasions are also common in accidents. Cuts, in contrast, are characterized by sharp and mostly well-adapting wound rims. Bite wounds in the facial area are rather rare.[24,25]

Wounds should be cleaned immediately and examined for associated injuries. Depending on the size of the wound and the patient's consent, this can happen during the initial examination or under general anesthesia. To achieve optimal healing, wounds should be treated within 8 hours after trauma (the so-called 8-hour rule). It is important to ensure that the wound is closed tissue layer by tissue layer, without application of tension. Monofilament suture sized 5–0 or smaller is recommended to decrease the risk of further damage and to produce a cosmetically favorable scar. To avoid distortions due to scar tissue, rim adaptation

Table 8.3 Other symptoms of orbital fractures, caused by associated injuries

Symptom	Associated injury
Malocclusion	Zygomatic bone fracture, LeFort fracture
Drawer effect	LeFort I–III fracture
Rhinoliquorrhea	Skull base fracture
Meningitis	Skull base fracture
Intracerebral air inclusions	Skull base fracture
Hematoma of the septum	Lesion of the septum
Anosmia	Degloving of the olfactory glands

should be as accurate as possible. Tension lines to the skin should be monitored.

8.6.2 Orbital Foreign Bodies

In leisure accidents but also in work- and sports-related accidents (in this case also in gunshot wounds) foreign bodies enter the orbit. Accidents at work mostly involve splinters of various materials (especially metal and glass), while leisure accidents often involve pieces of wood (see ▶ Fig. 4.6).[26,27,28] Depending on the material and size of the foreign body, extensive bulbar damage may occur despite very small entry wounds. Particularly in children, there are reported cases in which the foreign matter was found only after lengthy diagnostics (see Chapter 4).[29,30]

Treatment always involves surgical removal of the foreign body under general anesthesia. The removal of the whole of the foreign material must be ensured and orbit, eye, and skull base have to be inspected for associated injuries. In order to better localize the foreign body, surgical removal should be carried out using a computerized navigation system where possible.[31] The use of a magnet is helpful in the removal of metallic objects. Only in a very few cases, and only if a complete removal of metallic material involves a threat to patient's eyesight, can pieces be left in place.[32] Very pronounced orbital trauma with associated optic nerve injury, penetrating bulbar injury, or puncturing of the skull base may occasionally necessitate enucleation.

Complications and sometimes initial symptoms of intraorbital foreign bodies are orbital edema, cellulitis, and abscess, as well as meningitis and brain abscess in the case of skull base fractures.[33]

8.7 Orbital Wall Fractures

8.7.1 Medial Orbital Wall Fracture

Pathogenesis

The medial orbital wall is formed by the lamina papyracea, which separates the orbit from the ethmoidal cell system. As the name suggests, this is a paper-thin wall that fractures easily with only small force.

Symptoms

Medial orbital wall fractures present initial, self-limiting epistaxis. Since usually neither eye muscles nor periorbita are subject to incarceration, motility is preserved. Enophthalmos is generally mild but can lead to distracting diplopia.

Diagnostics

On suspicion of an isolated medial orbital wall fracture a CT scan is required alongside a clinical examination in order to rule out concomitant fractures.

Treatment

An isolated fracture of the medial orbital wall usually requires no treatment as patients are mostly symptom free. However, to avoid complications such as orbital emphysema the patient should refrain from nose blowing and physical activity.

Persistent diplopia due to enophthalmos or a cosmetically unacceptable enophthalmos can be treated surgically. In minor defects, the fracture piece can be endoscopically rotated and wedged.[34] If this fails, open surgery is necessary, for example, following the fronto-orbital approach based on Killian or the pericaruncular approach, or even endoscopically. Orbital contents can be supported by inserting absorbable materials such as PDS (polydioxanone) foil or copolymer plates made of D-lactic acids, L-lactic acids, and trimethylene carbonates[35] and also by inserting nonabsorbable material such as titanium mesh.[36]

8.7.2 Lateral Orbital Wall Fracture and Zygomatic Fracture (Lateral Midfacial Fracture)

Pathogenesis

Fractures of the lateral orbital wall and the zygomatic bone are caused by the impact of lateral and frontal forces. Isolated fractures of the lateral orbital wall are rather rare. This can be explained by the anatomy of the midface: To ensure the "lightweight" nature of the midface and sufficient stability at the same time, bony buttresses between a cavity system with thin bone lamellae are the force-absorbing elements (▶ Fig. 8.3). They aid the transmission of chewing forces onto the skull base as well as the absorption of external forces. The lateral orbital wall forms one of these pillars, explaining why heavy forces are necessary to cause a fracture in this area. If forces are sufficient to cause a fracture of the lateral orbital wall, further fractures of midfacial pillars are usually associated. In almost every case this includes the cheekbone. For anatomical reasons, the lateral orbital wall often

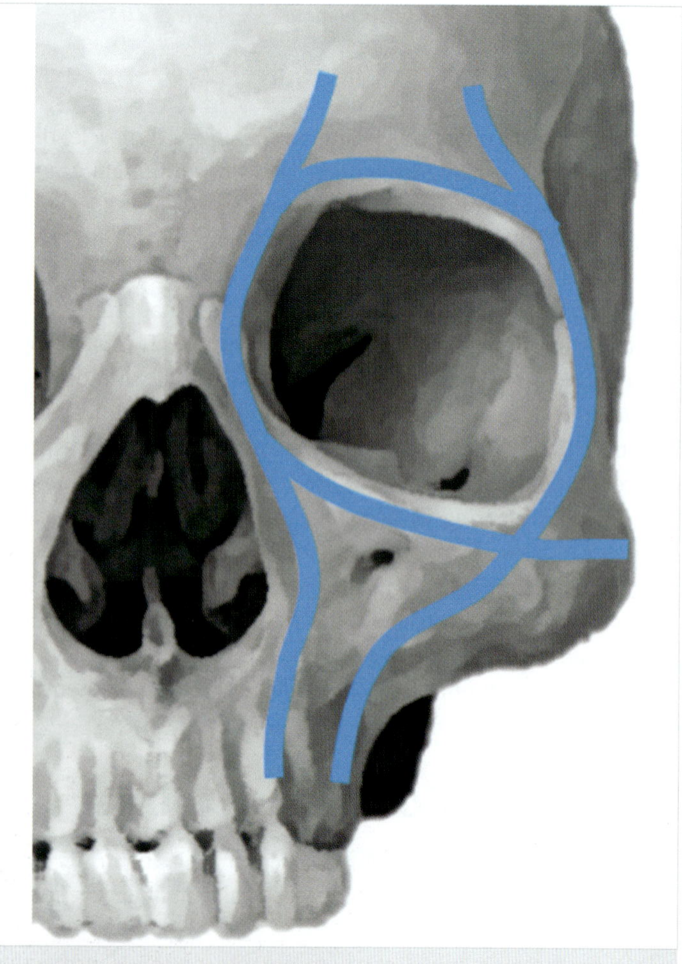

Fig. 8.3 Pillars of the midface (according to Schilli, 1980[37]).

Table 8.4 Classification of zygomatic fractures according to Becker and Austermann[38]

Classification	Type of fracture
I	Isolated zygomatic arch fracture
II	Nondislocated zygomatic bone fracture
III	Dislocated zygomatic bone fracture without diastasis at the lateral orbital rim • With medial rotation. • With lateral rotation (antral impaction).
IV	Dislocated zygomatic bone fracture with diastasis at the lateral orbital rim • With medial rotation. • With lateral rotation. • With dorsocaudal shearing.
V	Comminuted zygomatic bone fracture
VI	Type II–V fractures with fracture of the orbital floor

Table 8.5 Decision algorithm for lateral midfacial fracture treatment

Conservative treatment	Surgical treatment
Mouth opening and closing possible	Trismus
Unrestricted bulb motility	Diplopia/impaired eye bulb motility
Isolated sensitivity disorders	Cosmetically problematic enophthalmos
Nondisplaced fractures	Flattened facial contour
	Any displaced fracture
	Diastasis

exhibits destruction of the frontozygomatic structure instead of a fracture. Classification of fractures of the zygomatic bone is based on Becker and Austermann (▶ Table 8.4).

Clinical Examination

In addition to the typical hematoma and emphysema, which show significant decline starting around the third day after trauma, a disorder of mouth opening is an uncertain sign of fracture. While crepitation is usually not palpable due to the wedging of fragments, certain fracture signs often present palpable steps or diastases in the area of the zygomatic arch, the infraorbital rim, or the lateral orbital wall.

Radiological Imaging

CT imaging of both orbits as well as the midface is the diagnostic method of choice (▶ Fig. 8.4). In addition to the exclusion of a central midfacial fracture, the orbital floor can also be evaluated by CT. For an assessment of the zygomatic bone, especially if CT is contraindicated, sonography can be helpful. Discontinuities in the zygomatic arch and the zygomatic body as well as the lateral wall of the orbit can be detected sonographically.[20] A detailed sonographic localization of the fracture may be helpful even in cases of pronounced swelling and fracture steps that are not palpable, in order to support the planning of surgical treatment (determination of exact fracture location, length of fracture line).[39]

Therapy

Treatment depends on patient's symptoms, which require either clinical examination or CT imaging (▶ Table 8.5).

Conservative Fracture Treatment

Conservative treatment is indicated for nondisplaced fractures without formation of diastasis (type II) and complete preservation of function. Since the masseter muscle is attached to the zygomatic bone, causing caudal tension, additional tensile forces should be minimized to prevent defective healing with formation of a pseudarthrosis. To this end, detailed patient instructions on behavior (a soft diet, abstinence from sports, and entirely refraining from nose blowing) and consistent adherence to these is required for at least 6 weeks. There should also be regular, specialized medical checks to detect defective healing at an early stage and to initiate secondary surgical care where needed.

Surgical Fracture Treatment

Once a dislocation or impairment is present, surgical treatment is required within one week after trauma as already incipient healing processes can significantly complicate repositioning at a later stage. Depending on the type of fracture, surgery can be either percutaneous or open.

Percutaneous repositioning can be performed in type III fractures, classified according to Becker and Austermann (see

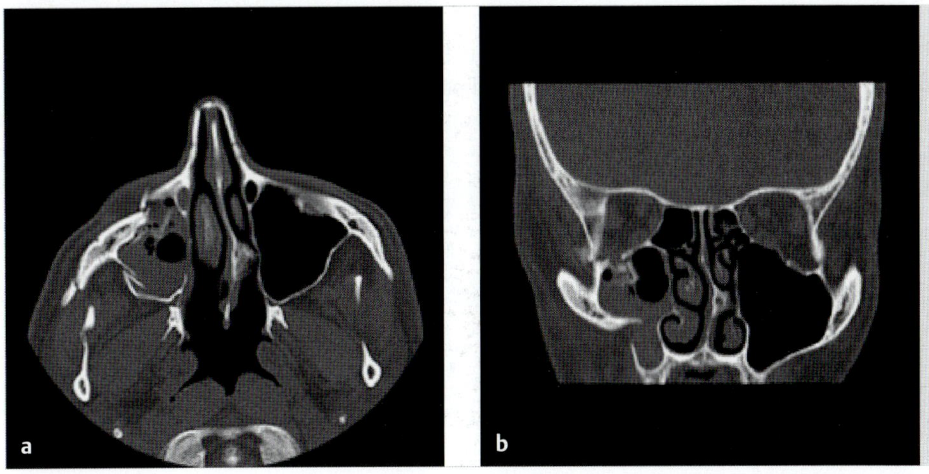

Fig. 8.4 CT scan with representation of an intrusion fracture on the right lateral midface: (a) coronal, (b) axial.

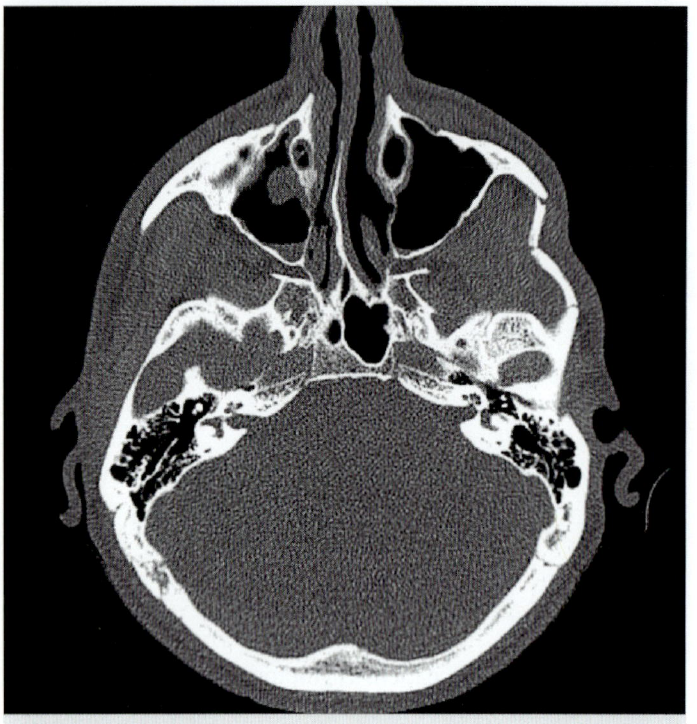

Fig. 8.5 Axial CT with representation of an isolated M-shaped zygomatic fracture (left).

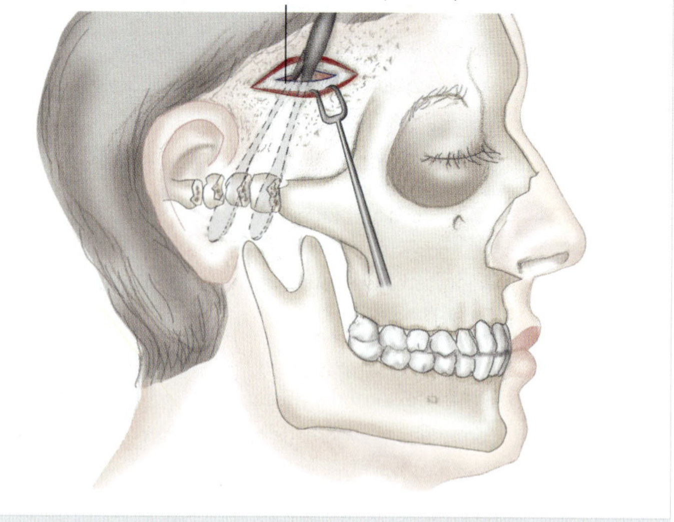

Fig. 8.6 Gillies approach for zygomatic fracture repositioning. Incision along the hairline and insertion of an elevator underneath the temporal fascia to the zygomatic arch. (Reproduced from Welkoborsky HJ. Traumatology. In: Strutz J, Mann W. eds. Practice of Otolaryngology, Head and Neck Surgery. Stuttgart: Thieme; 2009.)

▶ Table 8.4). For this purpose, a skin incision is made approximately 4 cm below the lateral orbital rim through which the orbit is entered using a single hook, inserted below the cheekbone, which is then repositioned under palpatory control. The zygomatic bone is securely reduced without osteosynthesis because fracture pieces are usually wedged together due to their often jagged edges. A similar procedure can be used in isolated zygomatic arch fractures (type I classification according to Becker and Austermann). Here, the single hook is directed through a small incision below the zygomatic arch to reach under the fracture pieces, which are then repositioned under application of slight tension. Another method for re-positioning an isolated zygomatic arch fracture includes using a small incision in the oral vestibule. The fractured zygomatic arch is usually dislocated in an M-shaped manner (▶ Fig. 8.5). Via this access point, an elevator is positioned underneath the fracture pieces to lift them upward. The same procedure is carried out in the Gillies approach with incision at the temporal hairline and following cranial elevation of the zygomatic arch (▶ Fig. 8.6).[40]

As in all percutaneous procedures, surgeons need to ensure that fractures are set in the correct position and remain stable. When destabilization of the fracture is observed, fixation through a small osteotomy is required. Patients must follow the same instructions as in conservative fracture treatment.

If there is no possibility for intraoperative radiography, positioning can be controlled using ultrasound.[39]

In all other cases, **open repositioning** is indicated. Here, the infraorbital plate is exposed through transconjunctival or subciliar incision, the lateral orbital wall via an incision in the lateral eyebrow considering skin tension lines, and the zygomatic arch, if necessary, through an incision above the fracture itself. In order not to jeopardize the zygomatic and temporal branches of the facial nerve, surgery with neuromonitoring of the facial nerve is recommended. Subsequently, repositioning can be performed under direct vision followed by osteosynthesis with mini-plates. This approach also offers the possibility of inspecting the orbital floor and medial orbital wall and, if necessary, treatment of the same (▶ Fig. 8.7). Surgical exposure of the zygomatic arch should only be carried out if it is not properly adjusted after repositioning.

In all surgical procedures, postoperative repositioning control using radiographic close-ups of the sinuses (see ▶ Fig. 4.2) and recording of the zygomatic arch in lateral projection is mandatory (▶ Fig. 8.8).

Complications

Complications of fractures of the zygomatic bone and zygomatic arch include infection, trismus, and emphysema as well as ophthalmic, neurogenic, and postoperative complications (see ▶ Table 8.6).

Table 8.6 Complications of zygomatic bone and zygomatic arch fractures

Ophthalmologic complications	Neurogenic complications	Postoperative complications	Other
Exophthalmos	Sensory deficits in the supply area of the infraorbital nerve	Intraorbital bleedings	Infections
Bulbus depression	Neuralgic pain	Bulbus injuries	Trismus
Proptosis		Ectropion	Soft tissue emphysema
Loss of vision		Keloid formation (rarely)	
Motility disorders			
Orbital emphysema			

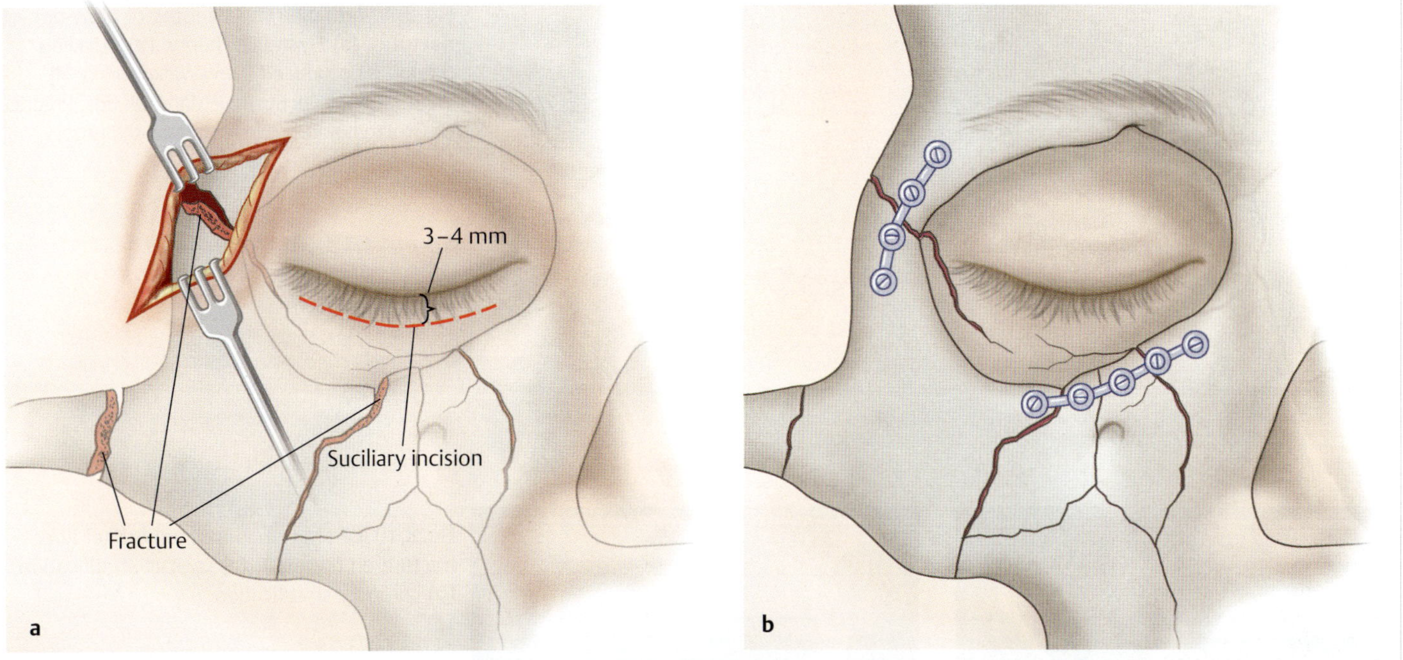

Fig. 8.7 Open surgical treatment of a lateral midface fracture. (a) Incision at the lateral eyebrow and subciliar incision. (b) Fixation with mini-plates. (Reproduced from Welkoborsky HJ. Traumatology. In: Strutz J, Mann W. eds. Practice of Otolaryngology, Head and Neck Surgery. Stuttgart: Thieme; 2009.)

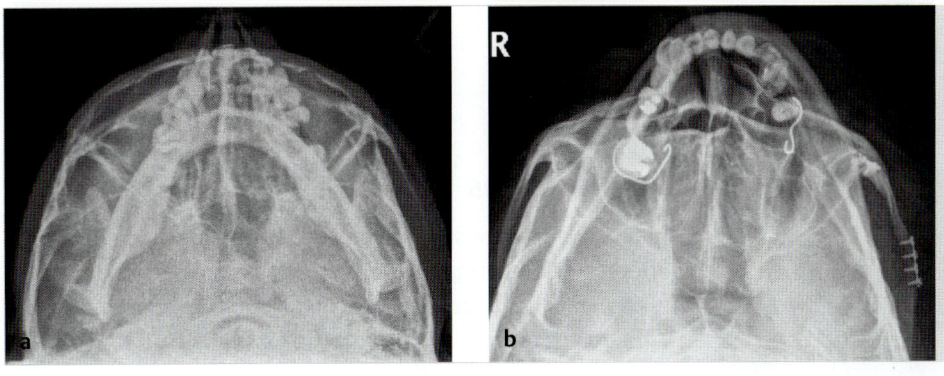

Fig. 8.8 Radiographs for repositioning control of the zygomatic arch. (a) Free repositioning of the zygomatic arch on the left side without osteosynthesis. (b) Treatment using mini-plate osteosynthesis on the left side.

8.8 Isolated Orbital Floor Fractures

8.8.1 Blow-out Fracture

Pathogenesis

In isolated orbital floor fractures, external force is usually not sufficient to impair the midface buttresses. Forces are transmitted to the parchmentlike orbital floor, leading to an isolated fracture in this area. Since fractures of the orbital floor usually continue into the maxillary sinus and bone fragments are often found there, they are also referred to as blow-out fractures. There are two origination theories for the fracture mechanism [41]:

- The **hydraulic theory** (▶ Fig. 8.9a) suggests a direct effect of force on the globe with closure of the orbit, where the bulb can only be displaced into the orbit. Here, orbital tissue serves as a form of hydraulic system. Since energy cannot escape otherwise, it fractures the weakest bone—the orbital floor. This is a typical mechanism, acting, for example, when a tennis ball directly strikes the eye.
- If force acts directly on the infraorbital rim, without resulting in fracture (e.g., in a blow or fall), energy is transmitted from the bone straight to the orbital floor, which cannot withstand the force, causing an isolated fracture. This mechanism is referred to as **bone transmission (buckling) theory** (▶ Fig. 8.9b).

In the literature, the occurrence rate of isolated orbital floor fractures in midface fractures is reported to be 11 to 13%.[11,42] Orbital involvement, particularly in cheekbone fractures, is observed in about 24% of cases.[2,43]

Investigative Imaging

On suspicion of an isolated orbital floor fracture or in cases representing a pendant drop in the occipitomental sinus radiograph (see ▶ Fig. 4.1), CT imaging is indicated, primarily to exclude further fractures. It also serves preoperatively in the determination of the fragment size and thus the planning of treatment. Despite coronary, axial, and sagittal stratification, the fragment size cannot always be determined conclusively in two-dimensional representation (▶ Fig. 8.10). 3D reconstruction can be helpful for this

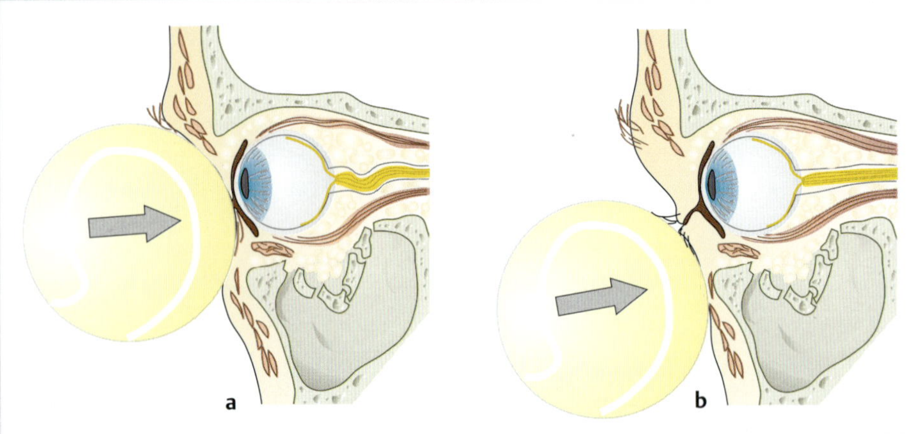

Fig. 8.9 Formation mechanisms of blow-out fractures. **(a)** Hydraulic theory. **(b)** Buckling theory. (Reproduced from Welkoborsky HJ. Traumatology. In: Strutz J, Mann W. eds. Practice of Otolaryngology, Head and Neck Surgery. Stuttgart: Thieme; 2009.)

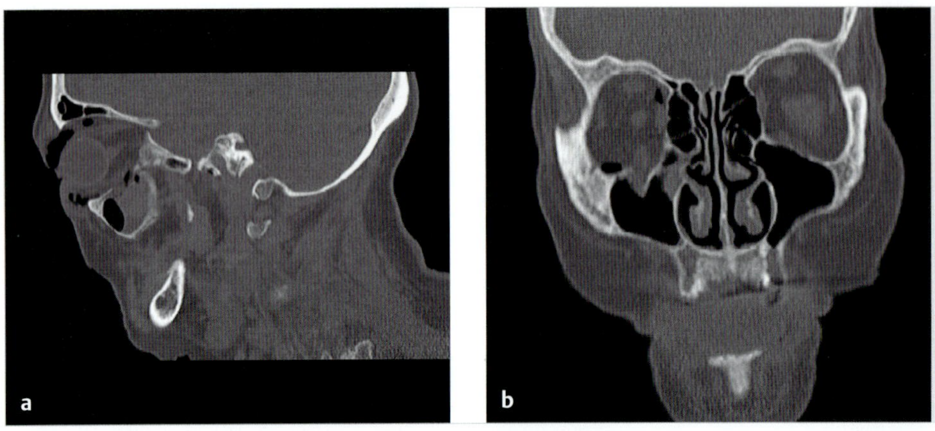

Fig. 8.10 CT scan of an isolated orbital floor fracture on the right: **(a)** sagittal stratification; **(b)** coronary stratification.

8

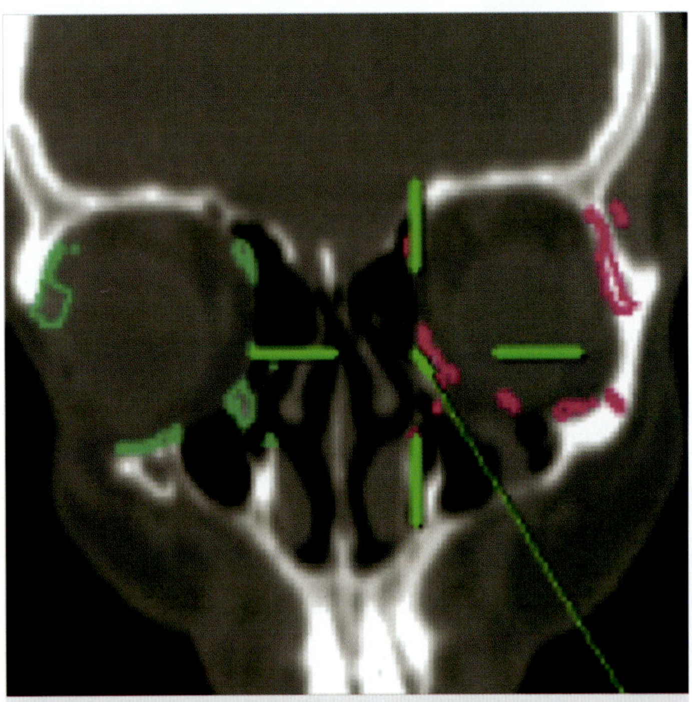

Fig. 8.11 CT navigation, mirroring the healthy orbital floor (right) onto the left fractured side.

purpose. In very large orbital floor fractures, the opposite orbital floor can be preoperatively mirrored onto the injured side using CT navigation in order to produce a precisely shaped titanium mesh (▶ Fig. 8.11), as reconstruction can be controlled using the mirrored image.[44,45]

Complications

Orbital floor fractures are often accompanied by complications common with paranasal sinus system involvement—namely, sinusitis. Also, pathogens may ascend from the paranasal sinuses leading to orbital cellulitis and abscesses. Furthermore, air can be forced out of the maxillary sinus into the orbit—a cause of emphysema.[46]

When a repositioning that is indicated is not carried out, the results are often cosmetically relevant enophthalmos, diplopia due to bulbar motility, disorders, and pseudoptosis, all of which may permanently affect the patient.

Since the fracture often involves the infraorbital nerve canal, one of the most common complications is sensory disturbance in the supply area of the infraorbital nerve, which patients get used to fairly quickly even though it may persist after surgical treatment. In most cases, sensory disturbances largely regenerate within 3 months.[47] Preoperative cases of sensory disturbance are described in 10 to 82% of cases. In a postoperative interval of 3 to 6 months, sensory disturbances are observed in only 8 to 25% of patients.[1,48,49,50,51]

Therapy

Decisions regarding **conservative therapy** should be based on the following criteria: absence of ocular symptoms (diplopia, enophthalmos), unbalanced risk–benefit ratio, or exclusive sensitivity disturbances (▶ Table 8.7). This specifically applies to elderly patients with increased intraoperative risk due to preexisting cardiovascular conditions as well as to patients suffering from

Table 8.7 Decision algorithm for the treatment of isolated orbital floor fractures

Surgical treatment indicated	Conservative treatment possible
Diplopia	Exclusive sensitivity disorders
Exophthalmos	Multi-morbid patients
Major defects	

dementia.[52] In either case, incarceration of the orbital muscle (inferior rectus muscle) must be prevented.

All other cases should be subject to **surgical treatment**. Incarceration of the inferior rectus muscle indicates treatment within 24 hours, as otherwise fibrosis occurs.[53] In all further cases surgery should be delayed until an accompanying swelling has decreased, guaranteeing notably improved interoperable visibility. Nevertheless, definitive surgical treatment must be carried out within 7 to 10 days following the trauma.

If surgical treatment is required, a transconjunctival or subciliar access to the orbital floor is recommended (see Chapter 18). In a subciliar access, the orbicularis oculi muscle is sought and forced apart, presenting the adjacent (intact) infraorbital rim. Now, eyeball and periorbita are pushed aside cranially. Prolapsed parts (periorbita, periorbital fat or possibly muscles) are then gradually removed from the fracture line and the fractured pieces are repositioned. Depending on the size and type of the fracture, its pieces are wedged into the orbital floor. After wedging the fragment of the fractured piece with the orbital floor, the contents of the orbit can be carried by this layer. In many cases this is not possible, requiring the bypassing of the defect. In small residual defects, endogenous material of the temporal fascia can be used,[54,55] but collagen membranes can also be used in fractures < 1 cm^2.[56] However, neither is stable enough to support the orbital content in larger defects. In such cases, a piece of PDS (polydioxanone) film is placed on the fracture edges (▶ Fig. 8.12).[57] Those edges are no longer sufficient as a supporting surface if the orbital floor is almost completely broken away. If this is the case, preformed titanium mesh can be used for reconstruction (▶ Fig. 8.13).[58] Here CT navigation mirroring the nonfractured orbital floor onto the traumatized side facilitates the localization of the correct position for the mesh (▶ Fig. 8.11).[44] Inserted material rarely causes problems and can therefore usually be left in place.[59]

It is recommended that subciliar cuts be performed laterally or medially to the pupillary line so as to prevent postoperative ectropion. Additionally, the tarsus and orbicularis oculi muscle should be largely spared.[60]

Caution: Neither mesh nor PDS foil should extend beyond the edge of the infraorbital rim, as they can otherwise cause irritation and pain.

8.8.2 Blow-in Fractures

Pathogenesis

In a so-called blow-in fracture the orbital floor fractures into the orbit. The supposed causal mechanism is direct exertion of force on to the frontal wall of the maxillary sinus. The frontal wall is not immediately fractured, but the thinner orbital floor yields and, due to the direction of the force, breaks into the orbit.[61,62] In most cases, the infraorbital rim remains intact. This fracture is comparatively rare. With 41 cases, Antonyshyn et al published the only major study in 1985.[63]

Symptoms

The clinical picture shows consequences common with the reduction of the orbital volume, namely, proptosis and motility disorders due to the compression of the eyeball, both leading to

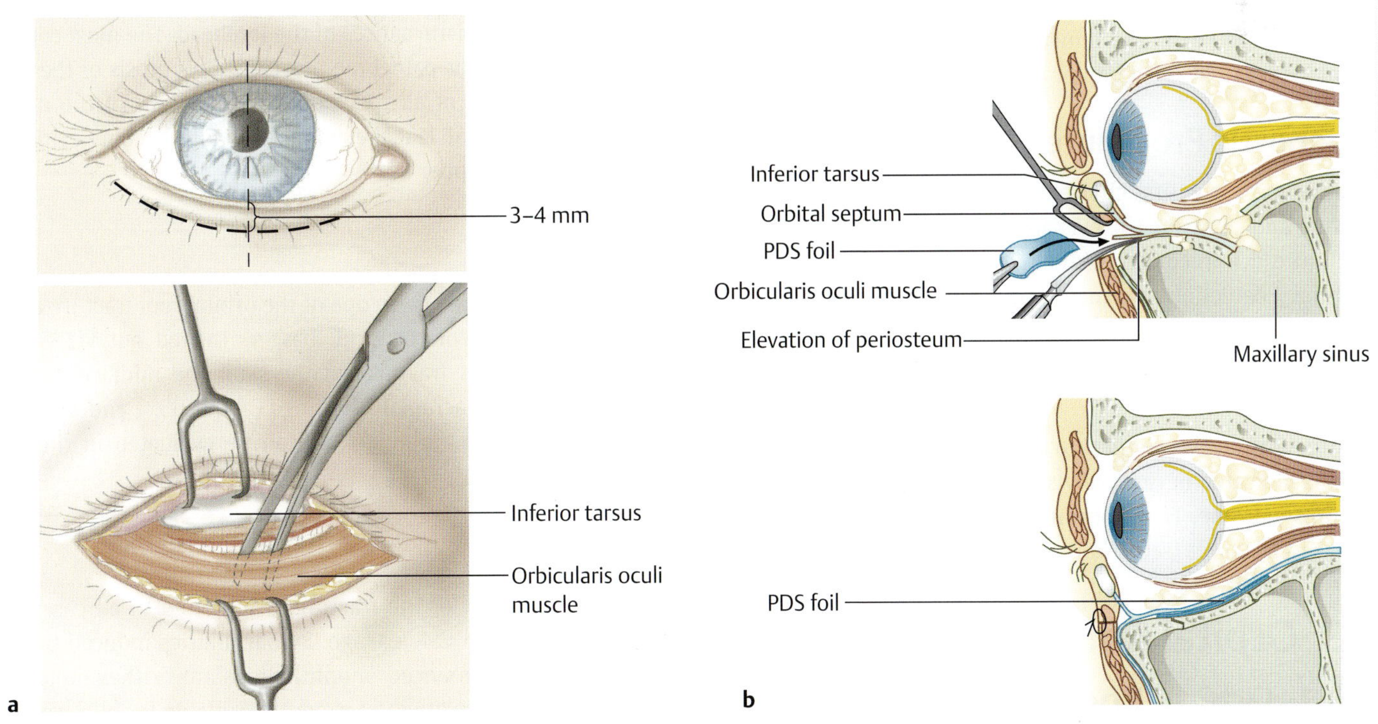

Fig. 8.12 Surgical treatment of an orbital floor fracture. (a) Subciliar incision and displacing of the orbicularis oculi muscle. (b) Insertion of PDS foil. (Reproduced from Welkoborsky HJ. Traumatology. In: Strutz J, Mann W. eds. Practice of Otolaryngology, Head and Neck Surgery. Stuttgart: Thieme; 2009.)

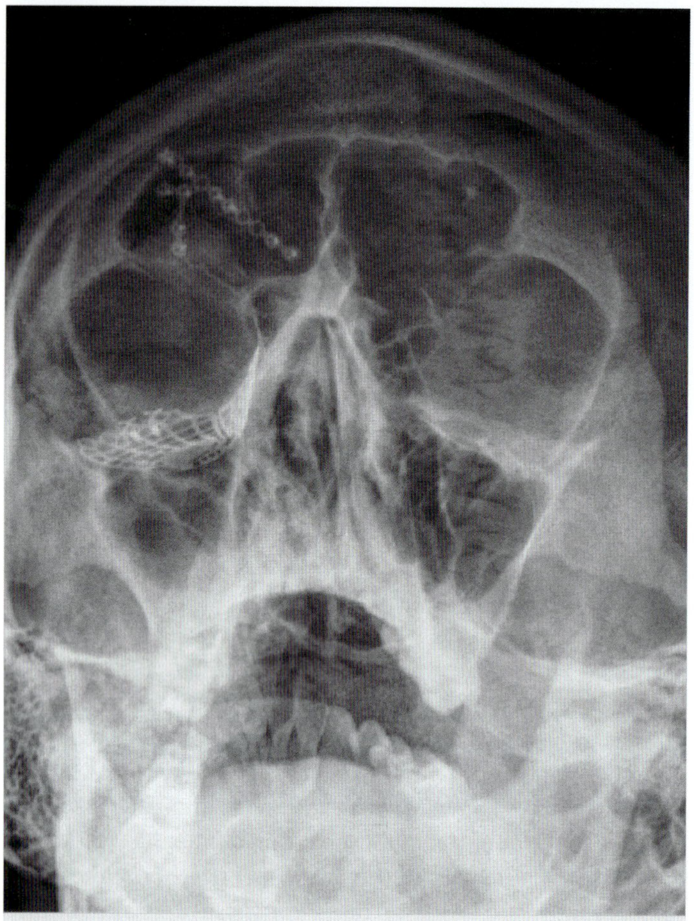

Fig. 8.13 Repositioning of the orbital floor on the right side using a titanium mesh, additionally frontal sinus repositioning by means of osteosynthesis on the right side.

double vision. A shift of the fragments into the orbit can result in the rupture of the eyeball, superior orbital fissure syndrome (paresis of cranial nerves III [oculomotor], IV [trochlear], VI [abducens] and the ophthalmic nerve [terminal branch of the trigeminal nerve (V)]), and injury of the optic nerve with consequent loss of sight (see Chapter 8.11).[63,64]

Diagnostic Procedures

CT scanning is the first choice for determining the extent of the fracture and assessing the eyeball, optic nerve, and superior orbital fissure.[64] Immediate ophthalmic co-assessment is necessary for timely detection of visual impairment or damage to the cranial nerves III, IV, or IV.

Therapy

Treatment is always surgical to avoid further damage. Immediate relief is indicated in cases of visual loss and with superior orbital fissure syndrome. The procedure is similar to that described for blow-out fractures (see "Therapy" in Chapter 8.8.1).[64]

8.9 Orbital Roof

8.9.1 Orbital Roof Fractures

Pathogenesis

Just like fractures of the lateral orbital wall, isolated orbital roof fractures are very rare. Only the application of larger forces

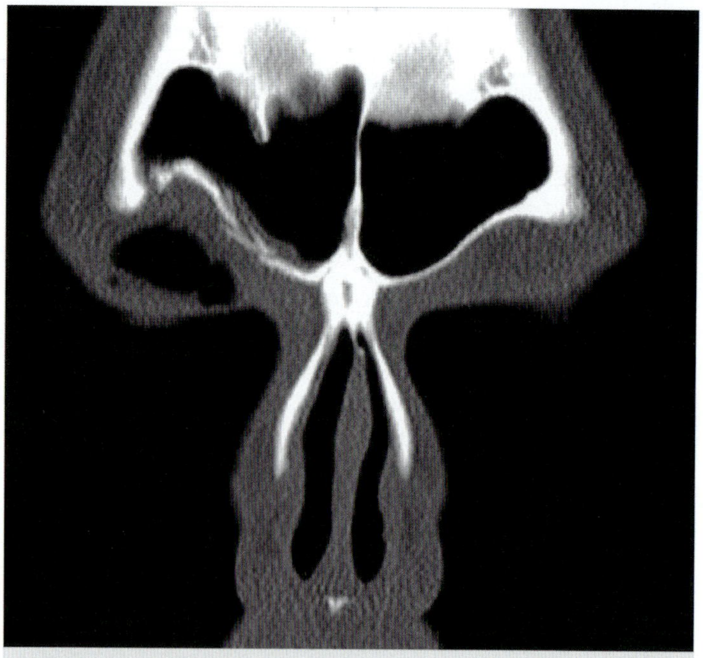

Fig. 8.14 CT imaging of a supraorbital rim/orbital roof fracture on the right side.

results in a fracture of the orbital roof, usually causing concurrent fractures in other parts of the midface and the skull base.

Clinical Symptoms

A fracture of the orbital roof may cause a clinically significant enophthalmos with diplopia, which can also develop as a sequela at a later stage if an orbital roof defect is not treated surgically.[65] A fracture of the supraorbital rim presents observable contour changes that are also palpable as a flattening of the same. An injury of the supraorbital nerve (sensitive terminal branch of the frontal nerve originating from the ophthalmic nerve V_1) can also result in sensory disturbances of the forehead. The most common injury of the levator palpebrae muscle shows ptosis of the upper eyelid. About 10% of all cases present an injury of the meninx accompanied by CSF leakage, which may also become evident by a swelling of the upper lid.[14]

Diagnostics

The determination of the scope of the orbital roof fracture as well as the evaluation of the skull base is carried out via CT-scan (▶ Fig. 8.14). Other fractures of the skull and midface (in about 85% of cases), intracranial bleedings (about 65%) and associated ophthalmic injuries (about 45%) can be evaluated in the same examination.[14]

Therapy

Surgical treatment of the fracture is indicated in all cases with meninx injury and CSF leakage. Bulbar injuries induced by bone fragments or pronounced enophthalmos are further indications for surgery. Conservative treatment is suitable for all cases with only slight dislocation.[14] Depending on the extent of the injury, an interdisciplinary treatment might be necessary.

Accessing the orbital roof via an extradural transfrontal approach provides for a good overview with the possibility of

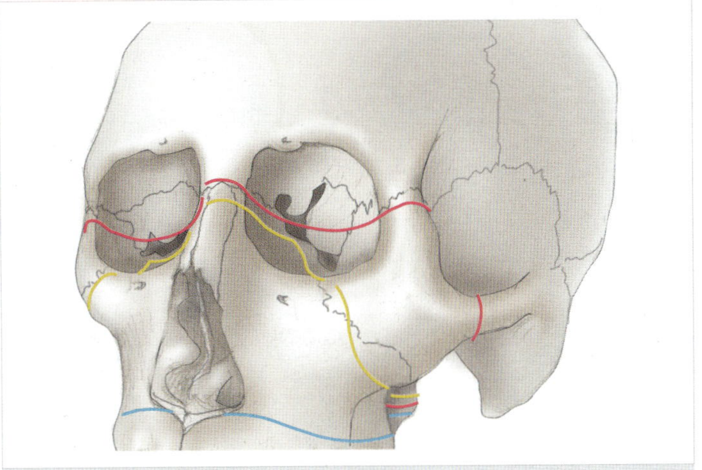

Fig. 8.15 Schematic representation of avulsion fractures classified by Le Fort. (Reproduced from Welkoborsky HJ. Traumatology. In: Strutz J, Mann W. eds. Practice of Otolaryngology, Head and Neck Surgery. Stuttgart: Thieme; 2009.)

intradural extension, if necessary. The fracture must be cleared and can be fixed with microplates. Then the leakage of spinal fluid can be treated. Minor injuries can be covered with temporal fascia, whereas a galea–periosteal flap provides secure coverage in large defects.[60]

Complications

Even after years, scar formation may lead to occlusion of the frontal sinus ostium. This causes recurrent sinusitis and the formation of mucoceles. Median drainage of the frontal sinus may be a prevention mechanism. Trauma itself or subsequent surgery may lead to an inability to smell, perceived as rather disturbing by patients.

8.10 Combined Fractures

8.10.1 Combined Fractures of Midface, Bony Orbit, and Skull Base

Pathogenesis

Viscerofacial and craniofacial fractures of the midface are caused by large forces applied frontally or frontolaterally,[66] presenting recurring fracture lines due to the system of bony buttresses and its absorption of energy with consequent fractures at sites of predilection.[37] Three fracture patterns are fairly common: a basal avulsion of the maxilla, a pyramidal avulsion of the maxilla with and without a fracture of the bony nasal framework, and a high avulsion of the facial skeleton originating from the neurocranium also with or without involvement of the osseous nasal structure. These fractures are classified according to Le Fort[67] (▶ Fig. 8.15, ▶ Fig. 8.16) and Wassmund,[68] in which schemes the Le Fort II and Wassmund II fractures correspond, as do Le Fort III and Wassmund IV fractures (compare ▶ Table 8.8). Fractures can occur unilaterally or bilaterally as well as in combination with each other.

Frontobasal fractures are usually the result of considerable violence in frontal trauma. In 62% of all cases they are associated with midfacial fractures,[69] and are classified according to Escher into types I–IV (▶ Table 8.9; ▶ Fig. 8.17). Rhinoliquorrhea is the main symptom in a defect of the anterior cranial fossa/skull base. Predilection sites for a CSF leakage are the posterior wall of the maxillary sinus, the lamina cribrosa, the roof of the ethmoidal cells, and the roof of the sphenoid sinus (▶ Fig. 8.18).[54,60]

Diagnostics

CT scans are useful to provide information on the fracture gradient (especially in 3D reconstruction). In addition to the paranasal sinuses and orbit, the neurocranium can also be evaluated that way. Consecutive intracerebral hemorrhage occurs frequently in these injuries, hence they always need to be excluded. In addition, intrathecal air pockets can indicate a skull base fracture. Rhinoliquorrhea is another essential finding that might still occur decades after a trauma (see Chapter 3.2).[71,72,73]

Treatment of Central and Centrolateral Midface Fractures

Conservative therapy is indicated only in nondislocated fractures, which are rather rare in central midface injuries. Skull base fractures, however, require surgical treatment only in case of heavy fragmentation or dislocation as well as with CSF leakage.[74]

Surgical treatment of these fractures is often an interdisciplinary task. In central and centrolateral midface fractures, the access route should be based on the fracture line. Coronal or lateral eyebrow incisions, a median canthus incision, or an access via the oral vestibule are all possible. Transconjunctival or subciliar sections are advisable for reaching the orbital floor. In case of malocclusion, the mandible must first be set in the correct occlusal plane and then fixed, for example, by using intermaxillary wiring. Mini- or micro-osteosynthesis systems should be used for the final osteosynthesis from caudal to cranial and from inside to outside (Markowitz rule).[75] A splint might be required, depending on the dental status.

Access routes to the skull base are dependent on the size and location of the defect. The endonasal endoscopic approach can be used in smaller and accessible defects. Larger defects, especially of the posterior wall of the frontal sinus, can be accessed via an

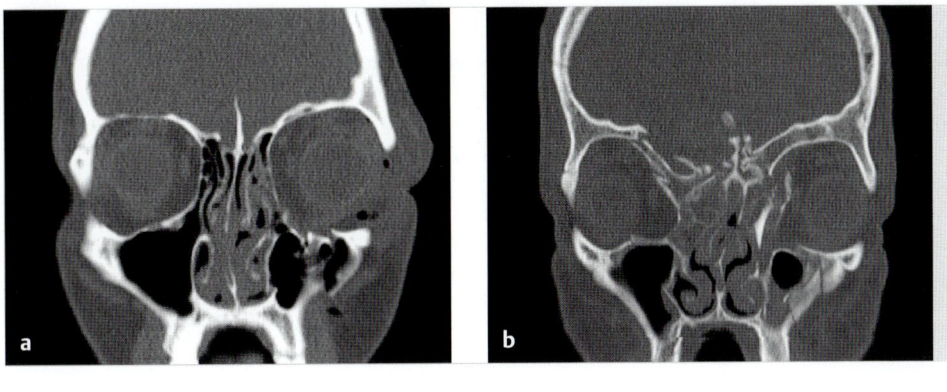

Fig. 8.16 (a) CT image of a midface fracture with LeFort II fracture (left). (b) CT image of a midface fracture with LeFort III fracture (right) and LeFort II fracture (left).

Table 8.8 Classification of central and centrolateral midface fractures according to LeFort[67] and Wassmund[68]

Classification	Description	Involved skeletal parts											
		Lateral nasal wall	Maxilla and maxillary sinus	Pterygoid process	Infraorbital rim	Vomer	Nasal septum	Lacrimal bone	Orbital floor	Frontal process (maxilla)	Lateral orbital wall	Zygomatic arch	Nasal root
Le Fort I	Basal avulsion of the maxilla	×	×	×			×						
Wassmund I	Pyramidal avulsion fracture of the whole maxilla excluding the bony nasal root		×	×	×	×	×	×	×				
Le Fort II/ Wassmund II	Pyramidal avulsion fracture of the whole maxilla including the bony nasal root		×	×	×	×	×	×	×				×
Wassmund III	High avulsion of the viscerocranium originating from the neurocranium excluding the osseous nasal root						×	×	×	×	×	×	
Le Fort III/ Wassmund IV	High avulsion of the viscerocranium originating from the neurocranium including the osseous nasal root						×	×	×	×	×	×	×

8

extradural transfacial/frontoethmoidal or transfrontal incision (Unterberger bow section). Extensive fractures with brain prolapse or abscess or with vascular lesions of the skull base as well as defects that cannot be reached via rhinosurgical methods must be approached neurosurgically. Decisions are always made on an individual case-by-case basis, with a possible combination of different approaches.[54]

Complications

Typical complications in midfacial fractures are permanent dysfunctions, cranial nerve involvement, cosmetic impairments, and rhinoliquorrhea. Complications associated with frontobasal fractures are intracranial and orbital infections, bleeding, olfactory dysfunctions, mucoceles, cephalalgia, and seizures (▶ Table 8.10).

8.11 Injuries of the Optic Nerve

8.11.1 Traumatic Optic Neuropathy (TON)

Pathogenesis

Traumatic optic neuropathy (TON) is a result of direct or indirect trauma to the orbit and thus to the optic nerve. Various pathogenetic mechanisms can cause TON [76]:

- **Shearing injury**: Especially in frontal and lateral trauma, significant shear forces can occur in the area of the exit point of the optic nerve within the optic canal, which can lead to the transection of individual axons.[22]
- **Pressure increase**: In trauma that results in retrobulbar or optic canal hemorrhage (hematoma of the optic nerve sheath), the pressure acting on the optic nerve can lead to a decline of visual acuity or even loss of vision. Posttraumatic edema may also result in increase of optic nerve canal pressure (Chapter 2).
- **Incarceration of bone fragments**: Fractures that run through the optic canal may result in incarceration of bone fragments in the nerve. The direct laceration of the axons then leads to a loss of vision.
- **Rupture of the nerve**: Trauma can lead to an instant rupture of the nerve (neurotmesis). This usually occurs directly at the scleronerval transition of the bulb.

Trauma jeopardizes the optic nerve especially in the area of the optic canal due to its tightness and anatomy (dura mater is adherent to the periosteum). Within the orbit the nerve is protected by its surrounding adipose tissue and in its intracranial course by its surrounding cerebrospinal fluid. Liquor and adipose tissue serve as a form of pressure pad.

Table 8.9 Classification of frontobasal fractures according to Escher[70]

Type according to Escher	I	II	III	IV
Description	High frontobasal fracture	Localized medial frontobasal fracture	Frontobasal fracture with avulsion of the facial bones	Lateral frontobasal fracture
Fractures	Comminuted fracture of the frontal bone	Lamina cribrosa	Impressions of the nasal root, crista galli and ethmoid bone into the anterior cranial fossa	Posterior wall of the frontal sinus
	Anterior and posterior wall of the frontal sinus	Crista galli		Orbital roof
	Anterior calvaria	Roof of the ethmoid and of the sphenoid bone		Lateral calvaria

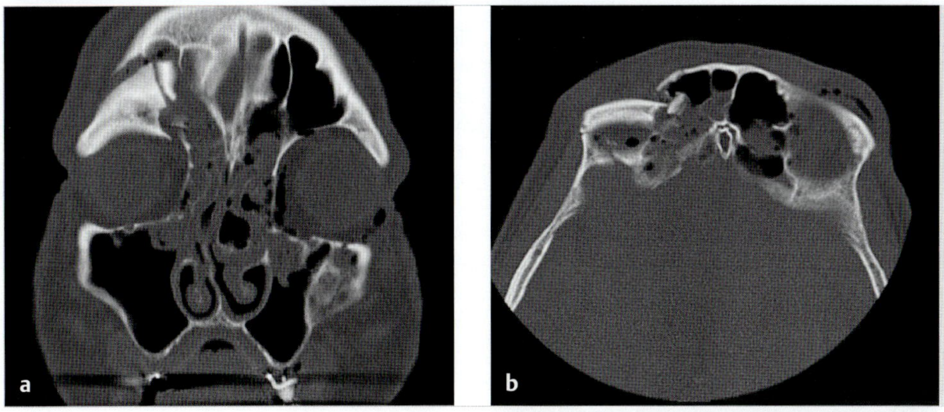

Fig. 8.17 CT scan of a lateral frontobasal fracture (Escher IV) to the right and simultaneous orbital floor fracture on the left: **(a)** coronal; **(b)** axial.

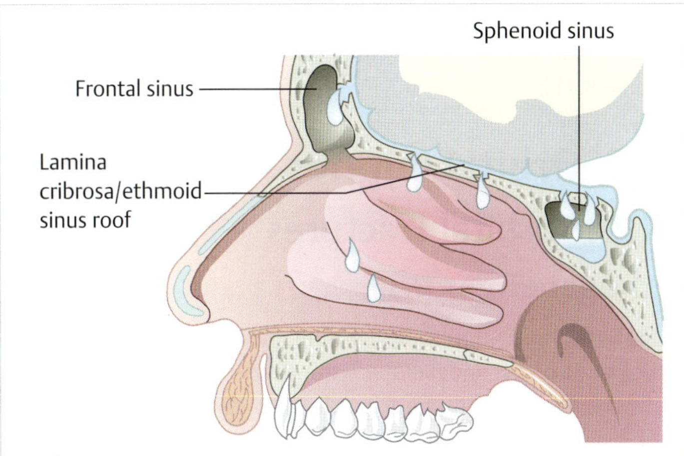

Fig. 8.18 Most common sites of CSF leakage in rhinoliquorrhea. (Reproduced from Welkoborsky HJ. Traumatology. In: Strutz J, Mann W. eds. Practice of Otolaryngology, Head and Neck Surgery. Stuttgart: Thieme; 2009.)

Table 8.10 Complications in viscerofacial and frontobasal fractures

Viscerofacial fractures	Frontobasal fractures
Rhinoliquorrhea	Meningitis
Meningitis	Cerebral abscess
Local osteomyelitis	Bleedings from branches of the maxillary and sphenopalatine arteries
Cranial nerve affections of cranial nerves I–VII	Orbital complications: • Visual loss (see Chapter 8.11) • Inflammatory orbit affection (see Chapter 6) • Orbital apex syndrome
Persisting dysfunctions	Dysosmia and ageusia
Cosmetic impairment due to scars	Sensory dysfunctions
	Paresis of cranial nerves II, IV, and VI
	Intracranial hematomas
	Recurring liquorrhea
	Mucoceles
	Chronic cephalgia
	Cerebral seizures
	Cosmetic impairment due to scars
	Osteomyelitis of the frontal bone

Clinical Investigation

Ophthalmic examination is the leading clinical investigation. In conscious patients this includes an assessment of the subjective perception of visual acuity as well as examination of the visual field. Pupillary response (afference defect), eye fundus, and eye motility should always be examined.

Instrumental Diagnostics

High-resolution CT of the skull and orbit, including a thin-film representation of the optic canal, facilitates the detection of incarcerated bone fragments (▶ Fig. 8.19) or a hematoma of the optic nerve sheath.

In addition, preoperative measurement of visual evoked potentials (VEP) is indicated in all patients. Along with pupillary responses, this facilitates the evaluation of the functioning of the optic nerve in comatose patients.[19] In some cases, a recovery of the potentials may already be observed during surgery after

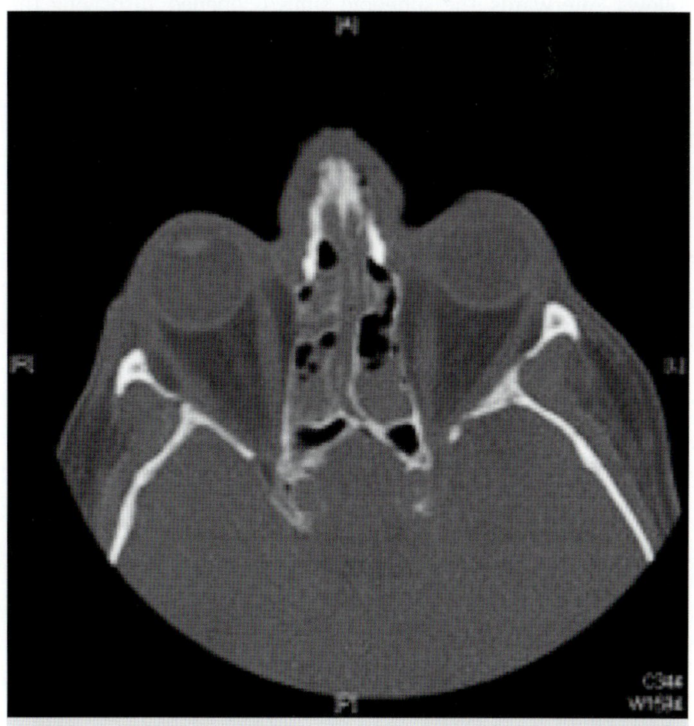

Fig. 8.19 Bone fragments in the left optic nerve canal (axial CT).

8

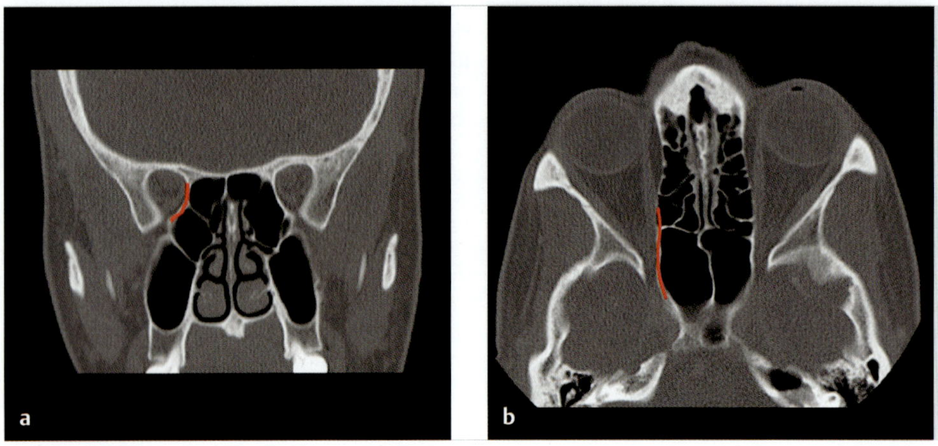

Fig. 8.20 Coronal and axial CT scans of an inconspicuous orbit and a normal sinus system. Bony areas that are to be removed in the microsurgical decompression of the optic nerve are marked in red.

slitting of the optic nerve sheath, suggesting a restoration of the functioning of the optic nerve.[76]

Therapy

There are currently no evidence-based treatment recommendations for TON.[77,78,79] However, the following procedure has proved to be useful: Penetrating bone fragments or a definite hematoma of the optic nerve sheath with consecutive loss of vision indicates surgical decompression of the optic nerve. Prompt surgical treatment is required to relieve the nerve even if there is the possibility of spontaneous remission.[79,80] Additional high-dose intravenous therapy with corticoids given for several days can improve the prognosis.[76]

CT-based interoperative navigation via an endonasal access is the most efficient approach for microsurgical decompression of the optic nerve. The middle turbinate is identified and medialized with the use of a microscope or endoscope. Now the removal of the ethmoidal cells as well as the exposition of the lamina papyracea follows. Afterwards, the sphenoid sinus is opened, displaying the lateral sphenoid sinus wall as well as the subjacent optic canal. The lamina papyracea is removed up to the sphenoid sinus. Then the lateral sphenoid sinus wall above the optic nerve is removed. After displaying 180° of the circumference of the nerve, the slitting of the periorbita as well as, if necessary, of the optic nerve sheath follows in order to achieve as much relieve as possible (▶ Fig. 8.20).

Prognosis

In about 50% of cases, visual acuity is expected to improve if consistent treatment is provided.[76,81,82] Prompt surgical treatment and intraoperative slitting of the nerve sheath have proved to be favorable to the prognosis. Complete blindness and a fracture line that runs through the optic canal seem to be rather unfavorable (▶ Table 8.11).

8.12 Orbital Injuries in Children

8.12.1 Orbital Fractures

Pathogenesis

Orbital walls in children are completely different from those in adults due to the undeveloped sinus system at birth. Only the lateral wall is roughly comparable. The pneumatization of the frontal sinus (cranial wall), the maxillary sinus (caudal wall), and the ethmoid sinus (medial wall) has not yet begun and only slowly progresses until adulthood.[83] For growth reasons, large parts of the visceral cranium are not yet ossified or provided with growth plates. This results in the fact that more energy can be absorbed and only high forces can cause fractures.[84] Due to the ratio of neurocranium to visceral cranium and the elasticity of the visceral cranium, fractures of the neurocranium are much more common than those of the visceral cranium.[85] Orbital fractures are comparatively rare in children (see ▶ Table 8.12).[86]

Table 8.11 Prognostic factors in patients with traumatic optic neuropathy[76]

Favorable prognosis	Unfavorable prognosis
Surgical treatment < 24 h, if possible < 8 h post trauma	Trauma more than 24 h previously
Residual visual function before surgery	Complete blindness before surgery
In case of hematoma of the optic nerve sheath, slitting of the sheath	Fracture of the optic canal

Table 8.12 Distribution of frequencies regarding structures involved in infantile midfacial fractures[86]

		Proportion of patients (n = 12,739)				
		5.7%	6.7%	14.3%	20.3%	53.0%
Fractured bone	Total frequency	0–1year of age	2–4 years	5–9 years	10–14 years	15–18 years
Mandible	33%	23%	21%	28%	30%	38%
Nasal bone	30%	35%	20%	25%	27%	34%
Maxilla	29%	32%	22%	24%	26%	32%
Orbit	20%	24%	22%	18%	22%	19%

The classification of midface and orbital fractures in children corresponds to that for adults.

Diagnostics

Since cooperation of the patient is usually lacking, important examination steps should precede subordinate ones, and potentially painful examinations should follow nonpainful ones. The loss of vision must be explicitly inquired about, because unilateral visual loss is not always autonomously reported by a child.[87]

For a precise representation of fractures and following surgical treatment, a CT scan of the orbit is the imaging method of choice if an orbital fracture is suspected.[87] However, where possible, the lens and the optic nerve as well as the brain should be shielded for protection from radiation exposure.[88] Additionally, the indication for a CT scan should be rather limited. Low-dose spiral CT or cone beam CT (CBC) could be an adequate alternative in the not too distant future.[89,90] Conventional radiographic imaging is an inferior diagnostic method especially in younger children, since vibrations occur frequently, resulting in limited validity. Nevertheless, a CT can provide precise information in course of a short anesthesia.[85] In zygomatic arch fractures and fractures of the infraorbital rim, however, studies have not provided any evidence suggesting a benefit of a CT scan compared to sonographic examination. Accordingly, ultrasonography should be the diagnostic measure of choice to exclude a fracture in this area in children.[91]

Therapy

Nondislocated fractures are common in children and require conservative treatment. For this purpose, such instructions as abstaining from sports and consistently refraining from nose blowing, as well as soft diet for 2–3 weeks, must be observed. Displaced orbital fractures in children require surgical care. To achieve the best possible results, all orbital fractures in children need immediate treatment.[92] The approach has to be as gentle as possible in order to preserve growth areas. However, growth impairments are observed in up to 40% of cases after severe trauma to the visceral cranium.[20,84]

References

[1] Rosado P, de Vicente JC. Retrospective analysis of 314 orbital fractures. Oral Surg Oral Med Oral Pathol Oral Radiol. 2012; 113(2):168–171

[2] Alvi A, Doherty T, Lewen G. Facial fractures and concomitant injuries in trauma patients. Laryngoscope. 2003; 113(1):102–106

[3] Erdmann D, Follmar KE, Debruijn M, et al. A retrospective analysis of facial fracture etiologies. Ann Plast Surg. 2008; 60(4):398–403

[4] Gadre KS, Halli R, Joshi S, et al. Incidence and pattern of cranio-maxillofacial injuries: a 22 year retrospective analysis of cases operated at major trauma hospitals/centres in Pune, India. J Maxillofac Oral Surg. 2013; 12(4):372–378

[5] Gassner R, Tuli T, Hächl O, Rudisch A, Ulmer H. Cranio-maxillofacial trauma: a 10 year review of 9,543 cases with 21,067 injuries. J Craniomaxillofac Surg. 2003; 31(1):51–61

[6] Klenk G, Kovacs A. Etiology and patterns of facial fractures in the United Arab Emirates. J Craniofac Surg. 2003; 14(1):78–84

[7] Lebeau J, Kanku V, Duroure F, Morand B, Sadek H, Raphaël B. Traumatismes faciaux au CHU de Grenoble. Etude épidémiologique de 961 dossiers sur une période de 365 jours. [Facial injuries treated in the Grenoble University Hospital. Epidemiological analysis of 961 patients managed in one year]. Rev Stomatol Chir Maxillofac. 2006; 107(1):23–29

[8] Maliska MC, Lima Júnior SM, Gil JN. Analysis of 185 maxillofacial fractures in the state of Santa Catarina, Brazil. Braz Oral Res. 2009; 23(3):268–274

[9] Prokop D, Boeckler HH. Morbiditätsanalyse von 1484 Gesichtsknochenfrakturen des Zeitraumes von 1968 bis 1987. [Morbidity analysis of 1484 facial bone fractures between 1968 and 1987]. Dtsch Z Mund Kiefer Gesichtschir. 1990; 14(4):287–292

[10] Afzelius LE, Rosén C. Influence of seat belt upon maxillofacial fractures. ORL J Otorhinolaryngol Relat Spec. 1980; 42(5):277–281

[11] Lee K. Global trends in maxillofacial fractures. Craniomaxillofac Trauma Reconstr. 2012; 5(4):213–222

[12] Pye G, Waters EA. Effect of seat belt legislation on injuries in road traffic accidents in Nottingham. Br Med J (Clin Res Ed). 1984; 288(6419):756–757

[13] Malara P, Malara B, Drugacz J. Characteristics of maxillofacial injuries resulting from road traffic accidents–a 5 year review of the case records from Department of Maxillofacial Surgery in Katowice, Poland. Head Face Med. 2006; 2:27

[14] Cossman JP, Morrison CS, Taylor HO, Salter AB, Klinge PM, Sullivan SR. Traumatic orbital roof fractures: interdisciplinary evaluation and management. Plast Reconstr Surg. 2014; 133(3):335e–343e

[15] Kim K, Ibrahim AM, Koolen PG, Lee BT, Lin SJ. Trends in facial fracture treatment using the American College of Surgeons National Surgical Quality Improvement Program database. Plast Reconstr Surg. 2014; 133(3):627–638

[16] Sharma B, Gupta R, Anand R, Ingle R. Ocular manifestations of head injury and incidence of post-traumatic ocular motor nerve involvement in cases of head injury: a clinical review. Int Ophthalmol. 2014; 34(4):893–900

[17] Bellamy JL, Mundinger GS, Reddy SK, Flores JM, Rodriguez ED, Dorafshar AH. Le Fort II fractures are associated with death: a comparison of simple and complex midface fractures. J Oral Maxillofac Surg. 2013; 71(9):1556–1562

[18] Lim LH, Lam LK, Moore MH, Trott JA, David DJ. Associated injuries in facial fractures: review of 839 patients. Br J Plast Surg. 1993; 46(8):635–638

[19] Schumann P, Kokemüller H, Tavassol F, et al. Optic nerve monitoring. Craniomaxillofac Trauma Reconstr. 2013; 6(2):75–86

[20] Jecker P. Ultraschalluntersuchung bei Erkrankungen der Nasennebenhöhlen, der Gesichtsweichteile, der Orbita und der knöchernen Strukturen des Gesichts. In: Welkoborsky H, Jecker P, Maurer J, Mann WJ, eds. Ultraschalldiagnostik Kopf-Hals. Stuttgart: Thieme; 2013:121–131

[21] Lin KY, Ngai P, Echegoyen JC, Tao JP. Imaging in orbital trauma. Saudi J Ophthalmol. 2012; 26(4):427–432

[22] Wilhelm H. Traumatische Optikusneuropathie. [Traumatic optic neuropathy]. Laryngorhinootologie. 2009; 88(3):194–203, quiz 204–207

[23] STIKO. Empfehlungen der Ständigen Impfkommission (STIKO) am Robert Koch-Institut: Stand August 2013. Epidemiologisches Bulletin 2013 Aug 26;(34)

[24] Bergmann J, Lee K, Klein R, Slonim CB. Upper face and orbit "degloving" dog bite injury. Ophthal Plast Reconstr Surg. 2009; 25(1):44–46

[25] Wladis EJ, Dewan MA. Periorbital trauma from pit bull terrier attacks. Orbit. 2012; 31(3):200–202

[26] Kim UR, Sivaraman KR. Penetrating orbital injuries from plant material during pond and river diving. Indian J Ophthalmol. 2013; 61(2):76–77

[27] Patel SN, Langer PD, Zarbin MA, Bhagat N. Diagnostic value of clinical examination and radiographic imaging in identification of intraocular foreign bodies in open globe injury. Eur J Ophthalmol. 2012; 22(2):259–268

[28] Shelsta HN, Bilyk JR, Rubin PA, Penne RB, Carrasco JR. Wooden intraorbital foreign body injuries: clinical characteristics and outcomes of 23 patients. Ophthal Plast Reconstr Surg. 2010; 26(4):238–244

[29] De León Tellado N, Tous H, Jiménez JC. Persistent caruncular hyperemia revealing unsuspected orbital foreign body. Bol Asoc Med P R. 2012; 104(2):74–76

[30] Gawdat TI, Ahmed RA. Orbital foreign bodies: expect the unexpected. J Pediatr Ophthalmol Strabismus. 2010; 47 Online:e1–e4

[31] Eggers G, Haag C, Hassfeld S. Image-guided removal of foreign bodies. Br J Oral Maxillofac Surg. 2005; 43(5):404–409

[32] Finkelstein M, Legmann A, Rubin PA. Projectile metallic foreign bodies in the orbit: a retrospective study of epidemiologic factors, management, and outcomes. Ophthalmology. 1997; 104(1):96–103

[33] Brandes A, Gehrke G. Fremdkörperentfernung an Orbita und Frontobasis. Mund Kiefer Gesichtschir. 1998; 2 Suppl 1:S113–S116

[34] Lee TH, Lee HM, Lee JM, Nam JG. Endoscopic reduction of orbital medial wall fracture using rotational repositioning of the fractured: lamina papyracea fragment. J Craniofac Surg. 2014; 25(2):460–462

[35] You JP, Kim DW, Jeon BJ, et al. Two-year follow-up on the use of absorbable mesh plates in the treatment of medial orbital wall fractures. Arch Plast Surg. 2013; 40(6):728–734

[36] Woo KS, Cho PD, Lee SH. Reconstruction of severe medial orbital wall fractures using titanium mesh plates by the pericaruncular approach. J Plast Surg Hand Surg. 2014; 48(4):248–253

[37] Schilli HW, Niederdellmann H. Verletzungen des Gesichtsschädels. [Injuries of the facial bones]. Aktuelle Probl Chir Orthop. 1980; 8:1–131

[38] Becker R, Austermann K. Frakturen des Gesichtsschädels. In: Schwenzer N, Grimm G, eds. Zahn-Mund-Kiefer-Heilkunde: Spezielle Chirurgie. Stuttgart: Thieme; 1981:464–584

[39] Soejima K, Sakurai H, Nozaki M, et al. Semi-closed reduction of tripod fractures of zygoma under intraoperative assessment using ultrasonography. J Plast Reconstr Aesthet Surg. 2009; 62(4):499–505

[40] Gillies HD, Kilner TP, Stone D. Fractures of the malar-zygomatic compound: with a description of a new x-ray position. Br J Surg. 1927; 14(56):651–656

[41] Waterhouse N, Lyne J, Urdang M, Garey L. An investigation into the mechanism of orbital blowout fractures. Br J Plast Surg. 1999; 52(8):607–612

[42] Arangio P, Vellone V, Torre U, Calafati V, Capriotti M, Cascone P. Maxillofacial fractures in the province of Latina, Lazio, Italy: review of 400 injuries and 83 cases. J Craniomaxillofac Surg. 2014; 42(5):583–587

[43] Motamedi MH. An assessment of maxillofacial fractures: a 5-year study of 237 patients. J Oral Maxillofac Surg. 2003; 61(1):61–64

[44] Essig H, Dressel L, Rana M, et al. Precision of posttraumatic primary orbital reconstruction using individually bent titanium mesh with and without navigation: a retrospective study. Head Face Med. 2013; 9:18

[45] Mustafa SF, Evans PL, Bocca A, Patton DW, Sugar AW, Baxter PW. Customized titanium reconstruction of post-traumatic orbital wall defects: a review of 22 cases. Int J Oral Maxillofac Surg. 2011; 40(12):1357–1362

[46] van Issum C, Courvoisier DS, Scolozzi P. Posttraumatic orbital emphysema: incidence, topographic classification and possible pathophysiologic mechanisms. A retrospective study of 137 patients. Oral Surg Oral Med Oral Pathol Oral Radiol. 2013; 115(6):737–742

[47] Schultze-Mosgau S, Krems H, Ott R, Neukam FW. A prospective electromyographic and computer-aided thermal sensitivity assessment of nerve lesions after sagittal split osteotomy and Le Fort I osteotomy. J Oral Maxillofac Surg. 2001; 59(2):128–138, discussion 138–139

[48] Bernal Sprekelsen M, Welkoborsky HJ. Fracturas del suelo de la órbita. Revisión a propósito de 346 casos. [Fractures of the orbital floor. Review of 346 cases]. Acta Otorrinolaringol Esp. 1991; 42(1):1–9

[49] Hwang K, Hwang JH. Do we have to dissect infraorbital nerve from periorbita in orbital floor fracture? J Craniofac Surg. 2009; 20(4):1260–1262

[50] Ozturk S, Sengezer M, Isik S, Turegun M, Deveci M, Cil Y. Long-term outcomes of ultra-thin porous polyethylene implants used for reconstruction of orbital floor defects. J Craniofac Surg. 2005; 16(6):973–977

[51] Schultze-Mosgau S, Erbe M, Rudolph D, Ott R, Neukam FW. Prospective study on post-traumatic and postoperative sensory disturbances of the inferior alveolar nerve and infraorbital nerve in mandibular and midfacial fractures. J Craniomaxillofac Surg. 1999; 27(2):86–93

[52] Zelken JA, Khalifian S, Mundinger GS, et al. Defining predictable patterns of craniomaxillofacial injury in the elderly: analysis of 1,047 patients. J Oral Maxillofac Surg. 2014; 72(2):352–361

[53] Lee JH. Complete reduction with traction of the infraorbital neurovascular bundle in a delayed patient with white-eyed blow-out fracture. J Craniofac Surg. 2014; 25(1):e54–e55

[54] Weerda H. Traumatologie der Frontobasis und Umgebung, einschließlich der endokraniellen Komplikationen. In: Kastenbauer ER, Tardy ME, Jr, eds. Gesicht, Nase und Gesichtsschädel, Pt II, 2nd revised ed. Stuttgart: Thieme; 1995:555–607

[55] Yan Z, Zhou Z, Song X. Nasal endoscopy-assisted reconstruction of orbital floor blowout fractures using temporal fascia grafting. J Oral Maxillofac Surg. 2012; 70(5):1119–1122

[56] Wahdan WS, Sleem HA. The use of collagen membranes in management of orbital floor fracture. Egypt J Oral Maxillofac Surg. 2014; 5(1):4–6

[57] Avashia YJ, Sastry A, Fan KL, Mir HS, Thaller SR. Materials used for reconstruction after orbital floor fracture. J Craniofac Surg. 2012; 23(7) Suppl 1:1991–1997

[58] Cho RI, Davies BW. Combined orbital floor and medial wall fractures involving the inferomedial strut: repair technique and case series using preshaped porous polyethylene/titanium implants. Craniomaxillofac Trauma Reconstr. 2013; 6(3):161–170

[59] Degala S, Shetty SK, Biddappa L. Reconstruction of post-traumatic internal orbital wall defects with titanium mesh. J Maxillofac Oral Surg. 2013; 12(4): 418–423

[60] Welkoborsky H. Traumatologie. In: Strutz J, Mann W, eds. Praxis der HNO-Heilkunde, Kopf- und Halschirurgie, 2nd revised extended ed. Stuttgart: Thieme; 2009:794–847

[61] Hwang K, Kim HJ, Lee HS. Blow-in fracture of the orbit. J Craniofac Surg. 2013; 24(5):1828–1829

[62] Lighterman I, Reckson C. “Blow-in” fracture of the orbit. Ann Plast Surg. 1979; 3(6):572–575

[63] Antonyshyn O, Gruss JS, Kassel EE. Blow-in fractures of the orbit. Plast Reconstr Surg. 1989; 84(1):10–20

[64] Elston JB, Ching JA, Hiro ME, Payne WG. Pure orbital floor blow-in fracture. Eplasty. 2013; 13:ic39

[65] Rha EY, Joo HS, Byeon JH. Orbital dystopia due to orbital roof defect. J Craniofac Surg. 2013; 24(5):e500–e504

[66] Cantini Ardila JE, Mendoza MÁ, Ortega VG. Sphenoid sinus and sphenoid bone fractures in patients with craniomaxillofacial trauma. Craniomaxillofac Trauma Reconstr. 2013; 6(3):179–186

[67] Le Fort R. Étude expérimentale sur les fractures de la machoire supérieure. Revue Chir Paris. 1901; 23:208–479

[68] Wassmund M. Frakturen und Luxationen des Gesichtsschädels. Berlin: Meusser; 1927

[69] Madhusudan G, Sharma RK, Khandelwal N, Tewari MK. Nomenclature of frontobasal trauma: a new clinicoradiographic classification. Plast Reconstr Surg. 2006; 117(7):2382–2388

[70] Escher F. Die Schädelbasisverletzungen Standpunkt des Otorhinologen. [The fractures of the basis of the skull: the standpoint of the oto-rhino-laryngologist (author's transl)]. Ther Umsch. 1974; 31(9):634–639

[71] Baker EH, Wood DM, Brennan AL, Baines DL, Philips BJ. New insights into the glucose oxidase stick test for cerebrospinal fluid rhinorrhoea. Emerg Med J. 2005; 22(8):556–557

[72] Kamochi H, Kusaka G, Ishikawa M, Ishikawa S, Tanaka Y. Late onset cerebrospinal fluid leakage associated with past head injury. Neurol Med Chir (Tokyo). 2013; 53(4):217–220

[73] Mantur M, Łukaszewicz-Zając M, Mroczko B, et al. Cerebrospinal fluid leakage–reliable diagnostic methods. Clin Chim Acta. 2011; 412(11–12):837–840

[74] Lin DT, Lin AC. Surgical treatment of traumatic injuries of the cranial base. Otolaryngol Clin North Am. 2013; 46(5):749–757

[75] Markowitz BL, Manson PN. Panfacial fractures: organization of treatment. Clin Plast Surg. 1989; 16(1):105–114

[76] Welkoborsky HJ, Möbius H, Bauer L, Wiechens B. Traumatische Optikusneuropathie. Langzeitergebnisse nach endonasaler mikrochirurgischer Dekompression des N. opticus. [Traumatic optic nerve neuropathy. Long-term results following microsurgical optic nerve decompression]. HNO. 2011; 59(10):997–1004

[77] Entezari M, Rajavi Z, Sedighi N, Daftarian N, Sanagoo M. High-dose intravenous methylprednisolone in recent traumatic optic neuropathy; a randomized double-masked placebo-controlled clinical trial. Graefes Arch Clin Exp Ophthalmol. 2007; 245(9):1267–1271

[78] Steinsapir KD. Treatment of traumatic optic neuropathy with high-dose corticosteroid. J Neuroophthalmol. 2006; 26(1):65–67

[79] Yu-Wai-Man P, Griffiths PG. Steroids for traumatic optic neuropathy. Cochrane Database Syst Rev. 2013(6):CD006032

[80] Levin LA, Beck RW, Joseph MP, Seiff S, Kraker R. The treatment of traumatic optic neuropathy: the International Optic Nerve Trauma Study. Ophthalmology. 1999; 106(7):1268–1277

[81] Li H, Zhou B, Shi J, Cheng L, Wen W, Xu G. Treatment of traumatic optic neuropathy: our experience of endoscopic optic nerve decompression. J Laryngol Otol. 2008; 122(12):1325–1329

[82] Zuo KJ, Shi JB, Wen WP, Chen HX, Zhang XM, Xu G. [Transnasal endoscopic optic nerve decompression for traumatic optic neuropathy: analysis of 155 cases]. [Article in Chinese]. Zhonghua Yi Xue Za Zhi. 2009; 89(6):389–392

[83] Oppenheimer AJ, Monson LA, Buchman SR. Pediatric orbital fractures. Craniomaxillofac Trauma Reconstr. 2013; 6(1):9–20

[84] Singh DJ, Bartlett SP. Pediatric craniofacial fractures: long-term consequences. Clin Plast Surg. 2004; 31(3):499–518, vii

[85] Ehrenfeld M, Cornelius CP. Traumatologie der Gesichtsweichgewebe, der Zähne und des Gesichtsschädels. In: Götte K, Nicolai T, eds. Pädiatrische HNO-Heilkunde. München: Elsevier, Urban & Fischer; 2010:357–369

[86] Imahara SD, Hopper RA, Wang J, Rivara FP, Klein MB. Patterns and outcomes of pediatric facial fractures in the United States: a survey of the National Trauma Data Bank. J Am Coll Surg. 2008; 207(5):710–716

[87] Kassam K, Rahim I, Mills C. Paediatric orbital fractures: the importance of regular thorough eye assessment and appropriate referral. Case Rep Emerg Med. 2013; 2013:376564

[88] Bernier MO, Rehel JL, Brisse HJ, et al. Radiation exposure from CT in early childhood: a French large-scale multicentre study. Br J Radiol. 2012; 85 (1009):53–60

[89] Morton RP, Reynolds RM, Ramakrishna R, et al. Low-dose head computed tomography in children: a single institutional experience in pediatric radiation risk reduction: clinical article. J Neurosurg Pediatr. 2013; 12(4):406–410

[90] Pindrik J, Huisman TA, Mahesh M, Tekes A, Ahn ES. Analysis of limited-sequence head computed tomography for children with shunted hydrocephalus: potential to reduce diagnostic radiation exposure. J Neurosurg Pediatr. 2013; 12(5):491–500

[91] Ogunmuyiwa SA, Fatusi OA, Ugboko VI, Ayoola OO, Maaji SM. The validity of ultrasonography in the diagnosis of zygomaticomaxillary complex fractures. Int J Oral Maxillofac Surg. 2012; 41(4):500–505

[92] Gerber B, Kiwanuka P, Dhariwal D. Orbital fractures in children: a review of outcomes. Br J Oral Maxillofac Surg. 2013; 51(8):789–793

Chapter 9

Pathology of the Orbit

9

9 Pathology of the Orbit

L. Wilkens

9.1 Introduction

9.1.1 General

Tissue formed from all three dermal layers is found in the orbit in a complex formation. As a result, nearly all types of inflammations and tumors can occur in this topographically narrowly restricted area.

This chapter is not meant to pass on detailed morphological knowledge but rather to provide those working in clinical practice with an overview of the diseases to be expected in the orbit and to illustrate how a pathologist names and classifies these. Thus, no detailed histological descriptions from the very comprehensive knowledge base will be presented, only an outline of what is essential. This is information that should enable anyone interested to acquire more in-depth knowledge and to be able to better understand the morphology.

To understand the pathologist's approach, one should be acquainted with the procedures used. Pathology originates from the dissecting room but its field of activity has expanded over the decades to encompass the microscopic examination of operation preparations and biopsies, which today account for 95% of the work. For histology, initially—with the knowledge of the patient's previous history—the tissue is examined with the naked eye—the macroscopic aspect. In this examination tissue samples are taken in a targeted manner. In contrast, small tissue biopsies are used in their entirety. Both kind of samples are then dehydrated and embedded in paraffin. Wafer-thin slices ~1 to 2 µm thick are prepared, mounted on microscope slides, and stained using various processes.

9

Histology is supplemented by cytology. In this technique, smears or cells obtained as fine needle aspirates are likewise mounted on slides and stained. In cytology the emphasis is on the assessment of individual cells, whereas in histology larger, functional cell groupings are considered. The preparations from these two complementary procedures are viewed under the microscope and, usually, a conclusion can reached at this stage.

If a conclusive assessment is not possible with the staining techniques already used, then immunohisto(cyto)chemistry is available. In this form of staining, there is no chemical reaction but an immunological antigen–antibody reaction is exploited. The antibodies that bind to the antigens in turn have reporter molecules, which only subsequently produce their own staining on the tissues in a second reaction.

There is now the possibility of further differentiation of the tissues by genetic procedures such as mutation analysis and gene expression analysis. A step by step diagnostic process is based on the results obtained via these diagnostic methods.

Pathomorphological examination of operation preparations and biopsies is likewise conducted with these complementary procedures.

9.1.2 Observations on Classification

The orbit is affected by diverse diseases with a significant emphasis on inflammatory reactive changes (▶ Table 9.1).

Although the terminology for inflammatory changes continues to be defined and refined, since the mid-1990s tumor pathology has developed considerably and become standardized. In the publications on tumor classification issued by the WHO, the tumor entities currently known are given standardized names and designated with a code (ICD-O key in the currently valid version). Both of these schemata are provided with the TNM classification for malignant epithelial tumors; the result is a comprehensive and mostly precise classification for every tumor. From this, in Anglo-Saxon countries the practice is to refrain from classical textual assessment and undertake the assessment in the form of tabular juxtapositions. This brings considerable advantages with regard to the completeness and accuracy of assessments. It is also beneficial for international comparability of research studies and comprehensibility of assessments across national borders.

Within the context of these classifications the tumors assessed are to be further assessed with regard to their biological significance. It is in this regard that **grading** of tumors is done. In principle the grading is as follows:

- G1: good differentiation; the histogenetic assignment of the tumor is without difficulty in the overview stainings. The differentiation of benign/malignant is somewhat difficult.
- G2: moderate differentiation; the histogenetic assignment is successful in the overview stainings. There is a discontinuity or "jump" in the differentiation, which clearly enables classification as a malignant tumor.
- G3: poor differentiation; the histogenetic assignment can only be done in the overview stainings to a limited extent or not at all. Immunohistochemical procedures may be necessary to enable assignment.
- G4: dedifferentiated malignant tumor. Here even immunohistochemistry may no longer help in the assignment.

In the grading of malignant tumors there are additional criteria for a number of entities that have proved to be important for the assessment of the biological behavior. In particular, FNCLCC (Fédération National des Centres de Lutte Contre le Cancer) standards apply for **sarcomas**. These are:

- Tumor differentiation (Score 1–3).
- Mitosis count (Score 1–3).
- Tumor necrosis (Score 1–3).

From these is derived the histological degree:

- Grade 1: total score 2, 3.
- Grade 2: total score 4, 5.
- Grade 3: total score 6, 7, 9.

Table 9.1 Distribution of orbital diseases (Rootman, 1988)

Disease	Percentage
Graves's disease	50%
Neoplasias	20%
Congenital diseases	15%
Inflammatory diseases	10%
Vascular diseases	3%
Degenerative diseases and depositions	2%

For **malignant melanomas** the TNM classification is supplemented with a series of histological parameters that, for example, are not (yet) required in carcinomas. From this there results a comprehensive assessment, which should contain the following points:

- Actual histological diagnosis.
- Tumor thickness (according to Breslow).
- Invasion level (according to Clark).
- Ulceration.
- Mitotic rate (per mm^2).
- Cell types (in different tumor cell groups).
- Regression.
- Tumor infiltration by lymphocytes (TIL).
- Evidence of plasma cells.
- Evidence of a neovascularization.
- Vascular invasion.
- Microscopically small satellites.
- Associated preexisting nevus.
- Margin of the resection edges.
- Additional parameters of the TNM classification (regional lymph nodes, remote metastases).

There results a breakdown as follows for a pathological–anatomical finding:

- Clinical findings.
- Macroscopic findings.
- Histologic findings.
- Assessment supplemented by the above-mentioned parameters; where necessary, commentary with an explanation (which should always be read and understood).
- Where applicable, tabular summary of all significant parameters.

9.2 Inflammations

An inflammation is the tissue's reaction to biological, chemical, or physical noxae. The nature of the inflammatory reaction permits some conclusions to be made about the influencing noxa (e.g., granuloma in the context of a mycobacteriosis). In the main, however, the appearance of the inflammation is unspecific.

In principle, an acute phase is followed by either healing (ad integrum) or the transition to chronic inflammation. Linked with this is a change in the inflammatory cells involved away from granulocytes to lymphocytes. The final stage of chronic inflammation is scar formation.

A primary chronic inflammation is also possible.

9.2.1 Acute Inflammations

► **Nonsuppurative (nonpurulent) inflammations.** These occur mostly as a spreading of inflammations from the sinuses.

► **Suppurative(purulent) inflammations.** These occur as purulent inflammations of the orbital soft tissue, mostly infection-induced. The most significant pathogens are staphylococci, often introduced as a result of wounds, with the recognized consequence of a phlegmonous inflammation; also phycomycosis occurs in the context of immunosuppression. The high mortality and grave local complications such as extensive thromboses are feared and difficult to prevent or treat. A distinguishing histologic feature is infiltration of the tissue through alternating densely packed granulocytes. These can be distributed diffusely through the tissue (phlegmonous) or be densely packed alongside each other, merging into necroses and an abscessing inflammation (► Fig. 9.1).

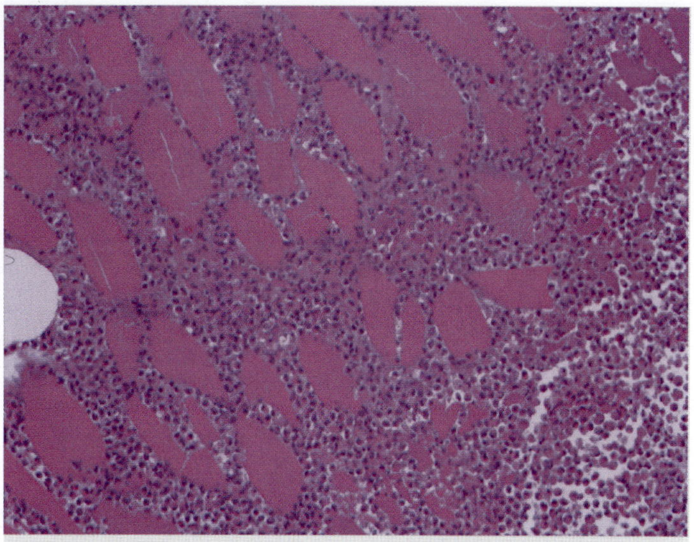

Fig. 9.1 Granulocytic inflammation. Dense infiltrations of granulocytes are located in the connective tissue and muscles. Some of the myocytes are necrotic and fragmented due to the inflammation (H&E staining, magnification 20 × 10).

9.2.2 Chronic Inflammations

► **Nongranulomatous inflammations.** Unspecific processes without known cause are most frequently in this form.

► **Granulomatous inflammations.** An important example of these is chalazion as a local inflammation of the meibomian glands (► Fig. 9.2). Granulomatous inflammations are commonly caused by pathogens that include in particular mycobacteria, treponemes, ***bartonella henselae***, fungi, and parasites (trichinosis, schistosomiasis). Autoimmune diseases can likewise feature granulomatous inflammation components (see below).

Cholesterol granulomas are the result of systemic or local metabolic disorders or lipid deposits (xanthelasma; see also xanthomatous tumors of the eyelids) in skin and soft tissue as the result of hematomas.

Systemic diseases such as sarcoidosis, Crohn's disease, and giant cell polymyositis often likewise lead to granulomas.

► **Local autoimmune inflammations.** Sjögren's syndrome is a disease of the lacrimal and salivary glands. There is a known close connection with the development of lymphomas (see below).

► **Idiopathic orbital inflammation (pseudotumor orbitae).** This is a protracted inflammatory lesion, which is difficult to differentiate from a "genuine" lymphoma in conventional stainings. The inflammation is located in the orbital soft tissue. Histologically, there is a lymphocytic infiltrate of varying density with similarly variable accompanying fibrosis. Classification as a reactive change has been considerably facilitated by new molecular pathology processes (clonality analysis).

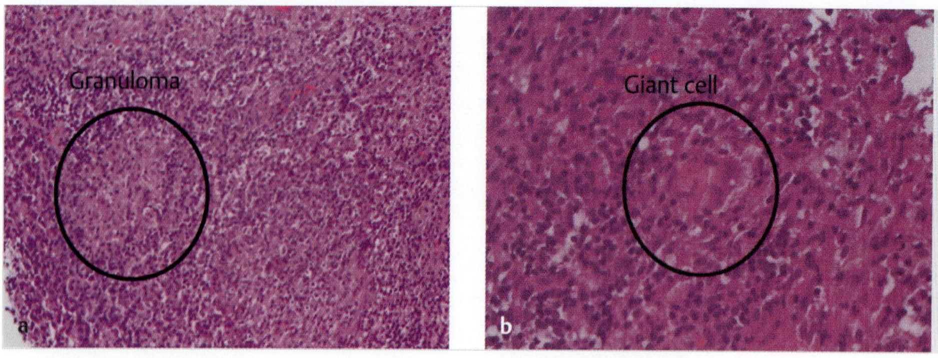

Fig. 9.2 Chalazion. Dense infiltrations of inflammatory cells beside clusters of epitheloid cells, which are grouped in granuloma pattern. **(a)** Granulomas (H&E staining, magnification 20 × 10). **(b)** Some giant cells occur in the lesion (H&E staining, magnification 40 × 10).

As radical removal does not affect survival and therefore a conservative approach is recommended, a reliable diagnosis becomes even more important.

9.3 Systemic Diseases Involving the Orbit

Basedow's disease is typical within the context of the Merseburg triad; however, the exophthalmos can also occur without tachycardia and struma. Caused by a cross reaction of antibodies, inflammatory changes are produced in the soft tissue of the orbit and with associated exophthalmos. With continual improvement in the treatment of the underlying disease and suppression of the unfavorable influencing factors (smoking), this disorder has become rare in its typical form.

Other systemic diseases that can occur with involvement of the orbit are myasthenia gravis, myotonia dystrophica, myotonia congenita, mitochondrial myopathy, and dermatomyositis.

9.4 Neoplasias (Arranged Topographically)

9.4.1 Tumors of the Optic Nerve

General

Approximately 5 to 8% of all tumors of the orbit grow in the optic nerve. Histogenetically, the tumors can be attributed to the actual nerve tissue, to the sheath tissue and to blood vessels (▶ Table 9.2). As nerve tissue is ultimately an outgrowth of the brain, tumors are of glial differentiation. In addition there are meningiomas deriving from meningeal cells as well as angiomas deriving from the blood vessels. As there are melanocytes in the meninges, the occurrence of melanocytic tumors can easily be understood. In addition, mesenchymal cells, like histiocytic cells, can lead to separate tumors.

Table 9.2 Tumors of the optic nerve

Benign	Uncertain biological behavior	Malignant
Meningioma	Hemangiopericytoma/SFT	Metastases
Pilocytic astrocytoma		Malignant astrocytoma
Melanocytoma		Malignant melanoma
Astrocytic hamartoma		
Hemangioma		
Juvenile xanthogranuloma		

In contrast, primary tumors of epithelial origin are not to be expected and occur in the optic nerve only as metastases. The primary origin of lymphomas is debatable but here too the assumption of metastasis is the rule.

Hence the variability of primary tumors of the optic nerve is fairly straightforward. Due to the unfavorable location of these tumors, irrespective of whether benign or malignant, they are without exception problematic. Thus tumors that in other locations of the body would simply be excised are treated conservatively in the optic nerve or even simply kept under observation.

Benign Tumors

Meningioma

Meningiomas are tumors of the arachnoid cells, which are situated in the arachnoidal villi of the nerve sheaths. Meningiomas represent the most frequent tumor group in the optic nerve and can occur in all sections of the nerve, but their most common location is the apex (~80%). The biological behavior is benign for the most part (WHO grade I). There are a series of morphological variants (▶ Fig. 9.3). Atypical and anaplastic variants (WHO grade II or III) are rare in contrast to intracranial meningiomas. In children these tumors grow much more aggressively. The tumor is nearly always unilateral and occurs somewhat more frequently in women than in men. The age distribution is given variously in the literature. An association with von Recklinghausen's disease has been reported very rarely.

Due to the very unfavorable location, if the vision is minimally affected a wait-and-see approach is discussed. Fractionated irradiation is performed in order to preserve the nerve. If sight is lost, surgical resection is performed. Recurrences are possible but rare.

Pilocytic astrocytoma

This is a benign tumor deriving from fibrous astrocytes. The frequently visible spindle cell–like offshoots of the tumor cells, which look like hairs, give the tumor its name. Of all tumors of the orbit 1 to 4% are pilocytic astrocytomas; 48% are found in the orbit, 28% in the intracranial section and 24% in both areas. Ninety percent of the tumors occur in the first two decades of life, but only rarely occur congenitally. Girls are more frequently affected (60/40). There is a known link with von Recklinghausen's disease; 30% of all tumor patients have this disease. These patients can also experience multicentric growth.

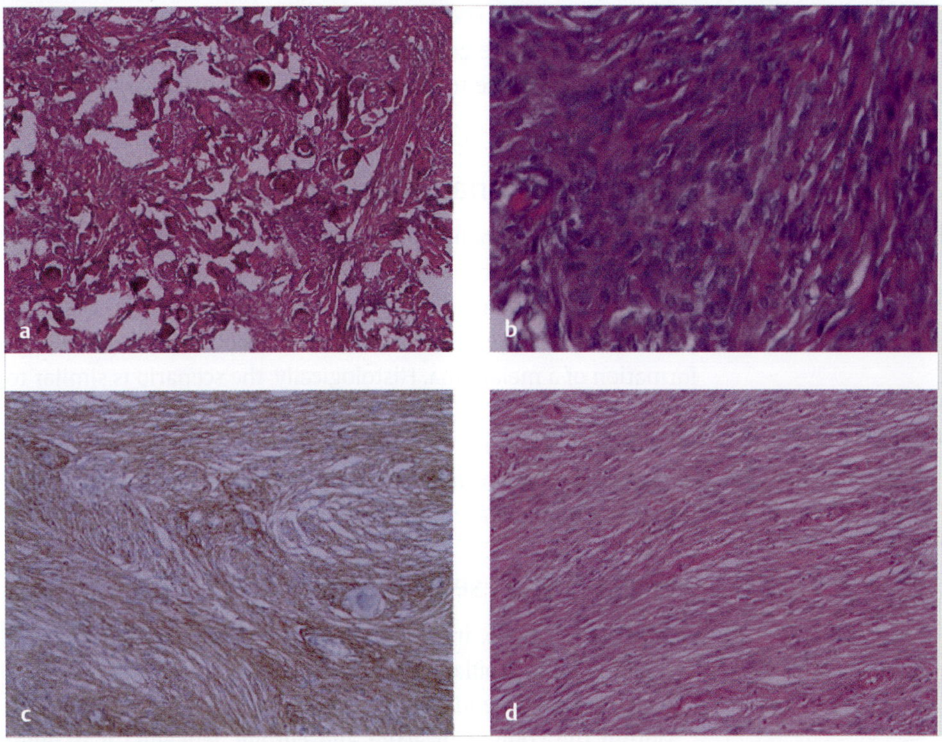

Fig. 9.3 Meningiomas. **(a)** Psammomatous meningioma: tumors cells are layered in a bundlelike pattern (H&E staining, magnification 10 × 10). **(b)** Psammomatous meningioma repeatedly displays so-called psammoma corpuscles in partly grouped pattern, representing a special kind of calcification (H&E staining, magnification 40 × 10). **(c)** The fibroblastic meningioma is also characterized by tumor cell bundles, which in this case resemble a fibroma (H&E staining, magnification 20 × 10). **(d)** Immunohistochemistry reveals positivity for EMA (epithelial membrane antigen), which helps to clarify the diagnosis (magnification 20 × 10).

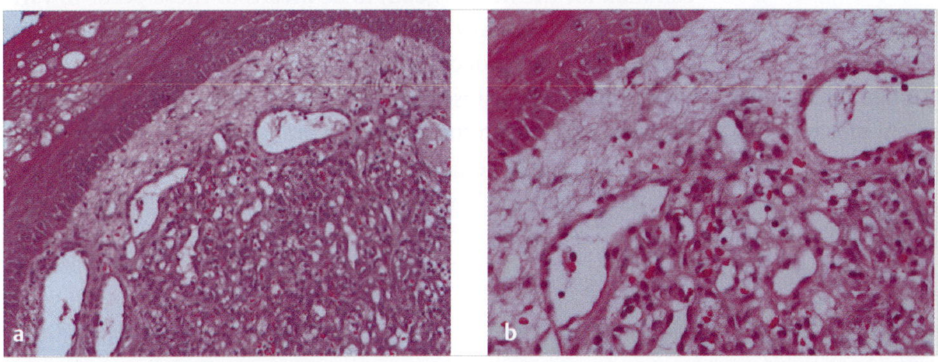

Fig. 9.4 Capillary hemangioma. Bundles of small blood vessels lined by a normal endothelium. Capillaries are layered in lobulelike pattern of different sizes. **(a)** H&E staining, magnification 20 × 10. **(b)** H&E staining, magnification 40 × 10.

Most pilocytic astrocytomas grow very slowly; some stop growing for some time and some show regression. Rapid growth and malignancy are an exception. Radiotherapy and surgical resection are possibilities. Growth in the chiasma or intracranially can lead to considerable difficulties in terms of curability.

Melanocytoma

Melanocytoma is a benign tumor, typically situated in the optic nerve, more rarely in the uvea and conjunctiva. Patients with dark pigmentation are more often affected. The tumor is constructed of densely packed melanocytic cells with a very prominent pigmentation with melanin.

Mostly only mild symptoms are reported and for the most part its discovery is by chance. A gray to black lesion is apparent opthalmoscopically on the optic nerve disc. It is very rare that both sides are affected.

For differential diagnosis, distinction from choroidal melanoma or necrotic juxtapapillary choroidal melanoma is important. Therapeutic inaction is justified in a significant proportion of the cases. Malignant transformation has been reported very rarely.

Astrocytic hamartoma

This is a benign and slow-growing tumorous of the optic disc and rarely of the surrounding retina. The tumor consists of spindle cells and squat astrocytes. There is a known association with tuberous sclerosis and neurofibromatosis (type 2).

Hemangioma

Capillary and cavernous hemangiomas arise at the optic disc and along the optic nerve. Capillary hemangiomas consist of small, densely packed vessels, lined with a flat endothelium without atypia (▶ Fig. 9.4). Capillary hemangiomas can grow endophytically and exophytically and into the vitreous humor and the head of the optic nerve. Sessile growth is also possible. There is a known link with von Hippel–Lindau disease. Capillary hemangiomas that feature fatty cells in the stroma and are associated with von Hippel-Lindau disease are termed *angiomatosis retinae*.

Juvenile xanthogranuloma

This is a benign and self-healing neoplasia with strikingly bluish/brownish and in part also reddish/yellow papules, sometimes as micronodular form or as nodules up to 20 mm. Histologically it is a mixed infiltrate of numerous histiocytes and Touton cells (giant cells) with sparse neutrophil and eosinophil granulocytes as well as lymphocytes. There is a known link with neurofibromatosis (Type 1 by far the majority). It most frequently occurs in the first year of life and is congenital in 5 to 17% of patients.

Tumors with Uncertain Biological Behavior

Hemangiopericytoma

(Current nomenclature is *solitary fibrous tumor, SFT.*) Origin in the cells of the meninges of the optic nerve is suggested. Histologically, there are bundles of spindle-shaped cells with irregularly shaped blood vessels running through them (▶ Fig. 9.5). The tumor tends to recur and in this respect the clinical behavior is not clearly benign. The tumor is noticed when it negatively affects the sight and CT shows a fusiform shape change of the optic nerve.

For a long time the designation of this tumor as a hemangiopericytoma and as a solitary fibrous tumor caused confusion. The latter designation was originally used for a mesenchymal tumor of the pleura. Since early this century it has been discovered that SFT occurs not only in the pleura but also at many other locations, including in the head area and there in the orbit and the nasal and sinus passages. It will be interesting to see how the designation of this tumor develops further.

Malignant Tumors

Malignant Astrocytoma

9

This is a malignant tumor that only rarely arises in the optic nerve. Histologically, atypical or pleomorphic tumor cells of glial differentiation are observable. Mitoses are numerous and necroses are repeatedly found. Those afflicted are mainly adults in the age range 20 to 80 years; the peak age is 52 years. Patients come to attention through a loss of sight; bilateral affliction via the chiasma occurs. Local destructive growth or infiltration of the dura accompany the growth of the tumor. The prognosis is poor, with a fatal outcome to the disease, mostly in the first year after diagnosis.

Primary malignant melanoma

Only rarely does a malignant melanoma occur as a primary in the optic nerve and the optic disc. The primary melanoma derives from melanocytes of the meninges. Correspondingly, a strong pigmentation of the nerve, as with a nevus ota, is associated with formation of a melanoma. Histologically, the scenario is similar to that in melanomas of other primary localization (▶ Fig. 9.6). By far the majority of melanomas in the optic nerve are the consequence of the involvement of juxtapapillary choroid melanomas or represent metastases. The prognosis is poor.

Metastases or secondary involvement

As described above, involvement of the optic nerve is possible through a juxtapapillary choroidal melanoma. Retinoblastomas can also metastasize in the optic nerve.

Within the context of acute and chronic leukemia it is quite common for the nerve (head) to be involved. These occur in various subtypes. Primary leukemias/lymphomas are extremely rare and are the subject of controversial debate.

Carcinoma metastases derive mainly from lung, breast, and stomach cancers. On the whole the prognosis of these metastases or secondary involvement is poor. Exceptions are leukemias/lymphomas. Prognosis has to be seen in relation to the underlying disease.

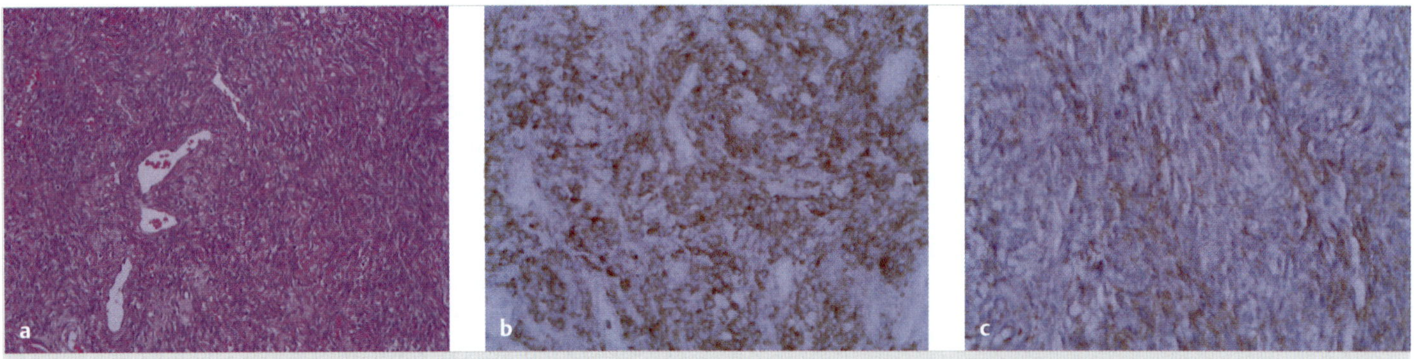

Fig. 9.5 Hemangiopericytoma. **(a)** The picture of a SFT (solitary fibrous tumor) is characterized by groups of longitudinal-oval cells that are arranged in storiform pattern (H&E staining, magnification 20 × 10). **(b)** The diagnosis is supported by immunohistochemistry, which reveals expression of BCL2 (magnification 40 × 10). **(c)** Immunohistochemistry reveals also expression of CD99 (magnification 40 × 10).

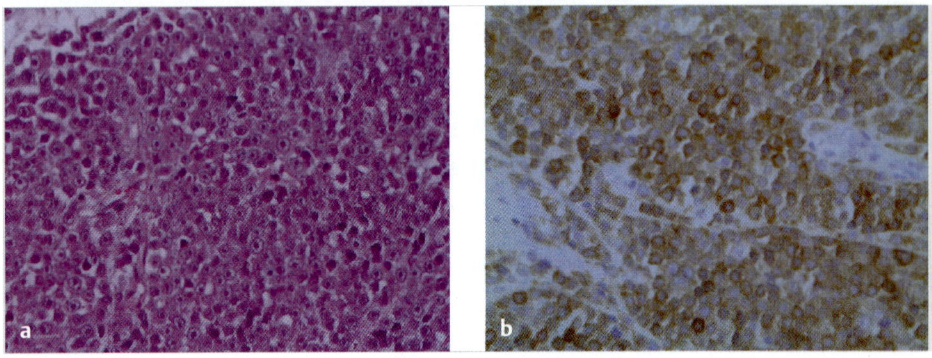

Fig. 9.6 Malignant melanoma. **(a)** Differentiation between a malignant melanoma and a diffuse large B-cell lymphoma is challenging due to lawnlike infiltration of large tumor cells with prominent nucleoli. **(b)** Positive staining with Melan A helps to clarify the diagnosis of a malignant melanoma (Melan A staining, magnification 40 × 10).

9.4.2 Tumors of the Conjunctiva and Caruncula

General

Tumors of the conjunctiva and caruncula, together with the tumors of the eyelids, constitute the most common tumors. A basic differentiation can be made between benign, premalignant, and malignant tumors. The most frequent tumors are epithelial, melanocytic, and lymphatic proliferates as well as choristomas, as reported in the case series of the AFIP and Doheny Eye Institute. Squamous cell carcinomas and their precursor lesions are reported to be the most common tumors in adults, while in children papillomas and choristomas represent the most significant tumor group (▶ Table 9.3).

In the melanocytic lesions, nevi represent the main group at 45%, but even so 36% have to be classed as melanomas (case series of the Doheny Eye Institute). Melanoses represent a further important group (with or without atypia).

Epithelial Tumors

Benign Tumours

Papillomas

Papillomas occur in all age groups but are more common in children. There is a close link to infection with the human papilloma viruses, in particular with serotypes 6, 11, and 16. Histologically, a deep, acanthotic squamous differentiated epithelium is laid over branching connective tissue branches.

Papillomas occur singly and in multiples. Both eyes can be affected. In children the place of origin is often the area around the caruncle, as well as around the semilunar fold on the inner canthus/fornix. In contrast, with adults the limbus is more often the primary site. Treatment for this is excision. Extensive and frequent recurrences can be treated, inter alia, with topically applied interferon.

Table 9.3 Tumors of the conjunctiva and caruncle

Benign	Uncertain biological behavior/ Precancerous lesions	Malignant
Epithelial		
Papilloma	Actinic keratosis	Squamous cell carcinoma
Keratoacanthoma	Conjunctival intraepithelial neoplasia	Basal cell carcinoma
Hereditary benign Intraepithelial dyskeratosis		Carcinoma of sebaceous glands
Epithelial cyst		
Unspecific keratinizing lesions		
Pseudoepitheliomatous hyperplasia		
Pterygium		
Melanocytic		
Nevus cell nevi	Primary acquired melanosis (PAM) with atypia and high risk	Malignant melanoma
• Junctional		
• Compound		
• Dermal		
Melanocytosis		
• Ocular		
• Oculodermal		
Blue nevus		
Spitz nevus		
Primary acquired melanosis (PAM)		
• Without atypia		
• With atypia and low risk		
Mesenchymal		
Vascular lesions • Telangiectasia • Malformations • Lymphangiectasia	Fibrous histiocytoma	Fibrous histiocytoma Rhabdomyosarcoma Kaposi's sarcoma
Myxoma		
Other tumors		
Dermoids		Lymphoma
Ectopic lacrimal glands		Plasmocytoma
Complex choristoma		Metastases

Keratoacanthoma

Keratoacanthoma is a very rapidly growing squamous cell epithelial lesion, very similar to a highly differentiated squamous cell epithelial carcinoma. The tumor typically grows in an undermining fashion while forming a so-called shoulder. The differential diagnosis from squamous cell epithelial carcinoma is very difficult and in particular barely possible from the biopsy. This makes the clinical results even more important. A favorite location is the sun-exposed conjunctiva. The lesion grows in a few weeks and then remains stationary or regresses. It is treated by excision.

Hereditary benign intraepithelial dyskeratosis

This is dyskeratosis and acanthosis of the conjunctival epithelium within the context of a very rare autosomal dominant hereditary disease (also known as Witkop–von Sallman syndrome). It affects squamous epithelium of the conjunctiva, which appears in childhood as a grayish coloration of both eyes. The thickened and inflamed epithelium often occurs interpalpebrally (nasally and temporally). The disease goes on to recur chronically. It is treated surgically. Relapses are frequent but malignant transformation has so far not been reported. The diagnosis of this very rare disease emerges not least from the family case history.

9

Epithelial cysts

Epithelial cysts are translucent, in part bluish, lesions. A few are congenital, but mainly they are acquired (e.g., as the result of inflammation and trauma). The most frequent localizations are lower fornix and nasal conjunctiva. A simple squamous epithelium, in part infiltrated by goblet cells, lines the cysts. Variations with a double-row epithelium are possible. A simple excision is carried out to treat them.

Unspecific keratinizing lesions

These constitute a malfunction of a benign nature in the maturation of the conjunctival epithelium. A series of changes are grouped under this term. Histologically, there are squamous metaplasia and hyperkeratosis, which can appear without an apparent reason. A link has been established with a vitamin A deficiency.

A histologically similar change occurs as the result of conjunctiva that is too dry as in Sjögren's disease, keratoconjunctivitis sicca, and following radiotherapy.

Pseudoepitheliomatous hyperplasia

Pseudoepitheliomatous hyperplasia is a reactive change of the epithelium in response to an inflammatory irritation. Histologically, there is a remarkable hyperplasia of the metaplastic squamous epithelium in which mitosis and dyskeratotic cells occur. This can make differentiation from squamous cell epithelium difficult (for this reason the name "pseudoepithelioma"). If granuloma occurs, one should think about a fungal infection in particular. After cessation of the cause the hyperplasia generally reduces in size.

Pseudoadenomatous hyperplasia

This is a benign glandlike proliferation that can be similar to a mucoepidermoid carcinoma.

Leukoplakia

The term leukoplakia ("white patch") is a clinical term under which many benign as well as malignant changes are grouped together. Leukoplakia is caused by a thickening of the squamous (metaplastic) epithelium and/or a fibrosis in the stroma. As a result, the fine blood vessels are seen to a lesser extent and the color changes from reddish to whitish.

Often leukoplakias are caused by light damage, in particular through UVB rays. This causes a squamous metaplasia with the formation of increased keratin and a degeneration of the basic structure of collagen fibers with increased deposition of collagen debris. Three such disorders are prevalent:

- *Solar elastosis* (no actual tumor formation): basophilic, stainable, clumpy degenerations are found in the stroma (▸ Fig. 9.7). A purely degenerative phenomenon and not spreading further beyond.
- *Pterygium*: The above-described changes of actinic elastosis and keratosis in alternation lead to this interpalpebrally located change involving the cornea (▸ Fig. 9.8).
- *Actinic keratosis*: see below under "Precancerous."

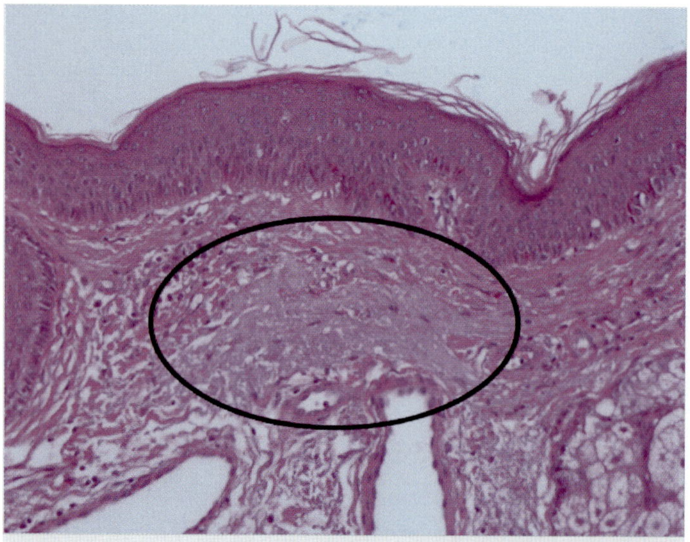

Fig. 9.7 Solar elastosis. Clumpy degenerative basophilic material represents degenerative elastic fibers. This degeneration is due to long-term extensive light exposure (H&E staining, magnification 20 × 10).

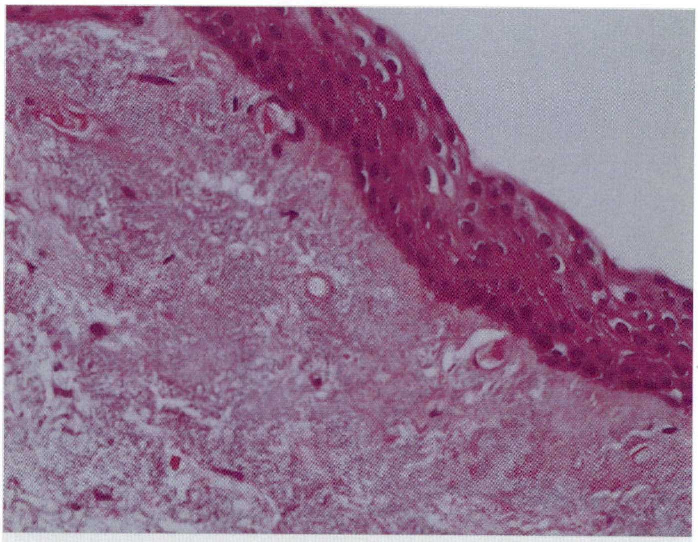

Fig. 9.8 Pterygium. Clumpy degenerates of basophilic material in the stroma are located underneath a metaplastic squamous epithelium, which resembles a cutaneous solar elastosis (H&E staining, magnification 40 × 10).

Precancerous

Actinic keratosis

Here the epithelium is damaged, nearly always showing *actinic elastosis*. Keratinization is disturbed. Dysplasias of different degrees can develop right through to a carcinoma in situ/Bowen's disease with possible transition to a squamous carcinoma.

Conjunctival intraepithelial neoplasias (IN)

Similarly to the concept of cervical intraepithelial neoplasia, the different stages of further neoplastic development of the conjunctival epithelium can be described in this terminology. Histologically, there is disruption in the structure of the squamous metaplastic epithelium. Slight, moderate, and severe dysplasias are distinguished in disruptions to the layers in the lower, in the lower and middle, and/or in all three parts of the epithelium. No clear distinction is made in the literature between severe dysplasia and carcinoma in situ or Bowen's disease, or they are used synonymously to some extent.

As in cervical IN, the human papilloma virus is known to be a trigger of conjunctival IN; there are also significant physical or chemical noxae known. Intensified light exposure (working in the open air), the effects of oil raffinates, cigarette smoke, and long-term treatment with chemotherapeutics such as cyclosporine (e.g., in transplantation patients). A link to conjunctival pigmentation is also known. At the very least, severe dysplasias are excised as these are precancerous with a high risk of malignancy. Recurrences are frequent; a "field effect" is recognized.

Malignant Tumors

Squamous epithelial carcinoma (SEC)

This malignant tumor develops from a conjunctival IN and also does so without preliminary stages. Here the preexisting layers of the squamous epithelial differentiated epithelium (▶ Fig. 9.9) are raised. The atypia of the cells can be very marked in different ways and determine the various histologic gradings (good, moderate, minimal; or G_1, G_2, G_3). A well-differentiated SEC can be difficult to distinguish from a marked squamous epithelial hyperplasia. The decisive point is the breakthrough into the stroma as the criterion of malignancy.

The risk factors of conjunctival IN obviously also apply for SEC. Actinic damage is the most frequent reason for the development of an SEC. Sun-rich countries have therefore a correspondingly higher incidence (3.5/100,000 in Uganda v. 0.03/100,000 in the United States). The genetically predetermined pigmentation is significant (higher incidence in whites). A higher incidence has been observed in HIV-positive patients (predominantly in Africa: the coupling of two risk factors—light and immunodeficiency). Further risk factors are xeroderma pigmentosum, albinism, and exposure to chemical and physical noxae. HPV is under consideration as the catalyst (bilateral lesions) for the factors named.

Surgical excision with a safety margin of 3 to 5 mm is the goal. An intraoperative check should be made of the resection edges. Recurrences are found in ~6%, depending on operability. With an incomplete resection, chemotherapy drugs are applied topically. If the SEC is not eradicated successfully, the destructive growth and metastases result in a disastrous progression.

Variants of SEC are spindle cell carcinoma, mucoepidermoid carcinoma, and adenosquamous carcinoma.0

Basal cell carcinoma

For this entity refer to the description for tumors of the eyelid in Chapter 9.4.3.

Carcinoma of the sebaceous glands

Infiltrations of the conjunctiva by cells with a sebaceous differentiation or a carcinoma of the meibomian glands are a rarity. The carcinoma first reveals itself as a chronic inflammation that evades diagnosis for some time. Histologically, there are carcinoma cells with a foamy cytoplasm, in small groups or solid groupings over the entire width of the conjunctiva. The tumor

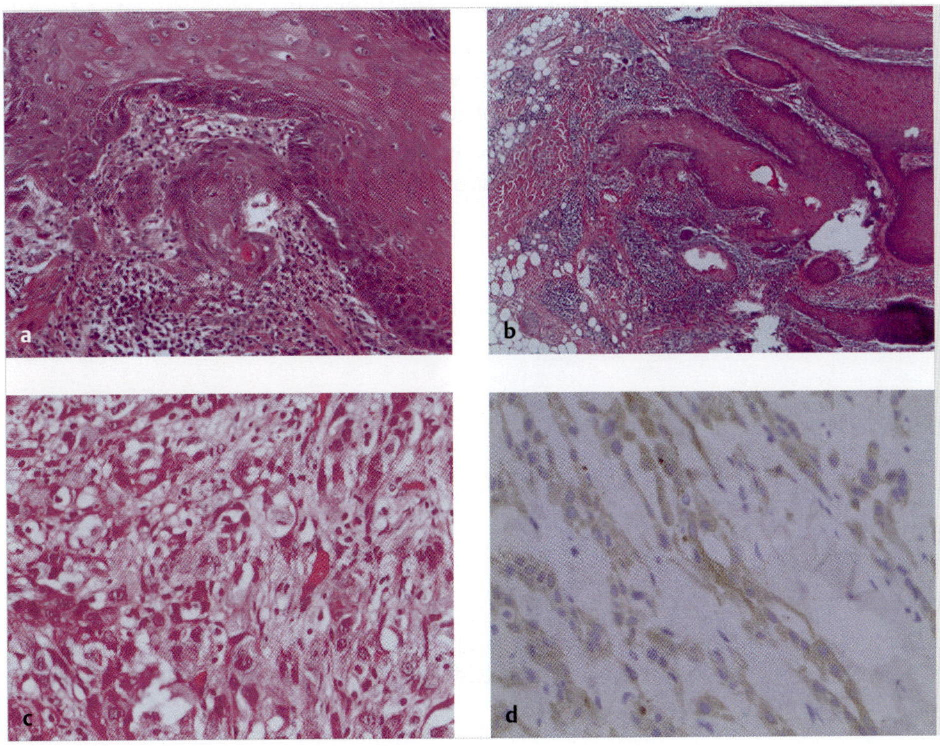

Fig. 9.9 Squamous cell carcinoma (SCC) can show a broad spectrum of degrees of differentiation. **(a)** In most cases the histiogenesis of the lesion is recognizable, but in some cases it is challenging. **(b)** An obvious infiltration of the tumor into the underlying tissue is recognizable only in particular areas in this case. **(c)** In the survey staining the differentiation between SCC and a sarcoma might be difficult in some tumors. **(d)** Immunohistochemistry reveals positive expression for CK 5/6 and helps to find the accurate diagnosis.

growth is mostly slow. Cryotherapy and surgical excision are treatment possibilities.

Melanocytic Lesions/Tumors

Benign Lesions/Tumors

Melanocytic lesions are collections of melanocytes in atypical differentiation and/or in an unusual place and/or in unusual numbers. Extremely important are distinguishing benign from malignant lesions and ascertaining precancerous changes.

Nevi are far and away the leaders among melanocytic lesions. These occur as the second most frequent tumors in the conjunctiva. The incidence is reported as 0.0012/100,000. Favored locations are the bulbar conjunctiva and the limbus in the area toward the interpalpebral region.

Typically the lesions appear in childhood and then become bigger. Multiple lesions are possible. Malignant degeneration of such changes is very rare, however, which is why these lesions are treated conservatively. In contrast, nevi that appear in adulthood require closer attention. It can be necessary to excise them, particularly when they change shape, show more blood vessel involvement, and change color.

Histologically, a distinction can be made between junctional, compound, and subepithelial nevi. Junctional nevi grow in the epithelium of the conjunctiva. Compound nevi are found in the epithelium as well as in the underlying stroma. Subepithelial nevi are correspondingly only found in the stroma. The latter are not pigmented in general and the designation as melanocytic lesion is therefore confusing. As with amelanocytic melanoma, it nevertheless implies the involvement of melanocytic cells but ones that have lost the property of forming melanin.

Subepithelial lesions include ocular melanocytosis and oculodermal melanocytosis. The latter differs from the former through an involvement of the surrounding skin in the area of the supplying trigeminal nerve branch (nevus of ota). There is indeed increasing incidence overall for melanomas, though not in the conjunctiva.

Further variants are the blue nevus (▶ Fig. 9.10) and the Spitz nevus. These nevi are similarly situated in the skin and have the same histological criteria as discussed in Chapter 9.4.3.

In some racial groups varying pigmentation occurs also on both sides. Likewise, pigmentation alterations may be consequences of metabolic influences as well as of systemic or locally acting noxae. Primary and secondary melanoses can appear unilaterally. These can be significant with regard to a further development into melanomas.

Primary acquired melanosis (PAM) is another variant. PAMs are overwhelmingly one-sided pigmentation disorders of the conjunctiva that are not infrequent (more than 30% of adults). The lesions occur in middle-aged patients as brown flecks that have a tendency to grow. Histologically, melanocytic cells are found in the epidermis. With further development of the condition, there follow hyperplasia of the melanocytes and the formation of cell clusters. A distinction is then made between PAM without atypia and PAM with atypia. The latter is further subdivided into PAM with low risk and those with high risk for developing further into melanoma. The frequency of development into melanoma is given at various rates in the literature (more than 10% of the "high risk" PAMs).

Excision is recommended as treatment where there is enlargement of pigment flecks or in general when the diameter is greater than 2 to 3 mm. Topical chemotherapy drugs are also administered.

Malignant Lesions/Tumors

Malignant melanomas

Of all malignomas of the eye, 2% are conjunctival melanomas. After SEC it is the second most common malignoma. One must differentiate between primary melanomas, melanomas from nevus cell nevi, and melanomas from primary acquired melanoses. Histologically, the same malignant cells are present as described in Chapter 9.4.3. Melanomas are very rarely found in children and patients with black skin. The peak age lies in the fifth decade of life. The most frequent places of origin are the interpalpebral region and the bulbar conjunctiva.

Treatment is surgical. This is combined with cryotherapy to achieve complete freedom from tumor in the resection edges as well. Radiotherapy and/or chemotherapy can then follow. The local recurrence rate is 25 to 55%. Enucleation is done mostly in the palliative context but even enucleation does not prevent metastases. The first sites of the metastasizing melanoma are preauricular lymph nodes as well as the intraparotidal nodes, followed by the submandibular and cervical nodes.

The Clark or Breslow classification system used for melanomas of the skin cannot be used for conjunctival melanomas. The absolute tumor thickness is decisive. From a thickness of 0.8 mm the prognosis deteriorates considerably. For tumors between 1 and

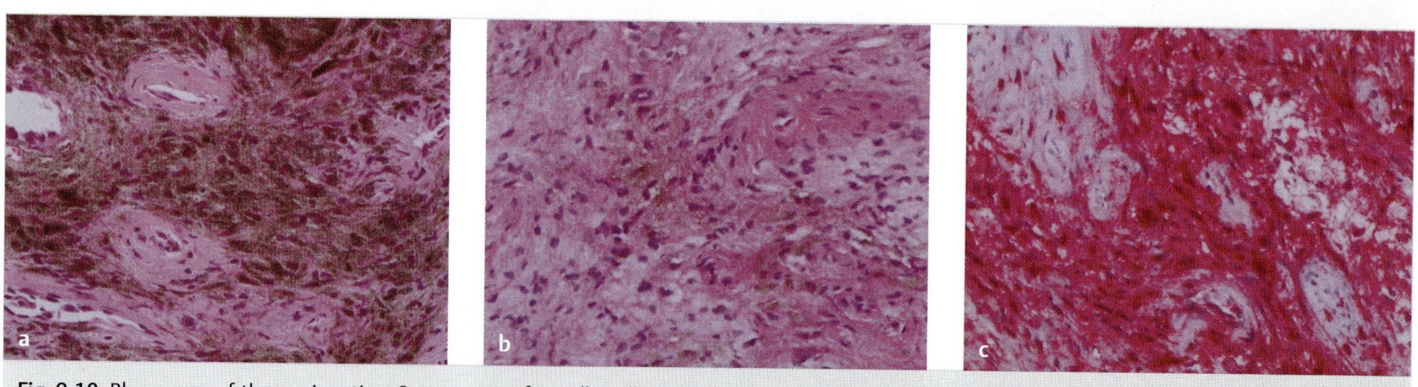

Fig. 9.10 Blue nevus of the conjunctiva. Some nests of spindle cells are layered between the collagen fibers of the dermis. **(a)** Cells showing strong pigmentation. **(b)** Bleaching of the specimen reveals a better identification of cell morphology. **(c)** Immunohistochemical staining with Melan A confirms the melanocytic origin of the cells (magnification 10 × 20).

9

4 mm, the mortality rate is increased by a factor of 2; if the melanoma is > 4 mm in thickness, the factor is 4. The 5-year survival rate lies between 77 and 86%; the 10-year survival between 64 and 73%. In producing or viewing the pathological findings one should pay attention to all of the numerous factors (refer to Chapter 9.1.2).

Mesenchymal Tumors

Benign

Vascular lesions

Benign lesions include capillary telangiectasias, vascular deformities, and lymphangiectasias. The last two mentioned also occur within the context of syndromes such as the Sturge–Weber syndrome and ataxia telangiectatica. Also to be considered are pyogenic granulomas/capillary hemangiomas, cavernous hemangiomas, and lymphangiomas. Their histological structure equates to those in other sites of the body.

Myxomas

Myxomas are rare benign tumors that occur in isolation or are seen within the context of the Carney complex. Histologically, there is tissue with relatively few cells comprising star-shaped cells with soft cytoplasmic offshoots. In between there is a substantial amount of myxoid substance. Myxomas are painless and well-defined tumors of the bulbar conjunctiva with a typical gelatinlike consistency.

Myxomas need to be differentiated from myxoid neurofibroma, nerve sheath myxoma, spindle cell lipoma, and lymphangioma. In children it must be differentiated from rhabdomyosarcoma. Simple excision is the treatment of choice. There are no reports of recurrences.

Malignant

Fibrous histiocytoma

Benign and malignant lesions are possible. Histiocytomas originate in the stroma of the conjunctiva and show the same histological structure as in other parts of the body. The most favored locations are the limbus and the epibulbar conjunctiva.

Treatment is surgical. Recurrences and metastases depend on the completeness of the excision and also on the histological degree.

Rhabdomyosarcoma

This malignant tumor of childhood occurs in the area of the conjunctiva, predominantly as a botryoid type. Histologically, there are spindle-shaped and round rhabdomyoblasts, which only exhibit cross-striation in a small number of cases. Large hyperchromatic cell nuclei are surrounded by an eosinophilic cytoplasm. In addition, there are smaller spindle tumor cells in the tumor matrix accompanied by cystic changes. Very typical is a ribbonlike infiltrate of several layers of tumor cells subepithelially, which is classed as a cambium layer. Quite often the tumor grows initially without any significant accompanying inflammation, which can lead to a delay in diagnosis. **Rapidly growing tumors in childhood are fundamentally suspicious and must be clarified.**

Primary chemotherapy and, where applicable, radiotherapy have decisively improved the chances of a cure in the last few decades and enabled the survival of many children.

Kaposi's sarcoma

Kaposi's sarcoma is a malignant tumor that appears in ~20% of patients suffering from AIDS. In 4 to 14% of AIDS patients it is the first clinical sign. A classification system has been suggested that makes it possible to assess diagnosis, postoperative management, and further clinical course better. Types I, II, and III are proposed, with a progressive clinical picture.

Local excision with a safety margin (1–2 mm) is aimed at, followed by cryotherapy. Radiotherapy and local injection of chemotherapy drugs and interferons are supplementary measures or alternatives.

Lymphomas

Primary benign and malignant lymphomas include a series of entities. These range from simple (follicular) lymphatic hyperplasia right through to aggressive, destructive lesions. The most frequent subtype is the extranodal marginal zone lymphoma (EMZL) originating from mucosa-associated lymphatic tissue (MALT). It is important to differentiate MALT lymphoma from follicular lymphoma, lymphoplasmacytic lymphoma, and chronic lymphatic leukemia of the B-cell type (B-CLL). Other lymphoma entities can occur but are very rare. Determination of the histological subtype is important for the prognosis and treatment. For example, while EMZL often shows an indolent growth (~70% remain without systemic spread), other lymphomas, such as the diffuse large cell B-cell lymphoma, are distinctly more aggressive and life-threatening (average survival 3 to 5 years).

Plasmocytoma

Plasmocytomas of the conjunctiva occur predominantly within the context of a multiple myeloma. It is rare to find a primary solitary plasmocytoma in the conjunctiva. Plasmocytomas are circumscribed reddish lesions that histologically consist of dense infiltrates of plasmacytoid cells. Various differentiation grades can occur. These tumors mostly occur in the fornix, bulbarly or tarsally. Usually the picture is of inflammation. Slow progression is reported with solitary plasmocytoma.

Metastases

Only rarely are metastases found in the conjunctiva, then mainly from breast and lung cancers as well as melanomas of the skin. Interestingly, metastasizing melanomas of the conjunctiva often have their primary in the lower extremities or the trunk. The prognosis is poor and accordingly treatment is palliative.

Congenital Tumorlike Lesions

Dermoid

Dermoids are cysts lined with layered squamous epithelium, sometimes with skin appendages in the cyst wall (▶ Fig. 9.11). Fatty tissue can also occur in the wall. A lining of conjunctival epithelium is also possible. The preferred location is at the inferotemporal limbus. Excision is the usual treatment.

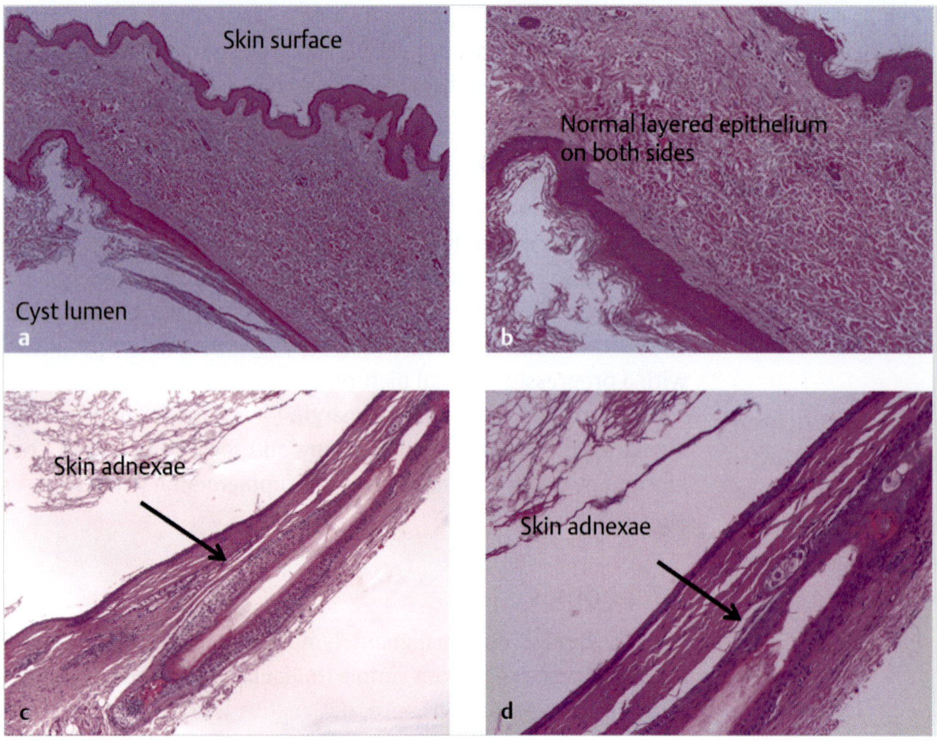

Fig. 9.11 Epidermal cyst/dermoid. **(a)** To one side the lesion is covered by the cutaneous epidermis (H&E staining, magnification 5 × 10). **(b)** The inner surface is lined by the same squamous epithelium, which does not show any atypia. Slight fibrosis occurs in the cyst's wall (H&E staining, magnification 10 × 10). **(c)** The second cyst shows skin adnexae in the wall (H&E staining, magnification 10 × 10). **(d)** A detail of (c) with higher magnification (H&E staining, magnification 20 × 10).

9

Ectopic lacrimal glands

The lesion's name is self-explanatory; in this condition the tear duct tissue is of normal form. It can be found in isolation, a combination with a choristoma is possible.

Complex choristoma

A choristoma arises from the proliferation of regular tissue in a location not typical for that tissue (e.g., adrenal cortex in the kidney). Tissue of the tear duct, cartilage, bone, brain tissue, and other tissue can be involved in a complex choristoma of the conjunctiva. Osseous choristoma is a bony lesion supratemporally between the superior rectus and lateralis muscles, and is situated ~5 mm behind the limbus.

9.4.3 Tumors of the Eyelids

General

Given the nature of the eyelids, tumors are found there that can also be found in other areas of the skin. Particular mention should be made basal cell carcinoma and squamous epithelium carcinoma, which often develop as a consequence of damage by light. Tumors can also develop from the skin adnexa. Some particular glands demonstrate similar differentiation in both their benign and their malignant variants (e.g., sebaceous gland adenomas and carcinomas). Melanocytic tumors should also be considered, which are classified analogously to those of the rest of the skin (▶ Table 9.4).

Epithelial Tumors (of the Outer Skin)

Benign

Seborrheic keratosis (verruca senilis, seborrheic warts, basal cell papilloma)

Histologically, these benign lesion of the skin are formed from an expanded squamous epithelium, in part of basal cellular differentiation (▶ Fig. 9.12). Horn pearls are found enclosed. Growth variants are possible (hyperkeratotic, acanthotic, adenoid). Intensified pigmentation makes it difficult to differentiate from basalioma among others. Inflammatory irritated forms can be difficult to classify histologically. Malignant transformation is not known. Excision is the treatment of choice.

Papillomas

Papilloma is the most frequent and benign tumor of the eyelid. Histologically, a folded papillary epithelium is seen over alternating widths of connective tissue septa, as described earlier for conjunctival papillomas. The epithelium matures and sometimes shows orthokeratosis. Papillomas can occur in isolation or in multiples. Excision is the treatment of choice. Recurrence (or a second papilloma) is possible.

Inverted follicular keratosis

This benign tumor appears as a small knotty lesion. Quite often there is enhanced pigmentation, which makes it difficult to differentiate from a melanocytic change. Histologically, lobular acanthosis is seen with the proliferation of partly basaloid, partly squamous, cells.

Benign lichenoid keratosis

This is a benign tumor that occurs predominantly as a single firm node. Histologically, the picture is similar to that in lichen planus, with a ribbonlike lymphocytic infiltrate under an irregular acanthotic epithelium. However, there is not hypergranulosis but there is parakeratosis.

Pseudocarcinomatous hyperplasia

The most varied of noxae can lead to a marked hyperplasia of the squamous epithelium. Here dyskeratoses and nuclear irregularities occur so that a differentiation from squamous epithelium carcinoma can be very difficult. A detailed reference to the case history and/or the clinical picture is important.

Table 9.4 Tumors of the eyelids

Benign	Uncertain biological behavior/Precancerous lesions	Malignant
Epithelial tumors/Tumors of the epidermis		
Seborrheic keratosis	Actinic keratosis	Bowen's disease/carcinoma in situ
Papilloma		SCC due to xeroderma pigmentosa
inverted follicular keratosis		Squamous cell carcinoma (SCC)
Benign lichenoid keratosis		Basal cell carcinoma (BCC)
Pseudocarcinomatous hyperplasia		
Keratoacanthoma		
Tumors of the sebaceous glands		
Sebaceous gland hyperplasia		Carcinoma of the sebaceous glands
Sebaceous gland adenoma		
Sebaceoma/sebaceous epithelioma		
Tumors of the eccrine and apocrine glands		
Chondroid syringoma		Mucinous sebaceous gland carcinoma
Eccrine acrospiroma		cutaneous adenoid cystic carcinoma
Moll's glands adenoma		Carcinoma of the eccrine sweat glands
		Adenocarcinoma of Moll's glands
Tumors of cutaneous pillar structures		
Trichoepithelioma		
Trichofolliculoma		
Trichilemmoma		
Pilomatrixoma		
Melanocytic tumors		
Lentigo simplex		Lentigo maligna
Lentigo solaris		Lentigo maligna melanoma
Ephelids		Superficial spreading melanoma
Nevus cell nevus • Dermal • Junctional • Compound		Nodular melanoma Melanoma ex nevi
Dysplastic nevus		
Congenital melanocytic giant nevus		
Kissing nevus		
Blue nevus		
Spitz nevus		
Vascular lesions		
Capillary hemangioma		Cutaneous angiosarcoma
Nevus flammeus		
Cavernous hemangioma		
Lymphangioma		
Glomus tumors/glomangioma		
Xanthomatous lesions		
Xanthelasma		
Fibrotic histiocytoma		
Tuberous xanthoma		
Juvenile xanthogranuloma		
Necrobiotic xanthogranuloma		
Mesenchymal tumors		
Nodular fasciitis	Juvenile fibromatosis	Merkel cell tumor
Granular cell tumor		
Intravascular papillary endothelial hyperplasia		
Other tumors		
		Malignant lymphoma

9

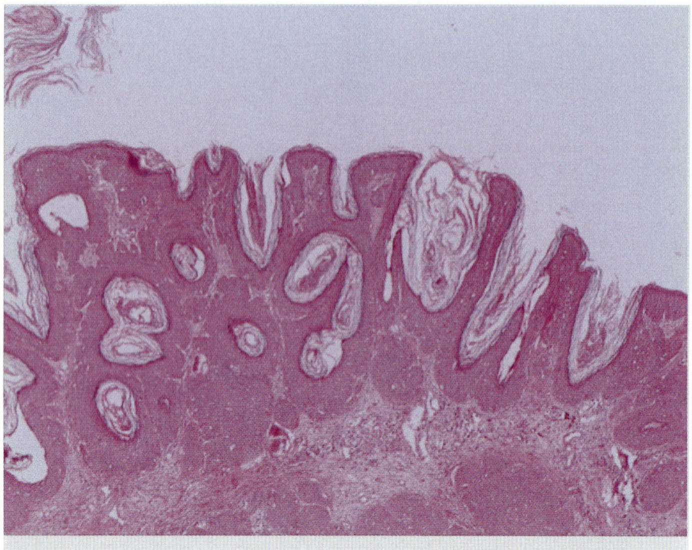

Fig. 9.12 Seborrhoic keratosis. Characteristic for this lesion is an enlarged squamous epithelium without any atypia and enclosed keratin pearls (H&E staining, magnification 5 × 10).

Keratoacanthoma

This benign tumor is distinguished by rapid growth and is often very difficult to differentiate from squamous epithelial carcinoma. Histologically, there is a round lesion consisting of squamous epithelium, which is covered on the margin by a "lip" or "shoulder." Keratin is found in the center. The basal membrane remains intact.

The rapid growth is alarming and often leads to an excision. Reliable differentiation from SEC is difficult as stated. Some authors see keratoacanthoma as a variation of a regressively developing SEC.

Premalignant and Malignant

Actinic keratosis

This is found predominantly in older patients with light skin color. The determining factor is long-term exposure to light, which leads to this disease. However, also in the context of long enduring inflammations, actinic keratosis appears visually similar to lichen ruber and lichen sclerosus. Histologically, there are numerous variants (hypertrophic, atrophic, acantholytic, and pigmented actinic keratosis). In general, an irregular orthokeratosis is manifest accompanied in some areas by a parakeratosis. The layering of the underlying squamous epithelium is disrupted to varying extents and can include all layers (Bowen's disease transition). Atypia and typically dyskeratoses occur. This is accompanied by a chronic inflammatory infiltrate as well as solar elastosis. In the hypertrophic variants the formation of a cornu cutaneum can result.

Excision is mostly practiced. As the light damage naturally affects broad areas of the (facial) skin, further foci are frequent.

Bowen's disease

Bowen's disease can develop from actinic keratosis, which is also regarded as a squamous cell carcinoma in situ. It is also quite possible as a development from other diseases or having no identifiable precursor lesion. Histologically, the layering of the squamous epithelium is raised. Considerable nucleic atypia, dyskeratoses, and mitoses can be seen, which move right up into the upper layers of the epithelium. The transition to SEC occurs with the breaking through of the basal membrane. Excision should be within the healthy tissue but this can be difficult for the same reasons as outlined for actinic keratosis.

Xeroderma pigmentosum with development of squamous epithelial carcinomas

In this disease a defect in a repair gene makes cells unable to repair double-stranded DNA breaks. As exposure to light can lead to such breaks, an accumulation of genetic damage is evident in exposed squamous epithelia. This leads to the development of multiple SEC with similar histology and later biological behavior as described previously for that condition.

Squamous epithelial carcinoma

As repeatedly described, this malignoma typically develops from squamous epithelia and the risk factors need not be described once again. Excision in the healthy tissue should always be the aim.

Basalioma

Basalioma is malignant tumor of advanced age resulting from actinic damage, especially by UV light. The tumor occurs frequently (150,000 new cases a year in Germany and about 1,600,000 cases per year in the US) and in over 90% of cases is found in a site exposed to light (in about 10% of cases this is not the case). The tumor grows slowly and infiltratingly with only a minimal tendency to metastasis (< 0.5%). Histologically, tumor cells probably derive from the outer root sheath layer. These cells are similar to the basal cells of the squamous epithelium. However, the karyoplasmic ratio is distorted and the number of mitoses is increased. The outer cells of the cell balls that form exhibit a palisade-like arrangement of the cell nuclei, which is very characteristic of basalioma (▶ Fig. 9.13). Growth variants are recognized: nodular, superficial, sclerodermiform, adamantoid.

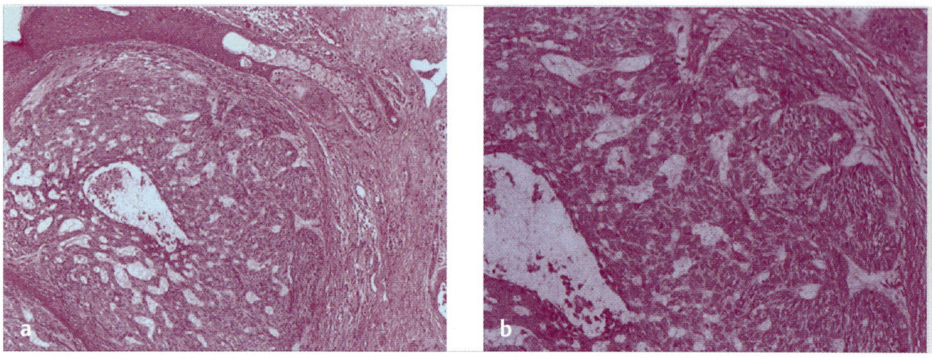

Fig. 9.13 Basal cell carcinoma (BCC). **(a)** Nests of basaloid differentiated cells, which are predominantly located in the subepithelial tissue layers, are characteristic for this tumor. Pseudocystic formations are possible (H&E staining, magnification 10 × 20). **(b)** A palisade-shaped pattern of tumor cell nuclei occurs in the periphery of the lesion (H&E staining, magnification 20 × 20).

There is a possible link to hereditary diseases or syndromes:

- Gorlin–Goltz syndrome
- Bazex–Dupré–Christol syndrome
- Dugois–Colomb–Berthon syndrome
- Rambo syndrome
- Xeroderma pigmentosum
- Oculocutaneous albinism

Treatment consists of complete local excision. An intraoperative check of the edges of the incision or prompt reappraisal within a day can be very helpful here. In particular, the sclerodermiform variation is known for small offshoots that can make a removal in healthy tissue very difficult.

Tumors of the Sebaceous Glands

Sebaceous glands are to be found in the eyelids and the caruncles, with some in the meibomian glands, some in the glands of Zeis, and some on infundibular structures. Benign and malignant tumors can develop from these sebaceous glands.

Benign

Sebaceous gland hyperplasia

This consists of nodular proliferation of sebaceous glands. Immunosuppression favors development. Histologically, sebaceous glands are found arranged around an infundibulum, and appear still immature toward the periphery. These structures mature toward the center and the sebum formed exits via the central infundibulum.

Sebaceous gland adenoma

Sebaceous gland adenomas are benign, mostly solitary nodules in older patients. Histologically, atypical sebaceous cells are identifiable that are laid down in lobules and are surrounded by rete ridges. Covering epithelium is often missing from the surface so that the tumor is covered by a scab. It likewise may be covered by a "horny plug" in the sense of a cornu cutaneum. A cystic growth can be an indication of Muir–Torre syndrome. Small lesions are difficult to demarcate from a sebaceous gland hyperplasia. Excision is the treatment of choice.

Sebaceous gland adenomas within the context of a Muir–Torre syndrome

Muir–Torre syndrome represents a phenotypic variant of hereditary non-polyposis colorectal cancer (HNPCC) syndrome. In this there is formation of multiple malignomas of the inner organs, in particular of colon carcinomas. Associated with this are keratoacanthomas and also sebaceous adenomas. This should be especially considered when sebaceous adenomas occur at a relatively young age, as multiple tumors, as tumors in unusual locations, or with keratoacanthomas in younger patients. Thus sebaceous adenomas can have an important indicator function.

Sebaceoma (sebaceous epithelioma)

These benign lesions occur in older patients and in women more often than in men. As a rule they appear as small nodules without ulceration. Histologically, there are groups of sebaceous gland cells of various sizes with basaloid differentiation. Embedded in these are secretory ducts, which can merge into cystic formations. The ordered structure as found in hyperplasia and adenoma is not found here. Due to the peculiar growth form, these tumors are listed separately and have been repeatedly renamed over the years. This tumor can be problematic because of the possibility of confusion with a basalioma with sebaceous differentiation.

Malignant

Sebaceous gland carcinoma

The points of origin of this rare malignant tumor of older patients in the area of the eyelid are the meibomian glands, the Zeis glands, and the sebaceous glands connected with the infundibula. Sebaceous gland carcinomas often occur clinically as prolonged inflammatory processes and there is often some delay in diagnosis. Their biological behavior is aggressive: about a third of them show recurrences and/or metastases after excision. Histologically, there are different degrees of differentiation of tumor cells, which show a more or less well developed sebaceous morphology. Some secretory ducts can be identified. The cells appearing as sebocytes exhibit increased mitoses, which differentiate these from benign cells. In some of these tumors sebaceous differentiation can be seen in very few cells only, making the diagnosis very difficult. Quite often there is a pagetoid growth in the neighboring epidermis. Excision in the healthy tissue should be achieved for the reasons mentioned.

Tumors of the Eccrine and Apocrine Glands

Benign

Syringoma

Syringoma is a benign, fairly common tumor of the sweat glands that occurs multiply and is yellow in color. It most frequently occurs in young women or during puberty. Histologically, groups of small ducts are found embedded in a fiber-rich stroma. The ducts are covered in a double-rowed epithelium. Myoepithelial cells are missing as margins of the ducts. Excision is the treatment of choice.

Chondroid syringoma

Chondroid syringoma is a benign tumor growing in the face area and back of the neck. An origin in the sweat glands is the subject of debate. As implied by the name, diversity characterizes the tumor histologically. Tubular formations with a double rowed arrangement of epithelial and myoepithelial cells are found in a mucoid matrix.

When tumors are growing, the pressure on neighboring structures causes damage. Excision is the treatment of choice. Complete removal can be difficult as the tumor tends to produce small satellites scattered in the surrounding tissue, which is why there are frequent recurrences.

Eccrine acrospiroma (clear cell hidradenoma, clear cell myoepithelioma, porosyringoma)

This benign tumor occurs as a single lesion situated in the dermis as a firm knot. Histologically, there are lobules, consisting of cells with a light cytoplasm. Some tumors do appear to exhibit a cystic growth pattern, however. Some tumor cells exhibit an eosinophilic cytoplasm and are round in shape. The cell nucleus is oval and exhibits a prominent nucleolus. Other tumor cells have light cytoplasm with well-defined cell boundaries. Here the nucleus is small and located eccentrically. Transitions occur between the two cell types. Typically, there are small vessels between the lobules, which are coated by an eosinophilic cuticle. Excision is the treatment of choice.

Adenoma of Moll's glands

This is a very rare benign tumor. To be sure of the diagnosis there needs to be a localization on the edge of the eyelid and clear-cut histology. This is based in particular on eosinophilia of the cytoplasm of the tumor cells, which still may show an active secretion.

Excision is the treatment of choice.

Malignant

Mucinous sweat gland carcinoma

This rare malignant tumor of the skin adnexa is more often found in men (around 60 years old). The tumor is convex with a firm consistency, but in part also cystic. Histologically, solid and trabecular formations of tumor cells "swim" in a mucinous substance. These are in turn separated from fibrovascular septa. In the solid formations are pseudo glands, which account for the sections of the tumor with a cystic aspect. Mitotic activity is relatively minimal.

9

Among carcinomas this tumor has a comparably good prognosis. Approximately 30% recur, ~10% put out metastases. Accordingly, excision is the treatment of choice.

Primary cutaneous adenoidcystic carcinoma

This is the rarest carcinoma with eccrine differentiation. Histologically, this tumor is like the adenoidcystic carcinomas of the saliva and lacrimal glands. Excision is the treatment of choice but it proves problematic that the carcinoma cells grow along nerve sheaths, which can make assured removal considerably more difficult.

Carcinoma of the eccrine sweat glands

This malignant tumor appears as a firm nodule with an undefined boundary. Histologically, tumor cells can be seen growing into the stroma in diffuse fashion, looking somewhat like a signet ring. Some tumor cells look as though they are in single file, not dissimilar to a lobular carcinoma of the breast. This is why a breast cancer metastasis should be excluded. Excision should be the aim.

Adenocarcinoma of Moll's glands

This is a rare tumor entity. See "Adenoma of Moll's glands" above: the basic differentiation of the tumor cells is likewise eosinophilic. The tumor cells are arranged as if in a gland and can exhibit a secretion.

Tumors of the Pilary Structures of the Eyelids

Benign

Trichoepthelioma

Trichoepthelioma is a benign tumor that can appear singly or multiply. When it occurs multiply it is possible that it is hereditary; if so, these appear in adolescence and exhibit continually increasing size. The tumors occur in the whole face including the eyelids. The scalp, back of the neck, and upper trunk are less often affected. The nodules are firm, raised, and often skin-colored. Histologically, numerous nests of basaloid cells can be seen under the formation of a cyst, the lumina of which are filled with keratin. It is sometimes difficult to distinguish it from a basalioma. A well-taken case history and clinical examination can identify the inherited form. With solitary lesions, excision leads to healing.

Trichofolliculoma

Trichofolliculoma is a benign tumor, appearing slightly raised, with a drawn in center that is a pore. Histologically, the pore is lined with a mature squamous epithelium and is linked directly to the epithelium of the skin's outer surface. Adjoining this pore are basaloid cells in a ribbonlike formation, which in the final analysis correspond to an abortive hair follicle. The lesion grows slowly up to ~5 mm in diameter. Excision cures it.

Trichilemmoma

Trichilemmoma is a benign tumor of the hair follicle, derived from the outer hair sheath. Histologically, glycogen-rich squamous epithelial cells can be seen as in an acanthosis. Lobules are formed that are bordered by a prominent basal membrane. Definitively distinguishing it from a basalioma can be problematic. It can also be confused with SEC, sebaceous gland carcinomas, and seborrheic keratoses as well.

Trichilemmoma occurs singly and remains small in size. In contrast to basalioma it is only rarely found on the edge of the eyelid. Excision is curative.

Pilomatrixoma (Malherbe calcifying epithelioma)

This is a benign tumor that almost always appears singly, that is well-defined, and that is found in the dermis and subcutis. Histologically, there are groups of small "blue" cells next to sections of "ghost cells," the number of which grows with the increasing age of the lesion. Calcifications occur repeatedly and not infrequently lead to allergic reactions. The blue cells can exhibit pleomorphia and considerable mitotic activity. Confusion with Merkel cell carcinomas has been reported. The tumor most often occurs in children and adolescents (60% before 20 years of age). Excision heals the lesion.

Melanocytic Tumors

Benign

Lentigo simplex

Lentigo simplex is a benign lesion 1 to 2 mm in diameter, flat, and brown in color. The lesions are clinically not distinguishable from junctional nevi. Histomorphologically, increased numbers of melanocytic cells are found in the basal epidermis as well as the papillary layer without atypia. The rete crests are partially lengthened.

Solar lentigo (senile lentigo)

This is a benign lesion, dark brown, mostly appearing multiply and somewhat irregularly defined. It predominantly appears in older patients. It is histologically similar to lentigo simplex:

increased melanocytic cells with increased melanin formation. The rete crests of the epithelium are elongated and partially irregular in structure.

Ephelides ("freckles")

This is a benign change in appearance that is widely familiar. Histologically, there are melanocytic cells with increased pigmentation in the basal epidermis. The rete crests are not elongated, however. In contrast to lentigo simplex, freckles become darker when exposed to light.

Nevocytic nevi (melanocytic nevi)

Nevocytic nevi (NCN) consist of nests or groups of melanocytic cells. There are the following subtypes according to the position of these cells. Dermal NCN: here the melanocytic cells lie only in the dermis. This NCN is the most frequent and exhibits the least tendency to malignant degeneration. Junctional NCN: this has melanocytic cells lying in the basal epidermis (▶ Fig. 9.14). Compound NCN is a lesion with both of these components. In principle there are no significant atypia of the melanocytic cells; there is "maturation" in depth, equating to the cells growing smaller; and the lesions are symmetrical.

Unfortunately, NCN occurs very often with a morphology that is not clearly definable and which can only be distinguished from melanomas with difficulty if at all. Trials of new molecular techniques (fluorescence in situ hybridization, comparative genomic hybridization) are being addressed to this purpose.

NCN can develop into melanoma. Its occurrence in large numbers is a particular problem. These patients require ongoing monitoring.

Dysplastic nevus

Dysplastic nevi are lesions with morphological abnormalities that do not justify classification as a melanoma and that behave as if benign. Because of this ambiguity there are difficulties in definite classification and therefore uncertainty in attribution of biological significance.

Congenital melanocytic giant nevus

This is an NCN with comparably large extent in the area of the eyelid and the surrounding skin and which, as the name indicates, occurs congenitally. Lesions of this kind in the head and neck area can be associated in general with clinically manifest epilepsy and mental retardation. Likewise, an association is recognized with leptomeningeal melanosis and primary melanomas of the leptomeninges or the brain.

A particularly striking variant of NCN is presented by "kissing nevus," in which the nevus has afflicted the upper as well as the lower eyelid. This is due to an event during development; the nevus forms during the fusion of the upper and lower lid during fetal development.

Blue nevus

Blue nevus is again a benign melanocytic tumor. These lesions mainly occur congenitally or in childhood. Clinically, nodules are found in a hemispherical shape, which are typically deep blue to black in color. Blue nevi are found severally and/or in groups. Histologically, groups of bipolar or dendritic and pigmented melanocytes are seen in the dermis. These lie singly or in groups between the collagen fibers of the dermis. The junction zone remains free. With the cell-rich blue nevus there are additionally groups of large, round melanocytes. These are only weak or not pigmented and exhibit a broad cytoplasm seam. In addition there are further histological variants, which will not be discussed further here (combined compound and epithelioid types).

Spitz nevus (juvenile melanoma)

As the synonym indicates, these tumors occur in childhood and exhibit a great similarity to melanomas. Biologically, however, the behavior is benign. This tumor entity described by Sophie Spitz appears before the 20th year of life in 80% of cases; congenital growth is also possible. Hemispherical nodules from light brown to red in color are seen, with the skin of the face as a favored location. Histologically, there are round to oval cells with a broad cytoplasmic margin and large nuclei. Nucleoli are repeatedly exhibited. Giant cells are mixed in. The cells are grouped in nests and appear in particular in the junction zone. In contrast to melanoma, the cells exhibit maturation in depth (cells become smaller). Mitoses can occur.

Distinguishing the Spitz nevus from melanoma can be one of the most difficult tasks in dermatopathology and requires the eye of an experienced dermatopathologist.

Malignant

Lentigo maligna

Flat lesion, not palpable, with irregular border and uneven color. The lesions can reach diameters of up to 7 cm and develop for more than 10 years until reaching the transition into the invasive phase. Histologically, atypical pleomorphic melanocytes are found in the basal layer of the epidermis.

Lentigo maligna melanoma

The later development of lentigo maligna, with which the invasive phase has begun and the melanoma cells cross the basal membrane.

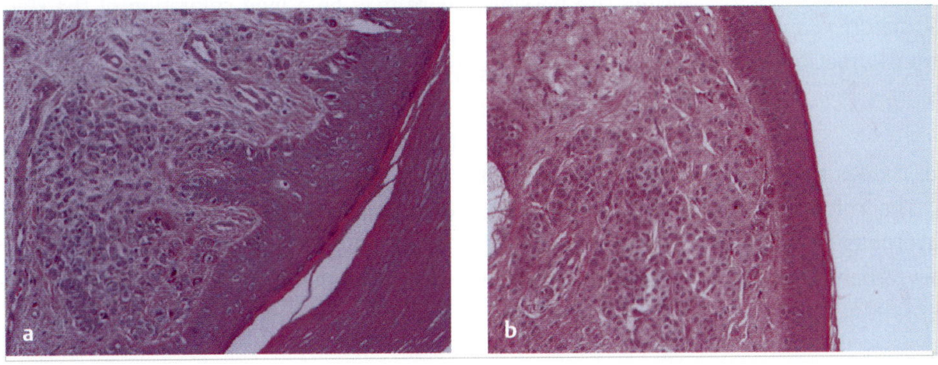

Fig. 9.14 Nevus cell nevi. **(a)** In this compound nevus, melanocytic cells occur in the epidermis as well as in the dermis. So-called maturation of the cells occurs in the deeper areas. Here the cells are getting smaller (H&E staining, magnification 20 × 10). **(b)** In dermal nevi melanocytic cells are limited to the dermis with the epidermis remaining unaffected. Maturation and high differentiation of cells is obvious in these benign lesions. (H&E staining, magnification 20 × 10).

Superficially spreading melanoma (SSM)

These melanomas are found in younger patients than is lentigo maligna, or mainly in the fifth decade of life. The diameter is generally smaller and they are mostly not found in places exposed to light. Whereas in lentigo maligna the atypical cells are found along the basal epidermis as if lined up, in SSM these cells ultimately appear as single cells or cell groups in all layers of the epidermis. The cells exhibit a certain uniformity and often look epithelioid. After transition to the vertical growth phase or into the invasive phase, the cells change and become polymorphic.

Nodular melanoma

This consists of mainly small blue-black nodules or amelanotic tumors, which are nearly always palpable when they are noticed. Patients 40 to 50 years old are the most frequently affected, men more than twice as often as women. Histologically, there are large anaplastic and epithelioid melanocytes; diagnosis usually takes place when it becomes invasive. Whether a horizontal phase has preceded this is debatable. Growth is more aggressive than in the previously mentioned forms.

Melanoma ex nevo

All melanomas can occur in association with a preexisting nevus. For SSM this can be identified in ~50% of cases; for the remaining variants it is considerably rarer. This acquires considerable significance in patients with multiple nevi. Close clinical checking is of crucial importance.

Vascular Tumors

Benign

Capillary hemangioma

This is a benign tumor with the same structure as capillary hemangiomas in other areas of the body. The tumor is common (1/200 children) and grows in the dermis as well as in the subcutis and musculature. There is evidence of significant mitotic activity. The edge of the eyelid is often affected as well. The hemangioma is apparent for the most part in the first two weeks after birth and can noticeably increase in size in the first 6 months. Thereafter, in the main, regression sets in: 30% of hemangiomas disappear completely within the first three years of life. At 7 years, some 70 to 90% of all hemangiomas have gone into complete regression. After regression, however, the covering skin shows coloration from reddish to grayish (skin colors with fine folds "like crepe paper"). It is important to distinguish this lesion from nevus flammeus.

Treatment is "wait and see" due to the normally expected regression and this only comes under question if function is affected or there are problems of a cosmetic nature. Capillary hemangioma does not exhibit any malignant transformation.

Nevus flammeus

This nevus is present at birth. When pressed, it does not grow paler, in contrast to capillary hemangioma. The color is also darker. Histologically, the vessels are rather cavernous. Its particular importance arises from the fact that the nevus flammeus can be seen as an indicator lesion for Sturge–Weber syndrome.

Cavernous hemangioma

This type of hemangioma mainly occurs in the second to the fourth decades and occasionally in the first decade of life. Histologically, fairly large dilated vessels can be seen, lined with a flat epithelium. Calcifications and phleboliths can occur as secondary changes. There are also fibrosis and lymphocytic infiltrates. In contrast to capillary hemangioma, cavernous hemangioma is bluish and can occur in deep-lying lesions without conspicuous coloring. Growth is slow and the delineation poor. A regression of the lesion does not happen. This is why a surgical intervention is often necessary. In children there is possible association with a thrombocythemia purpura in the sense of a Kasabach–Merritt syndrome. Here enlargement of the hemangioma quite often precedes the general symptoms. There is also an association with "blue rubber bleb nevus syndrome" and with Maffucci syndrome. Cavernous hemangioma does not exhibit malignant transformation.

Lymphangioma

Lymphangioma is a slowly growing lesion that can occur with shape anomalies in the conjunctiva and the face in general. There is no significant tendency to regression. Histologically, there are lymph vessels of various sizes lined with a flat endothelium. Lymphplasmocellular infiltrates in alternating cell-rich stroma are definitive. Lymphangiomas are differentiated between dermal, cavernous, and cystic. The latter is known as *hygroma colli* in the area of the back of the neck. In the orbit, cavernous lymphangioma is the most frequent type. Lymphangiomas do not communicate with the actual lymphatic system. Malignant transformation is reported is some cases.

Glomus tumor or glomangioma

This benign vascular tumor occurs singly or multiply and is noticeable by its purple color. Histologically, the glomus tumor is similar to the cavernous hemangiomas. Around the blood vessels there is a seam several layers thick of so-called glomus cells, which typically can be stained with smooth muscle–specific actin. Excision is the treatment of choice; malignant further development is not observed.

Malignant

Cutaneous angiosarcoma

This is quite a rare malignant tumor of the blood vessels on the eyelid. Most commonly the sarcoma occurs in the facial skin in older patients and, above all, on the skin of the head that was previously covered by hair. Single, multiple, or multicentric lesions are possible. There may be a livid coloration of the skin with accompanying inflammations and ulcerations as well as spontaneous bleeds. Histologically, irregular-shaped blood vessels are found, lined with an atypical endothelium. With increasing dedifferentiation the resulting image is of densely packed pleomorphic cells that only just permit an abortive vascular formation to be identified. Origin in a benign angioma is reported but this is rare.

Excision within the healthy tissue has to be attempted but is difficult. The mortality rate for angiosarcoma is high (over 40%).

Xanthomatous Tumors

Benign

Xanthelasma

Xanthelasma is benign lesion consisting of foamy cells (macrophages with a vacuolated cytoplasm) and is found in the dermis. There is an orientation along skin adnexa and blood vessels. Ultimately, lipids are deposited in the cytoplasm of the macrophages, which explains the yellow color of this reactive change (▶ Fig. 9.15). The flat to slightly raised lesions occur predominantly on both eyelids in middle-aged and older patients and are the expression of a disrupted metabolism.

In this connection, if other clinical circumstances are relevant, consider Erdheim–Chester disease. This can lead to the changes to the eyelid described. Excision is done essentially for cosmetic reasons.

Fibrous histiocytoma (dermatofibroma, sclerosing hemangioma)

This benign lesion is found in the subcutis and dermis. Histologically, a cell-rich change is noted that does not have clearly defined boundaries and consists of tracts of interwoven fibroblasts in a storiform arrangement. Scattered within in it are large histiocytes. Giant cells of the Touton type are common. The tumor is usually situated in the orbital soft tissue and less often in the skin of the eyelid.

Tuberous xanthoma

This is a benign reactive lesion that is often to be found in connection with hyperlipidemia types II and III. Histologically, there are foam-celled macrophages, enriched with giant cells of the Touton type. Extracellular cholesterol and moderate fibrosis and inflammation complete the picture. Favored locations are the buttocks, elbow, knee, and fingers. On the eyelid they are localized deeper than xanthelasmas.

Juvenile xanthogranuloma

Juvenile xanthogranuloma is a benign reactive lesion in children in the first and second years of life in which raised, reddish-brown single or multiple nodules are seen, which can also occur in a generalized form. Histologically, there is initially a monomorphic histiocytic infiltrate with admixed lymphocytes and eosinophils. Later, giant cells of the Touton type appear. Older lesions show increasing fibrosis. Juvenile xanthogranulomas in the iris are problematic; the prognosis for all other localizations is very good.

Necrobiotic xanthogranuloma

This benign change is associated with a paraproteinemia in ~80% of cases. Histologically, cell-rich granulomas are found in the dermis and subcutis, composed of foam cell histiocytes as well as multinucleated giant cells and lymphocytes. Necroses and negative imprints of cholesterol crystals are found in almost all cases.

Because of the small number of patients, there have not yet been any reliable studies on treatment.

Mesenchymal Tumors

Benign

Nodular fasciitis

This rapidly growing but benign tumor mostly grows on the eyelid in 4 to 8 weeks and leads to considerable anxiety. Histologically, it consists of fibroblastic aggregates of varying cellularity, some of which occur in clusters while others appear random.

The risk of confusion with a malignant process at clinical level and even histological level is great and must be avoided. It can be particularly difficult to differentiate between it and a fibrosarcoma; keeping this problem in mind is usually enough to avert the risk. Local excision is the initial treatment. Extensive excisions can be necessary for recurrences.

Granular cell tumor (also granular cell myoblastoma)

This benign tumor occurs in nearly all sites of the body, but mainly in the squamous epithelial coated mucous membrane of the oral cavity, the esophagus, and the skin. Histologically, there are groups of light cytoplasm-rich cells, which, in their immunohistochemistry, are positive for S100. Due to the frequently seen marked hyperplasia of the squamous epithelial coating there are frequent misdiagnoses as squamous epithelial carcinoma while the underlying lesion is overlooked. Excision is the first treatment of choice.

Intravascular papillary endothelial hyperplasia

This is a benign proliferation of endothelial cells via connective tissue septa of varying widths in blood vessels. Changes of this nature can occur within the context of hemangiomas and similar lesions or as the consequences of trauma, such as an injection into a vessel and the associated formation of thromboses. These are reactive hyperchanges of the endothelium and it is important that they are differentiated from neoplastic changes.

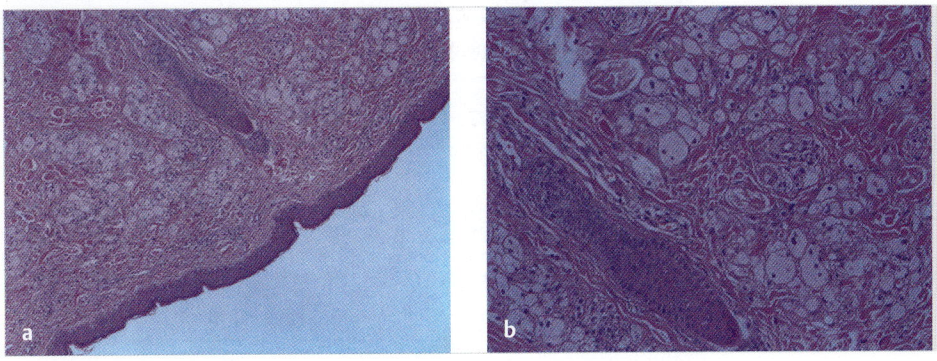

Fig. 9.15 Xanthelasma. **(a)** Clusters of macrophages with broad and bright cytoplasm. (H&E staining, magnification 10 × 10). **(b)** The foamy pattern of the cytoplasm is characteristic for foamy cell macrophages (H&E staining, magnification 20 × 10).

Unclear Biological Behavior

Juvenile fibromatosis

Juvenile fibromatosis constitutes a group of fibrous tumors in children and adolescents. The biological value is not always clear; there are recurrences. Histologically, there are proliferations of fibroblasts with indistinct delineation from the surrounding parenchyma.

Malignant

Merkel cell tumor

This malignant tumor of the Merkel tactile cells was described by Friedrich Merkel. Histologically, these are cell-rich tumors with rather small, uniformly shaped tumor cells that have a high mitotic activity. The tumor cells are positive for neuroendocrinal immunohistochemical markers such as CD56 and synaptophysin. The coexpression of cytokeratin 20 is typical. Due to the close morphological relationship, the Merkel cell tumor is described as a small-celled carcinoma of the skin. In fact it is important not to overlook metastasis through a small-cell carcinoma, in particular of the lung. The tumor exhibits aggressive growth; recurrences and metastases are frequent, even after a broad local excision.

Lymphomas

All kinds of lymphomas are possible in the eyelid and their description is well beyond the scope of this section. Here only mycosis fungoides is highlighted. This is a cutaneous T-cell lymphoma that can be found in three different stages: erythematous, plaquelike, and tumorous, which leads to a series of differential diagnoses. This is why knowledge of this actually very rare tumor is of significance.

9.4.4 Tumors of the Lacrimal Glands

General

Tumors of the lacrimal glands can primarily be divided into two groups: epithelial and nonepithelial. The latter group, accounting for two-thirds, heads the number of cases. Inflammatory changes or pseudotumors are included in this. In total, 5 to 18% of all tumors of the orbit are localized in the lacrimal gland (for overview see ▶ Table 9.5).

Given the similarity in structure to the salivary gland, tumors of the lacrimal glands are classified similarly by the WHO. Depending on the examination series, 21 to 39% of the tumors are graded as epithelial, and of those, 29 to 55% are in turn graded as malignant.

Table 9.5 Tumors of the lacrimal glands

Benign	Malignant
Epithelial tumors	
Papilloma	Squamous cell carcinoma
	Adenoid cystic carcinoma
	Mucoepidermoid carcinoma
Oncocytoma	Adenocarcinoma (NOS/not otherwise specified)
Other tumors	
	Malignant lymphoma
	Malignant melanoma

Epithelial tumors are very rare in children. The first cases are reported in the second decade of life, in particular pleomorphic adenomas and adenoid cystic carcinomas. Both tumor entities are subsequently also at the forefront in adulthood.

Epithelial Tumors

The histologic descriptions of the tumors listed are identical with those in the locations already listed. Their biological behavior is also similar and deviates only with regard to anatomical peculiarities.

Some tumors of epithelial origin that have so far not been listed for the other locations are listed here.

Benign

Pleomorphic adenoma

This is typically a tumor of the salivary glands that exhibits a similar structure in the lacrimal gland and a similarly benign biological behavior. Histologically, these are gland formations arising from a bland epithelium (▶ Fig. 9.16). Adjacent to sections with the formation of gland lumina there are solid growing tumor areas. These are accompanied by mesenchymal components as well, quite often with chondroid differentiation. A further characteristic is the strangulation of small satellite nodules into the neighboring tissue. This can hinder excision in healthy tissue and then is the cause of recurrences (or more accurately of residues). This can make control of the tumor impossible.

Oncocytoma

Oncocytoma is a benign tumor, histologically arising from larger, regular cells with a fine granulated and eosinophilic cytoplasm. The tumor cells exhibit great similarity with the epithelium lining the ducts in the glands. This tumor is predominantly found in the salivary glands. In the lacrimal glands this tumor (and its malignant counterpart, the oncocytic carcinoma) is found very rarely. Excision is the treatment of choice.

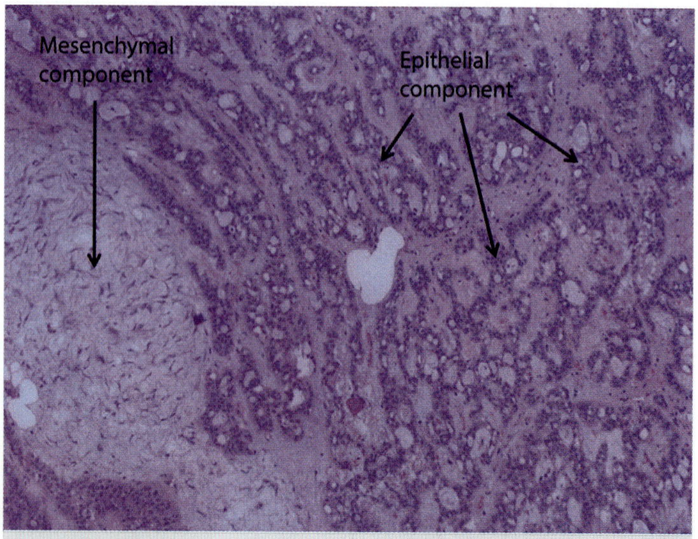

Fig. 9.16 Pleomorphic adenoma. The name of this tumor characterizes its polymorphic morphology, which comprises epithelial components as well as mesenchymal portions along with a "matrix" in which the tumor cells are embedded (H&E staining, magnification 10 × 10).

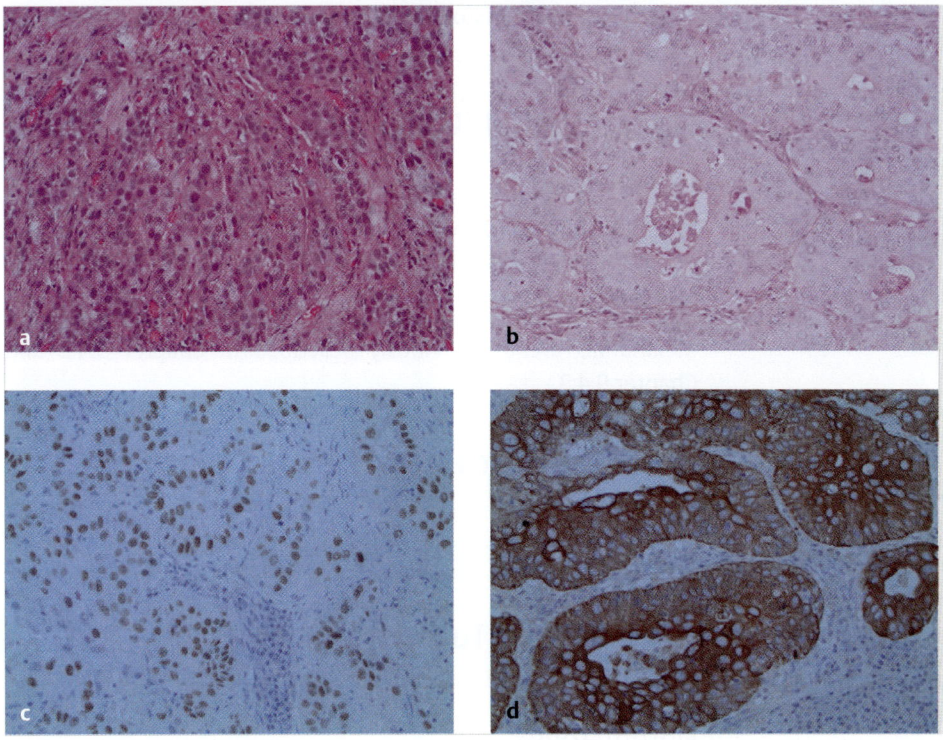

Fig. 9.17 Mucoepidermoid carcinoma. **(a)** Tumor cells of this low-grade malignant tumor show partly solid and adenomatous growth pattern (H&E staining). **(b)** PAS staining reveals slime formation of some cells without a typical differentiation into gland cells. **(c)** Immunohistochemistry also reveals a mixed differentiation with positive expression of squamous cell antigen (p63) **(d)** and also of adenomatous cell antigen (CK7). Magnification 20 × 10 in each panel.

Warthin's tumor

This benign tumor is likewise overwhelmingly found in the salivary glands and only rarely in the lacrimal glands. Histologically, there are oncocytic cells again, which are here accompanied by a lymphatic component in the interstitium. Excision is the treatment of choice.

Myoepithelioma

This is a rare benign tumor in the lacrimal glands. A common origin of pleomorphic adenoma and myoepithelioma is the subject of debate as these tumors differ only in the composition of the tumor cell components but not in the form of the tumor cells. Excision is the treatment of choice.

Malignant

Adenoid cystic carcinoma

Adenoid cystic carcinoma is a malignant epithelial tumor, composed of small pseudo glands that are arranged in groups of various sizes. Adenoid, trabecular, and basal variants occur. Necroses and bleeds as well as the mitotic activities and the basal-growing proportion determine the grading and also the prognosis. Particularly problematic is growth along nerve sheaths and in blood vessels: safe removal in healthy tissue is thereby made considerably more difficult and this leads to numerous recurrences that are then difficult to overcome.

Treatment is a matter of controversial debate. Prognosis is difficult on a whole and is still better for children than for adults.

Carcinoma ex pleomorphic adenoma

Carcinomas can arise from pleomorphic adenoma. The transition is generally abrupt as regards the histology. The prognosis is difficult and treatment needs to be discussed.

Mucoepidermoid carcinoma

This is a particular form of squamous epithelial carcinoma as previously described. Next to squamous epithelial solid tumor cell formations are found regions with formation of glandlike structures (▶ Fig. 9.17). Some 1 to 2% of all lacrimal gland tumors exhibit this differentiation.

Broad local excision is the aim; where necessary the local lymph nodes are removed at the same time. Treatment can be supplemented with radiotherapy.

Other carcinomas with minimal incidence are primary ductal carcinoma, acinus cell carcinoma, and sebaceous gland carcinoma.

Other Tumors and Tumorlike Lesions

The soft tissue of the orbit does not contain any lymph vessels or connected lymphatic tissue. For this reason it is not surprising that up to 90% of lymphomas of the orbit are localized in the lacrimal gland; conjunctiva and eyelids follow in decreasing frequency. Relatively, the number of lymphomas is high: ~50% of all malignant orbit tumors are lymphomas. In particular, these are mainly non-Hodgkin's lymphomas of the B-cell type. Again at the head of this group is the marginal zone lymphoma MALT (mucosa-associated lymphatic tissue). The median age is 65 years and women are more often affected than men. Treatment follows guidelines as published for different types of malignant lymphoma.

Tumorlike lesions

Tumorlike changes can occur within the context of chronically inflammatory processes. These can be associated with cell-rich aggregates of inflammatory cells or can form nodular scarring. Cysts and pseudocysts also arise within the framework of these processes.

Table 9.6 Tumors of the lacrimal duct system

Benign	Malignant
Epithelial tumors	
Papilloma	Squamous cell carcinoma
Oncocytoma	Adenoid cystic carcinoma
	Mucoepidermoid carcinoma
	Adenocarcinoma (NOS/not otherwise specified)
Other tumors	
	Malignant lymphoma
	Malignant melanoma

9.4.5 Tumors of the Lacrimal Duct System

General

The lacrimal duct system is lined with various epithelia. The canaliculus bears a nonkeratinizing squamous epithelium, whereas the tear sac and the nasolacrimal duct exhibit a highly prismatic, in part cilia-bearing, epithelium. Correspondingly, the differentiation of the emerging tumors in the areas mentioned is variable. Here too one should differentiate between benign and malignant variants. In addition, there are tumors that derive from the mesenchyme, which are rare. Melanomas also need to be considered (▶ Table 9.6).

9

On the whole, the number of occurrences of tumors of the tear duct system is minimal. The location of preference is the tear sac. The number of tumors in the other sites is apparently so low that they are not listed separately in studies.

Classification may be according to various criteria, primarily according to biological behavior (benign versus malignant) or according to the growth pattern (papillomas, papillomas with a transition into a carcinoma, carcinomas). These taxonomic approaches are not of primary relevance to the clinical approach.

Ultimately, the following distinctions can be made.

Epithelial Tumors

Benign

Papillomas and oncocytomas

These two entities look similar histologically and, ultimately, display similar clinical behavior to that described previously for these tumors. One should, however, qualify this by saying that in this localization the papilloma is in the transitional cell variant. As the designation indicates, in classical staining the overlying epithelium is similar to urothelium. With regard to clinical symptoms and therapy, behavior similar to that of other papillomas is seen.

Malignant

- Squamous epithelial carcinoma.
- Adenoid cystic carcinoma.
- Mucoepidermoid carcinoma.
- Adenocarcinoma (NOS).

Here too these entities exhibit the same histological aspect and a similar clinical behavior to that described previously for these tumor entities.

Again there is a histological carcinoma variant with transitional cell differentiation.

Nonepithelial (Lymphatic, Melanocytic)

Lymphomas

Lymphomas are as previously described in Chapter 9.4.4.

Melanomas

Melanomas are as previously described in Chapter 9.4.2 and Chapter 9.4.3.

9.4.6 Tumors of the Soft Tissue of the Orbit

An overview can be seen in ▶ Table 9.7.

Fibromatous Tumors

Benign

Fibromatous

Fibromatous development is random proliferation of fibroblastic cells that is ill-defined vis-à-vis the surrounding soft tissue. The poorly defined delineation can lead to considerable problems, as recurrences can happen despite the relatively good differentiation of the cells.

Various subtypes are known; here only infantile myofibromatosis is described. Overall these lesions occur predominantly in children and young adults. Local excision is the treatment to be pursued.

Nodular fasciitis

As already mentioned above, this is a benign proliferation of fibroblastic cells. It mainly affects young adults as well as children. The tumors grow quickly and lead to considerable anxiety in patients. This makes the distinction from a malignoma, in particular a fibrosarcoma, important but again also problematic. Spontaneous regressions do occur. Excision is the treatment of choice.

Fibroma

Fibroma is a benign proliferation of benign connective tissue cells without atypia. There is debate whether this is a matter of primarily reactive changes.

Tumors with Uncertain Biological Behavior/Malignant Tumors

Fibrous histiocytoma

Fibrous histiocytoma occurs as benign, locally aggressive, or malignant variants. The average patient's age for the disease is 43 years (2–85 years). Histologically, benign tumors are composed of fibroblasts arranged in storiform formation. Associated with this there can be found foam-celled macrophages and histiocytic giant cells. The surrounding matrix consists of collagen fibers, and in parts the tissue appears hyalinized. The locally aggressive variant shows infiltrative growth in its peripheral zone and

Table 9.7 Tumors of the orbital soft tissue

Benign	Uncertain biological behavior	Malignant
Fibromatous lesions		
Fibromatosis	Fibrous histiocytoma	Fibrosarcoma
Nodular fasciitis		
Fibroma		
Lipomatous tumors		
Lipoma		Liposarcoma
Myogenous tumors		
Leiomyoma		Leiomyosarcoma
Vascular leiomyoma		Rhabdomyosarcoma
Vascular lesions/mesenchymal tumors		
Capillary hemangioma	Solitary fibrous tumor (SFT)	Angiosarcoma
Cavernous hemangioma		
Lymphangioma		
Epithelioid hematogenous lesions		
Arteriovenous malformation (AVM)		
Intravascular papillary endothelial hyperplasia		
Nerve sheath tumors		
Neurofibroma		MPNST(malignant peripheral nerve sheath tumor)
Schwannoma (neurilemmoma)		
Granular cell tumor		
Bone tumors		
Fibrous dysplasia		Osteosarcoma
Ossifying fibroma		Mesenchymal chondrosarcoma
Histiocytosis		
		Langerhans cell histiocytosis
		Eosinophilic granuloma
Other tumors		
Epithelial cystic choristoma		Leucemia
Teratoma		Malignant lymphoma
Paraganglioma		Endodermal sinus tumor (yolk sac tumor = Dottersack tumor)
		Ewing sarcoma
		Malignant melanoma
		Alveolar soft tissue sarcoma
		Infiltration by tumors of anatomical structures adjacent to the orbit
		Metastases

exhibits hypercellular sections. However, necroses are not found such as are often seen in open malignant fibrous histiocytomas. there is a considerable pleomorphia of tumor cells, a raised number of mitotic cells, and also atypical nuclear division figures. A further subdivision of the malignant variant into neoplasias with storiform, pleomorphic, or myxoid growth is possible. The morphological picture correlates well with the biological behavior. Complete excision is the aim. Incomplete resection leads to recurrence. Locally aggressive or malignant tumors can compel exenteration. Fatal courses are possible. Metastases appear predominantly only after recurrences.

The histological differential diagnoses are broad. Malignant fibrous histiocytoma must be differentiated from other mesenchymal malignomas.

Fibrosarcoma

Fibrosarcoma is very rare malignant tumor that can occur in children, young people, and adults. Histology is similar to that of fibrosarcomas with other localization. It is important to differentiate between it and a rhabdomyosarcoma.

Lipomatous Tumors

Benign

Lipoma

Lipoma is a benign tumor with the same morphology as in other localizations. Excision is the treatment of choice.

Malignant

Liposarcoma

Liposarcoma is a malignant tumor in various histological variants. These include the well-differentiated, the dedifferentiated, the round-celled, and the pleomorphic liposarcoma.

Well-differentiated small liposarcomas have a thoroughly good prognosis after local excision. The remaining subtypes are associated with a poorer prognosis and when they recur can compel exenteration.

Myogenic Tumors

Benign

Leiomyoma

Leiomyoma is a benign tumor of the smooth musculature with the same histology as for other localizations. With this are found bundles of smooth muscle cells that are interwoven with each other. Significant atypia are not found, but occasionally a "disturbance." The nuclei of the cells are elongated and rounded off and provide a fairly typical aspect. The surrounding tissue is pushed to one side and is compromised. Excision is the treatment of choice. If resection is incomplete, recurrences are likely.

9

Vascular leiomyoma

This is a variant of leiomyoma with vessels situated between the myoma cells around which the tumor cells orientate themselves. The tumor can imitate a hemangioma in imaging processes. The tumor is well-defined vis-à-vis soft tissues. The Valsalva maneuver can cause pain and lead to protrusion. Incomplete excision can lead to recurrence.

Malignant

Leiomyosarcoma

Leiomyosarcoma is a malignant variant of tumors deriving from the smooth muscle cells. Mainly older patients are affected or the sarcoma is a consequence of radiation of a retinoblastoma. Histologically, smooth muscle cells are found with atypia of different degree and increased proliferation. Complete excision (where necessary with exenteration) is performed with additional chemotherapy and radiotherapy to treat it. Current literature should be monitored with regard to an optimization of treatment.

Rhabdomyosarcoma

As already detailed for rhabdomyosarcoma of the conjunctiva, this is a malignant tumor deriving from an undifferentiated mesenchyme in part with indications of differentiation of striated muscle cells. The tumor is subdivided histologically into the embryonal, alveolar, and pleomorphic variants. Tumors without identifiable differentiation or subtype are also designated as embryonal sarcomas. Rhabdomyosarcoma is assigned to the group of "small round blue cell" tumors.

Orbital rhabdomyosarcomas represent ~10% of all rhabdomyosarcomas. Patients' ages lie between 1 month and 68 years. Boys are more often affected than girls. Embryonal rhabdomyosarcomas occur predominantly in the first decade of life, while the alveolar variant is more often seen in adolescence. It takes a fulminant course and leads to a severe swelling and/or exophthalmos. The preferred location is the supranasal quadrant and the top half of the orbit; the alveolar variant, however, is more often to be found in the bottom half. The botyroid variant in contrast is mainly found in the conjunctiva. A primary located outside the orbit with the involvement of a secondary can occurs. Histologically, the variants listed above are found with a colorful multiplicity of tumor cell growth forms, the description of which is beyond the scope of this book. One should, however, mention that the embryonal variant and its subform, the botyroid variant, are the most common. Thereafter comes the alveolar variant, which is a typical cytogenetic aberration in the sense of a rearrangement of the *FKHR* gene with the *PAX3* or *PAX7* genes. Pleomorphic rhabdomyosarcoma is the rarest in occurrence.

Any suspicion of a rhabdomyosarcoma requires immediate histomorphologic investigation and accurate typing, where necessary with the assistance of a pathology reference service. Treatment is given in line with the current provisions or guidelines and has led to a dramatic improvement in the pediatric survival rate.

Vascular Tumors

Benign

Capillary hemangioma

As described in Chapter 9.4.3, this is a benign and common proliferation of small blood vessels. It represents 86% of all vascular lesions in children. Approximately one-third of all cases appear perinatally. Girls are more often affected than boys. Considerable growth can often be seen in the first few months. From the age of 2 years many cases witness a regression (~70%). About 30% of patients exhibit further cutaneous and/or visceral hemangiomas.

Excision is considered as for treatment for secondary problems. As hemangiomas can become large, this for the most part means growth pressing on sensitive tissue. Otherwise, monitoring of the clinical course is recommended. The diagnosis should be certain, however, and there should be no suspicion of a malignoma. Treatment with drugs can also be considered. Scarring can occur as a late consequence of a hemangioma that has changed due to regression.

Cavernous hemangioma

This is a benign, well-delineated vascular tumor, histologically constructed from vessels with a wide diameter. Two-thirds of patients are female, with a median age of 42 years. The clinical symptoms are a slow, painless exophthalmos and a loss of sight with the pressure on the optic nerve. Venous angioma is possibly a histological variant with the same clinical symptoms. Patients without clinical symptoms are monitored. Where there are clinical symptoms, excision is performed carefully. Recurrences are not reported. Venous angioma is difficult to remove, which is why complications are more frequent.

Lymphangioma

As in the other locations, this benign tumor is constructed from irregularly shaped lymph vessels. As lymph vessels are not normally found in the orbital soft tissue, this is a site disorder in the sense of a choristoma. These tumors are differentiated into superficial, deep, and combined subtypes. Superficial lymphangioma affects the conjunctiva and the eyelid. Due to its location, deep lymphangioma can lead to exophthalmos and deterioration in sight. Combined lymphangioma grows slowly and is difficult to eradicate completely by operation. Disfiguring complications and even loss of sight are possible. These complications are likewise problematic in treatment for the other two variants.

Epithelioid hemangioma

In this benign and rare tumor are found vessels lined with endothelial cells with an eosinophilic cytoplasm, in which there are in turn small vacuoles. It is important to differentiate between epithelioid hemangioendothelioma, epithelioid angiosarcoma, and bacillary angiomatosis. Complete excision is the treatment of choice.

Arteriovenous malformations (AVMs)

These benign vascular deformities are distinguished according to their flow characteristics (no blood flow, venous blood flow, arterial blood flow). AVMs can appear within the context of syndromes, of which the following should be mentioned: Klippel–Trenannay–Weber syndrome, "blue rubber bleb nevus" syndrome, Sturge–Weber syndrome, and Wyburn–Mason syndrome. Orbital varix nodes are generally regarded as congenital AVMs. Fresh thromboses and bleeds can simulate an acute tumor event. Histologically, there are various thick-walled, partly muscular vessels. Previous thromboses can take on the appearance of a papillary endothelial hyperplasia. Treatment is mostly conservative.

Intravascular papillary endothelial hyperplasia

This is a benign and/or reactive lesion in the sense of organized vascular damage and thrombus. Within the context of the recanalization of a thrombus, multiform papillary formations can develop, which can also exhibit irregular endothelia. The distinction from angiosarcoma is important.

Uncertain Biological Behavior

Solitary fibrous tumor

A solitary fibrous tumor is a mesenchymal tumor originally seen in the pleura that then manifests itself in a series of further localizations. In the orbit the biological behavior is graded as benign. Histologically, there are fibroblastic cells in a storiform growth pattern. Cells are positive for CD99, CD34, and S100. Malignant variants do occur, however, and then demonstrate high mitotic activity and a considerable cell pleomorphism.

The treatment of choice is excision. Recurrences have been reported, but it is difficult to make a reliable statement on this with the small number of cases so far (~20 cases). Note that, at the same time, earlier hemangiopericytoma has been identified as a solitary fibrous tumor. This can lead to confusion with regard to the terminology.

Malignant

Angiosarcoma

This is a malignant variant of vascular tumors. Histologically, there are different degrees of well-differentiated forms right through to highly pleomorphic tumors, which can only just be immunohistochemically identified. The course is very problematic and excision often not successful. Even with adjuvant therapy the prognosis does not change significantly.

Nerve Sheath Tumors

Benign

Neurofibroma

This is a benign tumor, histologically composed of nerve sheath cells or Schwann cells and endoneural as well as perineural fibroblasts. As an isolated neurofibroma, this entity appears as a single lesion that has well-defined boundaries, and does so in the third to fifth decades of life. The plexiform variant is to be regarded as pathognomonic for von Recklinghausen's disease type 1. The first symptoms appear in the first decade of life. This form of neurofibroma can spread to the other structures in the orbit. Neurofibromas with infiltrative and unclearly defined growth are designated as diffuse neurofibromas and do not have the close correlation with von Recklinghausen's disease. A malignant transformation has been described for the plexiform variant. Excision can be attempted and is promising in the isolated neurofibroma. This does not apply to the other forms, in particular in connection with von Recklinghausen's disease.

Schwannoma (neurilemmoma)

Benign tumors of the nerve sheath cells, these tumors occur sporadically in the main but they can occur multiply within the context of von Recklinghausen's disease type 2. Histologically, there are typically Antoni A areas (solid growth of the cells) as well as Antoni B areas (loose distribution of the cells in a mucinous matrix). Palisade-form positioning of the cell nuclei with cytoplasm offshoots in polar arrangement (Verocay bodies) is likewise typical. Old lesions exhibit degenerative changes. Distinguishing it from the morphologically very similar leiomyoma has been made easier with the introduction of immunohistochemical markers. Malignant transformation has been reported only in rare cases. Excision is the treatment of choice. If the excision is incomplete, recurrences are possible.

Granular cell tumor

As already described under mesenchymal tumors of the eyelids in Chapter 9.4.3, this is a benign tumor and is mentioned here for the sake of completeness. Local excision is the treatment of choice. Recurrences are possible.

Malignant

Malignant peripheral nerve sheath tumor (MPNST)

Synonyms for this tumor include the terms neurofibrosarcoma, perineural fibrosarcoma, malignant schwannoma, and neurogenic sarcoma. These synonyms indicate the histogenesis of this tumor. The designation as nerve sheath tumor covers the different cells of the nerve sheath tissue as the starting point, including the Schwann cells, the perineural cells, or the epineural and endoneural fibroblasts. Histologically, often a biphasic tumor is evident with pleomorphic spindle cells with clearly raised mitotic activity as well as epithelioid cells. Cell density varies.

Radical excision is the treatment of choice. Incomplete resection leads to a recurrence within a short time. Even with complete excision the prognosis is poor: 50% of patients die within the first 5 years of diagnosis.

Osseous Tumors

Benign

Fibrous dysplasia

This benign tumor exhibits a preference for the bones of the sphenoids, the maxilla, and the frontal os. Almost without exception the tumor occurs in children and adolescents as a solitary lesion. In imaging, the tumor is poorly defined and exhibits lytic and cystic stages. Histologically, there are bone trabeculae in a fiber-rich stroma. A border of osteoblasts is not seen. In structure the bone trabeculae appear to form "Chinese script." Typically there is an activating mutation in the *GNAS* gene, which does not always ensure a simple diagnosis in the overview staining.

Ossifying fibroma

In contrast to fibrous dysplasia, this tumor does not occur only in children and adolescents. The course is more aggressive and recurrences are reported. The tumor grows mainly in the frontal os and in the bones in the sphenoethmoidal area. Radiographically, there is a lesion that has a lighter center and exhibits sclerosed marginal segments. Histologically, there is a strongly vascularized fibrous stroma in which needlelike lamellar bones are found. These are surrounded by a border seam of osteoblasts. In part there is a psammomatous benign growth. These tumors are easily confused with meningiomas or with cementifying fibromas.

9

Malignant

Osteosarcoma

In the main, osteosarcoma develops in the sinuses and then breaks into the orbit. In children it occurs as a solitary lesion and appears without a prior lesion, in connection with a previous fibrous dysplasia, or as a consequence of radiation or even without any such in patients who have previously had a retinoblastoma. Treatment and prognosis is correspondingly problematic. Substantial resection accompanied by radiotherapy and chemotherapy may be necessary.

Mesenchymal chondrosarcoma

This is a malignant tumor growing in a bone or else extraskeletally, in which case it is mesenchymal variant. Histologically, there are segments that remind one of a hemangiopericytoma as well as segments with chondral differentiation. The former (hemangiopericytic) differentiation components can lead to metastases even after a considerable time.

Tumors in the Context of Leukemias and Lymphomas

As for other parts of the orbit, the soft tissue can be involved in the context of a leukemia or a lymphoma. Most frequently then, in childhood there can be found infiltrates of acute lymphatic leukemia and, in adulthood infiltrates of chronic lymphatic leukemia. A primary origin in the orbital soft tissue can be regarded as an absolute rarity. As therapy is nearly always systemic, the correct diagnosis is important to avoid inappropriate local treatment.

Here one should also note granulocytic sarcoma as an infiltrate of immature cells of granulocytic differentiation or within the context of a leukemia. These tumors quite often appear greenish on the cut surface due to the chlorine stored in the cells and this is also reason for the name chloroma.

Histiocytoses

Langerhans cell histiocytosis

This represents a group of diseases that result in infiltrates of atypical histiocytic cell, the so-called Langerhans cells. The most striking course is exhibited by Abt–Letterer–Siwe disease exhibiting acute symptoms, while eosinophilic granuloma (▶ Fig. 9.18) exhibits a chronic, rather indolent course. The orbit is afflicted mainly by the latter version. Here the bones are involved, mainly the supratemporal frontal. Children and adolescents are the groups most prone. A diagnosis can be reached using electron microscopy by displaying the Birbeck granules. Diagnosis has been significantly simplified by use of the antibodies for S100, CD1a, and langerin (CD207).

Other Tumors of the Orbit

Benign

Epithelial cystic choristomas

These are a group of malfunctions that lead to the development of cystic formations. Due to development-induced tissue scattering, dermoid or epidermal cysts arise as well as conjunctival cysts.

The best-known lesion is the dermoid cyst, which makes up ~30 to 50% of the operatively removed tumors of the orbit in childhood. These cysts are predominantly found supratemporally or supranasally in the front quadrants of the orbit. They are lined with keratinizing squamous epithelium. The keratin thus formed induces a considerable inflammation after a rupture. Skin appendages can be found in the cyst wall. Rarely, cuboidal and/or

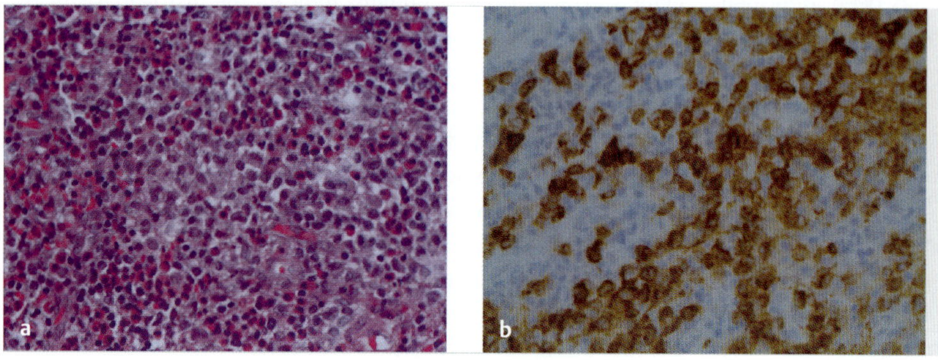

Fig. 9.18 Eosinophilic granuloma. **(a)** Dense groups of partly notched tumor cells along with an admixture of eosinophilic granulocytes. **(b)** Langerin staining confirms the origin of the tumor cells and the diagnosis of eosinophilic granuloma.

cilia-bearing epithelium is the lining, similar to that of the conjunctiva or respiratory epithelium.

Teratoma

Teratoma is rare in orbital soft tissue (~1% of the orbit tumors in childhood) and benign in behavior. It originates from scattered germ cells. Congenital occurrence is possible. Histologically, it is a delineated but not encapsulated lesion, consisting of the tissues of different germ layers. Malignant degeneration is very rare. Local excision is the treatment of choice.

Paragangliomas

Synonyms for paraganglioma are chemodectoma and glomus tumor. The tumor originates in the cells of the ciliary ganglion and exhibits benign behavior. Histologically, there are small vessels around which the similarly shaped tumor cells collect. A distinction is made between sustenticular cells and neurosecretory cells. Complete local excision is the treatment of choice. If removal is incomplete, recurrences are possible.

Malignant

Endodermal sinus tumor (yolk sac tumor)

This is a malignant tumor that derives from scattered germ cells in the area of the midline. Histologically, cuboidal embryonic cells are found arranged around vessels, forming so-called Schiller–Duval bodies. Cells exhibit considerable atypia and mitotic activity.

Ewing's sarcoma

This malignant tumor of childhood and adolescence is defined through a typical chromosomal translocation t(11;22) and variants. It is very rare that the orbit is the site of the primary; accordingly, one should first of all assume a metastasis. It is important to distinguish it from other "small blue cell" tumors, in particular lymphomas, rhabdomyosarcomas, and retinoblastomas. Histologically, the tumor cells exhibit a fine granular chromatin without nucleoli. The cytoplasm is mostly clear and stains in the PAS staining. The cells are typically positive for CD99 and vimentin.

The treatment is derived from a holistic view of the patient and is based on the current guidelines in the literature, which are continually being developed. It is important to confirm the diagnosis.

Primary melanoma

Refer to the histological descriptions already listed on this entity. Clinical symptoms indicate the direction of therapy. Primary melanomas in this localization occur in connection with melanosis oculi and nevus ota. Metastases and a local spread due to a melanoma of the uvea are likewise known. A primary melanoma in the soft tissue of the orbit represents less than 1% of all tumors in this localization.

Alveolar soft tissue sarcoma

This is a malignant tumor without known source cell population. In contrast to other localizations, the course in the orbit is indolent and recurrences are quite rare. The translocation t(11;22) is typical of this tumor. Histologically, there is a pseudoalveolar or organoid pattern.

Tumor metastases in the orbit

The majority of all secondary tumors in the orbit correspond to squamous epithelial carcinomas from the adjoining structures of the skin and conjunctiva as well as the sinuses. There is a similar situation with basaliomas. Meningiomas grow into the orbit from intracranial sites. Likewise, papillomas and lymphoepithelial carcinomas from the nasal passages and the sinuses are repeatedly observed. The same is valid for esthesioneuroblastoma and, an even rarer tumor, the ameloblastoma. Tumor metastases of the type described are one of the most frequent causes of exophthalmos.

Metastases

Metastases account for 3% of all orbit disease and 10% of all orbit neoplasias. Depending on whether a clinical investigation has been available or dissection studies have been conducted, the occurrence of orbit metastases is between 0.7 and 12%. The carcinomas most frequently mentioned in this connection are breast, lung, and prostate carcinomas in addition to melanomas of the skin. Surprisingly, 20% of these metastases represent the first manifestation of the underlying illness. Treatment is orientated on the basic illness.

9

9.4.7 Tumors of the Eyeball

General

Tumors of the eyeball and in particular of the uvea and retina are mentioned cursorily here. The absolute number of these tumors is low, but the number of entities is high. This not least due to the neural origin of significant parts of the structures named. For this reason only common tumors of the uvea and retina will be mentioned here (▶ Table 9.8).

Table 9.8 Tumors of the eye bulb

Benign	Uncertain biological behavior/ Precancerous lesions	Malignant
Tumors of the uvea		
Melanocytic lesions		
Nevus cell nevus		Malignant melanoma
• In the iris		• In the iris
• In the ciliary body		• In the ciliary body
• In the choroidea		• In the choroidea
Melanocytoma		
Other tumors		
Hemangioma	Solitary fibrous tumor (SFT)	Leiomyosarcoma
Leiomyoma	Fibrous histiocytoma	Leukemia
Neurofibroma		Malignant lymphoma
Schwannoma		Metastases
Osteoma		
Xanthomatous tumors		
Tumors of the retina		
		Retinoblastoma

Tumors of the Uvea

At the forefront are the melanocytic tumors, which in turn can be subdivided into benign and malignant lesions. The localization of the tumors also provides further differentiation. The description here is based on the anatomical details of the uvea with differentiation between lesions of the iris, of the ciliary body, and of the choroid.

Benign

Iris nevi

Collections of benign melanocytic nevi in the iris are found with plaquelike growth or intrastromal growth, with combinations of these, and also with diffuse growth in the stroma. The lesions occur mostly in the first three decades of life. Approximately 10 to 30% of all uveal nevi occur in the iris. A connection to choroidal melanomas and cutaneous melanomas has been described. The distinction from malignant melanomas of the uvea is not always simple and, after histological examination, can lead to a reclassification. Histologically, there are different types of melanocytic cells. These can be difficult to distinguish from cells of a low-malignancy spindle cell melanoma.

Treatment is conservative and is replaced by continuous check-ups. In only about 5% does an increase in size indicate possible malignant transformation.

Ciliary bodies

Melanocytic nevi often occur at the base of the ciliary body or accompany malignant melanomas. Less than 5% of the nevi of the uvea occur in this area and often remain undetected clinically. Large nevi can only be distinguished from malignant melanomas with difficulty and are a major diagnostic challenge. Here too treatment is initially conservative.

Choroid

More than 90% of all nevi appear in this tissue. Overall, the incidence of choroidal nevi is ~3% of the adult population. As the great majority of these, like the other nevi, do not occasion any relevant symptoms, they are only picked up in routine examinations. Histologically, there are four different cell types in various combinations. Again, distinguishing large nevi from melanomas is a considerable problem.

Melanocytoma

This is a nevus variant that is defined by its size. In the iris there are histologically melanocytic cells, which are mostly smaller than they are in other nevi. In the ciliary body and the choroid, in contrast, there are no differences from the nevi described above.

Once again, distinguishing between melanocytoma and a malignant melanoma is a problem, particularly as the size cannot be used as a criterion for making the distinction. Treatment of melanocytoma is conservative or wait-and-see.

Malignant

Iris melanomas

Approximately 5 to 15% of uvea melanomas grow in the iris. Biologically, these melanomas are graded as low malignancy. Metastases are possible (~5%). There is often a long back-story or a known pigmentation disorder, perhaps since childhood. It is noticeable that iris melanomas mainly occur in the bottom half of the iris. Iris melanomas are said to have a better course than the variants in the ciliary body and the choroid. Histologically, various cell types are known. Tumor cells with prominent nucleoli and diffuse growth patterns are said to be behind the other morphological variants from a prognostic point of view. Treatment needs to be adjusted for the individual; enucleation is typically not needed.

Ciliary body

Approximately 10% of uveal melanomas are located in this area. Melanomas are noticed through the deterioration of sight when the lens dislocates. Likewise, secondary glaucoma can be an indication of the melanoma. The histology is the same as in melanoma of the choroid. The prognosis is that 90% will be alive in 10 years' time. A local excision can be sufficient treatment.

Choroid

Melanomas of this localization are the most common malignant intraocular tumors in the adult. Only 1% of melanomas of the choroid occur in patients with a dark skin color; the great majority are found in blond and blue-eyed patients. Approximately 6 cases per 1 million inhabitants are observed in light-skinned populations. In addition, congenital melanosis, nevus ota, and nevi generally predispose to this disease. Familial forms are known but rare. Deterioration of the sight or restrictions in vision brings the patient to the doctor's office, but a considerable percentage of melanomas are discovered by routine eye tests. Histologically, various cell groups can be defined; these were described by Callender in 1931 but were later reclassified. In particular a distinction is made between different spindle cell variants and epithelioid tumor cells. The latter are reported to be associated with a poorer prognosis.

The metastasis rate is markedly higher than for the other melanomas described and is ~50% after 10 years. Adjustment of treatment in the light of this is the subject of debate. In addition to enucleation, radiotherapy and/or chemotherapy are considered as alternatives.

Nonmelanocytic Tumors

Nonmelanocytic tumors of the uvea include the following.

- Benign
  - Hemangiomas.
  - Leiomyomas.
  - Neurofibromas.
  - Schwannomas.
  - Osteomas.
  - Xanthomatous lesions.
- Unclear biological behavior
  - Solitary fibrous tumors.
  - Fibrous histiocytomas.
- Malignant
  - Leiomyosarcoma.
  - Lymphomas.
  - Leukemias.
  - Metastases.

These tumors are extremely rare and are histologically similar to those in the localizations already listed.

Tumors of the Retina

Malignant

Retinoblastoma

This is a malignant tumor of childhood, occurring both in a random manner but also in hereditary form. Retinoblastoma is by far the most significant tumor of the retina. Genetically, retinoblastoma can be attributed to the functional loss of both the alleles of the retinoblastoma gene (del13q14). Knudsen developed a model for this at the beginning of the 1970s that has contributed significantly to the understanding of malignant tumors.

The hereditary variant occurs in ~30 to 40% of cases. Some child patients exhibit somatic and mental problems. Hereditary retinoblastoma can occur bilaterally and/or multiply in one eye. The tumor occurs in the first three years of life but it can occur right through into adulthood, especially in the random forms.

Histologically, varying growth forms have been described: exophytic, endophytic, mixed, and diffuse. The tumor cells bear a large basophilic nucleus and only a narrow margin of cytoplasm. Intensive vascularization is observed, also intensive necrosis. Flexner–Wintersteiner rosettes are typical.

Tumor cells seed metastases along the optic nerve and also—via the vascular system—in the lung, bones, and CNS as the preferred locations. It spreads to the conjunctiva and the eyelids via the lymph system.

Treatment is based on numerous criteria or on staging. According to Rees and Ellsworth, patients are subdivided with regard to prognosis into very favorable, favorable, doubtful, unfavorable, and very unfavorable groups. As a result there is a broad spectrum of treatment options.

With the introduction of such treatment options, including radiotherapy and chemotherapy, the prognosis for children has improved considerably. More than 90% of children survive the disease for more than 5 years. Secondary tumors represent a problem and these are have to be discussed as a consequence of the treatment. In this context sarcomas, melanomas, and carcinomas must be considered. With the continual improvement in treatment, one can anticipate a reduction of these late complications.

Other tumors

Numerous other tumor entities can be seen in the retina, the following among others:

- Retinocytomas.
- Astrocytomas.
- Astrocytic hamartomas.
- Gliosis of the retina.
- Angiomatosis retinae.
- Cavernous hemangioma.
- Primary intraocular lymphoma.
- Neuroepithelial tumors.
- Medulloepithelioma.
- Metastases.

Suggested Further Readings

Standard Works

Dabbs D. Diagnostic Immunhistochemistry. 4th ed. Philadelphia, PA: Churchill Livingstone Elsevier; 2013

Fletcher DM, Bridge JA, Hogendoorn PCW, Mertens F, eds. WHO Classification of Soft Tissue and Bone. 4th ed. Lyon: WHO/International Agency for Research on Cancer (IARC); 2013

Font RL, Croxatto JO, Rao NA, for the American Registry of Pathology and the Armed Forces Institute of Pathology. AFIP Atlas of Tumor Pathology Series 4: Tumors of the Eye and Ocular Adnexa. Rockville, MD: ARP Press; 2006

Kerl H, Garbe C, Cerroni L, Wolff HH, Eds. Histopathologie der Haut [Histopathology of the Skin]. Berlin: Springer; 2003

Rootman J, ed. Diseases of the Orbit. Philadelphia: Lippincott; 1988

Yanoff M, Sassani JW. Ocular Pathology:Published. 6th ed. Philadelphia, PA: Mosby Elsevier; 2009

Studies Involving Different Topographies

Bonavolontà G, Strianese D, Grassi P, et al. An analysis of 2,480 space-occupying lesions of the orbit from 1976 to 2011. Ophthal Plast Reconstr Surg. 2013; 29(2): 79–86

Castillo BV, Jr, Kaufman L. Pediatric tumors of the eye and orbit. Pediatr Clin North Am. 2003; 50(1):149–172

Ho SF, Brown L, Bamford M, Sampath R, Burns J. 5 years review of periocular basal cell carcinoma and proposed follow-up protocol. Eye (Lond). 2013; 27(1):78–83

Lieb WE. [Tumors and tumor-like lesions of the orbit]. [Article in German]. HNO. 2010; 58(7):661–671

Pfeiffer ML, Savar A, Esmaeli B. Sentinel lymph node biopsy for eyelid and conjunctival tumors: what have we learned in the past decade? Ophthal Plast Reconstr Surg. 2013; 29(1):57–62

Rao AA, Naheedy JH, Chen JY, Robbins SL, Ramkumar HL. A clinical update and radiologic review of pediatric orbital and ocular tumors. J Oncol. 2013; 2013: 975908

Schittkowski MP, Fichter N. [Orbital neoplasia. Part I: Introduction, vascular and neurogenic tumors]. [Article in German]. Ophthalmologe. 2012; 109(10):1033–1044, quiz 1045

Schittkowski MP, Fichter N. [Orbital neoplasia. Part II: mesenchymal, leukemic, lymphoproliferative and bony tumors, metastasis]. [Article in German]. Ophthalmologe. 2013; 110(1):75–89, quiz 90–91

Shields CL, Shields JA. Ocular melanoma: relatively rare but requiring respect. Clin Dermatol. 2009; 27(1):122–133

Watanabe A, Sun MT, Pirbhai A, Ueda K, Katori N, Selva D. Sebaceous carcinoma in Japanese patients: clinical presentation, staging and outcomes. Br J Ophthalmol. 2013; 97(11):1459–1463

Weizman N, Horowitz G, Gil Z, Fliss DM. Surgical management of tumors involving the orbit. JAMA Otolaryngol Head Neck Surg. 2013; 139(8):841–846

Zembowicz A, Scolyer RA. Nevus/Melanocytoma/Melanoma: an emerging paradigm for classification of melanocytic neoplasms? Arch Pathol Lab Med. 2011; 135(3): 300–306

Orbitopathies (Locally and Systemically induced)

Nutting CM, Shah-Desai S, Rose GE, Norton AP, Plowman PN. Thyroid orbitopathy possibly predisposes to late-onset of periocular lymphoma. Eye (Lond). 2006; 20 (6):645–648

Wang Y, Smith TJ. Current concepts in the molecular pathogenesis of thyroid-associated ophthalmopathy. Invest Ophthalmol Vis Sci. 2014; 55(3):1735–1748

Tumors of the Optic Nerve

Chung EM, Specht CS, Schroeder JW. From the archives of the AFIP: Pediatric orbit tumors and tumorlike lesions: neuroepithelial lesions of the ocular globe and optic nerve. Radiographics. 2007; 27(4):1159–1186

Corrêa ZM, Augsburger JJ, Spaulding AG. Medulloepithelioma of the optic disc. Hum Pathol. 2011; 42(12):2047–2051

Edwards JR, Kulwin CG, Martin SE, Wilson S, Ho CY, Fulkerson DH. Temporal and optic pathway pilomyxoid astrocytoma mimicking dural-based lesion: case report and review of the literature. Pediatr Neurosurg. 2012; 48(4):253–257

Liu GT, Katowitz JA, Rorke-Adams LB, Fisher MJ. Optic pathway gliomas: neoplasms, not hamartomas. JAMA Ophthalmol. 2013; 131(5):646–650

Monteiro ML, Gonçalves AC, Siqueira SA, Gebrim EM. Optic nerve sheath meningioma in the first decade of life: case report and review of the literature. Case Rep Ophthalmol. 2012; 3(2):270–276

Rodriguez FJ, Lim KS, Bowers D, Eberhart CG. Pathological and molecular advances in pediatric low-grade astrocytoma. Annu Rev Pathol. 2013; 8:361–379

Sadighi Z, Slopis J. Pilocytic astrocytoma: a disease with evolving molecular heterogeneity. J Child Neurol. 2013; 28(5):625–632

Tumors of the Conjunctiva

Harooni H, Schoenfield LR, Singh AD. Current appraisal of conjunctival melanocytic tumors: classification and treatment. Future Oncol. 2011; 7(3):435–446

Kalogeropoulos C, Koumpoulis I, Papadiotis E, et al. Squamous cell papilloma of the conjunctiva due to human papillomavirus (HPV): presentation of two cases and review of literature. Clin Ophthalmol. 2012; 6:1553–1561

Kao AA, Galor A, Karp CL, Abdelaziz A, Feuer WJ, Dubovy SR. Clinicopathologic correlation of ocular surface squamous neoplasms at Bascom Palmer Eye Institute: 2001 to 2010. Ophthalmology. 2012; 119(9):1773–1776

Kenawy N, Lake SL, Coupland SE, Damato BE. Conjunctival melanoma and melanocytic intra-epithelial neoplasia. Eye (Lond). 2013; 27(2):142–152

Oellers P, Karp CL. Management of pigmented conjunctival lesions. Ocul Surf. 2012; 10(4):251–263

Shields JA, Shields CL, Mashayekhi A, et al. Primary acquired melanosis of the conjunctiva: risks for progression to melanoma in 311 eyes. The 2006 Lorenz E. Zimmerman lecture. Ophthalmology. 2008; 115(3):511–519.e2

Yousef YA, Finger PT. Squamous carcinoma and dysplasia of the conjunctiva and cornea: an analysis of 101 cases. Ophthalmology. 2012; 119(2):233–240

Tumors of the Eyelid

Actis AG, Actis G, De Sanctis U, Fea A, Rolle T, Grignolo FM. Eyelid benign and malignant tumors: issues in classification, excision and reconstruction. Minerva Chir. 2013; 68(6) Suppl 1:11–25

Bajaj MS, Khuraijam N, Sen S, Pushker N. Congenital melanocytoma manifesting as proptosis with multiple cutaneous melanocytic nevi and oculodermal melanosis. Arch Ophthalmol. 2009; 127(7):937–939

Boulos PR, Rubin PA. Cutaneous melanomas of the eyelid. Semin Ophthalmol. 2006; 21(3):195–206

Dekmezian MS, Cohen PR, Sami M, Tschen JA. Malignancies of the eyelid: a review of primary and metastatic cancers. Int J Dermatol. 2013; 52(8):903–926, quiz 922–923, 926

Esmaeli B, Youssef A, Naderi A, Ahmadi MA, Meyer DR, McNab A, Collaborative Eyelid Skin Melanoma Group. Margins of excision for cutaneous melanoma of the eyelid skin: the Collaborative Eyelid Skin Melanoma Group Report. Ophthal Plast Reconstr Surg. 2003; 19(2):96–101

Plowman PN. Eyelid tumours. Orbit. 2007; 26(3):207–213

Rosenberg C, Finger PT. Cutaneous malignant melanoma metastatic to the eye, lids, and orbit. Surv Ophthalmol. 2008; 53(3):187–202

Savage JA, Maize JC, Sr. Keratoacanthoma clinical behavior: a systematic review. Am J Dermatopathol. 2014; 36(5):422–429

Tumors of the Lacrimal Gland

Bagheri A, Amoohashemi N, Salour H, Yazdani S. Lacrimal gland lymphangioma: report of a case and review of literature. Orbit. 2012; 31(3):197–199

Bernardini FP, Devoto MH, Croxatto JO. Epithelial tumors of the lacrimal gland: an update. Curr Opin Ophthalmol. 2008; 19(5):409–413

Chawla B, Kashyap S, Sen S, et al. Clinicopathologic review of epithelial tumors of the lacrimal gland. Ophthal Plast Reconstr Surg. 2013; 29(6):440–445

Coupland SE, White VA, Rootman J, Damato B, Finger PT. A TNM-based clinical staging system of ocular adnexal lymphomas. Arch Pathol Lab Med. 2009; 133(8):1262–1267

Gurey LE, Brook CD, Parnes SM. Pleomorphic adenoma of the infratemporal fossa: case report and literature review. Laryngoscope. 2010; 120 Suppl 4:S151

Stacy RC, Jakobiec FA, Schoenfield L, Singh AD. Unifocal and multifocal reactive lymphoid hyperplasia vs follicular lymphoma of the ocular adnexa. Am J Ophthalmol. 2010; 150(3):412–426.e1

von Holstein SL, Coupland SE, Briscoe D, Le Tourneau C, Heegaard S. Epithelial tumours of the lacrimal gland: a clinical, histopathological, surgical and oncological survey. Acta Ophthalmol. 2013; 91(3):195–206

Tumors of the Tear Ducts

Domanski H, Ljungberg O, Andersson LO, Schele B. Oxyphil cell adenoma (oncocytoma) of the lacrimal sac. Review of the literature. Acta Ophthalmol (Copenh). 1994; 72(3):393–396

Eweiss AZ, Lund VJ, Jay A, Rose G. Transitional cell tumours of the lacrimal drainage apparatus. Rhinology. 2013; 51(4):349–354

Heindl LM, Jünemann AG, Kruse FE, Holbach LM. Tumors of the lacrimal drainage system. Orbit. 2010; 29(5):298–306

Montalban A, Liétin B, Louvrier C, et al. Malignant lacrimal sac tumors. Eur Ann Otorhinolaryngol Head Neck Dis. 2010; 127(5):165–172

Tumors in the Orbital Soft Tissue

Furusato E, Valenzuela IA, Fanburg-Smith JC, et al. Orbital solitary fibrous tumor: encompassing terminology for hemangiopericytoma, giant cell angiofibroma, and fibrous histiocytoma of the orbit: reappraisal of 41 cases. Hum Pathol. 2011; 42 (1):120–128

Poloschek CM, Lagrèze WA, Ridder GJ, Hader C. [Clinical and neuroradiological diagnostics of orbital tumors]. [Article in German]. Ophthalmologe. 2011; 108(6): 510–518

Tumors of the Eyeball (Uvea and Retina)

Coupland SE, Lake SL, Zeschnigk M, Damato BE. Molecular pathology of uveal melanoma. Eye (Lond). 2013; 27(2):230–242

Eagle RC, Jr. The pathology of ocular cancer. Eye (Lond). 2013; 27(2):128–136

Schoenfield L. Uveal melanoma: A pathologist's perspective and review of translational developments. Adv Anat Pathol. 2014; 21(2):138–143

Temming P, Lohmann D, Bornfeld N, Sauerwein W, Goericke SL, Eggert A. Current concepts for diagnosis and treatment of retinoblastoma in Germany: aiming for safe tumor control and vision preservation. Klin Padiatr. 2012; 224(6):339–347

Villegas VM, Hess DJ, Wildner A, Gold AS, Murray TG. Retinoblastoma. Curr Opin Ophthalmol. 2013; 24(6):581–588

Leukemias and Lymphomas

Bernardini FP, Bazzan M. Lymphoproliferative disease of the orbit. Curr Opin Ophthalmol. 2007; 18(5):398–401

Demirci H, Shields CL, Karatza EC, Shields JA. Orbital lymphoproliferative tumors: analysis of clinical features and systemic involvement in 160 cases. Ophthalmology. 2008; 115(9):1626–1631, 1631.e1–1631.e3

Sjo LD. Ophthalmic lymphoma: epidemiology and pathogenesis. Acta Ophthalmol 2009;87 Thesis 1:1–20. doi: 10.1111/j.1755-3768.2008.01478.x

Tanimoto K, Kaneko A, Suzuki S, et al. Long-term follow-up results of no initial therapy for ocular adnexal MALT lymphoma. Ann Oncol. 2006; 17(1):135–140

Chapter 10

Orbital Malformations

10

10 Orbital Malformations

Paul Schumann, Harald Essig, and Martin Rücker

10.1 Congenital Orbital Malformations

Malformations of the eyes, the orbits, and their surrounding tissues can be congenital or acquired. Congenital deformities occur in isolation, in combination, or as a component of broader, sometimes systemic, malformation syndromes. They can lead to a massive restriction in sight, or they may only pose a cosmetic problem, or may even cause no symptoms and either remain undetected or be diagnosed as incidental findings during routine examinations.[1,2] Congenital orbital anomalies have diverse causes such as genetic defects, numerical chromosomal aberrations, in utero exposure to exogenic teratogenic noxae (e.g., medicaments, infectious microorganisms), or peripartal complications (e.g., oligohydramnion).[2,3,4,5] The cause of many deformities lies in individual genetic defects leading to a series of anomalies, which in turn defines a sequence or a syndrome.[2,3]

10.1.1 Hypertelorism

10

In hypertelorism there is an enlarged interorbital and inner and outer canthal distance as well as an expanded interpupillary distance.[1,2,3] There can also be a defect in the *Lamina cribrosa* where applicable in connection with an anterior encephalocele. Hypertelorism has been documented in the context of over 550 cases. It is often misdiagnosed when the bridge of the nose is flat and there are epicanthal folds, exotropia, eyebrows wide apart, narrow palpebral fissures, and isolated canthal dystopias.[2,3]

Three basic mechanisms have been described for the formation of hypertelorism, each of which provides a plausible explanation for the occurrence of the orbital malformation in the context of syndromes. The first entails a premature ossification of the minor sphenoidal wing, which leads to the fixing of the orbits in the fetal position. The second involves a developmental disorder of the nasal capsule with consecutive protrusion of the primitive brain vesicle into the space thus created, with the result that further development of the eye position is blocked, as can be observed in a frontal encephalocele.[2,6] The third potential mechanism is represented by developmental disorders in the area of the base of the skull, which occur, for example, in craniosynostosis syndromes such as Apert's syndrome and Crouzon's syndrome or in midfacial malformations such as frontonasal dysplasia or craniofacial dysmorphia.[2,3,7,8]

As with hypotelorism, prenatal diagnosis can be made sonographically by measuring the interorbital distance when the 95th percentile curve is exceeded.[9,10] The operative correction is aimed at removing skeletal deformities and soft tissue changes simultaneously and is based on the concept of Tessier's combined intra- and extracranial method, which still today represents the basis of surgical treatment.[11,12] In this the interorbital distance is narrowed by means of a paramedian bone resection. After a frontal segment is removed, a circular osteotomy is performed at depth in the interior of the orbit socket and the paranasally expanded ethmoidal cells and other bony parts are resected up to the lamina cribrosa so that the eyeball can follow the correction made to the bone.[13,14]

10.1.2 Hypotelorism

Hypotelorism is a reduced distance between the medial orbit walls (interorbital distance) with likewise reduced inner and outer canthal distance.[1,2,3] It occurs most commonly in connection with a holoprosencephaly, a malformation of the cerebrum, in which an incomplete splitting of the forebrain occurs in the third to sixth embryonal week as the result of a defect in the area of the midline developmental field of the head.[2,15] Hypotelorism also occurs with other craniofacial malformations, which range from cyclopia—a rare malformation of the facial part of the skull in which the two eye primordia merge into one bony eye socket and which is often associated with holoprosencephaly—to a mild anomaly from a single central upper incisor in connection with unostentatious hypotelorism.[2,3]

Diagnosis can be made prenatally by means of sonography;[9,10] surgical treatment is based on the technique of the "functional orbit" of Tessier and Guiot as well as its diverse modifications.[12,16,17] The principle of transversal displacement, which was first described for hypertelorism, is accordingly reversed with hypotelorism. An osteotomy is performed on the medial orbit wall paranasally and the resection needed takes place in the area of the lateral orbital roofs. Removal of the lateral parts of the cheekbones can also be considered. The bony orbits are rotated laterally and the diastases at the side of the laminae cribriformes as well as in the area of the nose and the orbit sockets are bridged using osteoplastic techniques.[11]

10.1.3 Cyclopia and Synophthalmia

With these very rare facial malformations, which occur mainly in connection with holoprosencephaly, there is a joint orbit with two eyeballs lying next to each other (synophthalmia) or just one eye (cyclopia). Characteristic are a poor formation of the prechordal segment of the skull and an underdevelopment of the mouth–nose–throat area.[9] A severely abnormal development of the prosencephalon results in a partial or complete fusion of the optic vesicles.[18,19] As these malformations are usually associated with holoprosencephaly, their prognoses are mostly poor.[9]

10.1.4 Anophthalmia and Microphthalmia

Anophthalmia and microphthalmia are among the most common congenital ocular malformations and represent a significant factor in congenital blindness.[20,21] Reduced orbital growth is found not only with microphthalmia but also with anophthalmia.[9] They occur in isolation or in association with a syndrome. Microphthalmia designates a miniaturized eyeball, anophthalmia indicates a complete absence of the eye structure.[20]

Primary anophthalmia (absence of the eye structure) is characterized by a sporadic, non–syndrome-associated occurrence; it affects both eyes in approximately 75% of cases. Secondary anophthalmia results from a developmental defect of the entire neural tube. When there is a malformation or poor development of the optic vesicle after evagination from the diencephalon, one speaks of a degenerative anophthalmos, with which there is the possibility of evidence of neuroectodermal elements in the orbit.[18,20,21]

Microphthalmos can occur unilaterally or bilaterally and may be the expression of a primary ocular developmental disorder or may occur within the context of a craniofacial dysplasia and more extensive syndromes such as trisomy 13 and 18.[1,20,21] It also occurs in connection with ocular malformations such as persistent primary hyperplastic vitreous body, nuclear cataract, or coloboma.[1] Diverse genetic mutations associated with anophthalmia or microphthalmia have now been identified.[20,21,22]

Prenatal diagnosis is based on the evidence of an orbit that is too small with values under the 5th percentile curve along with evidence of a missing or too small eyeball; particular attention is given to comparison with the contralateral side in order to be better able to differentiate abnormalities in the area of the eyeball.[9] Satisfactory treatment for microphthalmos is usually possible with conformers or overlying prostheses. Expansion of the conjunctival sac with self-inflating hydrogel expanders leads to an earlier and better capability for accommodating prostheses and improving facial symmetry. With congenital clinical anophthalmos, first of all a stretching of the conjunctival sac is required with highly hydrophilic hydrogel expanders. Subsequently the use of self-inflating orbit expanders or a dermis fat transplant is recommended. In older children (> 5 years) with a contracted conjunctival sac incapable of taking a prosthesis and marked facial asymmetry, as well as patients who have previously undergone several operations, extensive orbital osteotomies and flap techniques have to be considered.[23]

10.1.5 Facial Clefts

In contrast to lip–jaw–palate clefts, the formation of clefts affecting the other parts of the face is very rare. There are diverse classifications for describing these rare facial clefts; for example, those according to Harkins, van der Meulen, or Tessier.[24,25,26]

Prediction can be made about the cleft formation to be anticipated based on the fusion lines of the embryo's facial bulges.[27] For example, an incomplete fusion in the pair of lower maxillary bulges leads to a median lower jaw cleft formation.[27]

The failure of an upper maxillary bulge to fuse with a lateral nasal bulge causes a diagonal facial cleft, which runs from the edge of the lower eyelid to the lower edge of the nasal opening wherein the nasolacrimal duct remains as an open groove. It can occur on one or on both sides and be combined with lip–jaw–palate clefts.[27,28]

Transverse facial clefts arise where the fusion of the upper and lower maxillary bulges is disrupted while the cheeks are being formed and the early primitive mouth cleft, which extends to the area of the ear structure, remains in various versions (macrostomy).[28]

The midfacial cleft can be construed as having been caused by a defective frontalization of nose and eyes during the fusion of the central nasal bulges. Here the medial facial furrows (e.g., between both processus globulares) fail to disappear.[28]

The rare facial clefts often influence orbital growth and are also often associated with malformations of the brain.[27]

10.1.6 Craniosynostoses

Craniosynostoses are caused by a premature closure of one or several cranial sutures and often exhibit a characteristic abnormal head shape.[27,29] Primary craniosynostoses have their origin in a disrupted ossification; the pathogenesis of secondary suture synostoses is very varied and includes, inter alia, metabolic and endocrinal disorders as well as poor brain growth.[27,30]

Primary craniosynostoses can be broken down further into nonsyndromal (85%) and syndromal forms (15%).[27] Nonsyndromal craniosynostoses usually manifest in a premature closure of a single cranial suture, whereas syndromal craniosynostoses are often characterized by multiple fused sutures and facial, brain, and other malformations. Apert's syndrome is usually associated with extensive syndactyly, Crouzon's syndrome with a market midface hypoplasia, exophthalmos and hypertelorism. Evidence of mutations in fibroblast growth factor receptor genes have been found with various syndromal craniofacial synostoses.[27]

Trigonocephaly

Trigonocephaly is caused by a premature ossification of the metopic suture. The craniosynostosis causes bulging in the area of the central forehead, which in many cases is identifiable as a distinct bony ridge. Due to the additional flattening of the frontolateral region, the frontal bone takes on the shape of a triangle in horizontal section. The forehead appears flat, narrow, and high with a clear broadening of the back of the head. There is hypotelorism with, for the most part, unaffected midfacial growth.[25,31,32]

Plagiocephalus

This malformation, which is often misinterpreted as birth-related or positional damage, is caused by a unilateral coronal or lambdoid synostosis. The forehead on the side affected is flat, the sagittal shortening of the skull goes right to the back of the head. The sphenoidal wing on the ipsilateral side is thickened, the anterior skull base is shortened. Characteristically, on the inside of the cranial vault there are impressiones digitatae (impressions of cerebral gyri) as an indication of a local constriction of the brain. The orbit socket is mainly flattened supraorbitally. Due to the growth in the direction of the suture affected, the facial axis deviates toward the healthy side, whereby the eye axis likewise tends toward the healthy side with a simultaneous contralateral descent of the occlusal plane.[31,32]

Oxycephaly

In oxycephaly there is a bilateral coronal suture synostosis, whereby a flat, high forehead develops as well as a skull that is shortened in the sagittal direction and broadened in the transversal direction. The anterior cranial fossa is distinctly shortened, the sphenoidal wing is markedly thickened, and intracranial pressure is often massively raised with consequent generalized impressiones digitatae. Due to a shortened orbit socket solely in the supraorbital area, it is only at this location that an exophthalmos occurs; the poorly marked nasofrontal angle is typical.[31,32]

Brachycephaly

Brachycephaly with its extreme form of cloverleaf skull is characterized by a premature coronal suture synostosis with a simultaneous fusion of the skull base sutures and possible involvement of viscerocranial sutures. As the growth of the sphenoid bone mass as a whole is constricted, the malformation does not remain restricted to the neurocranium but has massive effects on the viscerocranium right into the stomatognathic system. Clinically striking are a shortening of the skull and the base of the skull sagittally with bulges in the area of the forehead and temples, which results overall in a short, broad, and round skull. There is hypertelorism and the markedly flattened orbit sockets cause exophthalmos. The middle part of the face is markedly hypoplastic and, as a result of the inhibited rotation of the upper jaw, there is a circular open bite.[31,32]

Scaphocephaly

Premature ossification of the sagittal suture causes a transversal narrowing of the skull with compensatory increased growth sagittally giving the appearance of a long, narrow skull with a high forehead.[31,32]

The causes of rare secondary craniosynostoses are typically found in endocrinal and metabolic disorders such as renal osteodystrophy, hyperthyrosis, and hypophosphatasia, in which the physiological bone metabolism is disrupted. When hydrocephaly has been operated for, one may also observe secondary synostoses on occasion due to a premature easing of the natural growth pressure of the brain.[27,32]

An interdisciplinary process is obligatory in making a diagnosis, involving neuropediatrics, ophthalmology, and ENT. In the context of imaging diagnostics, transcranial sonography with the imaging of the brain sutures is indispensable. Conventional radiology can give indications of increased cerebral pressure through expanded emissary foramina.[32] However, CT with 3D reconstructions is the procedure of choice to ensure adequate preoperative planning and the capture of complex craniosynostoses. It allows a precise analysis of the skull malformation as well as possible intracranial changes, for example, of the ventricle system and other cerebral structures.[27,32,33] MRI is additionally indicated as an imaging investigation for syndromal craniosynostoses with associated cerebral anomalies.[27]

The surgical correction of cranial synostoses is often undertaken several times. If the orbits are involved, fronto-orbital advancement with its various modifications serves to correct the upper half of the orbit.[34,35,36] This is mostly conducted between the 6th and 12th months of life and is based on the repositioning of the fronto-orbital area by osteoplasty as well as ensuing osteosynthesis. It can be adjusted individually according to the positioning of the bone segments removed.[37,38] In the combined neurosurgical–facial surgical intervention, operative access is achieved via a coronal incision. Following the craniotomy, in standardized fronto-orbital advancement the osteotomy of the nasofrontal suture is conducted in the orbit sockets and from there via the orbit vault to the zygomaticofrontal suture after ventrally releasing the temple muscles from the temporal fossa while preserving the supra-orbital nerves. From here an osteotomy is performed in a bow shape to the coronal suture whilst forming a retention shape (tongue-in-groove technique) in the parietal area. Once the opposite side is reached along the coronal suture, the osteotomy is continued analogously. The resulting fronto-orbital section of bone is divided into a frontal and an orbital segment via a horizontal incision. First of all, the frontal bone flap is removed and then the orbital segment. The parts are extricated osteoplastically in accordance with their deformity and relocated forward using resorbable osteosynthesis material to fix them in a new position.[39] In this way space is created for the brain and the conditions are fulfilled for skull growth to be normalized by exploiting autoregulative forces, whereby not only functional but also aesthetic improvement is the aim.[38] For a comprehensive harmonization of the orbit shape as well as of the midface, an additional Le Fort II or Le Fort III distraction is indicated further down the line in many cases in order to give a final shape to the often hypoplastic midface underneath the zygomaticofrontal suture.

Apert's Syndrome

Apert's syndrome, also called acrocephalosyndactyly, is the most common syndromal craniosynostosis and is mainly characterized by brachyturricephaly, caused by a premature fusion of the coronal suture and possibly of the sagittal suture, as well as sometimes multiple symmetric syndactyly.[27,38,40] In its extreme form a cloverleaf skull can occur, which is characterized by a premature synostosis of all skull sutures with the exception of the metopic suture and the squamous suture. As regards the facial morphology, there is often marked hypoplasia of the midface, hypertelorism with an antimongoloid eyelid axis position, and strabismus.[38] Although most cases occur sporadically, an autosomal-dominant inheritance with complete penetrance and higher variance is documented. Specific mutations have been found in the fibroblast growth factor receptor gene (*FGFR2*), which plays a central role in the complex regulation of the morphogenesis of the skull and of the limbs.[27,41] Although 70% of the patients are of normal intelligence, associated cerebral anomalies such as agenesis of the corpus callosum or encephaloceles have been documented.[27]

Crouzon's Syndrome

Crouzon's syndrome, also known as dysostosis craniofacialis, is the second most common syndromal craniosynostosis [27,42] (▶ Fig. 10.1, ▶ Fig. 10.2). It displays autosomal-dominant inheritance with mutations in the *FGFR2* gene. The premature suture synostosis mainly affects the coronal suture, leading to a brachycephalic or an oxycephalic skull configuration. However, the lambdoid as well as the sagittal suture can just be equally affected.[38] The facial abnormalities are in particular maxillary retrognathia, strabismus divergens, exophthalmos, hypertelorism, and lateral slanting of the eyelid axes. Progressive hydrocephaly and malformations in the venous outflow belong, inter alia, to the associated intracranial anomalies.[27]

10.1.7 Syndromes of the First and Second Branchial Arches

Developmental disorders in the area of the first and second branchial arches as well as the first pharyngeal pouch can have complex deformities of the midface as consequences. The anomalies can occur unilaterally as well as bilaterally and can be extremely variable in their expression.[27]

The surgical treatment of these deformities is extremely complex and in nearly all cases requires a distraction of the midface

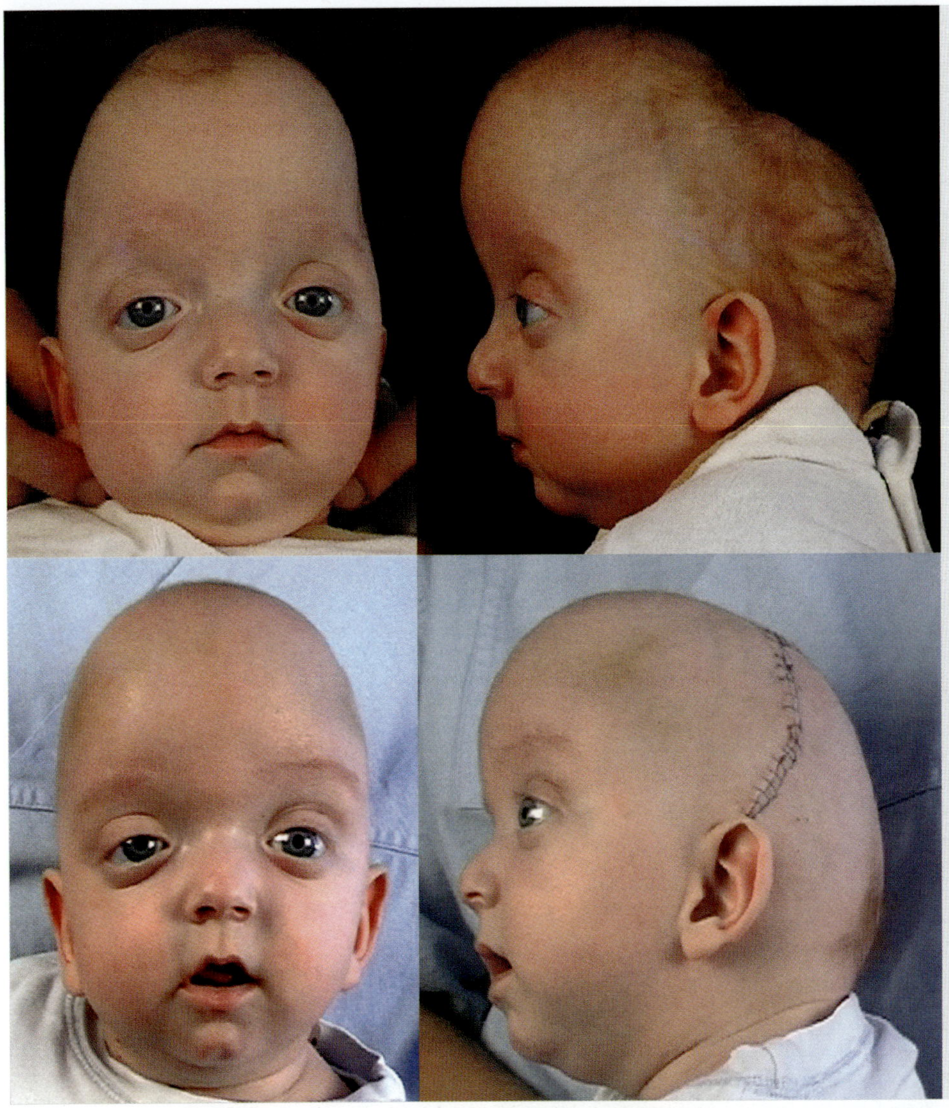

Fig. 10.1 Patient with Crouzon's syndrome before (top row) and after (bottom row) fronto-orbital advancement.

at Le Fort III level as well as a fronto-orbital advancement in order to correct the orbital any other midface anomalies. Furthermore, within the context of a multimodal treatment concepts such as an augmentative rhinoplasty, the closure of a cleft palate, or an orthodontic cotreatment are indicated.[43]

Goldenhar's Syndrome

Goldenhar's syndrome, also called oculo-auriculo-vertebral dysplasia or complex hemifacial microsomia, arises as a result of developmental disorders above all in the area of the first branchial arch and, as a rule, occurs unilaterally (▶ Fig. 10.3). Intrauterine ischemia of the corresponding tissues is assumed to be the cause.[27,44] The syndrome occurs sporadically in the main; in 1 to 2% there is an autosomal-dominant inherited element.[45]

Clinically, hypoplasia of the upper and lower jaw and of the cheekbone is apparent together with the deviation of the chin to the side affected and a microtia. In 92% of the patients there is an epibulbar dermoid; other ocular manifestations are colobomas, microphthalmia, and anophthalmia. In addition, hypoplasia's of the cervical vertebrae, heart defects, and kidney damage can also occur. Intracranial anomalies such as encephaloceles, holoprosencephaly, and dysgeneses of the corpus callosum have been documented.[27,45]

Diagnosis is made clinically in the majority of cases. Children with a marked lower jaw hypoplasia often suffer from a dangerous stenosis of the upper respiratory tracts, which makes a tracheotomy necessary in extreme cases. In such cases an early reconstruction with the aid of bone graft material (e.g., rib) or osteodistraction should be considered. An evaluation of the hearing by means of acoustic evoked potentials (AEP) is obligatory within the first 6 months in order to initiate further measures, such as speech therapy, promptly and in good time. Malformations of the outer ear can either be reconstructed autogenously or are given prostheses; associated malformations such as heart defects or renal anomalies can require further treatment.[45]

Treacher–Collins Syndrome

Treacher–Collins syndrome (synonyms: Franceschetti–Zwahlen syndrome, mandibulofacial dysostosis, dysostosis mandibulofacialis) arises as the result of bilateral symmetrical developmental disorders of the first branchial arch. Inheritance is autosomal-dominant with high penetrance and variable expressivity. The mutations can be localized in the *POLR1C*, *POLR1D*, or *TCOF1* genes, with a mutation in the *TCOF1* gene being responsible for the majority of the cases—approximately 90%.[27,46,47]

Characteristic facial dysmorphias are found in bilateral and symmetrical hypoplasia of the cheekbones, the infraorbital edges (80% of cases), and the lower jaw (78%), with marked hypoplasia of the soft tissue parts. Further symptoms are anti-mongoloid eyelid axes (89%) and colobomas of the lower lids (69%) with a

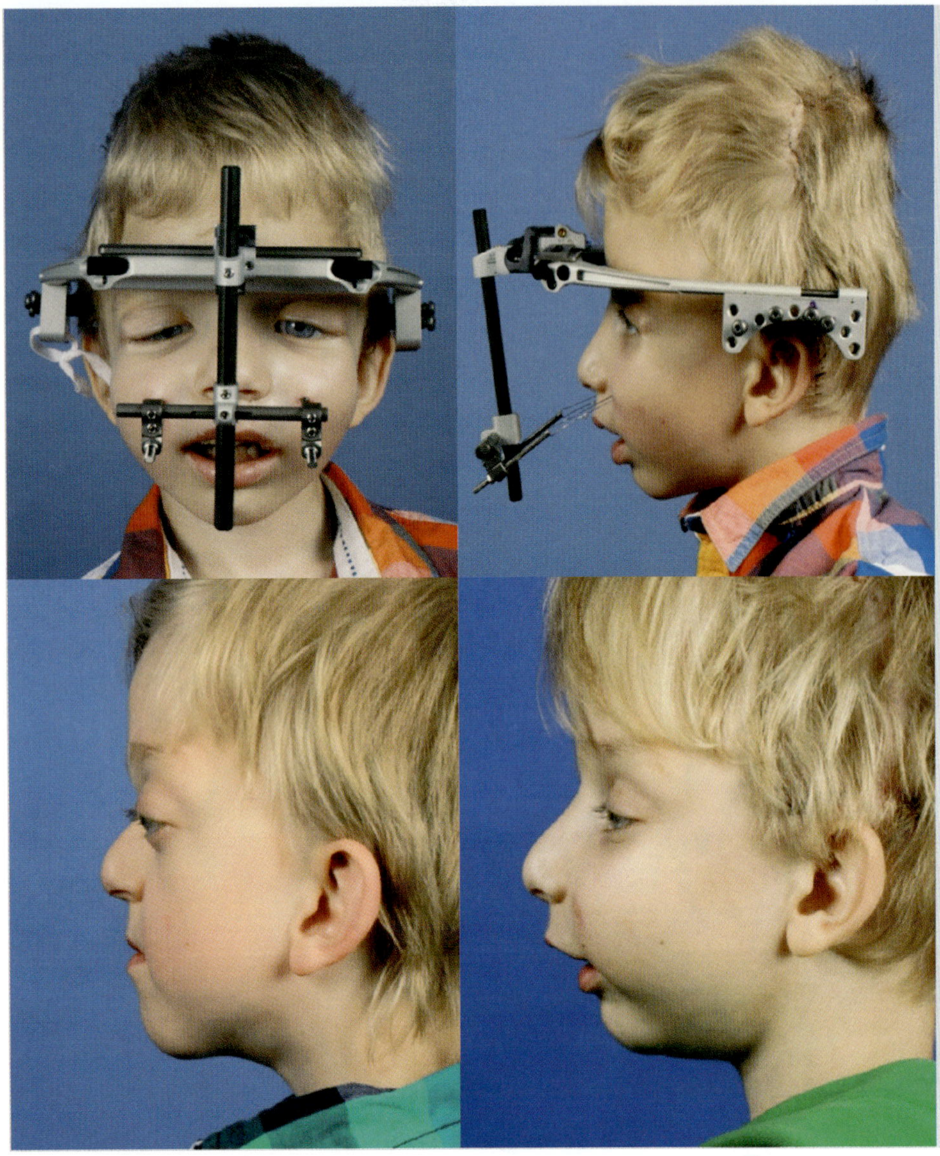

Fig. 10.2 Patient with Crouzon's syndrome. After fronto-orbital advancement performed in infancy, a Le Fort III distraction is conducted to harmonize the hypoplastic midface. Top row: postoperative status with attached RED (rigid external distraction) distractor. Bottom row: status before and after distraction.

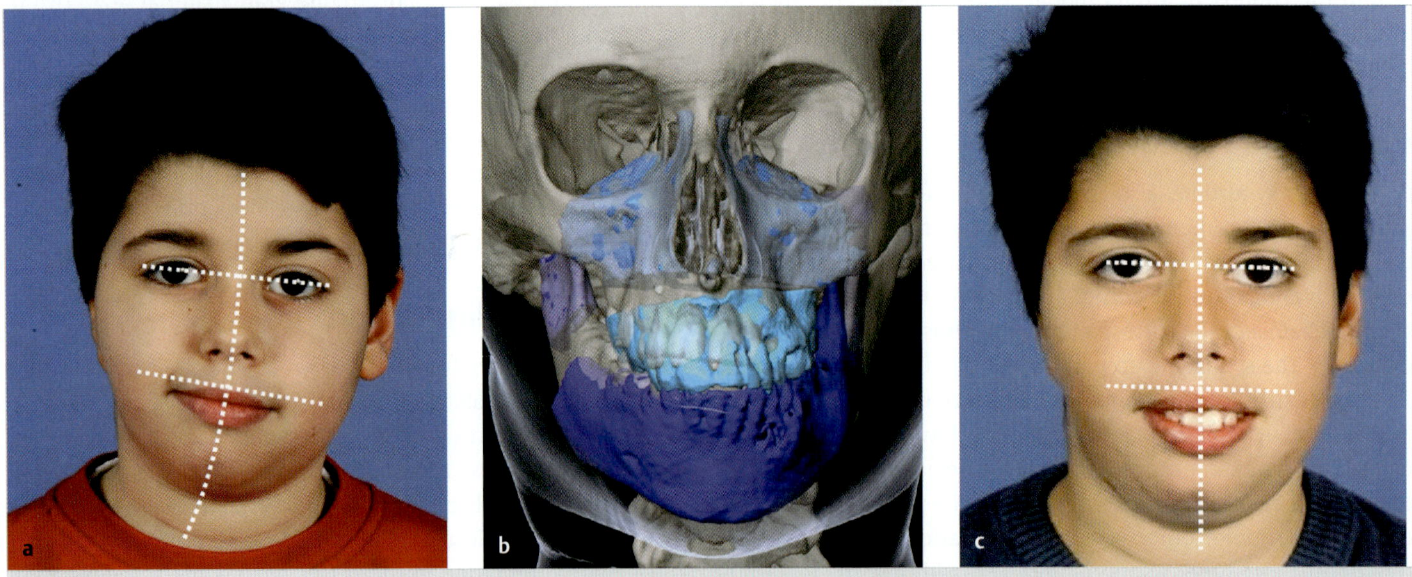

Fig. 10.3 Patient with Goldenhar's syndrome. **(a)** Preoperative starting point; **(b)** virtual planning of a monobloc distraction of upper and lower jaw; **(c)** postoperative result (right). Dotted lines: overlay of the facial axes to make clear the harmonization of the face.

lack of eyelashes in the outer third of the lower eyelid. Occasionally (28%) there is cleft palate, anomalies of the outer ear (for example, microtia or anotia); atresia of the outer ear canal and anomalies of the ossicular chain in the middle ear are common. Intelligence is normal as a rule.[47,48]

Diagnosis is made on a clinical and molecular genetic basis. Due to the complexity of the deformities, multidisciplinary care is obligatory. In individual cases a tracheotomy immediately after birth can be indicated. The marked bone hypoplasia requires constructive intervention with the assistance of osteodistraction or isogenic bone transplantation. The anomalies of the ear have to be reconstituted functionally (middle ear) and aesthetically (external ear). Potential hearing disorders have to be diagnosed as early as possible to achieve a normal development through adequate therapeutic measures.[48]

10.2 Acquired Orbital Malformations

Acquired malformations and deformities of the bony eye socket are mostly caused through trauma or space-occupying neoplasms. Here masses are mainly tumors of varying benignity/malignity ("dignity") and entity. In rare cases they can also occur within the context of an endocrine orbitopathy, the cause of which is assumed to lie in a hereditary autoimmune disease, which leads to an increase in volume of intraorbital muscle and fat tissue, causing a deformity of the orbit.[49] In what follows the acquired orbital malformations concerned are dealt with.

10.2.1 Trauma-Induced Orbital Malformations

Trauma-induced deformities of the bony orbit arise as the direct or indirect effect of force on the bony facial support structures or the displacement of the orbital tissue by direct force. In comparison with the orbit vault and the massive lateral orbit wall, the particularly filigree bony structures of the medial and inferior orbit wall (orbital floor) mostly tend to yield to such stress and are particularly prone to fractures.

Clinically, dystopia of the eyeball can present due to the post-traumatic relative alteration in intraorbital volume. A clinically relevant eyeball displacement mostly causes double vision. This is caused partly by the altered position of the eyeball and also by the altered force vectors of the outer eye musculature. In some cases a mechanical limitation due, for example, to bony fragments that have been dislodged into eye muscles or so-called trapdoor effects, also lead—especially in children—to eye motility limitations. Due to the risk of incarceration, trapped eye muscles (trapdoor fractures) represent an emergency case indication, and necessitate an acute surgical intervention.

With isolated orbital wall fractures, the increase in the intraorbital volume is often indicated by a posterior displacement of the eyeball (enophthalmos) and, when the orbit floor is involved, by a displacement caudally (hypoglobus). Should the outer facial support structures also be affected (combined cheekbone/orbit wall fracture), this can also lead to a constriction of the intraorbital volume so that, clinically, exophthalmos is observed.

Orbital deformations with the above-mentioned clinical symptoms are seen not only directly after the imposition of force but also after inadequate operative care or lack of operative care. Depending on the time delay after the primary traumatic incident, changes and physiological adjustments of the soft tissues make the possibilities of surgical reconstruction (secondary reconstruction) more difficult. With misalignments of bony orbit walls or deformities that have existed for weeks and months, the reconstruction of a normal periorbital soft tissue situation is distinctly more difficult.

As well as a comprehensive case history and clinical examination with detailed recording of ophthalmologic findings (eyeball motility, position of eyeball/exophthalmometry, vision, pupil reaction, anthropometric measurements such as pupillary distance, and so on), three-dimensional imaging above all belongs to the basic diagnostic techniques of bony deformities of the orbit. With modern digital operation simulation platforms, deviations from an idealized mirror symmetry of the facial skull can be detected. At the same time, three dimensional analysis of the imagery produced enables the assessment of the extent of necessary repositioning (primary reconstruction) or necessary displacement of bony viscerocranial parts (osteotomy, secondary reconstruction; ▶ Fig. 10.4).

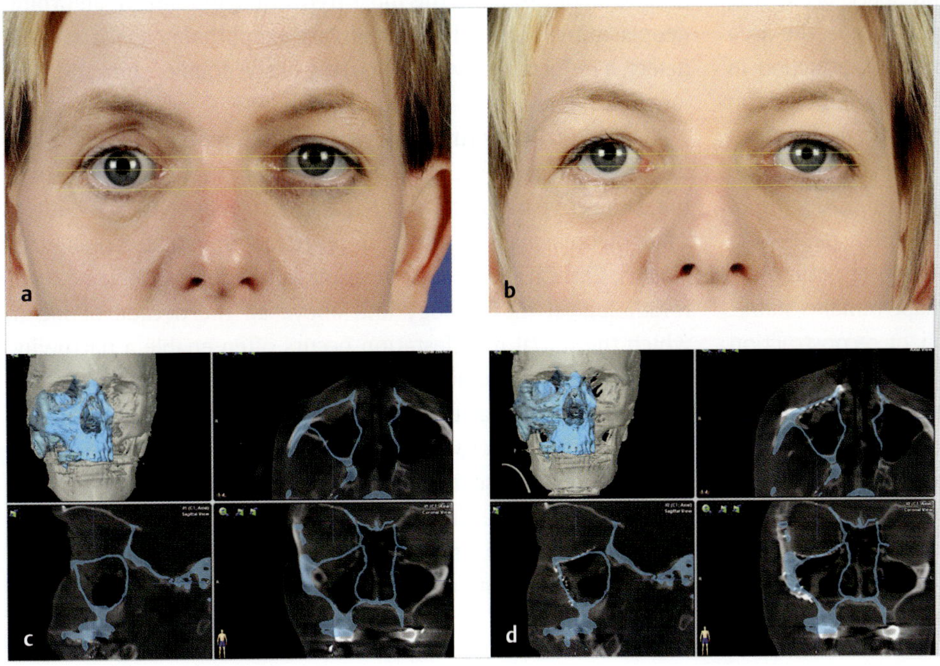

Fig. 10.4 Secondary corrective osteotomy of cheekbone and simultaneous reconstruction of the orbit after inadequately treated fracture of the lateral midface right. Preoperative clinical situation with hypoglobus, deepened supratarsal crease, displacement of the cheekbone prominence, and eyelid retraction **(a)** with corresponding preoperative imagery **(c)** and overlay of the virtual mirroring of the unaffected side (blue). Postoperative situation 4 weeks after corrective osteotomy via transoral and transconjunctival access **(b)**. A slightly raised position of the eyeball can still be seen as well as an improved lower lid position. **(d)** Overlay of the preoperative planning with the actual postoperative result as quality control.

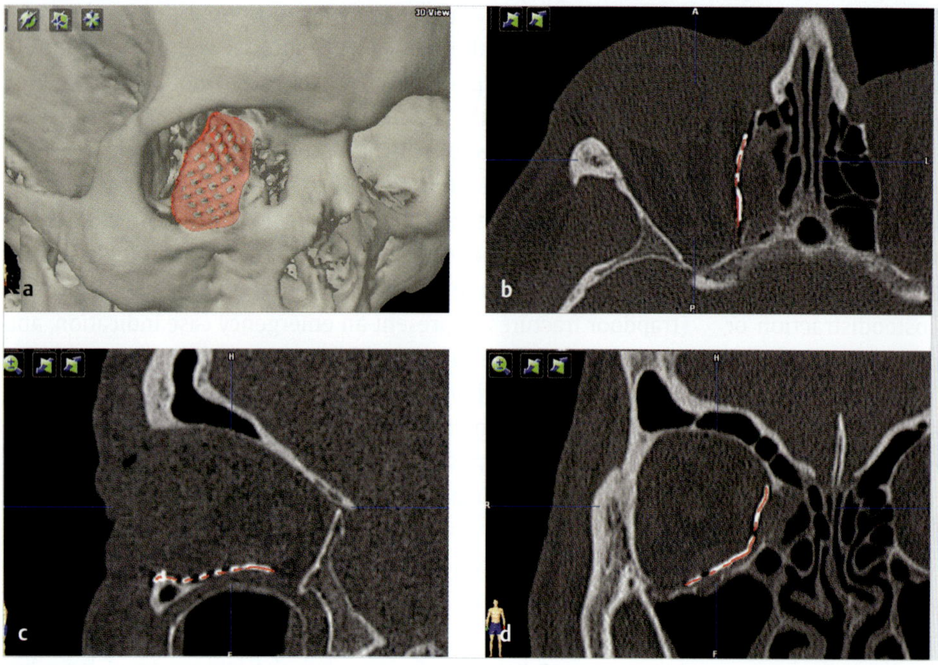

Fig. 10.5 Reconstruction of a complex orbit multiple wall fracture right with patient-specific titanium implant produced by laser sintering process. Overlay of the postoperative imagery with the computer-assisted preoperative planning including virtual implant (red) in three dimensional reconstruction **(a)**, as well as in axial **(b)**, sagittal **(c)**, and coronal **(d)** planes.

Indications for a surgical correction should give due regard not only to an improvement in functional terms but also to aesthetic aspects. The principle first of all consists in the restitution of normal anatomical conditions (true-to-original reconstruction). Insofar as the bony foundation exhibits its original position, then in the primary reconstruction the periorbital and intraorbital soft tissues follow so that, as a rule, the position of the eyeball is normalized and motility is achieved. From this is also derived the requirement for a prompt repositioning of dislodged bony fragments of relevant facial supporting structures. However, even those orbit walls which, due to their filigree form, are in need of a primary reconstruction but cannot always be repositioned so that their shape is stable (medial and inferior orbit wall), should be treated for prompt reconstruction if clinical symptoms are present or, for example, after regression of a concealing swelling, are to be expected with great probability.

The ideal point in time for treating a traumatic orbit deformity depends on various factors. An emergency intervention is indicated for aggravating accompanying symptoms, chief among which are entrapment of the eye muscle and space-occupying retrobulbar bleeds,[50] which lead to a rise in pressure in the area of the optic nerve and thus can result in immediate reduction in vision right through to blinding. A prompt operative intervention is indicated for combined fractures of the orbit walls and fractures of the central and lateral midface in order to prevent the bone healing in a misaligned position by an adequate repositioning of the dislodged fragments. A repositioning of the often paper-thin walls should indeed be the general intention but it often cannot be achieved in such a way that the repositioned shape remains stable. However, reconstruction through the insertion of reconstruction material is not restricted only to emergencies.

For decades there has been heated debated about suitable reconstruction material for orbit wall fractures. The use of resorbable materials such as poly(*p*-dioxanone) (PDS foils) as ideal is advocated by some for the reconstruction of even complex orbit multiple wall fractures;[51,52] others advocate the use of form-stable, nonresorbable materials such as titanium implants [53,54,55] for reconstruction, which also allow direct visualization of the reconstruction by means of 3D imaging (volume tomography, computed tomography).

The particular selection of a suitable reconstruction material and a suitable surgical access seems to have considerable influence on the long-term results after orbit reconstruction. Preoperatively, the reconstruction can be planned in advance in virtual form (computer-assisted surgery) and the corresponding reconstruction material required can be produced in a patient-specific manner (▶ Fig. 10.5). Intraoperatively, the use of navigation and intraoperative imagery (3D C-arc, DVT, CT) allows a position check.

Particularly complex is the reconstruction of the anophthalmic orbit (see “Post-enucleation Syndrome” below in the next subsection) to create the ability to accommodate a prosthesis.

10.2.2 Tumor-Induced Orbital Deformities

Various entities of neoplasms of differing dignity can lead to orbital deformity. One-third of all neoplasms in the orbit exhibit signs of malignancy. Among the most frequent symptoms of an orbital neoplasm mentioned in the main are exophthalmos, a facial field defect, a reduction in vision, starting to see double, pain, and conjunctival edema.

Basically, primary tumors have to be differentiated from secondaries of the orbit.[56] Depending on the location with respect to the connective tissue cone of the four straight eye muscles, intraconal neoplasms are also differentiated from extraconal neoplasms. Clinical symptoms, location in relation to the cone, neuroradiological morphology and above all the decade of life in which the initial manifestation occurs often enable a narrowing down of the variable differential diagnoses.[57]

However, as well as the primary intraorbital neoplasms, tumors in neighboring structures can also spread into the orbit.[58] Among benign tumors these are above all tumors of the ancillary structures, tumors of the sinuses, hemangiomas, and lymphangiomas, as well as primary intracranial tumors such as meningiomas and gliomas grade 1. Among malignant tumors with the possibility of spreading into the orbit are also—as well as the corresponding

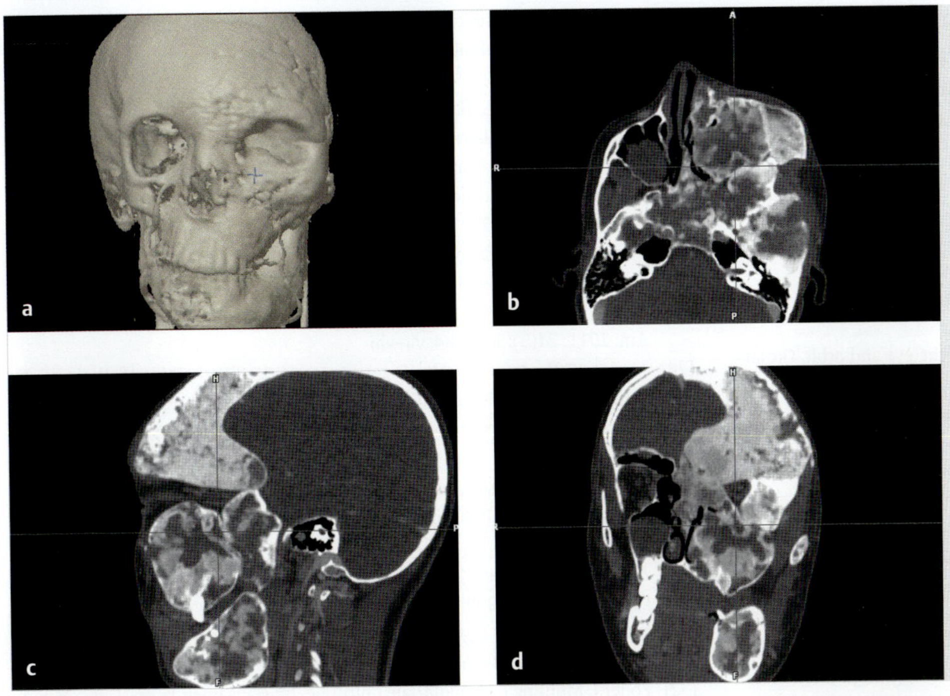

Fig. 10.6 Extensive fibrous dysplasia in three-dimensional reconstruction (a), as well as in axial (b), sagittal (c), and coronal (d) planes.

malignant versions of the tumors mentioned above—periorbital skin tumors such as melanomas, bone tumors of the cerebral and visceral cranium, and soft tissue tumors of the head.

Therapy depending on the entity and dignity. Therapy modalities encompass operative resection, radiotherapy, interventional embolization, and medication. With malignant processes, occasionally various modalities are used in combination. The reconstruction of the orbit often presents a major challenge as here it is not only a matter of bony deformities or defects but functional and aesthetically significant soft tissue parts also have to be replaced.

Preoperative planning is necessary in particular after enucleation or exenteration, and this should have in mind the later prosthetic care desired. Here, a combination of bony reconstruction with local flap plastics or microvascular anastomosed remote flap plastics are mostly used.

Tumorlike Malformations of the Orbit

Disorders of the musculoskeletal system can likewise lead to a deformity of the orbit. in particular fibrous dysplasia, a malformation that occurs mainly in childhood and adolescence and is associated with massive new bone formation, can lead to a grotesque deformation of the orbit. The usually painful bone swelling and the resulting stenosis of the foramina of the bony orbit often then leads to a compression of the optic nerve with the risk of blindness (▶ Fig. 10.6).

Fibrous dysplasia is regarded as a self-limiting disease that is mainly active in childhood and puberty and stabilizes in later adulthood.[59] Hence the treatment philosophy essentially depends on the age of the patient. Surgical treatment in the sense of a remodeling osteotomy for decompression purposes is recommended only if cosmetic disfigurement, pain that cannot be controlled by medication, or compression syndromes arise.[60] Radical resection of fibrous dysplasia, which still favored in the 1980s, is now the subject of much debate. With monostotic forms some authors report a definitive treatment with good functional and aesthetic results.[61] There is no current guideline in place at the time of writing (as of 2016).

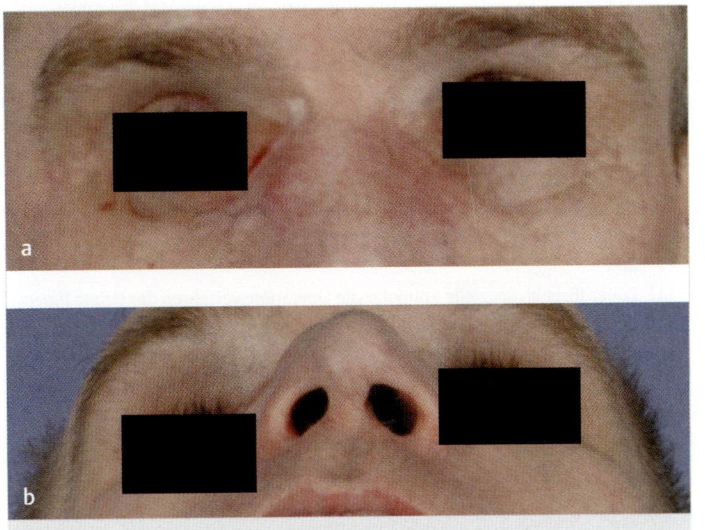

Fig. 10.7 Post-enucleation syndrome with clinical indications of an anophthalmic enophthalmos, a deepened supratarsal crease, and low position of the eye prosthesis.

Post-enucleation Syndrome

After exenteration of the orbit (removal of the contents of the eye socket including the eyeball), so-called post-enucleation syndrome often develops, which is noticeable clinically due to “enophthalmos” of the eye prosthesis and a deepened supratarsal eyelid fold (▶ Fig. 10.7). The correction of these clinical symptoms in a mild case of post-enucleation syndrome can be achieved for a certain time by adjusting the eye prosthesis. This masking effect generally reduces over time through relaxation of the eyelid structures, which can then no longer provide the support needed for movement by the eye prosthesis, with potential luxation. Secondary ptosis results.

Treatment for this intraorbital lack of volume and the decreasing functionality of the eyelid structures constitutes a major challenge not only for the surgeon but also for the eye prosthesis itself.[62] While the lack of volume can be compensated for by the use of fat tissue or by the insertion of alloplastic materials, often it becomes necessary to tighten the eyelid mechanism. For this, techniques are mainly used that can tighten the overstretched eyelid ligament (e.g., a laterally pedicled Tenzel flap or a bridge flap à la Tripier) and thus are able to give the eye prosthesis sufficient support.

References

[1] Levin AV. Congenital eye anomalies. Pediatr Clin North Am. 2003; 50(1):55–76

[2] Guercio JR, Martyn LJ. Congenital malformations of the eye and orbit. Otolaryngol Clin North Am. 2007; 40(1):113–140, vii

[3] Dollfus H, Verloes A. Dysmorphology and the orbital region: a practical clinical approach. Surv Ophthalmol. 2004; 49(6):547–561

[4] Epstein CJ. The new dysmorphology: application of insights from basic developmental biology to the understanding of human birth defects. Proc Natl Acad Sci U S A. 1995; 92(19):8566–8573

[5] Opitz JM. The developmental field concept in clinical genetics. J Pediatr. 1982; 101(5):805–809

[6] Cohen MM, Jr, Lemire RJ. Syndromes with cephaloceles. Teratology. 1982; 25 (2):161–172

[7] Guion-Almeida ML, Richieri-Costa A, Saavedra D, Cohen MM, Jr. Frontonasal dysplasia: analysis of 21 cases and literature review. Int J Oral Maxillofac Surg. 1996; 25(2):91–97

[8] Saavedra D, Richieri-Costa A, Guion-Almeida ML, Cohen MM, Jr. Craniofrontonasal syndrome: study of 41 patients. Am J Med Genet. 1996; 61(2):147–151

[9] Merz E. Kopffehlbildungen Malformations of the head [in German]. In: Merz E, ed. Geburtshilfe [Obstetrics]. 2nd completely revised edition. Stuttgart: Thieme; 2001:234f. Merz E, ed. Sonographische Diagnostik in Gynäkologie und Geburtshilfe [Sonographic Diagnostics in Gynecology and Obstetrics]; vol 2

[10] Burns NS, Iyer RS, Robinson AJ, Chapman T. Diagnostic imaging of fetal and pediatric orbital abnormalities. AJR Am J Roentgenol. 2013; 201(6):W797–808

[11] Zöller JE, et al. Spezielle kraniofaziale Operationsverfahren der Orbita [Special craniofacial operating procedures on the orbit]. In: Zöller JE, Kübler AC, Lorber WD, Mühling J, eds. Kraniofaziale Chirurgie: Diagnostik und Therapie kraniofazialer Fehlbildungen [Craniofacial Surgery: Diagnostics and Treatment of Craniofacial Malformations]. Stuttgart: Thieme; 2003:132–149

[12] Tessier P, Guiot G, Rougerie J, Delbet JP, Pastoriza P. Hypertelorism: cranio-naso-orbito-facial and subethmoid osteotomy. Panminerva Med. 1969; 11(3): 102–116

[13] Saffar M. Ergebnisse der operativen Therapie von Orbitadystopien [Results of operative treatment of orbit dystopies]. In: Der Heidelberger Dokumentenserver [the Heidelberg Document Server]. Heidelberg: University Library. URL: http://www.ub.uni-heidelberg.de/archiv/998. Accessed August 25, 2016

[14] Muhling J, Zöller J, Saffar M, Reinhart E, Reuther J. Results of surgical therapy of bony orbit dystopies. [Article in German]. Mund Kiefer Gesichtschir. 1998; 2 Suppl 1:S94–S97

[15] Golden JA. Holoprosencephaly: a defect in brain patterning. J Neuropathol Exp Neurol. 1998; 57(11):991–999

[16] Converse JM, McCarthy JG. Orbital hypertelorism. Scand J Plast Reconstr Surg. 1981; 15(3):265–276

[17] Jackson IT, Tanner NS, Hide TA. Frontonasal encephalocele–"long nose hypertelorism". Ann Plast Surg. 1983; 11(6):490–500

[18] Smith CG, Gallie BL, Morin JD. Normal and abnormal development of the eye. In: Crawford JS, Morin JD, eds. The Eye in Childhood. New York, NY: Grune and Stratton; 1982:1–18

[19] Torczynski E, Jakobiec FA. Cyclopia and synophthalmia, In: Jakobiec FA, ed. Ocular Anatomy, Embryology and Teratology. Philadelphia, PA: Harper and Row; 1982:143

[20] Gujar SK, Gandhi D. Congenital malformations of the orbit. Neuroimaging Clin N Am. 2011; 21(3):585–602, viii

[21] Verma AS, Fitzpatrick DR. Anophthalmia and microphthalmia. Orphanet J Rare Dis. 2007; 2:47

[22] Fitzpatrick DR, van Heyningen V. Developmental eye disorders. Curr Opin Genet Dev. 2005; 15(3):348–353

[23] Schittkowski MP, Gundlach KK, Guthoff RF. [Congenital clinical anophthalmia and blind microphthalmia]. [Article in German]. Ophthalmologe. 2003; 100 (7):507–517

[24] Harkins CS, Berlin A, Harding RL, Longacre JJ, Snodgrasse RM. A classification of cleft lip and cleft palate. Plast Reconstr Surg Transplant Bull. 1962; 29:31–39

[25] van der Meulen JC, Mazzola R, Vermey-Keers C, Stricker M, Raphael B. A morphogenetic classification of craniofacial malformations. Plast Reconstr Surg. 1983; 71(4):560–572

[26] Tessier P. Anatomical classification facial, cranio-facial and latero-facial clefts. J Maxillofac Surg. 1976; 4(2):69–92

[27] Baxter DJ, Shroff M. Congenital midface abnormalities. Neuroimaging Clin N Am. 2011; 21(3):563–584, vii–viii

[28] Modul 19 Verdauungstrakt [Digestive tract], 19.8 Pathologie [Pathology]. In: Online Embryologiekurs für Studierende der Medizin [Online Embryology Course for Students of Medicine]. Switzerland: Universities of Fribourg, Lausanne, and Bern. http://www.embryology.ch/allemand/sdigestive/patholdigest01.html. Accessed August 25, 2016

[29] Albright AL, Byrd RP. Suture pathology in craniosynostosis. J Neurosurg. 1981; 54(3):384–387

[30] Alden TD, Lin KY, Jane JA. Mechanisms of premature closure of cranial sutures. Childs Nerv Syst. 1999; 15(11–12):670–675

[31] Marchac D, Renier D. Craniofacial surgery for craniosynostosis. Boston, MA: Little, Brown; 1982

[32] Zöller J, Mühling J. Kraniofaziale Chirurgie. In: Hausamen JE, et al.,eds. Mund-, Kiefer- und Gesichtschirurgie Operationslehre und Atlas [Mouth, Jaw and Facial Surgery Operating Techniques]. 4th fully revised ed. Berlin, Heidelberg: Springer; 2012:417–438

[33] Badve CA, K MM, Iyer RS, Ishak GE, Khanna PC. Craniosynostosis: imaging review and primer on computed tomography. Pediatr Radiol. 2013; 43(6):728–742, quiz 725–727

[34] Raulo Y, Tessier P. Fronto-facial advancement for Crouzon's and Apert's syndromes. Scand J Plast Reconstr Surg. 1981; 15(3):245–250

[35] Ortiz-Monasterio F, del Campo AF, Carrillo A. Advancement of the orbits and the midface in one piece, combined with frontal repositioning, for the correction of Crouzon's deformities. Plast Reconstr Surg. 1978; 61(4):507–516

[36] Marchac D, Cophignon J, Neulen JV, Bouchta M. [Osteotomy for advancement of the face and skull]. [Article in French]. Ann Chir Plast. 1974; 19(4):311–323

[37] Bernardy M, Donauer E, Neuenfeldt D. Premature craniosynostosis. A retrospective analysis of a series of 52 cases. Acta Neurochir (Wien). 1994; 128(1–4):88–100

[38] Bottler T. Katamnesen nach chirurgischer Versorgung prämaturer Nahtsynostosen: eine retrospektive Analyse [Catamneses after surgery on premature suture synostoses]. In: Eberhard Karls Universität Tübingen, University Library Publication System. URL: http://nbn-resolving.de/urn:nbn:de:bsz:21-opus-27834. Accessed August 25, 2016

[39] Zöller JE. Kraniofaziale Fehlbildungen [Craniofacial malformations]. In: Schwenzer N, Ehrenfeld M, eds. Mund-Kiefer-Gesichtschirurgie [Mouth-Jaw-Facial Surgery]. 4th, fully revised and expanded edition. Stuttgart: Thieme; 2010:263–280

[40] Kim H, Uppal V, Wallach R. Apert syndrome and fetal hydrocephaly. Hum Genet. 1986; 73(1):93–95

[41] Blaser S, Armstrong D. Congenital malformations of the face. In: King SJ, Boothroyd AE, eds. Pediatric ENT Radiology. Berlin, Heidelberg: Springer; 2002:99–118

[42] Turvey TA, Long RE, Jr, Hall DJ. Multidisciplinary management of Crouzon syndrome. J Am Dent Assoc. 1979; 99(2):205–209

[43] Richardson D, Thiruchelvam JK. Craniofacial surgery for orbital malformations. Eye (Lond). 2006; 20(10):1224–1227

[44] Santos DT, Miyazaki O, Cavalcanti MG. Clinical-embryological and radiological correlations of oculo-auriculo-vertebral spectrum using 3D-CT. Dentomaxillofac Radiol. 2003; 32(1):8–14

[45] Heike CL, Hing AV. Craniofacial microsomia overview. In: Pagon RA, et al., eds. GeneReviews. Seattle, WA: University of Washington; 1993

[46] Dixon MJ. Treacher Collins syndrome. J Med Genet. 1995; 32(10):806–808

[47] Katsanis SH, Jabs EW. Treacher Collins syndrome. In PagonRA, et al., eds. GeneReviews. Seattle, WA: University of Washington; 1993

[48] Posnick JC. Treacher Collins syndrome: perspectives in evaluation and treatment. J Oral Maxillofac Surg. 1997; 55(10):1120–1133

[49] Kamer L, Noser H, Kirsch E, Hammer B. Anatomy-based surgical concepts for individualized orbital decompression surgery in graves orbitopathy. II. Orbital rim position and angulation. Ophthal Plast Reconstr Surg. 2012; 28(4):251–255

[50] Zimmerer R, Schattmann K, Essig H, et al. Efficacy of transcutaneous transseptal orbital decompression in treating acute retrobulbar hemorrhage and a literature review. Craniomaxillofac Trauma Reconstr. 2014; 7(1):17–26

[51] Hidding J, Deitmer T, Hemprich A, Ahrberg W. [Primary correction of orbital fractures using PDS-foil]. [Article in German]. Fortschr Kiefer Gesichtschir. 1991; 36:195–196

[52] Merten HA, Luhr HG. [Resorbable synthetics (PDS foils) for bridging extensive orbital wall defects in an animal experiment comparison]. [Article in German]. Fortschr Kiefer Gesichtschir. 1994; 39:186–190

[53] Essig H, Dressel L, Rana M, et al. Precision of posttraumatic primary orbital reconstruction using individually bent titanium mesh with and without navigation: a retrospective study. Head Face Med. 2013; 9(1):18

[54] Schramm A, Suarez-Cunqueiro MM, Rücker M, et al. Computer-assisted therapy in orbital and mid-facial reconstructions. Int J Med Robot. 2009; 5(2): 111–124

[55] Ellis E, III. Reconstruction of orbital floor defects. J Oral Maxillofac Surg. 2012; 70(10):2255

[56] Eckardt AM, Rana M, Essig H, Gellrich NC. Orbital metastases as first sign of metastatic spread in breast cancer: case report and review of the literature. Head Neck Oncol. 2011; 3:37

[57] Smolarz-Wojnowska A, Essig H, Gellrich NC, Klein CM. [Orbital tumours in children and adolescents. Differential diagnostics and clinical symptoms]. [Article in German]. Ophthalmologe. 2010; 107(6):543–548

[58] Hassler W, Unsöld R, Schick U. Raumforderungen der Orbita. [Masses in the orbit]. Dtsch Arztebl. 2007; 104:A496–A501

[59] Maran AGD, Lund VJ. Clinical Rhinology. Stuttgart: Thieme; 1990

[60] Dämmrich TD, Knapp FB, Boedeker CC, et al. Kraniofaziale Fibröse Dysplasie: Observieren oder Operieren? [Craniofacial fibrous dysplasia: observe or operate?]. Laryngorhinootologie. 2007; 86(3):184–192

[61] Valentini V, Cassoni A, Marianetti TM, Terenzi V, Fadda MT, Iannetti G. Craniomaxillofacial fibrous dysplasia: conservative treatment or radical surgery? A retrospective study on 68 patients. Plast Reconstr Surg. 2009; 123(2):653–660

[62] Rana M, Essig H, Rücker M, Gellrich NC. Development and demonstration of a novel computer planning solution for predefined correction of enophthalmos in anophthalmic patients using prebended 3D titanium-meshes–a technical note. J Oral Maxillofac Surg. 2012; 70(11):e631–e638

Chapter 11

Tumors of the Orbit and the Eye

11 Tumors of the Orbit and the Eye

11.1 Malignant Tumors of the Eye

B. Wiechens

Depending on their origin, tumors of the orbit can be divided into primary, secondary, and metastatic lesions. While primary tumors originate directly from different types of tissue in the orbit, secondary tumors represent a transmission from neighboring anatomical structures such as the eye, the sinuses, the skull base and the eyelids. Metastases can also occur from primary tumors arising in other sites than the orbit but also in the eye itself. The vast majority of these tumors are carcinomas. Sarcomas, however, metastasize less frequently into the orbit.[1] In general, more than 50% of orbital neoplasms are nonprimary orbital tumors.[2]

11.1.1 Tumors of the Eye with Potential Orbital Involvement

Retinoblastoma

Epidemiology

The retinoblastoma is the most common intraocular tumor in childhood, with an incidence of approximately one new case in 18–20,000 live births/year. Thus in Germany there are 60 new cases per year, 200 to 300 in the United States,[3] and worldwide there are some 5,000 to 8,000 new cases per year.[4]

11

The incidence is very similar in all western countries. There is no predilection with regard to sex or ethnic origin. Since the tumor consists of primitive retinal cells, which as a result of differentiation disappear in the first few years of life, the vast majority of retinoblastomas occur before the fifth to eighth year of life.[4] Later manifestations are possible, but very rare. Within the last 100 years the mortality rate of retinoblastoma has decreased from 95% to below 5%.[1] However, it must be emphasized that even today an *untreated* tumor is nearly always fatal as spontaneous regression occurs very rarely (see "Retinoma" below).

Symptoms

Leukocoria is a pathognomonic symptom indicating, among others, retinoblastoma (▸ Fig. 11.1). When an examination light is shone through the pupil, a red-orange reflection from a healthy ocular fundus is normal; a white-yellow reflection is caused by pathologic intraocular changes such as white retinoblastoma tissue. Due to the frequently associated visual impairment, secondary strabismus can occur. If the duration of these symptoms is unclear, the parents of affected children should be asked for old photographs from which to check whether a squint or leukocoria had been present before. In advanced stages of the disease, secondary glaucoma can occur. Because leukocoria is not present in every case of retinoblastoma, bilateral funduscopy (dilated pupil) should be carried out in every newly diagnosed case of strabismus in young children. Orbital extension with proptosis and a unilateral unresponsive pupil is a potential complication and carries a poor prognosis, especially in developing countries. Immediate investigation is strongly recommended to differentiate retinoblastoma from other sight threatening diseases such as congenital cataract, retinopathy of prematurity (ROP), idiopathic primary hyperplastic vitreous (PHPV), or Coats's disease.

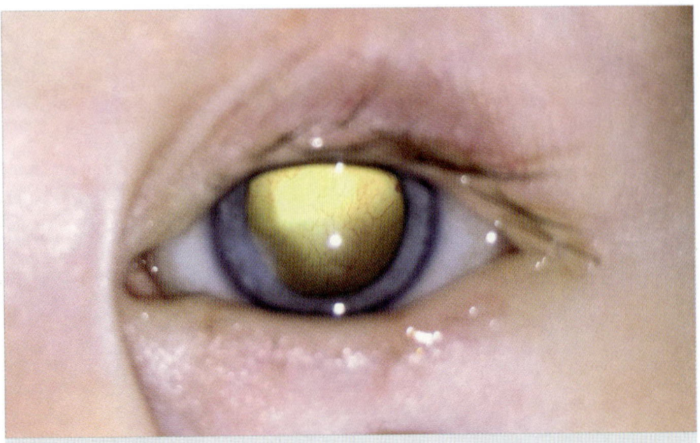

Fig. 11.1 Leukocoria (left eye).

Depending on the symptoms and findings at initial presentation, an ophthalmologic and strabological examination (in case of strabismus) has to be made. A binophthalmoscopic funduscopy is mandatory. As retinoblastoma is most frequently diagnosed within the first 2 years of life (bilateral retinoblastoma is usually detected 10–12 months earlier than unilateral retinoblastoma because of bilateral symptoms) an urgent presentation in a specialized eye hospital for an examination under a general anesthesia with ultrasonography should be arranged if retinoblastoma is suspected.[5]

Retinoblastomas can arise unilaterally or bilaterally, unifocally or multifocally. The growth pattern of retinoblastomas is either exophytic (i.e., under the retina), endophytic (i.e., in the vitreous chamber with secondary involvement of the anterior chamber), or mixed. Vitreous seeding can take place in an early stage of the disease, when the tumor is still rather small. In cases with diffuse infiltration of the vitreous or the aqueous humor ("pseudohypopyon"), these findings can be falsely interpreted as an intraocular inflammation. In this event an echography should be carried out. Intraocular calcifications give a hint for the diagnosis of retinoblastoma. In assumed retinoblastoma, intraocular biopsy should be **avoided** to prevent seeding of retinoblastoma tumor cells with considerable deterioration of the prognosis. If a retinoblastoma is suspected or confirmed, patient must be presented to a national reference center for the treatment of retinoblastoma (in Germany, e.g., the Department of Ophthalmology, University Hospital Essen).

Genetics

The genesis of retinoblastoma is triggered by the inactivation of both alleles of the retinoblastoma gene (*RB1*, chromosome 13q) in still-undifferentiated retinal precursor cells. About 45% of patients have a heritable form of retinoblastoma (heritable retinoblastoma); in ~55% of patients there is a nonheritable form, which frequently occurs unilaterally.[6,7]

Investigation of the genetics of retinoblastoma was pioneered by A.G. Knudson in 1971. He was the first to describe the two-mutation theory, confirmed later by genetic studies.[8] According to this theory a new mutation of the *RB1* gene (tumor suppressor gene, chromosome 13) occurs in the germ cells of one of the parents (germinal mutation). Thus all body cells carry the genetic mutation in the form of an inactivated allele. If, during the course of embryological development in the immature retinal precursor cells, the second allele is lost, then the development of retinoblastoma is the result. This is the reason for the bilateral appearance of heritable retinoblastoma. Multifocal tumor growth is typical.

In the nonheritable form of retinoblastoma both mutations required for tumor development occur in body cells (somatic mutation). Both mutations have to be present in the same cell. This being a very rare event, usually only one eye is affected with a predominantly monofocal growth pattern.

In heritable retinoblastoma, in family members usually both eyes are affected.[9] These members are at risk of passing on the mutated *RB1* gene in ~50% to their offspring. However, with incomplete penetrance, the risk of developing the disease is lower. In some of these families, only unilateral and unifocal retinoblastomas occur as a result of reduced expression.

When a retinoblastoma has been conclusively diagnosed, genetic testing and counseling of the family must always be undertaken to identify the carriers of an *RB1* gene mutation. Patients may continue to develop new tumors for a few years after diagnosis and treatment; for this reason, they need to be examined frequently.

The classification of retinoblastoma was elaborated in the decades after the Reese–Ellsworth classification was developed in the 1960s. As this classification does not contain a classic staging system, new classifications, such as the ABC classification, are now being developed that follow current therapeutic guidelines.

Trilateral Retinoblastoma

In approximately 5 to 10% of children with heritable retinoblastoma, a simultaneous pineoblastoma can develop. This rare event is associated with a very poor prognosis. Pineal gland cyst detected by MRI must be distinguished from these malignant tumors.

Retinoma

Retinoma or retinocytoma is a retinoblastoma that has spontaneously regressed. However, this condition is only found in ~2% of family members of children suffering from retinoblastoma. Clinically, this tumor presents like a retinoblastoma in regression.[9] Patients with a retinoma should likewise have regular clinical and ophthalmologic check-ups and be provided with genetic counseling.

Orbital Involvement of Retinoblastoma

The earlier the diagnosis of a retinoblastoma is made, the better the prognosis with respect to life expectancy and visual acuity. As in all malignant tumors, retinoblastoma bears the risk of tumor invasion and spread. Depending on the tumor's location, it can spread into all areas of the eye, predominantly into the choroid, the ocular vessels, and the optic nerve. It should be noted that extraocular tumor growth via the posterior ciliary circulation or the other vascular systems is rather rare. Most often extraocular tumor growth occurs along the optic nerve.[10] Tumors that extend beyond the lamina cribrosa are usually associated with a poor prognosis. If there is evidence for optic nerve involvement after enucleation, further imaging and cytopathologic diagnosis is necessary including assessment of the cerebrospinal fluid. As well as the local tumor invasion into the orbit, there is a risk for distant metastases depending on the duration of the disease. Today the prognosis of the disease and the risk for other relatives to be affected can be determined by pathological and molecular genetic examination of fresh tumor specimen and of serological samples.

Treatment of Unilateral Retinoblastomas

Because of mild symptoms the diagnosis of unilateral retinoblastomas is often delayed, so that at the initial examination the disease can be in an advanced stage. Treatment options are mainly guided by the localization of the tumor or tumors and how the prognosis is assessed. Enucleation of the affected eye is the treatment of choice if the tumor is at an advanced stage with de facto blindness, or if the primary tumor has developed in such an unfavorable location that usable visual acuity cannot be achieved by another form of treatment.[5]

An attempt of eye-saving treatment is indicated for solitary tumors, for those tumors in favorable location, and if an acceptable visual acuity can be preserved. Therapeutic approach consists of brachytherapy using ruthenium 106/rhodium 106, iodine 125, or iridium 192 plaques or of repeated photocoagulation and cryocoagulation of very small tumors. Treatment options should be discussed in detail with the parents of the patient.

Patients should be monitored lifelong with ophthalmologic and medical examination.

Treatment of Bilateral Retinoblastomas

Treatment of bilateral (heritable) retinoblastomas usually combines surgical and medical therapeutic approaches. Percutaneous radiotherapy, which was often carried out in earlier times, has been abandoned due to the high risk of subsequent neoplasms (such as osteogenic sarcoma) occurring at a later age.[5]

Primary polychemotherapy in combination with local photocoagulation, transpupillary laser hyperthermia, or cryocoagulation can be associated with a higher recurrence rate. For this reason the treatment strategy must be determined in each case individually, according to the findings of both eyes, and discussed with the parents.

If seeding of tumor cells into the vitreous body of the more affected eye has occurred and this eye is virtually blind, attempts to preserve the eye are usually unsuccessful and primary enucleation is inevitable. However, if significant tumor regression can be expected following chemotherapy even in the more severely affected eye, and if there is the potential for visual improvement, enucleation can be postponed until final tumor regression can be assessed. If preservation of the eye and of a useful visual acuity is then an option, subsequent brachytherapy (e.g., ruthenium 106/rhodium 106) or treatment by adjuvant photocoagulation and/or transpupillary laser hyperthermia can be given.

In the less affected eye (i.e., the eye with better visual acuity), monitoring of the effect of polychemotherapy, followed by local therapy (brachytherapy, photocoagulation, etc.) if necessary, is justified. In all cases, however, close follow-up is mandatory as recurrences are to be expected.

Recently, at the Departments of Ophthalmology and Pediatrics at the University of Essen, Germany, a successful outcome to primary treatment was achieved in 75% of the eyes by administration of a chemotherapy regimen modified from an established protocol using cyclophosphamide, vincristine, etoposide, and carboplatin. Although tumors in categories A and B were controlled in 75% (of 56 eyes) and 85%, respectively, the failure rate was significantly higher (83%) in larger tumors of categories D/E.[11] Recently, Abramson and coworkers from the Memorial Sloan Kettering Cancer Center in New York published the 2-year results of intra-arterial chemotherapy with melphalan, topotecan, and carboplatin (superselective intra-arterial chemotherapy, 76 eyes of 67 patients).[12] With this therapeutic approach the rate of enucleation could be significantly reduced and eyes could be salvaged in 83%.

Treatment of Retinoblastoma with Orbital Involvement

Orbital involvement of a retinoblastoma is a rare occurrence in developed countries. A transscleral spread is regarded as an extraocular manifestation because the risk of a further spread of the tumor into the meninges, the brain, and the cerebrospinal fluid. The risk of distant metastases is significantly elevated, accompanied by a poor prognosis. There are no proven treatment protocols for orbital retinoblastoma. An individual multimodal therapeutic approach is needed. According to the recommendations of the National Cancer Institute in the United States, surgical treatment should be postponed until the response to polychemotherapy can be assessed. Further treatment options are surgery (enucleation of the eye, orbital exenteration), additional chemotherapy, and external beam radiation therapy (40–45 Gy).[13]

Follow-ups and Prognosis

Once the treatment has been completed, regular ophthalmological and pediatric-oncologic check-ups should be performed (approximately on a 4-weekly basis, where applicable under general anesthesia). If a recurrence is diagnosed early, the tumor can be brought under control by means of local treatment. Depending on the findings and the age of the patient, the follow-up intervals can then be extended. Regular check-ups, however, should take place up to the fifth year of life. These should always include binophthalmoscopic fundus examinations. Additionally, in patients with heritable retinoblastoma, regular MRI follow-up images should be obtained in collaboration with the pediatric and radiological departments to exclude trilateral retinoblastoma.

As mentioned above, the chances of curing a retinoblastoma have dramatically improved over the recent decades due to the development of interdisciplinary treatment strategies and close controls. Today, through early diagnosis, adequate interdisciplinary therapy, and regular follow-ups, success rates of over 95% can be achieved.

Choroidal Melanoma

Epidemiology

Choroidal melanoma is the most common primary malignant intraocular tumor in adults. While it is extremely rare in blacks, the incidence in whites is between 6 (USA) and 8 (Scandinavia) new cases per year and 1,000,000 inhabitants.[5,14] There is no clear gender predilection. Whereas females under the age of 40 years are affected more frequently, more males are affected in the older age group.[14] Choroidal melanoma is rarely found in children or young adults. The prevalence in patients under the age of 20 years is 1.1%.[15] From the fifth decade of life onward, choroidal melanoma occurs more often, reaching its maximum between sixth and eighth decades. Thus it is a typical, most commonly unilateral tumor of middle and older age.

Etiological factors for choroidal melanomas are unclear. In particular, risk factors for cutaneous melanoma (e.g., exposure to UV radiation) have not been shown to be significant for the development of choroidal melanoma.[16,17,18] The two tumors are distinct from each other. The risk for transformation of choroidal nevi into a choroidal melanoma depends on the prominence of the lesion (> 2 mm), the presence of subretinal fluid, clinical symptoms, orange pigment, and tumor margins within 3 mm of the optic disc.[19] There are reports of isolated cases of higher familial clustering. Occupational and chemical exposure may increase risk in certain professions,[20] as well as a presumed pathogenetic relevance of exposure to electromagnetic radiation.[21]

Symptoms

The extent and course of the symptoms depend considerably on the location of the tumor and concomitant diseases. Melanomas located in the ciliary body and in the peripheral retina may remain without symptoms for a long time, whereas patients notice visual disturbances earlier if the macula is involved, due to direct tumor growth or serous detachment. Thus, peripheral melanomas are often discovered accidentally during a routine examination or at an advanced stage when either the optical axis is obscured or a compression-induced cataract develops. Often patients indicate only nonspecific symptoms of visual deterioration, while pain is not a typical complaint related to melanoma unless intraocular inflammation, extraocular growth, or neovascular glaucoma occur in advanced stages. There is previous history of malignancy in 6 to 10% of all patients with choroidal melanoma. Patients should therefore be asked whether they have had other neoplasms in the past.[14]

Binophthalmoscopic funduscopy can be regarded as the standard procedure for diagnosis. More than 90% of choroidal melanomas can be identified with this technique (▶ Fig. 11.2). Typical

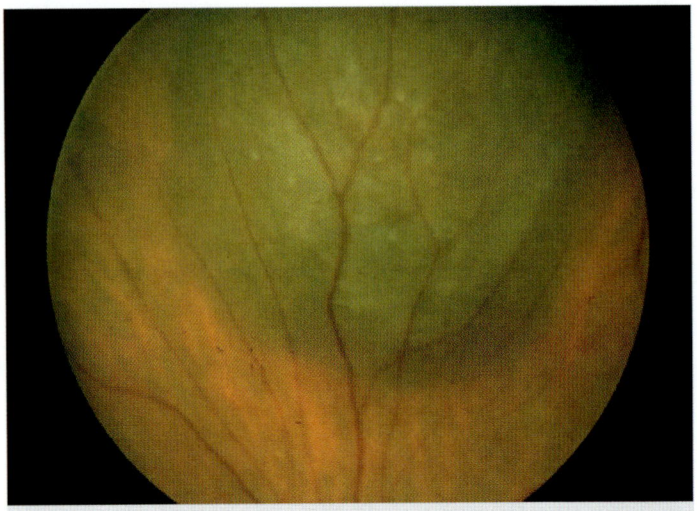

Fig. 11.2 Uveal melanoma.

characteristics are pigmentation on the tumor´s surface, "orange pigment," and the occasional visualization of the tumor's own vascular system as well as an accompanying serous detachment in melanomas with a prominence more than 3 to 4 mm. Dilatation and increased tortuosity of episcleral veins can be observed in peripheral melanomas, predominantly in the ciliary body. If a ciliary body melanoma is suspected, gonioscopy can help to evaluate whether the tumor has already infiltrated the iridocorneal angle. In ophthalmoscopy, and more so in ultrasound, a mushroom or collar-button shape of the tumor is pathognomonic. Unfortunately, however, there are melanomas that do not present this typical form.

Genetics

Usually choroidal melanomas are genetically homogeneous with specific cytogenetic aberrations.[14] Several studies have shown that these variations in the primary tumors influence their metastasizing potential. In some tumors monosomy of chromosome 3 has been demonstrated.[22] This particular chromosomal aberration correlates with a higher risk of distant metastases and with a poor survival rate. Today it is possible to predict this risk by means of molecular-genetic investigations and chromosomal analyses.[23] It must be discussed whether patients wish the results of this analysis to be disclosed.[5]

Diagnostics

In most cases clinically suspected choroidal melanoma can be confirmed by A- and B-mode ultrasonography. In A-mode-sonography choroidal melanomas demonstrate a typical medium to low internal echoes with sound attenuation as well as vascular pulsations. Whereas the measurement of the thickness can often be determined more precisely in A-mode sonography, B-mode sonography is advantageous to assess the dimensions of the tumor.

Further investigations such as fluorescein or ICG (indocyanine green) angiography or optical coherence tomography are only occasionally needed. Currently the role of magnetic resonance imaging for diagnosis has not been definitively clarified. It can be helpful in those cases, in which clinically and sonographically an older, prominent subretinal hemorrhage alone or camouflaging a melanoma cannot be differentiated from a melanoma alone.

Occasionally a transretinal biopsy of the tumor has to be performed, especially in amelanotic melanomas, which can mimic intraocular metastases or chorioretinal inflammatory processes. The risk of tumor cell seeding caused by the biopsy itself appears very low,[24,25,26] however, surgeons should refrain from transscleral biopsies of the tumor base.[5]

Orbital Involvement of the Choroidal Melanoma

Melanomas can lead to orbital involvement by spreading via the emissary vessels and along the optic nerve.[27] Extrascleral spread occurs in 10 to 15% of patients with choroidal melanoma,[10] associated with a significantly increased risk of distant metastases. Although fewer than 2% of patients have distant metastases at the time of diagnosis only, 40 to 50% of all patients will eventually die of distant metastases over the course of the disease. Most common sites of metastases are the liver (~90%), lungs (~24%), and bones (~16%).[28] If metastases occur in the liver, the average survival time is about 6 months, with a chance of survival of 15 to 20% for 1 year and ~10% for 2 years.[29,30] The prognosis is poor if extraocular growth and orbital involvement are present at the time of diagnosis (mortality rate between 73 and 81%).[31]

Therapy

The earlier hypothesis that primary enucleation of the affected eye improves the survival rate of the patients was not supported by many studies. According to these studies there is no statistically significant difference for the survival rate among those patients being enucleated, with and without accompanying radiotherapy,[32] and those with primary enucleation or globe-preserving brachytherapy.[33] Poor prognosis of choroidal melanoma is associated with multiple factors, such as older age at presentation, male sex, larger tumor basal diameter and thickness, ciliary body location, diffuse tumor configuration, melanocytosis, extraocular tumor extension, advanced tumor staging, epithelioid cell type, high mitotic activity, higher microvascular density, higher expression of IGF-1 receptor and HLA-class-I- and -II, monosomy 3, and other factors.[34] Depending on the size and location of the tumor as well as the prognosis in regard to visual acuity, eye-preserving treatment—if possible—should be discussed with the patient. However, the patient must be made aware that this form of treatment is more time-consuming and requires lifelong follow-up examinations.

A wait-and-see approach along with regular follow-ups is justified in patients with small tumors and suspected melanoma, depending on the localization and the clinical symptoms. If progression becomes evident treatment has to be initiated.

Treatment options in small tumors are photocoagulation,[35] photodynamic therapy,[36] transpupillary thermotherapy,[37] and brachytherapy.[38,39] Additional treatment options for tumors with a thickness of up to 6 mm is brachytherapy using ruthenium 106/rhodium 106, iodine 125, or palladium 103 plaques (cobalt 60, strontium 90, and cesium 131 have also been used), percutaneous radiation therapy with protons and helium ions, as well as the Leksell Gamma knife.[40,41,42,43]

11

For tumors with a thickness exceeding 6 mm, iodine 125 applicators have to be used. Due to the greater thickness and the higher dose of radiation, a higher incidence of radiogenic complications such as optic nerve atrophy, cataract, secondary glaucoma, and radiation retinopathy have to be reckoned with when treating larger tumors.[44,45] It is recommended that the scleral dose should not exceed 1,500 Gy. Further therapeutic options are transscleral local resection of the tumor in deep arterial hypotony as well as endoresection combined with adjuvant radiotherapy.[46,47,48] If an extraocular growth is suspected at the time of presentation, a combined radiotherapy and modified enucleation with tenonectomy or orbital exenteration should be planned depending on the nature of the extraocular growth (flat, nodular, suspicion of involvement of the vortex veins).[49] If an extrascleral spread of the choroidal melanoma is discovered during the operation upon inspection of the enucleated globe, likewise a modified enucleation with tenonectomy and subsequent radiotherapy has to be carried out. A similar treatment modality is followed if extraocular involvement is not discovered until the histological examination of the enucleated eye.

Potential extension of the treatment with subsequent radiotherapy must always be discussed with the patient prior to surgery.

Follow-ups and Prognosis

Today's operating procedures and radio-oncological methods enable better local tumor control. Despite these efforts, the survival rate of patients with choroidal melanoma has basically not changed over the last 30 years. If distant metastases develop or if they already exist at initial presentation, chemotherapy is the only therapeutic option. In spite of oncologic therapy, life expectancy in metastatic melanoma is about 6 to 9 months only. However, one should bear in mind that patients with asymptomatic metastases have a slightly longer survival time than symptomatic patients. Accordingly it should be discussed with the patient whether the limited benefits of chemotherapy outweigh the serious side effects and the reduced quality of life.

In those patients in whom local tumor control has been achieved, lifelong follow-examinations with oncologic check-ups (including ultrasonography of the liver) are recommended.

11.1.2 Intraocular Metastases

Epidemiology

In the United States, like in other western industrial countries, after heart disease (614,348 deaths), malignancies are the second most common cause of death (591,699 deaths).[50] In the United States, there will be an estimated 1,685,210 new cancer cases with an estimated 595,690 cancer deaths in 2016. The most frequent cancer types are breast cancer with a total of 249,260 new cases per year and lung/bronchial cancer with a total of 224,390 new cases in 2016, followed by prostate (180,890 new cases/year) and colorectal cancer (134,490 new cases/year).[51] Estimated deaths in 2016 are 158,080 due to lung/bronchial cancer, 49,190 due to colorectal cancer, and 40,890 due to breast cancer.[51]

11

The eye and its adnexa can be affected either by metastases of a distant primary tumor or by invasion of primary tumors from adjacent anatomical structures such as the paranasal sinuses, the eyelids, the surface of the eye, or the orbit. Most frequently ocular metastases occur by hematogenous tumor cell seeding. In rare cases the eye can also be involved indirectly in paraneoplastic syndromes or by toxic adverse effects from chemotherapy.

First descriptions of a choroidal metastasis [52,53] were given by Horner (1864) and later by Perl (1872). In an evaluation of 8,712 cancer patients, Gottfredsen reported only 6 cases (0.07%) with choroidal metastases.[54] Accordingly, in the first half of the 20th century the frequency of intraocular metastases was regarded as relatively low. However, by systematic examination of autopsy material, in the second half of the century a markedly higher incidence of intraocular metastases was found. In their pioneering histological examination of autopsy material from 230 patients with metastasizing carcinomas, Bloch and Gartner discovered choroidal metastases in 10% of cases.[55] Four years prior to that, Albert and colleagues had found choroidal metastases in 2.0% (bronchial carcinoma) and in 7.7% (breast cancer) by ophthalmological examinations on 213 asymptomatic patients with known metastasizing tumors.[56] The authors concluded that the risk of choroidal metastases is apparently higher than hitherto has been assumed in the literature.[56,57] In further studies by Nelson and coworkers as well as by Eliassi-Rad et al, previous estimates of incidence rates could be confirmed (9.3% and 12.6%).[58,59]

Most often (82%) intraocular metastases derive from carcinoma, whereas sarcomas are less frequently the primary tumors.[60]

Breast Cancer

Between 40 and 49% of all choroidal metastases are caused by breast carcinoma.[60,61,62] As would be expected, women are affected most often, whereas choroidal metastases in men caused by breast cancer are extremely rare.[60]

The risk of metastases to the choroid is lower than into other organs such as bones, brain, kidneys, and other internal organs. The incidence is reported to be 0.07 to 37%.[63] The risk of intraocular metastases rises from 5% to 11% in asymptomatic patients if more than one organ contains metastases.[64]

Lung Cancer

The second most frequent primary tumor prone for intraocular metastasis is lung carcinoma. The prevalence varies between 14 and 30%.[60,61,62] The vast majority of patients are male (67.3%);[60] of these, 78.3% are smokers. According to a study by Singh et al, adenocarcinomas are the most frequent cause of choroidal metastases, followed by squamous cell carcinomas and small cell bronchial carcinomas.[65]

Other Primary Tumors

Other primary tumors bearing the risk of ocular metastasis are neoplasms of the gastrointestinal tract (~4%), of the kidneys (~2–4%), of the skin (0–2%), and of prostate (1.3–3.6%), cutaneous melanoma (0–4.5%), as well as others (5–20.9%).[60,61,62]

In asymptomatic cancer patients (e.g., breast and lung cancer or other primary tumors) intraocular metastases may be discovered before the actual primary tumor is diagnosed. The ensuing search for tumor can finally lead to the diagnosis. Nevertheless, in their study of 420 patients with choroidal metastases, Shields et al. did not find a primary tumor in 17% of patients (73 of 520 eyes).[60]

Clinical Findings

The most frequent intraocular site of metastases is the uvea. Although the iris or the ciliary body is involved in 4–11% of patients, the vast majority of metastases arise in the posterior choroid (88 to > 90%).[59,60,61]

Anterior Uvea (Iris and Ciliary Body)

Many primary tumors are able to metastasize into the iris and the ciliary body. Regardless of the histology of the primary malignancy, choroidal metastases appear relatively similar as yellowish-orange to brownish lesions, sometimes with exact margins, but often with unclear boundaries to the surrounding iris stroma (▶ Fig. 11.3, ▶ Fig. 11.4, ▶ Fig. 11.5). Metastases in the ciliary body and the iridocorneal angle can lead to a subsequent occlusion of epibulbar vessels. If congestion of scleroconjunctival vessels cannot be attributed to an extraocular disease, one should always search for an intraocular malignancy. In the initial stage of the disease this can quite often only be assessed by gonioscopy or ultrasound biomicroscopy. Occasionally metastases of the ciliary body, and even more so iris metastases, can be associated with symptoms such as an anterior chamber hematoma (hyphema), pseudohypopyon (▶ Fig. 11.6, ▶ Fig. 11.7), rubeosis iridis, anterior and posterior synechiae, displacement of the iridocorneal angle with ocular hypertension and uveitis.

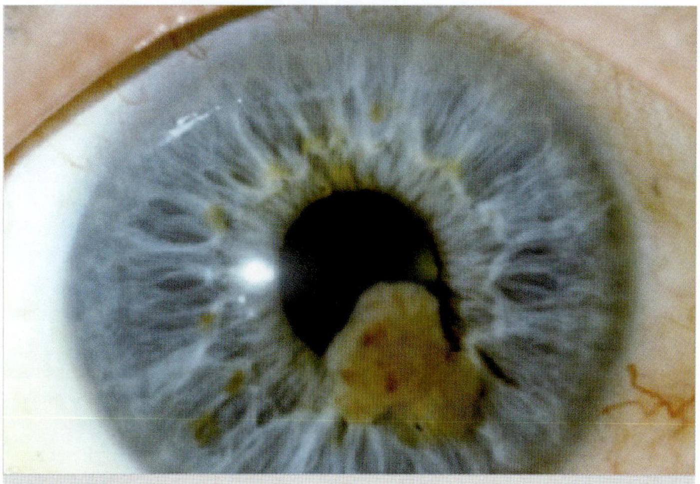

Fig. 11.3 Metastasis of lung cancer in the iris.

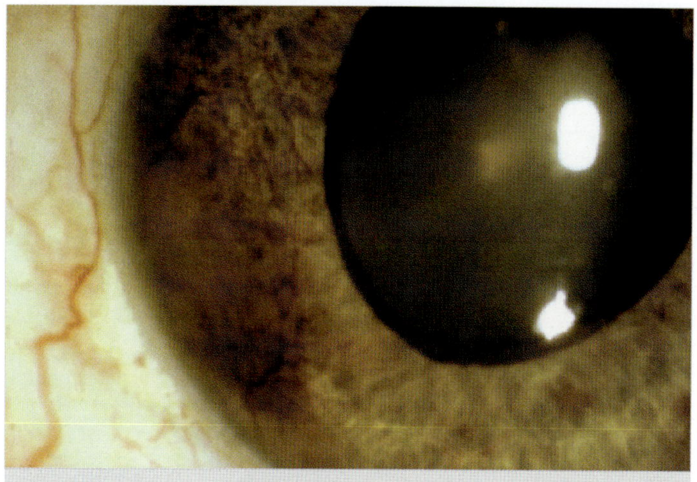

Fig. 11.4 Metastasis of hypernephroid carcinoma in the iris.

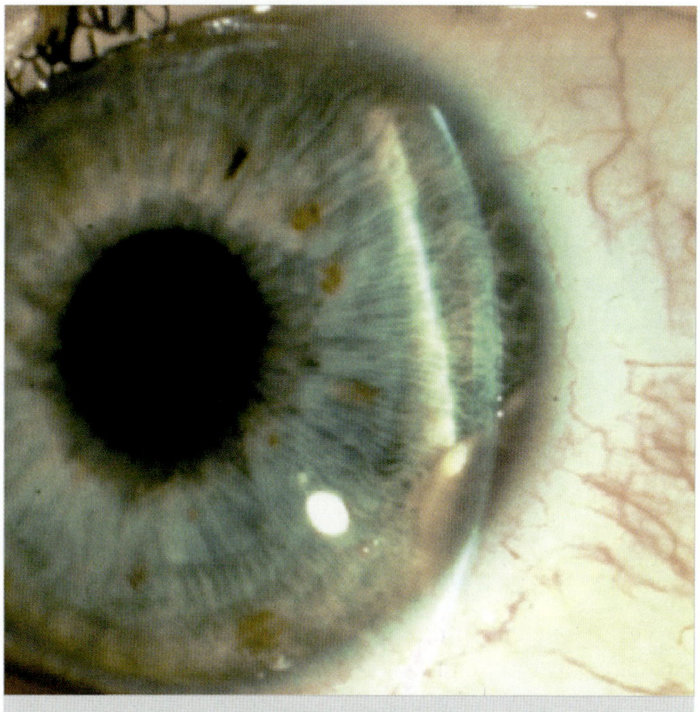

Fig. 11.5 Metastasis of breast cancer in the iris.

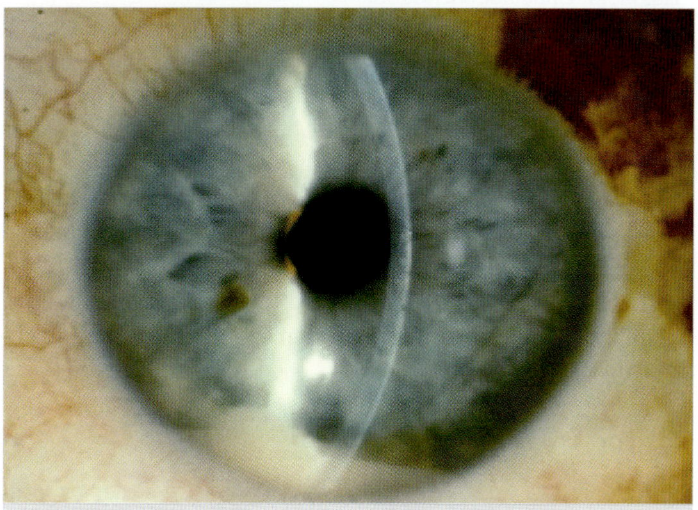

Fig. 11.7 Pseudohypopyon due to metastasis of malignant non-Hodgkin lymphoma.

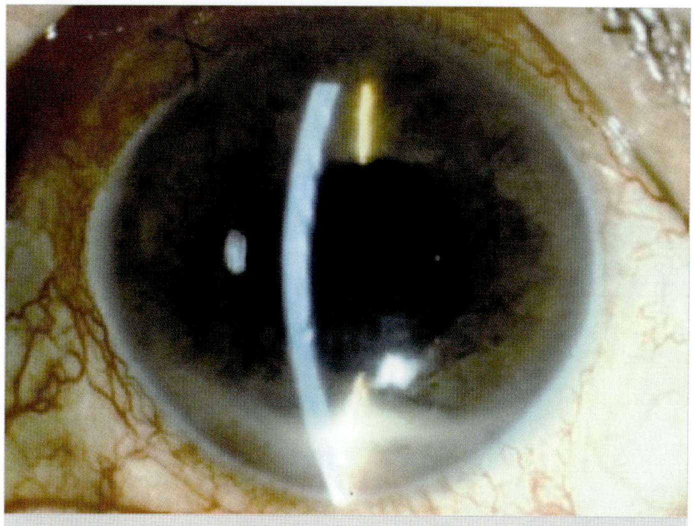

Fig. 11.6 Pseudohypopyon due to a metastasis of breast cancer.

Depending on the history and the age of the patient, there should be consideration of primary iris and ciliary body tumors such as amelanotic melanoma, iris cysts, or retinoblastoma; inflammatory diseases such as a granulomatous uveitis; and granulomas after foreign body injury.

Posterior Uvea (Choroid)

As mentioned earlier, in the vast majority of cases metastases occur in the posterior choroid. Although choroidal metastases occur more frequently than previously thought (5–9%), the majority of patients report a painless impairment of vision and defects in the visual field.

Irrespective of the underlying primary tumor most choroidal metastases are flat or slightly prominent and of gray-whitish to yellow-whitish and plaquelike appearance. They can occur monofocally or, quite often, multifocally or confluently, unilaterally or bilaterally; they usually exhibit only minimal pigment changes; and they are rarely associated with retinal or vitreous hemorrhage (▶ Fig. 11.8, ▶ Fig. 11.9, ▶ Fig. 11.10). In a study by Shields et al[60] choroidal metastases were accompanied by an exudative retinal detachment in 73% of eyes. While even an extensive associated retinal detachment can remain without any clinical

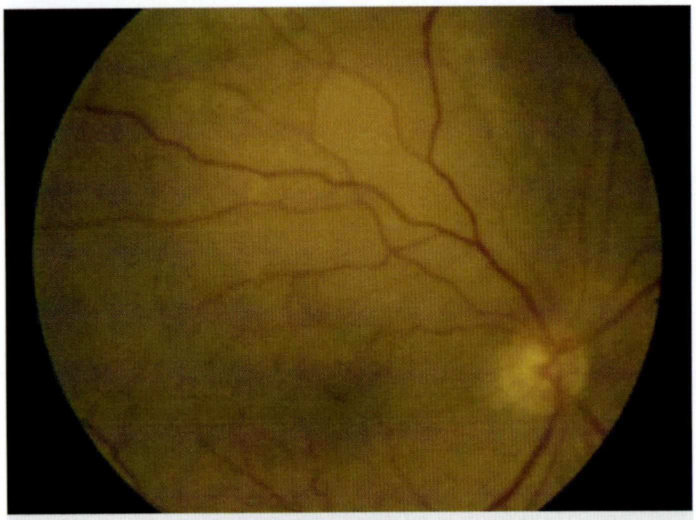

Fig. 11.8 Monofocal choroidal metastasis of lung cancer.

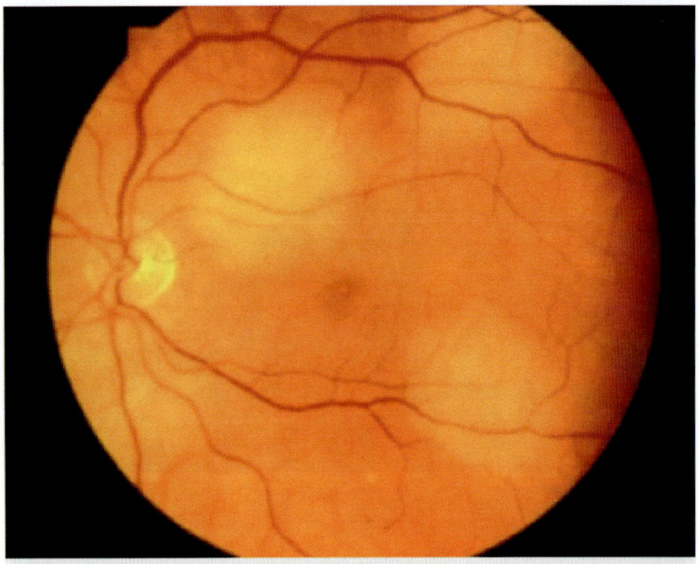

Fig. 11.9 Multifocal choroidal metastases of breast cancer.

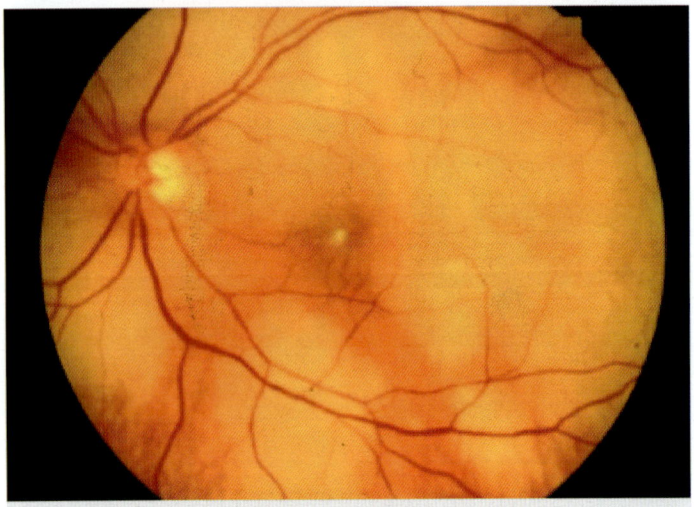

Fig. 11.10 Confluent choroidal breast cancer metastases.

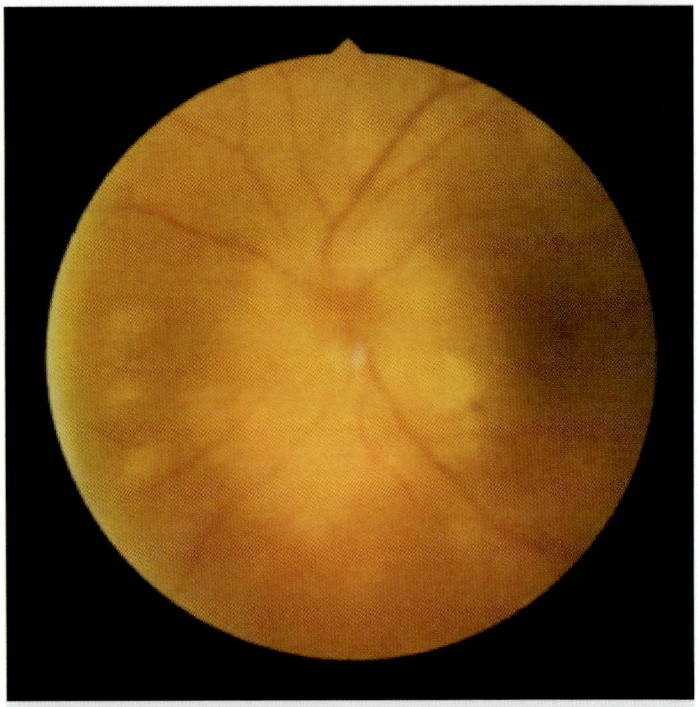

Fig. 11.11 Optic disc metastasis.

symptoms if located in the periphery, minimal accumulation of subretinal/intraretinal fluid in the center of the retina can lead to early visual deterioration. After regression of choroidal metastases, often lesions with fuzzy margins and overlying pigment epithelial changes or subretinal fluid remain funduscopically visible.

Differential diagnosis should include, among other possibilities, inflammatory diseases (e.g., granulomatous uveitis, chorioretinitis, Vogt–Koyanagi–Harada syndrome, *Pneumocystis carinii* infection) as well as osteoma, choroidal hemangioma, amelanotic melanomas, and nevi.

Optic Disc and Optic Nerve

Metastases of the optic disc/nerve are rather rare at ~4.5% of cases.[65] Beside a primary involvement of the optic disc or the spread of a metastatic lesion from the choroid into the disc and into the optic nerve or, vice versa, an intraocular extension of a metastasis primarily located in the optic nerve to the disc is also possible. Shields et al observed an associated juxtapapillary choroidal lesion in 74% of eyes.[65]

Symptoms and the clinical picture are usually nonspecific. Hence many patients complain of a gradual, sometimes even acute deterioration of vision and visual field defects as well as of color vision disturbances. A relative afferent pupillary defect occurs quite often. Clinical signs are an edematous optic disc with flamelike hemorrhages and tortuosity of congested venous blood vessels (▶ Fig. 11.11, ▶ Fig. 11.12). In late stages, atrophy of the optic disc can develop.

Differential diagnosis comprises optic neuritis, acute anterior ischemic optic neuropathy, papilledema, optic disc drusen, and capillary hemangiomas.

Retina

Retinal metastases are extremely rare. They arise either by local infiltration of choroidal metastases or by direct hematogenous tumor cell seeding into the retina. Usually they appear as circumscribed, mostly whitish lesions, occasionally with accompanying retinal hemorrhages, adjacent vitreoretinal changes such as

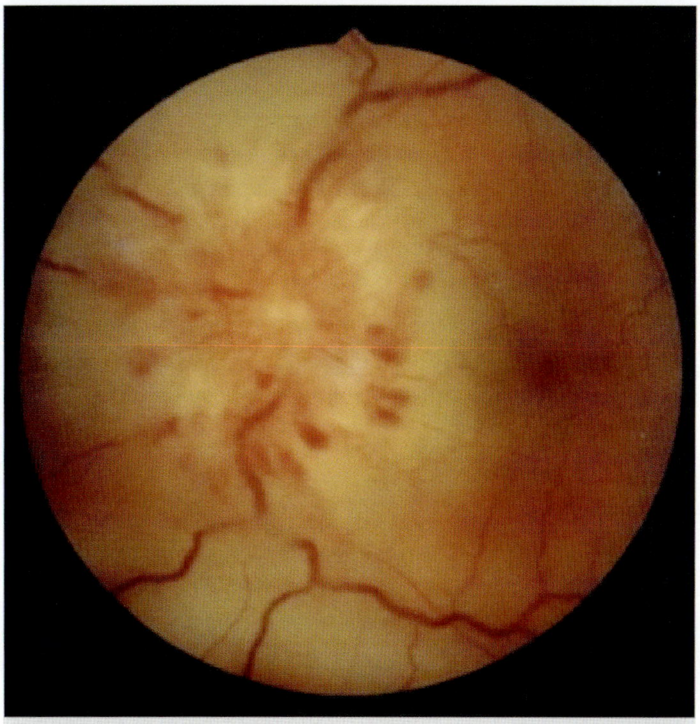

Fig. 11.12 Significant papilledema and optic disc hemorrhage due to metastasis.

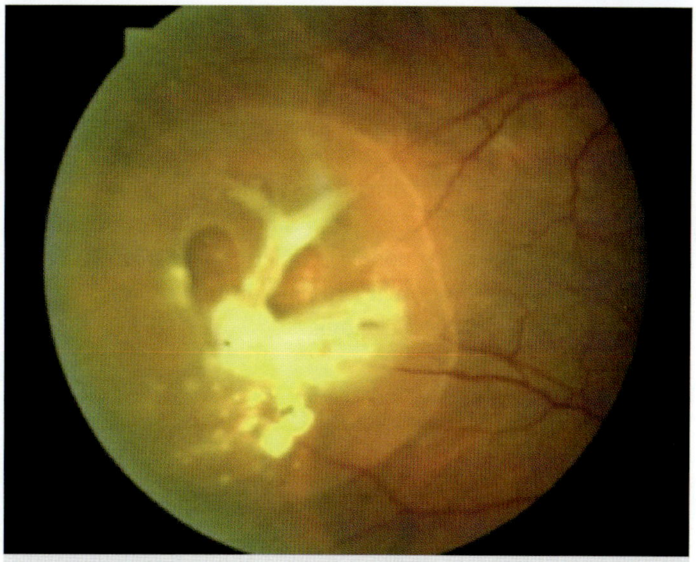

Fig. 11.13 Retinal metastasis of breast cancer.

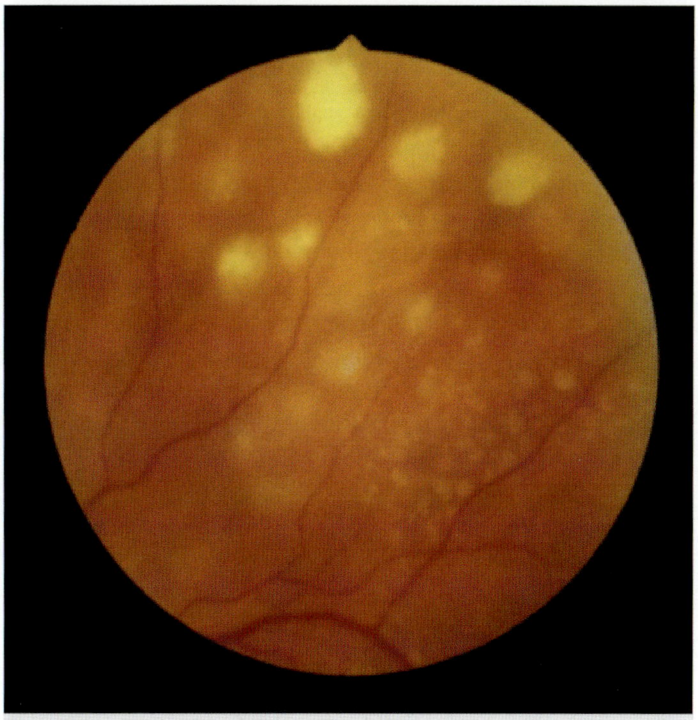

Fig. 11.14 Non-Hodgkin lymphoma (chorioretinal infiltrates).

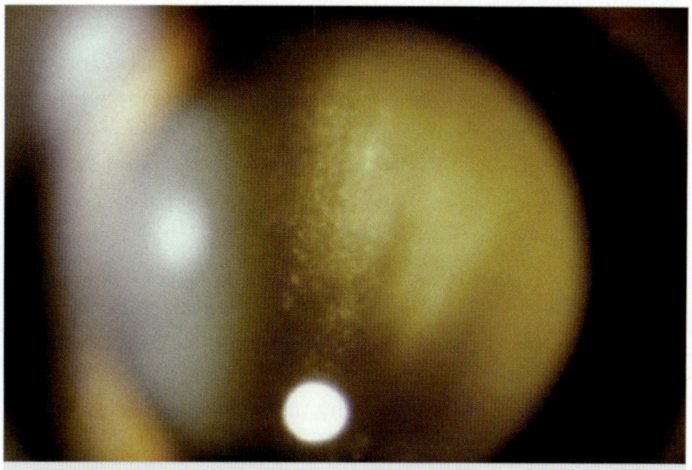

Fig. 11.15 Non-Hodgkin lymphoma in the vitreous body.

periretinal membrane formation, and vitreous body infiltration/hemorrhage, as well as traction and exudative retinal detachment (▶ Fig. 11.13, ▶ Fig. 11.14).

Retinitis, proliferative vitreoretinopathy with traction retinal detachment, and retinal vessel occlusions have to be considered in the differential diagnosis.

Vitreous Body

Tumor cell infiltration of the vitreous body can occur secondary to a ciliary or retinal metastasis. Also primary hematogenic tumor cell seeding of the vitreous body associated with, for example, skin melanoma or non-Hodgkin's lymphoma have been described (▶ Fig. 11.15). Occasionally, secondary vitreous hemorrhages can occur after intraocular metastases.

Differential diagnosis may be challenging especially in those cases, where no involvement of other ocular structures is evident. Intravitreal inflammatory disorders such as endophthalmitis, posterior uveitis, or iridocyclitis should be considered. Sometimes a diagnostic vitrectomy with cytopathologic investigation of the vitreous cell aspirate may be mandatory in order to be able to make the correct diagnosis.

Metastases of the Conjunctiva, the Sclera, and the Eyelids

In rare cases (< 1%) metastases can manifest in the conjunctiva; they usually present as yellowish-orange prominent lesions.

Primary metastases of the sclera are extremely rare, but the sclera may be secondarily involved after invasion or spread of intraocular or intraorbital tumors.

Likewise metastases of the eyelids are rare and constitute only 0.3–1.1% of lid tumors. In a study conducted by Mansour et al, metastatic lid lesions were discovered earlier than the underlying primary tumors in 45% of cases.[66] Clinically, these lesions frequently appear as isolate nodular epidermal tumors with occasional ulcerations. The primary tumors are often breast cancer, lung cancer, or cutaneous melanoma.

Diagnosis

Because patients present with rather nonspecific symptoms such as vision loss, photophobia, metamorphopsia, or vitreous floaters (mouches volantes), obtaining a thorough history, especially of previous cancer, is crucial. The complete ophthalmologic examination can be supplemented in patients with suspected intraocular metastases by further investigational procedures such as A- and B-mode ultrasonography, ultrasound biomicroscopy, fluorescein/ICG angiography, and optical coherence tomography (OCT).

Ultrasonographic Examination

Ultrasonography provides an important means if opaque optic media and unclear retinal/choroidal lesions are present, particularly if space-occupying intraocular disease processes are being masked by associated hemorrhages, exudations, or exudative retinal detachment. Ultrasonography is a rapid and simple method and has the advantage of minimal stress for the patients, suitability for follow-up examinations, and low cost. Due to the minimal thickness of intraocular metastases, it can be challenging with ultrasound evaluation to depict the internal characteristics of suspected lesions even when the investigator is very experienced. Normally they show a high internal and frequently irregular reflectivity pattern. These sonographic patterns differ significantly from those of other intraocular tumors, such as choroidal melanoma. In A-mode sonography the latter typically shows an initial prominent spike, followed by a homogenous low-to-medium internal reflectivity and typical sound attenuation. Vascular pulsations can be seen as fine oscillations of the internal spiking pattern within the lesion. In B-mode ultrasound, occasionally the typical collar-button or dome-shape of choroidal melanoma can be depicted.

Ultrasound biomicroscopy can be helpful to investigate disease processes in the iris and the ciliary body. A major drawback is the low penetration depth (e.g., to distinguish cystic from solid structures) so that examination of subjacent structures is limited.

Fluorescein and ICG Angiography

Fluorescence angiography can be helpful in distinguishing between intraocular metastases, inflammatory processes, and other chorioretinal pathologies, such as choroidal neovascularization. In contrast to primary ocular neoplasms, intraocular metastases are often hypofluorescent in the early stages of the angiogram. Depending on the ophthalmoscopic findings (presence of pigment epithelial changes) in the course of the angiogram, an inhomogeneous, sometimes pinpoint leakage can develop associated with blockage phenomena. In late stages, frequently a diffuse hyperfluorescence may be present in the area of the lesion. Indocyanine green (ICG) angiography often reveals nonspecific subtle, occult lesions.

Because of frequent nonspecific angiographic findings, fluorescein angiography often has only documentary value in patients with intraocular metastases. Nevertheless, it can provide significant differential diagnostic information in particular cases.[67,68]

Further Diagnostic Procedures

Further diagnostic procedures include computed tomography, MRI, and positron emission tomography (PET). For further diagnostic purposes, fine needle aspiration biopsy or tissue biopsy are suitable.

Therapy

The type and scope of the treatment depend strongly on the size, number, and localization of intraocular metastases. When discussing therapy of intraocular metastases the basic oncologic therapy (the chemotherapy and radiotherapy modality), the age of the patient and the prognosis must be taken into account. The therapeutic decision is therefore influenced by many individual factors.

If chemotherapy is administered, usually a response should be awaited. Often, metastases (e.g., in breast or prostate carcinoma) regress over the course of chemotherapy.[69] Even without treatment, choroidal metastases can remain stable and asymptomatic for a long time.

Further treatment options are available if metastases are unresponsive to medical therapy or show progression and if the patient is compromised by ocular symptoms or visual disturbances.[70]

A promising treatment modality is available with percutaneous radiotherapy (external beam radiotherapy, EBRT), which is effective, cost-effective, and, as a rule, less stressful for patients. Because local EBRT does not treat the primary tumor, a precise interdisciplinary therapy schedule should be elaborated in order to coordinate the different treatment modalities. Usually, percutaneous radiotherapy is applied with a linear accelerator in the lateral portal with a target volume dose of 30–40 Gy in fractions of 2–3 Gy. Local tumor control can be achieved in 33 to 89% of cases,[71] depending on the underlying primary tumor. For a comprehensive review of radiation therapy see Chapter 14.

In most studies it was possible to achieve stabilization or even improvement of visual acuity as frequently the exudative retinal detachment responds very well to radiotherapy.[72] Radiogenic cataract formation, radiation retinopathy, and dry eyes are known side effects. After regression of choroidal metastasis, in many cases there is atrophy of the choroid and of the retinal pigment epithelium, combined with pigment epithelium accumulation.

Brachytherapy is a treatment option in solitary metastases, particularly if they are localized in the periphery of the choroid. Regression in 94% of cases can be achieved.[73] In the posterior eye segment, ruthenium 106 and iodine 125 plaques are particularly used; for tumors of the anterior segment, cobalt 60 plaques have been widely used.

Further therapeutic options include transpupillary thermotherapy, or in exceptional cases, local resection of a solitary metastasis in combination with brachytherapy.[72,74,75]

In cases of advanced metastatic disease with severe vision loss or pain caused by secondary glaucoma, enucleation should be discussed with the patient if an improvement of the situation cannot be expected. The indication for enucleation should be discussed in terms of the general prognosis. If life expectancy is only a few months and the progression is minimal, patients can be treated by alternative modalities such as a retrobulbar alcohol injection, sparing them from the psychological trauma of enucleation.

Prognosis

Metastases probably represent the most common intraocular malignancy. The prognosis in patients with intraocular metastases depends on the nature of the primary tumor and the extent of metastatic disease. Median survival time of 2–32 months after diagnosis of metastases is reported.[61,76,77,78,79,80] Survival time for patients with breast carcinoma is reported to be the longest, at 18–32 months, while it is significantly less in patients with gastrointestinal and lung cancer, with an average of 5 months.[71,77,81]

As asymptomatic metastases, in particular choroidal metastases, occur more often than previously thought, all patients with malignancies should routinely have ophthalmologic check-ups. Diagnosis of intraocular metastases can be made by means of a slit lamp examination and by simple binocular ophthalmoscopy. Further diagnostic investigations and interdisciplinary collaboration can be initiated if the ophthalmologic work-up has disclosed intraocular metastases.

11.2 Tumors of the Lacrimal Glands and Lacrimal Ducts

H.-J. Welkoborsky

Tumors of the lacrimal glands are rare. Only 0.1% of all tumors occurring in people are localized in the lacrimal glands or ducts.[82] Their incidence amounts to ~0.07 per 100,000.[83] It is necessary to differentiate between pseudo tumors, benign and malignant epithelial tumors, and malignant lymphomas.

11.2.1 Tumors of the Lacrimal Glands

Pseudo Tumors

Pseudo tumors include the **dermoids** or dermoid cysts most commonly. In the true meaning of the word these are not tumors of the lacrimal glands themselves; dermoids are rather congenital lesions that are often localized in the area of the orbital edge and here in particular in the upper outer quadrant. They often arise in places, in which embryonal clefts close and cystic lesions can result through the migration of epithelium from the epidermis; however, a traumatic origin is also possible. They can contain hair, several layers of squamous cell epithelium, or callus material. The tumors appear in early childhood and, due to their typical clinical appearance together with the ultrasound diagnostic findings, do not cause any diagnostic difficulties. Dermoids appear as smooth circumscribed, firm elastic space-occupying lesions that can often be easily moved. Sonography (see Chapter 4.6) exhibits a circumscribed, anechoic space-occupying mass with dorsal enhancement. Depending on the nature of the contents of the cyst there may be some intralesional echoes, which correspond to the callus material or cell debris in the cyst's fluid. A displacement of the eye globe occurs only in very extensive lesions. Treatment consists of complete excision. The prognosis is good.

Sjögren's disease is an autoimmune disease. Women over 40 years of age are mostly affected. Clinically, there is a reduced tear and saliva production with dryness of the mouth and eyes in the foreground. The large salivary glands and the lacrimal glands are mostly swollen on both sides and can thus simulate a tumor. The histological characteristic is a lymphocytic and plasma cellular infiltration of the salivary and lacrimal glands, which are then destroyed by this. As a rule, diagnosis presents no difficulties due to the very typical clinical signs and the characteristic sonographic finding. Treatment consists in giving corticosteroids. Sjögren's syndrome is associated in some cases with lymphoproliferative diseases.

Benign Tumors

Essentially the same benign tumors occur in the lacrimal glands as in the salivary glands. The most common benign tumor is the **pleomorphic adenoma**, which forms over 50% of all tear gland tumors.[84,85] Clinically, a unilateral, coarse, easily movable space-occupying mass appears on the lateral upper lid. A displacement of the eye globe occurs in the nasal caudal direction only in extended tumors (▶ Fig. 11.16). As with pleomorphic adenomas of the large salivary glands, the etiology of the tumor is currently unknown. Molecular genetic studies indicate numerical and structural aberrations in diverse chromosome areas, predominantly on the short arm of chromosome 9 (9p23-p22.3). The PLAG1 oncoprotein, among others, is coded in this area.[86] Sonographically a well-defined anechoic space-occupying mass appears that is often circumscribed and polycyclic, with dorsal enhancement. Magnetic resonance imaging can be used for further diagnostics. Here the tumor spread, in particular toward the dorsal orbital compartments, can be assessed. Treatment consists of complete tumor resection. Since the tumors are surrounded by a fine capsule, which at the same time often exhibits small eversions, particular care is indicated in preparation. An injury to the capsule that opens up the tumor can lead to tumor cell seeding, with the result of recurrences.[84]

Other benign tumors are **Warthin's tumor**, **myoepithelioma**, **oncocytic adenoma**, and **basal cell adenoma**; these, however, are rarities. The clinical signs and treatment are the same as those for pleomorphic adenoma.

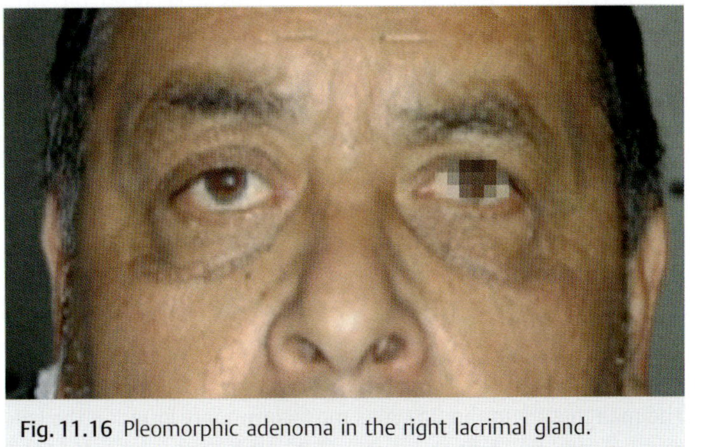

Fig. 11.16 Pleomorphic adenoma in the right lacrimal gland.

Malignant Tumors

The most common malignant epithelial tumor of the lacrimal glands is **adenoid cystic carcinoma**, followed by **adenocarcinoma, carcinoma ex pleomorphic adenoma**, **mucoepidermoid carcinoma**, and **myoepithelial carcinoma**.[84,87,88,89] Adenoid cystic carcinoma develops from glandular tissue. The etiology is so far unclear, but genomic imbalances and mutations of oncogenes, such as *PLAG1*, and an activation of the *MYB* gene have been shown.[90,91] The significance of these research results for clinical symptoms is so far unclear. The histological differentiation between pleomorphic adenomas and adenoid cystic carcinomas does occasionally cause difficulties and is only possible using immunohistochemical investigations.[84,89] Here both tumor entities differ significantly with regard to the expression of the Ki67 proliferation marker as well as of the p53, PLAG1, Survivin, and MYB oncoproteins.[91,92] Clinically, with malignant tumors of the lacrimal glands, a slowly progressing unilateral space-occupying mass appears in the area of the lateral upper lid. In some cases there is infiltration of the skin of the lid, occasionally with the formation of a fistula. Infiltration of the outer eye muscles or of the eye bulb leads to a disruption to the motility of the globe with double vision or displacement of the globe. A peculiarity with adenoid cystic carcinoma is its tendency to infiltration of the perineural sheaths, which is why a complete removal of the tumor is often not possible. The diagnosis is made by clinical examination; moreover, adenoid cystic carcinomas often cause pain.[91] Sonographically guided fine needle aspiration biopsy with cytological examination has proved invaluable. The infiltration of the deeper lying orbit structures or of the eye globe is best identified by magnetic resonance imaging. Metastasis into local lymph nodes is rare; the parotideal or submandibular lymph nodes are affected in under 10% of cases.[83] Nevertheless sonography of the salivary glands as well as of the soft tissues of the neck should be carried out within the context of the staging examinations. With adenoid cystic carcinomas, a CT of the thoracic organs is additionally necessary, as a pulmonary metastasis can quickly develop.[83]

11

Treatment of malignant lacrimal gland tumors consists of complete tumor excision. Depending on the situation and size of the tumor, a frontal orbitotomy via an eyebrow and orbital edge incision or a lateral orbitotomy can be indicated as the approach. Orbital exenteration should be discussed if the eye bulb or the intraorbital muscles have been infiltrated. Postoperative radiotherapy is usually indicated.[82,83] Recently, studies on radiotherapy alone and on neutron radiotherapy for adenoid cystic carcinomas showed promising results.[82,93] The latter achieved a 5-year tumor control rate of 80%.[93] Some studies have been recently published on the adjuvant use of cytostatic drugs, applied either systemically or intra-arterially and produced encouraging results with regard to long-term tumor control.[94]

Distant metastases of tumors with another provenance are rare in the lacrimal glands and mostly derive from primary tumors of other glandular organs.[95] In the treatment of distant metastases the indication of surgery, in particular of mutilating interventions, is to be discussed very conservatively and critically.

Malignant Lymphoma

The malignant lymphoma types most commonly found in the lacrimal glands are **diffuse large cell B-cell lymphoma** and **MALT lymphoma**.[96] They mostly appear in the seventh to eighth decades of life. Diagnosis can only be made on the basis of histological and immunohistological investigations. Most malignant lymphomas of the lacrimal glands are low-grade tumors. However, a change in the *MYC* oncogene expression and of the nuclear factor κB1 (NF-κB1) signal pathway is an indication of high aggressivity.[97,98] In the context of staging investigations it must be clarified whether there are further lymphoma manifestations, for example, in the area of the eyelid or conjunctiva ("salmon pink" coloration with MALT lymphoma) and in the other regional lymph nodes. Whereas diffuse large cell B-cell lymphoma mostly appears unilaterally, with MALT lymphoma a diffuse spread predominates.[96] With a local manifestation, treatment is radiotherapy; with a systemic manifestation, it is chemotherapy; and with MALT lymphoma, it is chemotherapy in a combination with rituximab.[82,96] The 5-year survival rate of malignant lymphomas of the lacrimal glands is around 70%.

11.2.2 Tumors of the Lacrimal Ducts

Tumors of the lacrimal ducts are extremely rare. In a series of 502 endonasal dacryocystorhinostomies, Tanweer et al found 5 tumors that were responsible for the indication-determining lacrimal duct stenosis.[98]

Among the **benign** tumors **pleomorphic adenomas** are the most common. A rare tumor that can occur exceptionally in the lacrimal sac and the nasolacrimal canal is **transitional cell papilloma**, which develops from the transitional cell epithelium, which can also be found in the ureter.[99]

Malignant tumors of the lacrimal sac and the tear ducts are mostly adenoid cystic carcinomas, followed by **adenocarcinomas, mucoepidermoid carcinomas**, and **lymphoepithelial carcinomas**.[87]

Clinical symptoms consist in a slowly progressing swelling in the area of the lacrimal sac on and underneath the medial canthus of the eye with epiphora. For this reason, when making a differential diagnosis, benign cicatricial stenoses of the tear ducts with consecutive dacryocystitis must be considered. Treatment consists in a complete tumor resection, where necessary followed by adjuvant radiotherapy.[99,100]

Malignant lymphomas of the tear ducts, in line with the malignant lymphomas of the lacrimal glands, are mostly **diffuse-large-cell B-cell lymphomas** or **MALT lymphomas**. In contrast to the malignant lymphomas of the lacrimal glands, highly aggressive tumors are more often encountered.[96,101] The diagnostics and treatment are the same as those for malignant lymphomas of the lacrimal glands. The prognosis is markedly poorer, however, with a 5-year survival rate of 20 to 40%.[96]

11.3 Tumors of the Sinuses with Spread to the Orbit

H.-J. Welkoborsky

Due to the close proximity to the orbit, tumors in the paranasal sinuses often involve the bony walls of the orbit or the intraorbital structures. These tumors are designated as secondary orbital tumors.[102] In detail, differentiation should be made between three large tumor groups:

Table 11.1 WHO classification of tumors of the paranasal sinuses[11]

Tumor	Benign	Malignant
Epithelial tumors	Papillomas (inverted, oncocytic, exophytic); salivary gland tumors (e.g. pleomorphic adenomas, oncocytomas)	Squamous cell carcinomas; lymphoepithelial carcinoma; sinonasal undifferentiated carcinoma (SNUC), adenocarcinomas; salivary gland tumors (adenoid cystic carcinomas, mucoepidermoid carcinoma, etc.); neuroendocrine tumors
Mesenchymal tumors	Myxoma; leiomyoma; hemangioma; schwannoma; meningioma; neurinoma	Sarcomas (fibrosarcoma; leiomyosarcoma, rhabdomyosarcoma, angiosarcoma); malignant peripheral nerve sheath tumor
Tumors of bones and cartilage tissue	Chondroma, osteoma, chondroblastoma, osteochondroma, osteoblastoma, chondromesenchymal hamartoma, giant cell tumor	Chondrosarcoma; osteosarcoma; chordoma
Hematolymphoid tumors		Extranodal T-cell lymphoma (natural killer cell lymphoma); diffuse-large-cell B-cell lymphoma; extramedullary plasmocytoma; extramedullary myeloid sarcoma; histiocytic sarcoma
Neuroectodermal tumors		Ewing's sarcoma; primitive neuroectodermal tumor; olfactory neuroblastoma; melanotic neuroectodermal tumor of childhood; mucosal melanoma
Germ cell tumors	Dermoid cysts; teratoma	Teratoma with malignant transformation; sinonasal teratocarcinoma
Secondary tumors		Metastases of tumors of another provenance

- Pseudo tumors.
- Benign tumors.
- Malignant tumors.

While primaries—tumors emanating from the orbital structures—are very rare and mostly benign, secondary tumors, which spread from the paranasal sinuses to the orbit, are often malignant.[102,103] According to the WHO classification, tumors of the paranasal sinuses are divided into epithelial and mesenchymal tumors, tumors emanating from bones and cartilage, hematolymphoid tumors, neuroectodermal tumors, germ cell tumors, and secondary tumors (metastases)[104] (▶ Table 11.1).

11.3.1 Symptoms

The symptoms of tumors and pseudo tumors of the paranasal sinuses with orbital involvement are nonspecific and often depend on the tumor entity. Thus, for example, mucoceles of the ethmoid bone or the frontal sinuses lead to a mostly painless displacement of the soft tissue in the orbit without destroying the function of nerves, whereas there can often be a painful swelling or motoric limitations with malignant tumors.[105,106] ▶ Table 11.2 provides a general overview of frequent nasal and orbital symptoms in tumors of the paranasal sinuses in our own group of patients.

As can be seen from ▶ Table 11.2, nasal symptoms (i.e., nasal obstruction, epistaxis, nasal hypersecretion – often unilateral) are the most frequent symptoms; orbital symptoms follow later but with a clear interval.[107]

11.3.2 Pseudo Tumors

In addition to cysts and mucoceles, fibro-osseous lesions and nasal polyposis are also pseudo tumors of the paranasal sinuses, which can cause orbital symptoms.

Mucoceles and Cysts

Mucoceles and cysts of the paranasal sinuses are caused by the retention of secretion in sealed-off spaces lined with mucosa. The cause of retained secretion is mostly a preceding operation, an injury, or an inflammation. The difference between a mucocele and a cyst is that the first tends more to progression and can lead to a rarefaction of osseous structures with consecutive spreading into neighboring organs due to internal pressure.[108]

Cysts in the area of the ethmoid bone, the maxillary sinus, or the frontal sinus only rarely lead to orbital symptoms, and if then to nonspecific phenomena such as epiphora, a diffuse feeling of peri- and retrobulbar pressure or subjective blurred vision. Treatment consists of an endonasal clearing-out of the sinus affected with removal or drainage of the cyst via endoscopy or microscopy into the main nasal cavity.

Mucoceles of the nasal cavities and paranasal sinuses can reach considerable dimensions.[108] Depending on the sinus affected they lead to a displacement of the internal structures of the orbit

Table 11.2 General overview of symptoms of patients with tumors of the paranasal sinuses in the authors' own patient cohort ($n = 178$)

Symptom	Frequency
Nasal obstruction	56%
Epistaxis	35%
Swelling of the cheeks	24%
Head and/or facial pain	23%
Mostly unilateral nasal hypersecretion	20%
Exophthalmos	16%
Facial deformities	12%
Epiphora	12%
Diplopia/loss of sight/globe motility impairment	9%
Paresthesias	8%

(▶ Fig. 11.17). It is mostly the frontal sinuses and the ethmoidal cells that are affected, with previous operations or trauma representing predisposing factors. Thus they are often localized in the upper inner quadrants of the orbit.[109] Subjective complaints can be eyeball motility impairment and, due to the pressure on the optic nerve, impairment of visual acuity as well as an exophthalmos. As with cysts, treatment consists of functional endoscopic or microscopic paranasal sinus surgery with drainage or removal of the mucocele.[110] In that one must take care that the mucocele sac is removed as much as possible or a that wide drainage of the mucocele is performed, otherwise recurrences are frequent. In some cases an operation is necessary via an external approach to ensure the removal of the mucocele.

Fibro-osseous Lesions of the Paranasal Sinuses

Fibro-osseous lesions of the paranasal sinuses include fibrous dysplasia, ossifying fibroma, osseous dysplasia (which mostly occurs in the region of the lower jaw and only infrequently in the area of the paranasal sinuses),[111] and the rare giant cell granuloma.[112] Within this group **fibrous dysplasia** with an occurrence of 37 to 56% is the most common disease, followed by ossifying fibroma (~33%) and osseous dysplasia (11–25%).[113,114,115] The etiology of the disease is essentially unknown[116] but a defect of progenitor cell differentiation is being discussed[117] along with defects of the *APC* and *CTNNB1* genes, which are responsible for β-catenin formation. Aberrant or lacking β-catenin formation has been documented in numerous osseous lesions and odontogenic tumors.[118] The disease is benign; malignant degeneration in a leiomyosarcoma has been reported.[119] Fibrous dysplasia is mostly localized in the area of the maxillary bone or the mandible. The frontal sinuses, ethmoidal cells, sphenoidal sinuses, or clivus are significantly less often affected,[120,121] although the disease can be very extensive and affect almost the entire skull base.[122] Orbital symptoms occur when the bony orbital walls are affected or, in the event of a localization in the clivus or in the sphenoid bone, as a sight impairment through compression of the optic nerve, or as pain in the form of neuralgia by compression of the maxillary nerve when the foramen rotundum is affected.[122] CT and MRI will provide guidance for the diagnosis[120,123] (see Chapter 4). However, diagnosis ultimately has to be reached histologically.[124]

The treatment for fibro-osseous lesions is based on the spread and symptomatology of the findings. With smaller asymptomatic lesions a wait-and-see approach with MRI or CT check-ups might be indicated.[121] Extensive and/or symptomatic processes should be cleaned out surgically. Many operating procedures have been described for this, which range from locally circumscribed operative procedures right through to a complete craniofacial resection with reconstruction of the skull base and the orbital walls.[122,125] These operations are usually conducted on an interdisciplinary basis. If the optic nerve is being compressed within the context of a fibrous dysplasia then an optic nerve decompression has to be done. Identification of the nerve is often made difficult due to the bone having been altered by fibrous dysplasia so that the decompression is only possible with the assistance of a computerized navigation system.

Nasal Polyposis

Nasal polyposis is a chronic inflammatory disease of the paranasal sinuses. The etiology of the disease is so far unclear, but a disorder of the arachidonic acid metabolism of the mucous cells has been suggested as the cause of polyp development. Nasal polyps are not true neoplasias. Although some become a substantial size (▶ Fig. 11.18), they are still only reactions of the mucous membrane to a chronical inflammation stimulus. To what extent an allergic rhinopathy or sinupathy predisposes to the formation

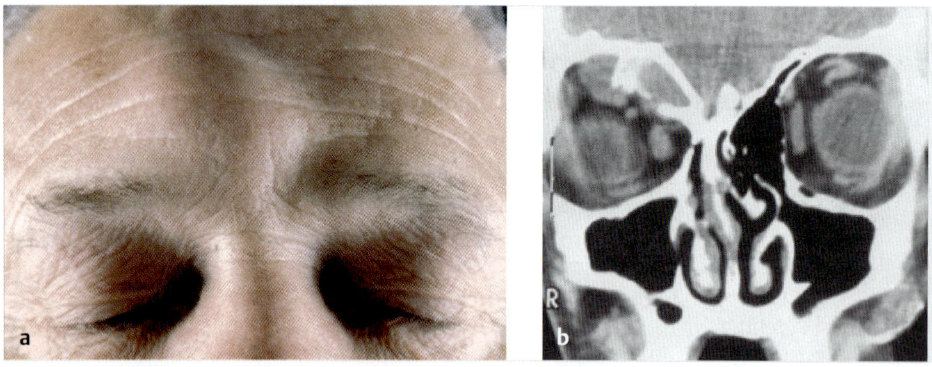

Fig. 11.17 (a, b) Mucocele of the frontal sinus with intraorbital extension. The mucocele led to a rarefaction of the bone along with caudal displacement of intraorbital structures.

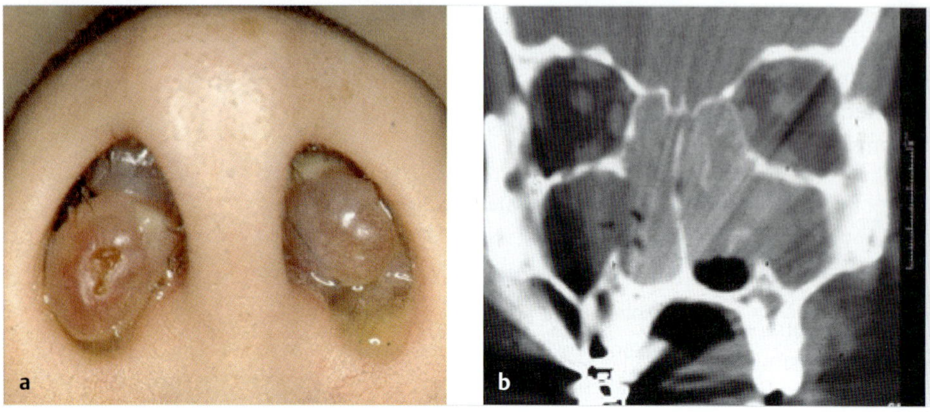

Fig. 11.18 Nasal polyposis: **(a)** clinical view; **(b)** CT scan.

of polyps is the subject of some debate and no clear cut connection has yet been established.[126] Together with bronchial asthma and subjective anosmia, nasal polyposis is pathognomonic for nonsteroidal analgesic intolerance syndrome (NSAIS) (so-called Samter's triad: polyposis nasi, bronchial asthma, nonsteroidal analgesic intolerance syndrome). The symptoms of chronic polypoid pansinusitis with nasal polyposis are far-reaching, covering nasal breathing impairment marked by a feeling of pressure, nasal obstruction, cephalgias, and nasal or retronasal secretion. Orbital symptoms are epiphora, a diffuse periorbital and, where the sphenoid bone is also affected, also a retroorbital feeling of pressure, occasionally with subjective blurred vision. There is usually no pain. Nor do any eyeball motility disruptions occur. The bony walls of the orbit are preserved even with the most marked disease (▶ Fig. 11.18). Treatment consists in the endonasal functional paranasal sinus operation with the removal of the polyps. Consistent postoperative follow-up treatment with topical corticoids is important in order to prevent a polyposis recurring.[103,127] The recurrence rate is ~20%.

11.3.3 Benign Tumors of the Paranasal Sinuses with Orbit Involvement

Inverted Papillomas

Inverted papillomas represent genuine neoplasias of the paranasal sinus mucous membrane. The etiology is unknown; an association with an infection through the human papilloma virus is under discussion. At 30% they are the most common tumor in the nasal cavity and paranasal sinuses.[103] The tumor consists of mature respiratory epithelium and cylindrical cells. Squamous cell epithelial metaplasias are common. Their place of origin is mostly the medial wall of the sinus maxillaris in the maxilloethmoidal recess. In decreasing frequency there follow the ethmoid bone and the frontal sinus.[128] Inverted papillomas of the sphenoid sinus are in contrast markedly less frequent. The tumor mostly occurs unilaterally; at 4% synchronous bilateral inverted papillomas are rare.[103,128]

The clinical symptoms are nonspecific, as with nasal polyps. However, nasal breathing impairment is marked only unilaterally as a rule. The tumor is visible endoscopically, and looks like a nasal polyp. Further symptoms can be an epistaxis, purulent unilateral rhinorrhea, and pressure in the head. Clinical peculiarities of inverted papillomas include firstly its tendency to recur, which is given as 15 to 20%.[128] Beside this there is a transition to a squamous cell carcinoma in 1 to 7% of cases.[103] Diagnosis can only be achieved by means of a histological examination. The constellation of symptoms—unilateral nasal breathing impairment, visible polypoid structures in the nasal cavity, and unilateral soft tissue shading in the CT image—prompts the suspicion of the existence of such a tumor. Nevertheless, many tumors are only discovered as an accidental finding in the histological examination of the tissues of patients who were primarily operated on under the diagnosis of nasal polyposis. Inverted papillomas grow to cause local displacement and occasionally lead to bone erosion.[127] With invasion of the orbit the internal orbital structures can be compressed, with a displacement of the eyeball.[129] The periorbita is as a rule intact and can be identified in the CT or MRI as fine tissue lamella between tumor and orbital contents.

Treatment of the inverted papilloma consists of its complete surgical removal, for which oncosurgical conditions have to be applied.[103,128] Depending on the location and the extent of the tumor, an endonasal access can be used in most cases. If tumor resection via an endonasal endoscopic approach is not possible, a midfacial degloving or lateral rhinotomy[110,129] might be appropriate. An intraoperative frozen-section analysis of the margins to check for tumor freedom has proved favorable.

Paragangliomas

Paragangliomas originate from nonchromaffin cells, whose existence in the mucous membrane of the nose and the paranasal sinuses has been demonstrated. These are primarily benign tumors; however, clinical and cellular biological examinations indicate that these tumors are clinically malignant in ~50% of cases with infiltration of the skull base and the orbit as well as potential for metastatic development.[130,131] Symptoms are determined by the localization of the tumor. In the area of the nasal cavity a unilateral nasal breathing impairment occurs. As the tumors are very densely perfused, there is often a recurring epistaxis in the forefront. CT and the MRI show the extent of the tumor and the possible bone erosions (▶ Fig. 11.19). The treatment consists of complete surgical removal of the tumor. The approach needs to be selected such that the tumor can be well exposed so that any bleeds occurring can be coagulated and supplying vessels can be tied as much as possible. When the tumor is located in the area of the anterior skull base and the paranasal sinuses, a bifrontal approach or an endoscopic approach may be indicated. Other possible approaches are midfacial degloving in tumors located in the area of the middle or posterior skull base or even lateral rhinotomy. Angiography with possible superselective embolization of the supplying tumor vessels should be performed 24 hours preoperatively.

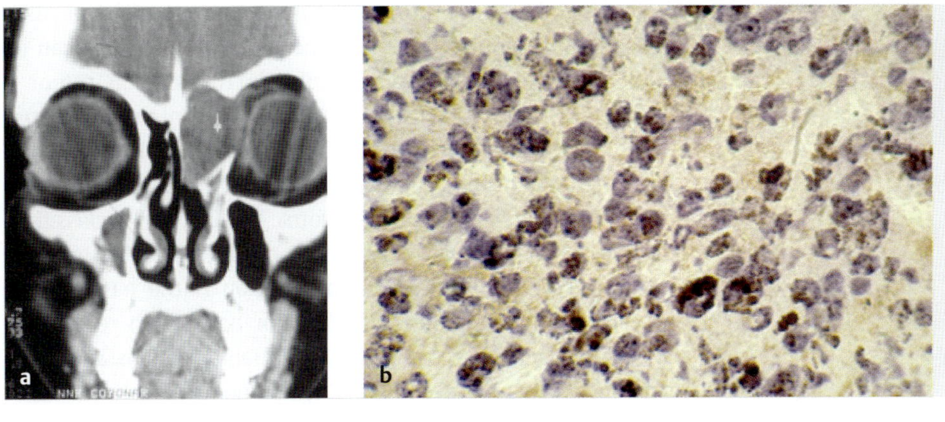

Fig. 11.19 Paraganglioma in the anterior ethmoid cells with erosion of the medial bony orbital wall: (a) CT; (b) histology.

Osteomas

Osteomas are benign tumors of the osseous matrix. They grow very slowly and are mostly localized in the area of the frontal sinuses (80%) and in the ethmoid bone (20%).[127] Men are afflicted twice as often as women. Asymptomatic osteomas are often discovered as accidental findings in radiographs or CT images of the paranasal sinuses. Symptoms consist of cephalgias from local pressure or blocking of the drainage pathway of the sinus concerned, with subsequent inflammation. Orbital symptoms are rare and only occur once growth advances into the orbit's internal structures in the form of a crowding of the orbital contents. On CT the tumor is seen as a characteristic bone-dense mass (see Chapter 4). Therapeutically one should aim to remove the tumor entirely. With small tumors, especially in the ethmoid bone, an endoscopic nasal approach can be sufficient; larger tumors in the area of the frontal sinus are removed via a transfrontal osteoplastic approach.[127]

11.3.4 Malignant Tumors of the Paranasal Sinuses with Orbit Involvement

Malignant tumors of the nasal cavity and the paranasal sinuses make up 1 to 3% of all malignomas in people.[103,132,133,134] Their incidence is given as 1:100,000.[135] There are regional and gender-specific differences: In an evaluation of the cases of sinonasal carcinomas in the Dutch cancer register, the incidence in men reduced from 15/1 million in the years 1973–1995 to 11/1 million in the years 1996–2009. In women, meanwhile, it rose from 5/1 million in the years 1973–1995 to 7.5/1 million in the years 1996–2009, which was attributed to, amongst other things, an increasing nicotine consumption on the part of women.[136]

11

With regard to the tumor entities, **squamous cell carcinoma** occupies first place at 48 to 60%, followed by adenocarcinoma at 9 to 15% (▶ Table 11.3). Sarcomas are common in children.[137] There also seem to be regional differences in the incidence of tumor entities. Reno et al in 2000 gave the percentage of squamous cell carcinomas as 82%,[138] while in our group of patients it lies at around 60%. In turn adenocarcinomas and malignant non-Hodgkin's lymphomas are markedly more commonly observed in our patient group. Neuroendocrine tumors, with the exception of malignant melanoma are reported by some authors at over 5%;[139] however. in our own group of patients we have seen only isolated cases.

Epithelial tumors of the maxillary sinus and the nasal cavity as well as of the ethmoid sinuses are classified by means of a TNM classification adjusted to the anatomical conditions.[140] There is infiltration of the orbit in stages T3, T4a, and T4b.

Table 11.3 Relative frequency of malignant tumors of the nose and the paranasal sinuses

Tumor entity	Frequency
Squamous cell carcinoma	60%
Adenocarcinoma	12%
Adenoid cystic carcinoma	4%
Malignant lymphomas	8%
Malignant melanomas	1%
Sarcomas	3%
Other (including metastases)	12%

Squamous Cell Carcinomas

Squamous cell carcinoma is the most common tumor. Approximately 3% of all malignomas in the head–neck area are squamous cell carcinomas of the nose and in the paranasal sinuses.[141] This tumor occurs primarily in the nasal cavity, in the maxillary sinus, and in the ethmoid cells. Risk factors for this are tobacco smoke and exposure to nickel or chromates.[103,105,136] Men are afflicted approximately 2 to 3 times more often than women, and the tumor mostly occurs after the age of 60 years.[141] Ethnic differences also seem apparent: in an American study the incidence rose between 2003 and 2009 in African Americans, while it fell in the white population.[141] If the tumors are localized in the area of the paranasal sinuses, they cause problems only relatively late in the form of impairing nasal breathing, recurrent epistaxis, or even pain, in particular if nerve structures are being affected by the tumor. Extensive tumors are visible endoscopically in the nasal cavity; likewise the penetration of the upper jaw by a tumor (see Chapter 3.2). Regional lymph node metastases are seen in approximately only 10% of cases.[105,133]

Adeno- and Adenoid Cystic Carcinomas

Adenocarcinomas originate in the glandular tissue of the mucosa. The etiology is unknown, but the lesion often occurs in patients who have been exposed to hardwood dusts. Men are afflicted 6 to 8 times more often than women. The tumor is mostly localized in the area of the nasal cavity, on the roof of the nose, or in the ethmoid sinus. The symptoms are similar to those of squamous cell carcinoma.

Adenoid cystic carcinomas are a type of salivary gland tumor and likewise originate in the glandular tissue of the mucosa. The tumor grows relatively slowly, but infiltration of the perineural sheaths is pathognomonic, and makes the complete surgical removal of the tumor difficult. As well as perineural sheath infiltration, distant metastases, in particular in the lung, are often also to be found even with relatively small tumors.

Mucoepidermoid carcinomas are seldom found in the area of the nose and paranasal sinuses. They do, however, cause pain even in early stages.[142] The other symptoms equate to those of squamous cell carcinomas.

Malignant Melanomas

Malignant melanoma consists of melanocytes, which are found in mucous membrane of the respiratory system. In ~70% of cases these are amelanotic tumors or amelanotic tumor parts can be established.[143] With an incidence of 0.05/100,000 this tumor is very rare.[134] The etiology is to a great extent unknown because risk factors that have been established as predisposing for malignant melanoma of the skin (including direct UV irradiation) cannot play any role in mucosal melanoma. The Clark level classification used for melanomas of the skin is not applicable for mucosal melanomas.[144] The favored tumor location is the nasal cavity. Even after complete removal the tumor has a high recurrence rate. At the start of treatment ~4% of patients have distant metastases and 10 to 20% have regional lymph node metastases.[103]

Neuroendocrine Tumors

Within the group of neuroendocrinally differentiated tumors (with the exception of malignant melanoma) **olfactory neuroblastoma** (synonym esthesioneuroblastoma) is the most common type. The tumor originates from undifferentiated neuroectodermal tissue of the olfactory epithelium.[139] Correspondingly, the favored tumor site is the roof of the nose in the region of the olfactory rim, the upper nasal septum as well as the ethmoid plate. Infiltration along the olfactory fibers through the skull base is common. Extensive olfactory neuroblastomas reach the orbit cranially and are mostly localized there in the craniomedial quadrants. Correspondingly, the eye globe is displaced in a lateral-caudal direction. An impairment to eye bulb motility is only found when the orbital muscles are infiltrated, in particular the superior rectus, superior oblique, and medial rectus muscles.

Malignant Lymphomas

The malignant lymphomas are mostly non-Hodgkin's lymphomas. They can originate in the orbit primarily or in the paranasal sinuses. While lymphomas in the orbit are mostly malignant B-cell lymphomas (with the diffuse large cell lymphoma as the most common), in the nasal area they are mostly T-cell lymphomas.[145,146] In the orbit they lead to an infiltration of the soft tissue structures and of the osseous walls accompanied by proptosis, chemosis, diplopia, epiphora, and ultimately vision loss. The indication exists for an operation to obtain a tissue sample for histological confirmation and subtyping of the lymphoma. A rapid loss of sight due to pressure on the optic nerve can make a microsurgical optic nerve decompression necessary. Once histological confirmation has been obtained, as a rule extensive staging investigations must take place in order to detect further manifestations. Treatment consists of chemotherapy and, where applicable, of local radiotherapy (see Chapter 14).

Metastases

Distant metastases of tumors of another provenance can occur in the area of the nose, the paranasal sinuses, and the orbit. Non-small cell and light-cell adenocarcinomas particularly— for example, from breast, kidney, pancreas, colon, or bronchial cancers— often metastasize in this area.[147] To a great extent the symptoms correspond to those of primary tumors of the paranasal sinuses. In staging investigations, intracerebral metastases are also always to be excluded and, if it is not known, the primary tumor is to be sought, for which PET-CT has proved invaluable in many cases (see Chapter 4). As they are hematogenic distant metastases, treatment should be evaluated with a particularly critical eye. In particular, a conservative approach should be taken with regard to extensive, perhaps even mutilating, interventions.[103,105]

Sinonasal Undifferentiated Carcinoma

Sinonasal undifferentiated carcinoma (sinonasal undifferentiated carcinoma, SNUC) is a very aggressive tumor of the paranasal sinuses. The orbit is infiltrated in early stages of the tumor. The tumor mostly originates in the ethmoid sinus and attacks the posterior, intraconal parts of the orbit, occasionally also the orbital apex.[148,149] Accordingly, as well as chemosis, exophthalmos, and displacement of the eyeball there are also motility impairment due to an infiltration of cranial nerves III, IV, or VI and sight problems.

Table 11.4 Stages of orbital infiltration through malignant tumors of the nasal cavity and the paranasal sinuses (modified according to Maroldi[151])

Stage	Description
I	Tumor reaches the orbital walls; bone erosion without involvement of the orbital contents
II	Tumor causes bone erosion with involvement of the orbital structures; infiltration of the periorbita; the latter is still intact, however
III	Tumor has broken through the bony walls and the periorbita and led to a circumscribed infiltration of the orbit's internal structures (e.g., extraocular muscles)
IV	Diffuse infiltration of the orbit

11.3.5 Infiltration of the Orbit

In line with the close interconnections due to the proximity between the nasal cavity, paranasal sinuses, and orbit, the tumors in question often attack the internal structures of the orbit. With squamous cell carcinoma of the maxillary sinus, the rate of orbital involvement is ~29%.[150] With the primary localization of the tumor in the maxillary sinus, first of all the orbital floor is infiltrated; with the seat of the tumor in the ethmoid sinus, the medial parts of the orbit and the medial part of the orbital floor are infiltrated; and with localization of the tumor in the frontal sinus, the orbital roof is infiltrated.

By means of CT or MRI, infiltration of the orbit can be allocated to stages I to IV, where stage I signifies bone erosion without involvement of the orbit, and stage IV a diffuse orbital infiltration[151] (▶ Table 11.4; ▶ Fig. 11.20).

11.3.6 Treatment of Malignant Tumors

The treatment of malignant tumors of the paranasal sinuses with involvement of the orbit depends on the tumor entity, the tumor stage, and the tumor localization. With squamous cell carcinomas, adenocarcinomas, olfactory neuroblastoma, and malignant melanomas the focus is on surgery to remove the tumor.[143] The approach depends on the tumor localization and tumor extent. With smaller tumors, an endonasal operation controlled endoscopically or microscopically can bring the tumor under control.[110,152] More extensive findings have to be removed via a midfacial degloving approach, a lateral rhinotomy, a bifrontal access, or a transfrontal extradural and intradural approach.[153] The complication rate for the extensive open surgical approaches is reported as 23%, for endoscopic approaches ~6%.[154] Modern surgical concepts have the preservation of the eye as their aim.[150,155] However, if there is a diffuse infiltration of intraorbital structures or of the entire orbit, then orbital exenteration often cannot be avoided.[135] The rationale for an orbital exenteration here is that the area of the tumor can be more easily controlled, and the radiotherapy that usually follows does not have to take special care over radiation-sensitive tissue such as the lens.[156]

As lymph node metastases are found only in ~10% of cases,[103,105,133] a simultaneous neck dissection is only indicated if there is a suspicion sonographically of a metastasis.[103,105]

11

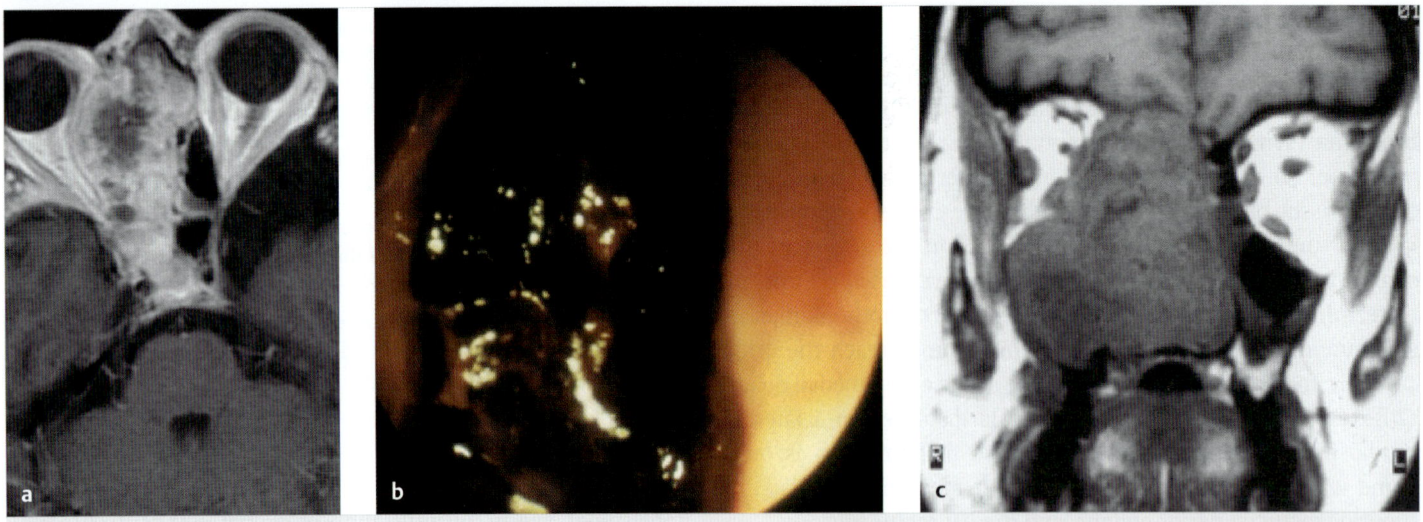

Fig. 11.20 Stages of orbital infiltration by malignant tumors of the paranasal sinuses. (a) Adenocarcinoma with orbital infiltration stage II, MRI. (b) Adenocarcinoma with orbital infiltration stage II, endoscopic view. (c) Orbital infiltration stage III-IV, MRI.

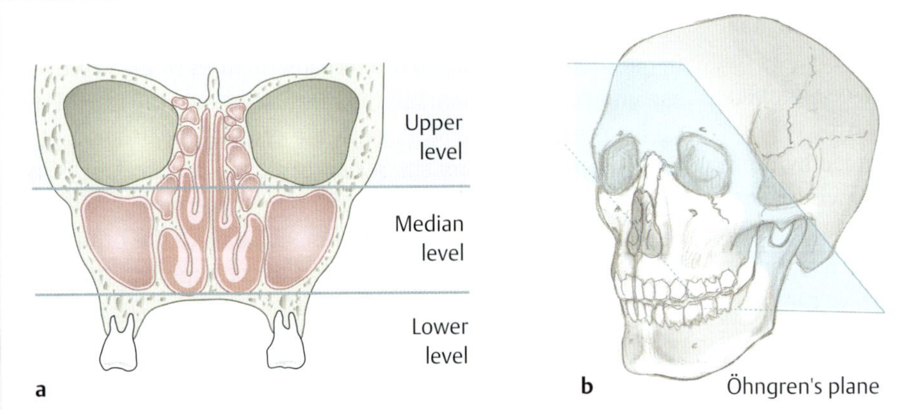

Fig. 11.21 (a) Sebileau levels and (b) Öhngren planes for estimating the prognosis of malignant paranasal sinus tumors. (Reproduced from Strutz J, Mann W, eds. Praxis der HNO-Heilkunde, Kopf- und Halschirurgie. 2nd ed. Stuttgart: Thieme; 2010. Figs. 10.16 e, f.)

With squamous cell carcinoma postoperative radiotherapy is recommended.[103,157] Even with malignant melanomas postoperative radiotherapy seems to have a favorable effect on the prognosis.[143,158] With adenocarcinomas the therapeutic use of radiotherapy with regard to the prognosis is debatable.[132]

11.3.7 Prognosis

The prognosis for malignant tumors in the paranasal sinuses with infiltration of the orbit depends on tumor entity, tumor localization, and tumor extent. As early as 1906, Sebileau described three levels, according to which the prognosis becomes poorer the further cranially the tumor is localized.[159] Öhngren defined a plane somewhat parallel to the skull base and ascribed a prognostic significance to this. If a tumor is located on the cranial side of this plane then the prognosis is significantly poorer than for tumors that are localized caudally to it[159] (▶ Fig. 11.21). These parameters largely based on anatomical conditions. Today, however, they have only historical significance. In particular, the T stage is significantly more closely linked to the prognosis then the anatomical tumor localization.[160,161] Infiltration of the skull base, the orbital apex, or the cavernous sinus or a diffuse infiltration of the orbit are indicators for a poor prognosis.[158,160,162,163]

In total the 5-year survival rates for squamous cell carcinoma and for adenocarcinoma are ~40%.[103,157] Malignant melanomas have a poorer prognosis, mainly due to their high rate of local recurrences.[143,158] The 3-year and 5-year survival rates are reported as 44% and 24–27%.[134,158] After surgical removal, the 5-year survival rate for olfactory neuroblastomas is over 55%.[139,162,164]

References

[1] Jakobiec FA, Rootman J, Jones IS. Secondary and metastatic tumors of the orbit. In: Jones IS, Jakobiec FA, eds. Diseases of the Orbit. Hagerstown, NY: Harper & Row; 1979:503ff

[2] Henderson JW. Orbital Tumors. Philadelphia, PA: WB Saunders; 1973: 444–494

[3] http://www.cancer.net/cancer-types/retinoblastoma-childhood/statistics

[4] Bornfeld N, Schüler A, Bölöni R, et al. Retinoblastom. [Retinoblastoma]. Ophthalmologe. 2006; 103(1):59–76, quiz 77–78

[5] Bornfeld N, Anastassiou A, Fitzek M, et al. Perspektiven der Ophthalmoonkologie. [Article in German]. Dtsch Arztebl. 2004; 101:A2526–A2535

[6] Lohmann D. Die Genetik des Retinoblastoms. Was wissen wir und wie hilft es den Patienten und seiner Familie. WIR Informationsschrift der Aktion für krebskranke Kinder e.V. (Bonn) 2007;1:31–33

[7] Lohmann D. Retinoblastoma. Adv Exp Med Biol. 2010; 685:220–227

[8] Knudson AG, Jr. Mutation and cancer: statistical study of retinoblastoma. Proc Natl Acad Sci U S A. 1971; 68(4):820–823

[9] Jurklies C. Das Retinoblastom—Diagnose und Therapie. WIR Informationsschrift der Aktion für krebskranke Kinder e.V. (Bonn) 2007;1:26

[10] Rootman J. Neoplasia. In: Rootman J, ed. Diseases of the Orbit. A Multidisciplinary Approach. 2nd ed. Philadelphia, PA: Lippincott Wilkins & Williams; 2003:322–324

[11] Künkele A, Jurklies C, Wieland R, et al. Chemoreduction improves eye retention in patients with retinoblastoma: a report from the German Retinoblastoma Reference Centre. Br J Ophthalmol. 2013; 97(10):1277–1283
[12] Abramson DH, Marr BP, Dunkel IJ, et al. Intra-arterial chemotherapy for retinoblastoma in eyes with vitreous and/or subretinal seeding: 2-year results. Br J Ophthalmol. 2012; 96(4):499–502
[13] Natl. Cancer Inst., NIH, USA 12/06/2013. http://www.cancer.gov/cancertopics/types/retinoblastoma
[14] Singh P, Singh A. Choroidal melanoma. Oman J Ophthalmol. 2012; 5(1):3–9
[15] Shields CL, Shields JA, Milite J, De Potter P, Sabbagh R, Menduke H. Uveal melanoma in teenagers and children. A report of 40 cases. Ophthalmology. 1991; 98(11):1662–1666
[16] Dolin PJ, Foss AJ, Hungerford JL. Uveal melanoma: is solar ultraviolet radiation a risk factor? Ophthalmic Epidemiol. 1994; 1(1):27–30
[17] Schmidt-Pokrzywniak A, Jöckel KH, Bornfeld N, Sauerwein W, Stang A. Positive interaction between light iris color and ultraviolet radiation in relation to the risk of uveal melanoma: a case-control study. Ophthalmology. 2009; 116(2):340–348
[18] Singh AD, Rennie IG, Seregard S, Giblin M, McKenzie J. Sunlight exposure and pathogenesis of uveal melanoma. Surv Ophthalmol. 2004; 49(4):419–428
[19] Shields CL, Furuta M, Berman EL, et al. Choroidal nevus transformation into melanoma: analysis of 2514 consecutive cases. Arch Ophthalmol. 2009; 127 (8):981–987
[20] Stang A, Ahrens W, Baumgardt-Elms C, et al. Cooking and uveal melanoma risk: results from two German case-control studies. Cancer Causes Control. 2003; 14(4):377–380
[21] Guénel P, Laforest L, Cyr D, et al. Occupational risk factors, ultraviolet radiation, and ocular melanoma: a case-control study in France. Cancer Causes Control. 2001; 12(5):451–459
[22] Prescher G, Bornfeld N, Hirche H, Horsthemke B, Jöckel KH, Becher R. Prognostic implications of monosomy 3 in uveal melanoma. Lancet. 1996; 347 (9010):1222–1225
[23] Metz CH, Lohmann D, Zeschnigk M, Bornfeld N. [Uveal melanoma: current insights into clinical relevance of genetic testing]. [Article in German]. Klin Monatsbl Augenheilkd. 2013; 230(7):686–691
[24] Abi-Ayad N, Grange JD, Salle M, Kodjikian L. Transretinal uveal melanoma biopsy with 25-gauge vitrectomy system. Acta Ophthalmol. 2013; 91(3):279–281
[25] Augsburger JJ, Shields JA, Folberg R, Lang W, O'Hara BJ, Claricci JD. Fine needle aspiration biopsy in the diagnosis of intraocular cancer. Cytologic-histologic correlations. Ophthalmology. 1985; 92(1):39–49
[26] Fastenberg DM, Finger PT, Chess Q, Koizumi JH, Packer S. Vitrectomy retinotomy aspiration biopsy of choroidal tumors. Am J Ophthalmol. 1990; 110(4): 361–365
[27] Shields CL, Shields JA, Yarian DL, Augsburger JJ. Intracranial extension of choroidal melanoma via the optic nerve. Br J Ophthalmol. 1987; 71(3):172–176
[28] Collaborative Ocular Melanoma Study Group.. Assessment of metastatic disease status at death in 435 patients with large choroidal melanoma in the Collaborative Ocular Melanoma Study (COMS): COMS report no. 15. Arch Ophthalmol. 2001; 119(5):670–676
[29] Bedikian AY. Metastatic uveal melanoma therapy: current options. Int Ophthalmol Clin. 2006; 46(1):151–166
[30] Diener-West M, Reynolds SM, Agugliaro DJ, et al. Collaborative Ocular Melanoma Study Group. Development of metastatic disease after enrollment in the COMS trials for treatment of choroidal melanoma: Collaborative Ocular Melanoma Study Group Report No. 26. Arch Ophthalmol. 2005; 123(12): 1639–1643
[31] Rootman J. Neoplasia. In: Rootman J, ed. Diseases of the Orbit. A Multidisciplinary Approach. 2nd ed. Philadelphia, PA: Lippincott Wilkins & Williams; 2003:324–326
[32] Hawkins BS, Collaborative Ocular Melanoma Study Group. The Collaborative Ocular Melanoma Study (COMS) randomized trial of pre-enucleation radiation of large choroidal melanoma: IV. Ten-year mortality findings and prognostic factors. COMS report number 24. Am J Ophthalmol. 2004; 138(6): 936–951
[33] Hawkins BS. Collaborative ocular melanoma study randomized trial of I-125 brachytherapy. Clin Trials. 2011; 8(5):661–673
[34] Kaliki S, Shields CL, Shields JA. Uveal melanoma: estimating prognosis. Indian J Ophthalmol. 2015; 63(2):93–102
[35] Aaberg TM, Jr. Laser for choroidal melanoma. Int Ophthalmol Clin. 2006; 46 (1):15–26
[36] Lang GE, Mennel S, Spital G, et al. [Different indications of photodynamic therapy in ophthalmology]. [Article in German]. Klin Monatsbl Augenheilkd. 2009; 226(9):725–739
[37] De Potter P, Levecq L. [Transpupillary thermotherapy in the treatment of choroid melanoma]. [Article in French]. J Fr Ophtalmol. 2001; 24(9):937–943
[38] American Brachytherapy Society–Ophthalmic Oncology Task Force. Electronic address: paulfinger@eyecancer.com, ABS–OOTF Committee. The American Brachytherapy Society consensus guidelines for plaque brachytherapy of uveal melanoma and retinoblastoma. Brachytherapy. 2014; 13(1): 1–14
[39] Foerster MH, Bornfeld N, Wessing A, Schulz U, Schmitt G, Meyer-Schwickerath G. [Treatment of malignant melanomas of the uvea with 106-ruthenium applicators. Report on the first 100 Essen cases]. [Article in German]. Klin Monatsbl Augenheilkd. 1984; 185(6):490–494
[40] Gragoudas ES, Seddon J, Goitein M, et al. Current results of proton beam irradiation of uveal melanomas. Ophthalmology. 1985; 92(2):284–291
[41] Linstadt D, Castro J, Char D, et al. Long-term results of helium ion irradiation of uveal melanoma. Int J Radiat Oncol Biol Phys. 1990; 19(3):613–618
[42] Modorati G, Miserocchi E, Galli L, Picozzi P, Rama P. Gamma knife radiosurgery for uveal melanoma: 12 years of experience. Br J Ophthalmol. 2009; 93 (1):40–44
[43] Schönfeld S, Cordini D, Riechardt AI, et al. Proton beam therapy leads to excellent local control rates in choroidal melanoma in the intermediate fundus zone. Am J Ophthalmol. 2014; 158(6):1184–1191
[44] Bechrakis NE, Bornfeld N, Zöller I, Foerster MH. Iodine 125 plaque brachytherapy versus transscleral tumor resection in the treatment of large uveal melanomas. Ophthalmology. 2002; 109(10):1855–1861
[45] Finger PT. Radiation therapy for choroidal melanoma. Surv Ophthalmol. 1997; 42(3):215–232
[46] Damato BE, Foulds WS. Surgical resection of choroidal melanomas. In: Ryan SJ. Retina. St. Louis, MO: Mosby; 2001:762–772
[47] Foulds WS. Local resection and other conservative therapies for intraocular melanoma. Curr Opin Ophthalmol. 1995; 6(3):62–69
[48] Rice JC, Stannard C, Cook C, Lecuona K, Myer L, Scholtz RP. Brachytherapy and endoresection for choroidal melanoma: a cohort study. Br J Ophthalmol. 2014; 98(1):86–91
[49] Shields JA. Intraocular Tumors. A Text and Atlas. Philadelphia, PA: WB Saunders; 1992:175
[50] Center for Disease Control and Prevention, 2014. https://www.cdc.gov/nchs/fastats/deaths.htm
[51] National Cancer Institute. https://cancerstatisticscenter.cancer.org/?_ga=1.153190392.1951915466.1483126234#/
[52] Horner JF. Carcinom der Dura mater und Metastase der Mm. recti mit Exophthalmus. [Article in German]. Klin Monatsbl Augenheilkd. 1864; 2–1:86–1–90
[53] Perl M. Contribution to pathology of tumors. Virchows Arch Pathol Anat. 1872; 56:445–448
[54] Godtfredsen E. On the frequency of secondary carcinoma of the choroid. Acta Ophthalmol. 1944; 22:394–400
[55] Bloch RS, Gartner S. The incidence of ocular metastatic carcinoma. Arch Ophthalmol. 1971; 85(6):673–675
[56] Albert DM, Rubenstein RA, Scheie HG. Tumor metastasis to the eye. I. Incidence in 213 adult patients with generalized malignancy. Am J Ophthalmol. 1967; 63(4):723–726
[57] Albert DM, Rubenstein RA, Scheie HG. Tumor metastasis to the eye. II. Clinical study in infants and children. Am J Ophthalmol. 1967; 63(4):727–732
[58] Eliassi-Rad B, Albert DM, Green WR. Frequency of ocular metastases in patients dying of cancer in eye bank populations. Br J Ophthalmol. 1996; 80(2): 125–128
[59] Nelson CC, Hertzberg BS, Klintworth GK. A histopathologic study of 716 unselected eyes in patients with cancer at the time of death. Am J Ophthalmol. 1983; 95(6):788–793
[60] Shields CL, Shields JA, Gross NE, Schwartz GP, Lally SE. Survey of 520 eyes with uveal metastases. Ophthalmology. 1997; 104(8):1265–1276
[61] Ferry AP, Font RL. Carcinoma metastatic to the eye and orbit. I. A clinicopathologic study of 227 cases. Arch Ophthalmol. 1974; 92(4):276–286
[62] Freedman MI, Folk JC. Metastatic tumors to the eye and orbit. Patient survival and clinical characteristics. Arch Ophthalmol. 1987; 105(9):1215–1219
[63] Weiss L. Analysis of the incidence of intraocular metastasis. Br J Ophthalmol. 1993; 77(3):149–151

[64] Wiegel T, Kreusel KM, Bornfeld N, et al. Frequency of asymptomatic choroidal metastasis in patients with disseminated breast cancer: results of a prospective screening programme. Br J Ophthalmol. 1998; 82(10): 1159–1161

[65] Shields JA, Shields CL, Singh AD. Metastatic neoplasms in the optic disc: the 1999 Bjerrum Lecture: part 2. Arch Ophthalmol. 2000; 118(2):217–224

[66] Mansour AM, Hidayat AA. Metastatic eyelid disease. Ophthalmology. 1987; 94(6):667–670

[67] Augsburger JJ. Fluorescence angiography of choroidal and retinal tumors. In: Tasman W, ed., Jaeger EA, assoc. ed. Duane's Foundations of Clinical Ophthalmology. CD-ROM ed. Vol. 2. Hagerstown, NY: Lippincott Williams & Wilkins; 2006

[68] Heimann H, Kellner U, Foerster MH. Atlas of Fundus Angiography. Stuttgart: Thieme; 2006:90–91

[69] Kreusel KM, Wiegel T, Stange M, Bornfeld N, Foerster MH. [Intraocular metastases of metastatic breast carcinoma in the woman. Incidence, risk factors and therapy]. [Article in German]. Ophthalmologe. 2000; 97(5):342–346

[70] Chen CJ, McCoy AN, Brahmer J, Handa JT. Emerging treatments for choroidal metastases. Surv Ophthalmol. 2011; 56(6):511–521

[71] Small W, Jr. Management of ocular metastasis. Cancer Contr. 1998; 5(4):326–332

[72] Shah SU, Mashayekhi A, Shields CL, et al. Uveal metastasis from lung cancer: clinical features, treatment, and outcome in 194 patients. Ophthalmology. 2014; 121(1):352–357

[73] Shields CL, Shields JA, De Potter P, et al. Plaque radiotherapy for the management of uveal metastasis. Arch Ophthalmol. 1997; 115(2):203–209

[74] Puri P, Gupta M, Rundle PA, Rennie IG. Indocyanine green augmented transpupillary thermotherapy in the management of choroidal metastasis from breast carcinoma. Eye (Lond). 2001; 15(Pt 4):515–518

[75] Romanowska-Dixon B, Kowal J, Pogrzebielski A, Markiewicz A. [Transpupillary thermotherapy (TTT) for intraocular metastases in choroid]. [Article in Polish]. Klin Oczna. 2011; 113(4–6):132–135

[76] Brady LW, Shields JA, Augsburger JJ, Day JL. Malignant intraocular tumors. Cancer. 1982; 49(3):578–585

[77] Lommatzsch AP. Metastastische Tumoren der Aderhaut und der Netzhaut. In: Lommatzsch PK, eds. Ophthalmologische Onkologie. Stuttgart: Enke;1999:374–380

[78] Martín Martorell P, Marí Cotino JF, Insa A. Choroidal metastases from lung adenocarcinoma. Clin Transl Oncol. 2009; 11(10):694–697

[79] Merrill CF, Kaufman DI, Dimitrov NV. Breast cancer metastatic to the eye is a common entity. Cancer. 1991; 68(3):623–627

[80] Shields JA, Shields CL, Kiratli H, de Potter P. Metastatic tumors to the iris in 40 patients. Am J Ophthalmol. 1995; 119(4):422–430

[81] Shakin EP, Shields JA. Metastatic cancer to the eye and adnexa. In: Tasman W, ed., Jaeger EA, assoc. ed. Duane's Ophthalmology. CD-ROM ed. Vol. 5. Philadelphia, PA: Lippincott Williams & Wilkins; 2006. http://www.oculist.net/downaton502/prof/ebook/duanes/pages/v5/v5c034.html. Accessed August 25, 2016

[82] Marwaha G, Macklis R, Singh AD. Radiation therapy: orbital tumors. Dev Ophthalmol. 2013; 52:94–101

[83] Skinner HD, Garden AS, Rosenthal DI, et al. Outcomes of malignant tumors of the lacrimal apparatus: the University of Texas MD Anderson Cancer Center experience. Cancer. 2011; 117(12):2801–2810

[84] Chawla B, Kashyap S, Sen S, et al. Clinicopathologic review of epithelial tumors of the lacrimal gland. Ophthal Plast Reconstr Surg. 2013; 29(6):440–445

[85] Gupta A, Khandelwal A. Lacrimal gland pleomorphic adenoma: an inconceivable diagnosis in a child. BMJ Case Rep. 2013; 2013:bcr2013009138

[86] von Holstein SL, Fehr A, Persson M, et al. Lacrimal gland pleomorphic adenoma and carcinoma ex pleomorphic adenoma: genomic profiles, gene fusions, and clinical characteristics. Ophthalmology. 2014; 121(5):1125–1133

[87] Schwarcz RM, Coupland SE, Finger PT. Cancer of the orbit and adnexa. Am J Clin Oncol. 2013; 36(2):197–205

[88] Moret A, Tabareau-Delalande F, Joly A, de Muret A, Goga D, Laure B. [Myoepithelial carcinoma of the lacrimal gland]. Rev Stomatol Chir Maxillofac Chir Orale. 2014; 115(3):172–177

[89] Kubota T, Moritani S, Ichihara S. Clinicopathologic and immunohistochemical features of primary ductal adenocarcinoma of lacrimal gland: five new cases and review of literature. Graefes Arch Clin Exp Ophthalmol. 2013; 251(8): 2071–2076

[90] von Holstein SL, Fehr A, Persson M, et al. Adenoid cystic carcinoma of the lacrimal gland: MYB gene activation, genomic imbalances, and clinical characteristics. Ophthalmology. 2013; 120(10):2130–2138

[91] Mendoza PR, Jakobiec FA, Krane JF. Immunohistochemical features of lacrimal gland epithelial tumors. Am J Ophthalmol. 2013; 156(6):1147–1158.e1

[92] Mulay K, Puthyapurayil FM, Mohammad JA, Hasnat Ali M, Honavar SG, Reddy VA. Adenoid cystic carcinoma of the lacrimal gland: role of nuclear survivin (BIRC5) as a prognostic marker. Histopathology. 2013; 62(6):840–846

[93] Gensheimer MF, Rainey D, Douglas JG, et al. Neutron radiotherapy for adenoid cystic carcinoma of the lacrimal gland. Ophthal Plast Reconstr Surg. 2013; 29(4):256–260

[94] Tse DT, Kossler AL, Feuer WJ, Benedetto PW. Long-term outcomes of neoadjuvant intra-arterial cytoreductive chemotherapy for lacrimal gland adenoid cystic carcinoma. Ophthalmology. 2013; 120(7):1313–1323

[95] Boecker W, Stenman G, Loening T, et al. K5/K14-positive cells contribute to salivary gland-like breast tumors with myoepithelial differentiation. Mod Pathol. 2013; 26(8):1086–1100

[96] Rasmussen PK. Diffuse large B-cell lymphoma and mantle cell lymphoma of the ocular adnexal region, and lymphoma of the lacrimal gland: an investigation of clinical and histopathological features. Acta Ophthalmol 2013;91 Thesis 5:1–27. doi: 10.1111/aos.12189

[97] Hother C, Rasmussen PK, Joshi T, et al. MicroRNA profiling in ocular adnexal lymphoma: a role for MYC and NFKB1 mediated dysregulation of microRNA expression in aggressive disease. Invest Ophthalmol Vis Sci. 2013; 54(8): 5169–5175

[98] Tanweer F, Mahkamova K, Harkness P. Nasolacrimal duct tumours in the era of endoscopic dacryocystorhinostomy: literature review. J Laryngol Otol. 2013; 127(7):670–675

[99] Eweiss AZ, Lund VJ, Jay A, Rose G. Transitional cell tumours of the lacrimal drainage apparatus. Rhinology. 2013; 51(4):349–354

[100] Qiu B, Lin YB, Cai QQ, et al. Primary lymphoepithelioma-like carcinoma of ocular adnexa: clinicopathologic features and treatment. Curr Oncol. 2013; 20 (2):e113–e122

[101] Zhu D, Ikpatt OF, Dubovy SR, et al. Molecular and genomic aberrations in Chlamydophila psittaci negative ocular adnexal marginal zone lymphomas. Am J Hematol. 2013; 88(9):730–735

[102] Weisman RA, Kikkawa D, Moe KS, Osguthorpe JD. Orbital tumors. Otolaryngol Clin North Am. 2001; 34(6):1157–1174, ix–x

[103] Hosemann W. Innere Nase und Nasennebenhöhlen. In: Strutz J, Mann W, eds. Praxis der HNO-Heilkunde, Kopf- und Halschirurgie. 2nd ed. Stuttgart: Thieme; 2010:402–454

[104] Barnes L, Eveson JW, Reichart P, et al. Pathology and Genetics of Head and Neck Tumors (WHO organization classification of tumors). Lyon, France: IARC Press; 2005

[105] Hosemann W, Dammer R, Bloss HG, Fietkau R. [Therapy of malignant tumors in the area of the paranasal sinuses]. [Article in German]. HNO. 2002; 50(6): 578–592, quiz 593–595

[106] Lee KY, Seah LL, Tow S, Cullen JF, Fong KS. Nasopharyngeal carcinoma with orbital involvement. Ophthal Plast Reconstr Surg. 2008; 24(3):185–189

[107] Keche P, Nitnaware AZ, Mair M, Sakhare P, Satpute S. A study of tumours giving rise to unilateral proptosis. Indian J Otolaryngol Head Neck Surg. 2013; 65 Suppl 1:6–13

[108] Galiè M, Mandrioli S, Tieghi R, Clauser L. Giant mucocele of the frontal sinus. J Craniofac Surg. 2005; 16(5):933–935

[109] Bonavolontà G, Strianese D, Grassi P, et al. An analysis of 2,480 space-occupying lesions of the orbit from 1976 to 2011. Ophthal Plast Reconstr Surg. 2013; 29(2):79–86

[110] Lund VJ, Stammberger H, Nicolai P, et al. European Rhinologic Society Advisory Board on Endoscopic Techniques in the Management of Nose, Paranasal Sinus and Skull Base Tumours. European position paper on endoscopic management of tumours of the nose, paranasal sinuses and skull base. Rhinol Suppl. 2010; 22(22):1–143

[111] Owosho AA, Potluri A, Bilodeau EA. Osseous dysplasia (cemento-osseous dysplasia) of the jaw bones in western Pennsylvania patients: analysis of 35 cases. Pa Dent J (Harrisb). 2013; 80(6):25–29

[112] Damera NC, Vallabhaneni KC, Tripuraneni SC, Madala S, Diddi RR. Non malignant maxillary lesions: our experience. Indian J Otolaryngol Head Neck Surg. 2013; 65 Suppl 1:74–79

[113] Selva D, White VA, O'Connell JX, Rootman J. Primary bone tumors of the orbit. Surv Ophthalmol. 2004; 49(3):328–342

[114] Muwazi LM, Kamulegeya A. The 5-year prevalence of maxillofacial fibro-osseous lesions in Uganda. Oral Dis. 2015; 21(1):e79–e85

[115] Phattarataratip E, Pholjaroen C, Tiranon P. A clinicopathologic analysis of 207 cases of benign fibro-osseous lesions of the jaws. Int J Surg Pathol. 2014; 22 (4):326–333

[116] Carini F, Saggese V, Porcaro G, Baldoni M. Treatment of craniofacial fibrous dysplasia: a case report. Minerva Stomatol. 2014; 63(1–2):43–49

[117] Foster BL, Ramnitz MS, Gafni RI, et al. Rare bone diseases and their dental, oral, and craniofacial manifestations. J Dent Res. 2014; 93(7) Suppl:7S–19S

[118] E Horvai A, C Jordan R. Fibro-osseous lesions of the craniofacial bones: β-catenin immunohistochemical analysis and CTNNB1 and APC mutation analysis. Head Neck Pathol. 2014; 8(3):291–297

[119] Garg MK, Bhardwaj R, Gupta S, Mann N, Kharb S, Pandit A. Sarcomatous transformation (Leiomyosarcoma) in polyostotic fibrous dysplagia. Indian J Endocrinol Metab. 2013; 17(6):1120–1123

[120] Chourmouzi D, Psoma E, Drevelegas A. Ground-glass pattern fibrous dysplasia of frontal sinus. JBR-BTR. 2013; 96(6):378–380

[121] Wong G, Randhawa P, Stephens J, Saleh H. Fibrous dysplasia of the nasal bone: case reports and literature review. J Laryngol Otol. 2013; 127(11): 1152–1154

[122] Bowers CA, Taussky P, Couldwell WT. Surgical treatment of craniofacial fibrous dysplasia in adults. Neurosurg Rev. 2014; 37(1):47–53

[123] Fusconi M, Conte M, Pagliarella M, et al. Fibrous dysplasia of the maxilla: diagnostic reliability of the study image. Literature review. J Neurol Surg B Skull Base. 2013; 74(6):364–368

[124] Wick MR, McDermott MB, Swanson PE. Proliferative, reparative, and reactive benign bone lesions that may be confused diagnostically with true osseous neoplasms. Semin Diagn Pathol. 2014; 31(1):66–88

[125] Coulter C, Richards R, Peterson D, Collier J. Parietal skull reconstruction using immediate PEEK cranioplasty following resection for craniofacial fibrous dysplasia. J Plast Reconstr Aesthet Surg. 2014; 67(8):e208–e209

[126] Welkoborsky HJ, Portmann K, Hoffmann F, Jacob R, Mann WJ, Amedee RG. Proliferative activity and cytometric characteristics in polyps of the nasal cavity and paranasal sinuses. Am J Rhinol. 2000; 14(2):87–91

[127] Kühnel T, Hosemann W. Chirurgische Therapie. In: Strutz J, Mann W, eds. Praxis der HNO-Heilkunde, Kopf- und Halschirurgie. 2nd ed. Stuttgart: Thieme; 2010:455–469

[128] Kim DY, Hong SL, Lee CH, et al. Inverted papilloma of the nasal cavity and paranasal sinuses: a Korean multicenter study. Laryngoscope. 2012; 122(3): 487–494

[129] Saldana M, Wearne M, Beigi B, Petrarca R. Inverted papillomas of the nasal and paranasal sinuses that involve the ocular/adnexal region. Orbit. 2013; 32 (6):366–369

[130] Welkoborsky HJ, Gosepath J, Jacob R, Mann WJ, Amedee RG. Biologic characteristics of paragangliomas of the nasal cavity and paranasal sinuses. Am J Rhinol. 2000; 14(6):419–426

[131] Papaspyrou K, Welkoborsky HJ, Gouveris H, Mann WJ. Malignant and benign sinonasal paragangliomas. Laryngoscope. 2013; 123(8):1830–1836

[132] Van Gerven L, Vander Poorten V, Jorissen M. Adenocarcinomas of the sinonasal tract: current opinion. B-ENT. 2011; 7 Suppl 17:15–20

[133] Pickhard A, Durst F, Staudenmaier R, Reiter R. Management und Prognose von Patienten mit Plattenepithelkarzinomen der Nasenhaupt- und Nasennebenhöhlen. [Management and prognosis of patients with squamous cell carcinomas of the nasal cavity and the paranasal sinuses]. Laryngo-rhino-otol. 2012; 91(10):627–632

[134] Gal TJ, Silver N, Huang B. Demographics and treatment trends in sinonasal mucosal melanoma. Laryngoscope. 2011; 121(9):2026–2033

[135] Gras Cabrerizo JR, Sarandeses Garcia A, Montserrat I, Gili JR, Orus Dotu C. Revision of carcinomas in paranasal sinuses. Acta Otorrinolaringol. 2007; 58(6): 266–275

[136] Kuijpens JH, Louwman MW, Peters R, Janssens GO, Burdorf AL, Coebergh JW. Trends in sinonasal cancer in The Netherlands: more squamous cell cancer, less adenocarcinoma. A population-based study 1973–2009. Eur J Cancer. 2012; 48(15):2369–2374

[137] Yi JS, Cho GS, Shim MJ, Min JY, Chung YS, Lee BJ. Malignant tumors of the sinonasal tract in the pediatric population. Acta Otolaryngol. 2012; 132 Suppl 1:S21–S26

[138] Reino AJ. Factors in the pathogenesis of tumors of the sphenoid and maxillary sinuses: a comparative study. Laryngoscope. 2000; 110(10 Pt 2) Suppl 96:1–38

[139] Mitchell EH, Diaz A, Yilmaz T, et al. Multimodality treatment for sinonasal neuroendocrine carcinoma. Head Neck. 2012; 34(10):1372–1376

[140] Wittekind C, Klimpfinger M, Sobin LH. TNM-Atlas. 5th ed. Heidelberg: Springer; 2005

[141] Ansa B, Goodman M, Ward K, et al. Paranasal sinus squamous cell carcinoma incidence and survival based on Surveillance, Epidemiology, and End Results data, 1973 to 2009. Cancer. 2013; 119(14):2602–2610

[142] Wolfish EB, Nelson BL, Thompson LD. Sinonasal tract mucoepidermoid carcinoma: a clinicopathologic and immunophenotypic study of 19 cases combined with a comprehensive review of the literature. Head Neck Pathol. 2012; 6(2):191–207

[143] Jangard M, Hansson J, Ragnarsson-Olding B. Primary sinonasal malignant melanoma: a nationwide study of the Swedish population, 1960–2000. Rhinology. 2013; 51(1):22–30

[144] Welkoborsky HJ, Sorger K, Collo D. Klinische, histologische und immunhistochemische Charakteristika der Schleimhautmelanome der Nase und Nasennebenhöhlen. [Malignant melanoma of the mucous membranes of the upper aerodigestive tract. Clinical, histological and immunohistochemical characteristics]. Laryngorhinootologie. 1991; 70:302–306

[145] Cuadra-Garcia I, Proulx GM, Wu CL, et al. Sinonasal lymphoma: a clinicopathologic analysis of 58 cases from the Massachusetts General Hospital. Am J Surg Pathol. 1999; 23(11):1356–1369

[146] Abbondanzo SL, Wenig BM. Non-Hodgkin's lymphoma of the sinonasal tract. A clinicopathologic and immunophenotypic study of 120 cases. Cancer. 1995; 75(6):1281–1291

[147] De Potter P, Disneur D, Levecq L, Snyers B. [Ocular manifestations of cancer]. J Fr Ophtalmol. 2002; 25(2):194–202

[148] Spitellie PH, Jordan DR, Brownstein S, Gooi P, Burns B. Sinonasal undifferentiated carcinoma with a frozen globe. Ophthal Plast Reconstr Surg. 2008; 24 (3):225–227

[149] Wallace S, Pilon A, Kwok P, Messner LV, Hitchcock Y. Ophthalmic manifestations of an undifferentiated sinonasal carcinoma. Optom Vis Sci. 2008; 85(4): 226–229

[150] Nishino H, Takanosawa M, Kawada K, et al. Multidisciplinary therapy consisting of minimally invasive resection, irradiation, and intra-arterial infusion of 5-fluorouracil for maxillary sinus carcinomas. Head Neck. 2013; 35(6):772–778

[151] Maroldi R, Farina D, Battaglia G, Maculotti P, Chiesa A. [Magnetic resonance and computed tomography compared in the staging of rhinosinusal neoplasms. A cost-effectiveness evaluation]. Radiol Med (Torino). 1996; 91(3): 211–218

[152] Karligkiotis A, Appiani MC, Verillaud B, Herman P. How to prevent diplopia in endoscopic transnasal resection of tumors involving the medial orbital wall. Laryngoscope. 2014; 124(9):2017–2020

[153] Zhang TM, Fang JG, Chen XH, Zhang JL, Li Y, Zhao JW. [Trans-cranio-naso-orbital approach in treatment of ethmoid sinus malignant tumors: analysis of 39 cases]. Zhonghua Yi Xue Za Zhi. 2007; 87(5):304–307

[154] Suh JD, Ramakrishnan VR, Chi JJ, Palmer JN, Chiu AG. Outcomes and complications of endoscopic approaches for malignancies of the paranasal sinuses and anterior skull base. Ann Otol Rhinol Laryngol. 2013; 122(1):54–59

[155] Tiwari R, Quak J, Egeler S, et al. Tumors of the infratemporal fossa. Skull Base Surg. 2000; 10(1):1–9

[156] Frunză A, Slăvescu D, Zamfirescu D, et al. Orbital exenteration—a salvage procedure? Rom J Morphol Embryol. 2013; 54(4):1161–1167

[157] Ren B, Cui Y, Chen J. [Analysis of the late curative effect of 432 cases with advanced squamous cell carcinoma of the maxillary sinus]. Zhonghua Er Bi Yan Hou Ke Za Zhi. 1999; 34(4):201–203

[158] Koivunen P, Bäck L, Pukkila M, et al. Accuracy of the current TNM classification in predicting survival in patients with sinonasal mucosal melanoma. Laryngoscope. 2012; 122(8):1734–1738

[159] Ohngren G. Malignant disease of the upper jaw (Section of Laryngology and Section of Otology). Proc R Soc Med. 1936; 29(11):1497–1514

[160] Cantú G, Solero CL, Mariani L, Mattavelli F, Pizzi N, Licitra L. A new classification for malignant tumors involving the anterior skull base. Arch Otolaryngol Head Neck Surg. 1999; 125(11):1252–1257

[161] Kreppel M, Scheer M, Beutner D, et al. Stage grouping in tumors of the ethmoid sinuses and the nasal cavity using the sixth edition of the UICC classification of malignant tumors. Head Neck 2013;35:257–264

[162] Albu S, St Florian I, Szabo I, Băciuţ G, Băciuţ M, Mitre I. Craniofacial resection for malignant tumors of the paranasal sinuses. Chirurgia (Bucur). 2011; 106 (2):219–225

[163] Ye M, Tu GY. [Proposal on T staging of maxillary sinus cancer]. Zhonghua Zhong Liu Za Zhi. 1988; 10(2):129–131

[164] Michel J, Fakhry N, Santini L, Mancini J, Giovanni A, Dessi P. Nasal and paranasal esthesioneuroblastomas: clinical outcomes. Eur Ann Otorhinolaryngol Head Neck Dis. 2012; 129(5):238–243

Suggested Further Readings

Singh N, Kulkarni P, Aggarwal AN, et al. Choroidal metastasis as a presenting manifestation of lung cancer: a report of 3 cases and systematic review of the literature. Medicine (Baltimore). 2012; 91(4):179–194

Augsburger JJ, Shields JA. Fine needle aspiration biopsy of solid intraocular tumors: indications, instrumentation and techniques. Ophthalmic Surg. 1984; 15(1):34–40

Cohen VML. Ocular metastases. Eye (Lond). 2013; 27(2):137–141

Kreusel KM, Wiegel T, Stange M, Hinkelbein W. Aderhautmetastasen bei metastasiertem Bronchialcarcinom–erste Ergebnisse einer klinischen Studie. [Article in German]. Der Ophthalmologe. 1997 Suppl. 1:S:160

Kreusel KM, Bechrakis N, Wiegel T, Emmerlich T, Foerster MH. Klinische Charakteristika der Aderhautmetastasierung. [Clinical characteristics of choroidal metastasis]. Ophthalmologe. 2003; 100(8):618–622

Mewis L, Young SE. Breast carcinoma metastatic to the choroid. Analysis of 67 patients. Ophthalmology. 1982; 89(2):147–151

Sassmannshausen J, Bornfeld N, Foerster MH, Sauerwein W, Schreiber T, Wessing A. Metastasen maligner extraokularer Tumoren in der Aderhaut. Diagnose und fraktionierte Strahlentherapie. [Article in German]. Fortschr Ophthalmol. 1990; 87(1):69–73

Shields JA, Shields CL, Donoso LA. Management of posterior uveal melanoma. Surv Ophthalmol. 1991; 36(3):161–195

Shields JA, Shields CL, De Potter P, Cu-Unjieng A, Hernandez C, Brady LW. Plaque radiotherapy for uveal melanoma. Int Ophthalmol Clin. 1993; 33(3):129–135

Shields JA, Shields CL, Eagle RC, Jr, Gündüz K, Lin B. Diffuse ocular metastases as an initial sign of metastatic lung cancer. Ophthalmic Surg Lasers. 1998; 29(7): 598–601

Shields JA, Shields CL, Eagle RC, Jr, McNamara JA. Lung cancer presenting as vitreous hemorrhage from choroidal metastasis. Retina. 2004; 24(1):168–170

Stephens RF, Shields JA. Diagnosis and management of cancer metastatic to the uvea: a study of 70 cases. Ophthalmology. 1979; 86(7):1336–1349

Klimek T, Atai E, Schubert M, Glanz H. Inverted papilloma of the nasal cavity and paranasal sinuses: clinical data, surgical strategy and recurrence rates. Acta Otolaryngol. 2000; 120(2):267–272

Chapter 12

Tumors of the Fronto-orbital Skull Base, the Optic Nerves, and the Intracranial Optic Pathways

12

12 Tumors of the Fronto-orbital Skull Base, the Optic Nerves, and the Intracranial Optic Pathways

I. E. Sandalcioglu and U. Sure

12.1 Introduction

Orbital tumors are rare, while tumors localized at the medial and lateral frontobasal skull base involving and infiltrating the orbital structures are common. These tumors are divided into primary and secondary orbital tumors depending on their dignity and localization, which can cause different clinical symptoms and require various treatment strategies.[1] In contrast to inflammatory or vascular orbital lesions, orbital tumors present with slow progressive symptoms such as proptosis and incomplete eyelid occlusion. Another major symptom is the slow progressive impairment of vision, which can also deteriorate acutely in a progressive condition.

Proptosis due to local mass effect and consequent decrease of the mobility of the eye can cause additional symptoms such as double vision. Visual function can also be impaired by direct neuronal and muscular damage due to lesions inside or adjacent to the orbit. The most frequent reasons for neuronal dysfunctions are tumorous processes infiltrating the anatomical pathways of the orbit, such as the superior and inferior orbital fissure and the optic canal.

The different tumors of the orbit, the fronto-orbital skull base, and the optic pathways are described according to their clinical importance and frequency in the following.

12

Memorize M!

Orbital tumors can occur within the orbit or adjacent to the orbit with secondary infiltration. Painless proptosis and impairment of visual acuity are the leading symptoms.

12.2 Meningiomas of the Frontal Skull Base and the Orbit

Intracranial meningiomas are very common, accounting for 25 to 30% of all primary intracranial tumors; they frequently involve the orbital structures or grow intraorbitally.[2,3,4]

Meningiomas commonly arise intracranially from the frontal skull base and are classified according to their localization and dural attachment and as well as to their histological differentiation. Histologically they are mostly benign tumors classified as grade I and infrequently as grade II tumors (atypical meningiomas). Malignant meningiomas are rare and classified as grade III tumors (anaplastic meningioma) and are characterized by a poor prognosis.[5]

The most common localization with orbital involvement is the medial and lateral **sphenoid wing**, the **anterior clinoid process**, the **tuberculum sellae**, and the **frontal skull base**. In contrast to these localizations, meningiomas of the **orbit** and **optic sheath meningiomas** are rare.[2,4,6,7,8,9,10]

Whereas meningiomas arising from the sphenoid wing, the anterior clinoid process, and optic sheath result in unilateral symptoms, midline tumors arising from the sellar tubercle or sphenoidal plane lead frequently to bilateral symptoms and visual impairment due to their close correlation and affection of both optic nerves and the optic chiasm.[9]

Imaging studies and intraoperative findings show infiltration of the optic canal, optic nerve involvement, or infiltration of the cavernous sinus by meningiomas with "en plaque" growth pattern[7,11,12,13] (▶ Fig. 12.1).

Tumors arising from the sphenoid wing with extension to the lateral orbital wall are defined as spheno-orbital meningiomas. These tumors grow slowly with absent or minor symptoms, but they can achieve enormous sizes and consequently involve important neurovascular structures[14] (▶ Fig. 12.2). Radical resection of these tumors is related to high risks, so that an incomplete resection is preferred to preserve neurovascular functions.[2,3,7,9,11,13] Magnetic resonance imaging (MRI) is the most important diagnostic method for imaging of meningiomas. These tumors are characterized by a mass with clearly defined borders and typical homogeneous contrast enhancement (▶ Fig. 12.3 and ▶ Fig. 12.4). Meningiomas of the sphenoid wing can infiltrate the osseous structures or can grow entirely intraosseously. The osseous elements with tumorous infiltration appear enlarged and can involve the lateral orbital wall. High-resolution computed tomography with three-dimensional reconstruction is recommended in these cases for the delineation of the osseous structures involved and for surgical planning of osseous resection and preoperative planning of necessary cranio-orbital reconstruction.

Memorize M!

Meningiomas are mostly benign tumors and can reach large sizes due to their slow growth pattern. If they are localized in the optic canal, they can cause loss of visual acuity in the early onset of the disease.

Optic canal tumors can grow in the circumference of the optic nerve. These tumors can be approached and resected via the subfrontal route. If necessary, the complete course of the optic nerve can be delineated and decompressed.

Complete tumor resection is achieved and both optic nerves, the chiasm, and the contralateral internal carotid artery are delineated after meticulous mobilization of the tumor and decompression of the optic nerve (▶ Fig. 12.1d). Both optic nerves, the optic chiasm, and the contralateral internal carotid artery are exposed (▶ Fig. 12.1e).

12.3 Malignant Tumors of the Frontal Skull Base and the Orbit

Carcinomas of the paranasal sinuses, metastases, esthesioneuroblastomas, sarcomas and malignant melanomas are the most common malignant tumors of the frontal skull base with infiltration of the orbit.[15,16]

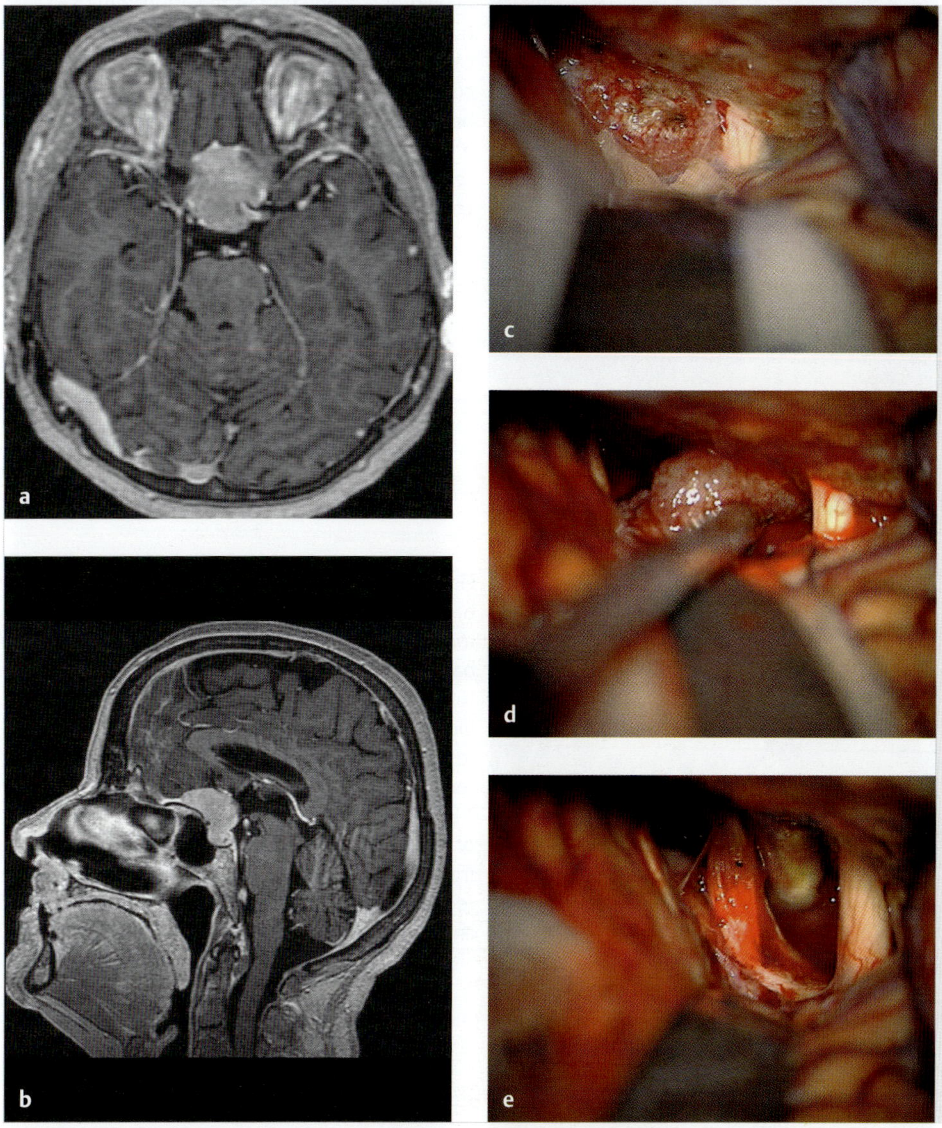

Fig. 12.1 Tuberculum sellae meningioma with optic nerve involvement. **(a, b)** MRI of a tuberculum sellae meningioma with extension to the sphenoidal plane and distinct compression of the optic chiasm. Homogeneous contrast enhancement is characteristic of the circumscribed tumor with contact with the dural matrix and invasion into the sellar region. **(c–e)** Intraoperative delineation of the tumor after right-sided frontal craniotomy and subfrontal approach. The surgeon reaches the surface of the tumor after exposure of the cisterns and release of CSF **(c)**. The tumor causes significant medial compression of the ipsilateral optic nerve within optic canal. The orbital roof can be exposed extradurally and intradurally with this approach.

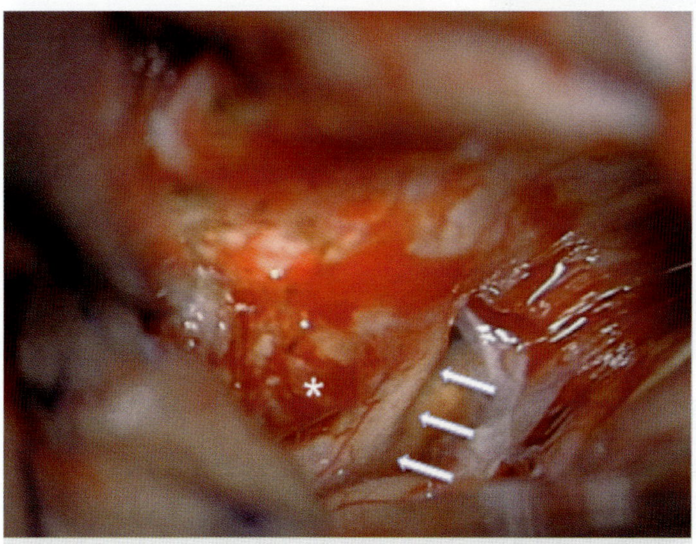

Fig. 12.2 Meningioma of the left anterior clinoid process with optic canal infiltration. Intradural delineation of a left-sided meningioma (*asterisk*) laterally to the optic nerve (*arrows*) arising from the anterior clinoid process after left-sided supraorbital "keyhole" craniotomy. Note the compression of the left optic nerve in the proximity and within the optic canal by the meningioma. Although the tumor has a size of a few millimeters, it affects the optic nerve by compression at the entrance to the orbit, with visual impairment and visual field disturbance.

Both orbits can be involved and infiltrated because of their close anatomical relationships, so that surgical resection can be significantly aggravated.[17] Contrast-enhanced MRI and high-resolution CT are the diagnostic methods of imaging with sagittal and coronal reconstructions and are employed for proper surgical planning. The possibilities and the dimension of surgical resection should be evaluated very precisely and discussed thoroughly with the patient as part of an interdisciplinary treatment protocol with the focus on the risks to visual function and the prognosis.

The resection of tumorous osseous structures such as the orbital roof or the lateral orbital wall is not associated with resulting functional deficits. In contrast, a higher functional risk is seen in tumors with infiltration of the periorbita or the ocular muscles. The osseous elements can be reconstructed using various methods and materials. Autologous tissues can be used, such as calvarial split bone of the healthy tabula interna of a frontal bone flap, or industrially produced materials such as titanium mesh or computer-aided design implants.

Malignant tumors often infiltrate the frontobasal dura, so that meticulous duraplasty and cranioplasty should be undertaken maximally (▶ Fig. 12.5, ▶ Fig. 12.6).[17]

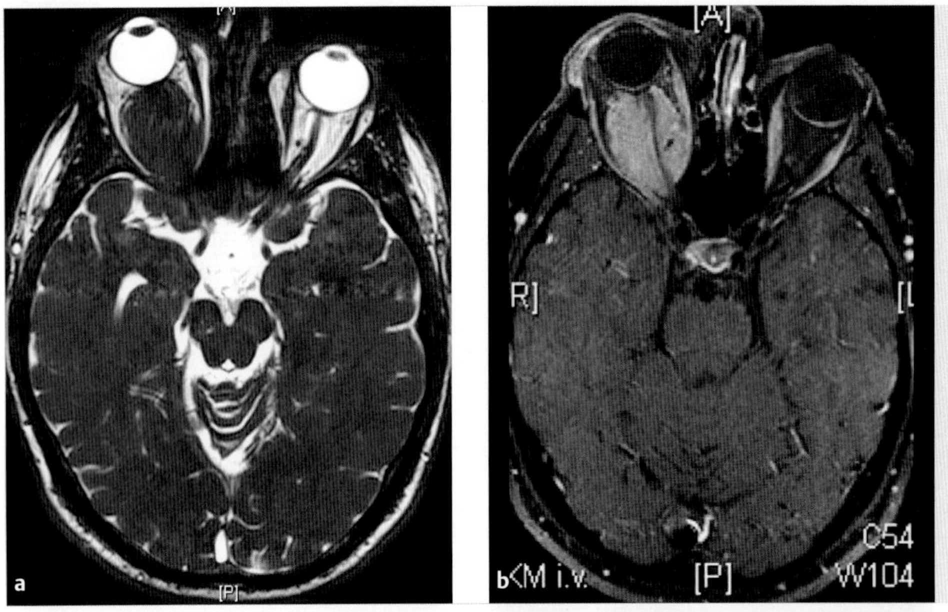

Fig. 12.3 Optic sheath meningioma. **(a)** MRI of a patient with an optic sheath meningioma with hypointense depiction in the T2-weighted transversal slices. Note the distinct proptosis caused by the intraorbital mass effect. **(b)** The contrast enhanced sequences show the typical homogeneous enhancement of the tumor. The affected and compressed optic nerve can be seen in the center of the tumor inside the complete intraorbital course.

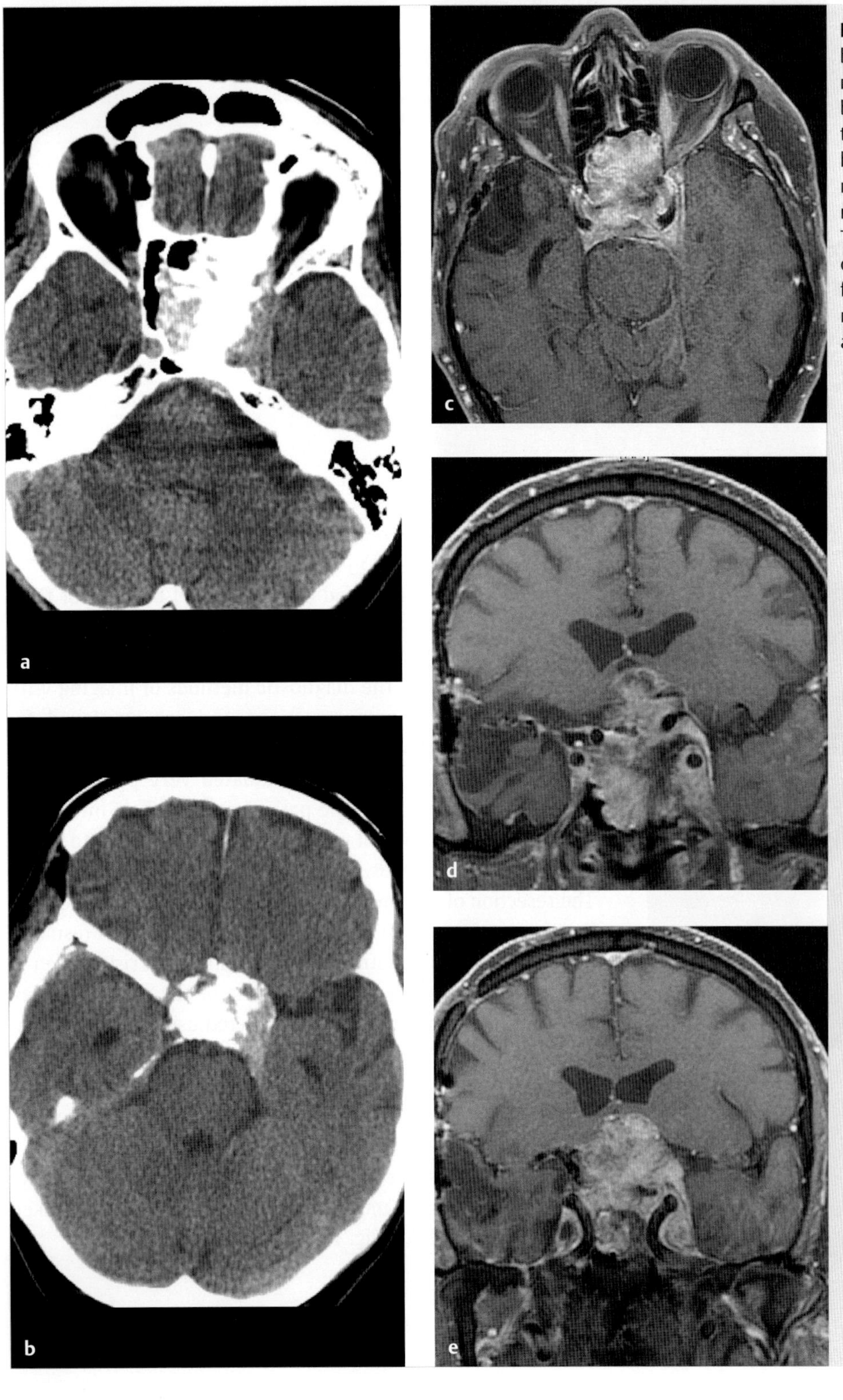

Fig. 12.4 Invasive meningioma of the frontal base. **(a, b)** Amaurotic patient with an invasive meningioma of the anterior and middle skull base with demonstrated calcification of the tumor. Calcifications with this pattern tend to be high risk, so that an extended biopsy or partial resection with optic canal decompression is recommended. The transversal **(c)** und coronal T1-weighted MRI slices **(d, e)** show the extension of the tumor after contrast enhancement on the frontal skull base spreading to the suprasellar region with infiltration of the cavernous sinus and surrounding of the internal carotid artery.

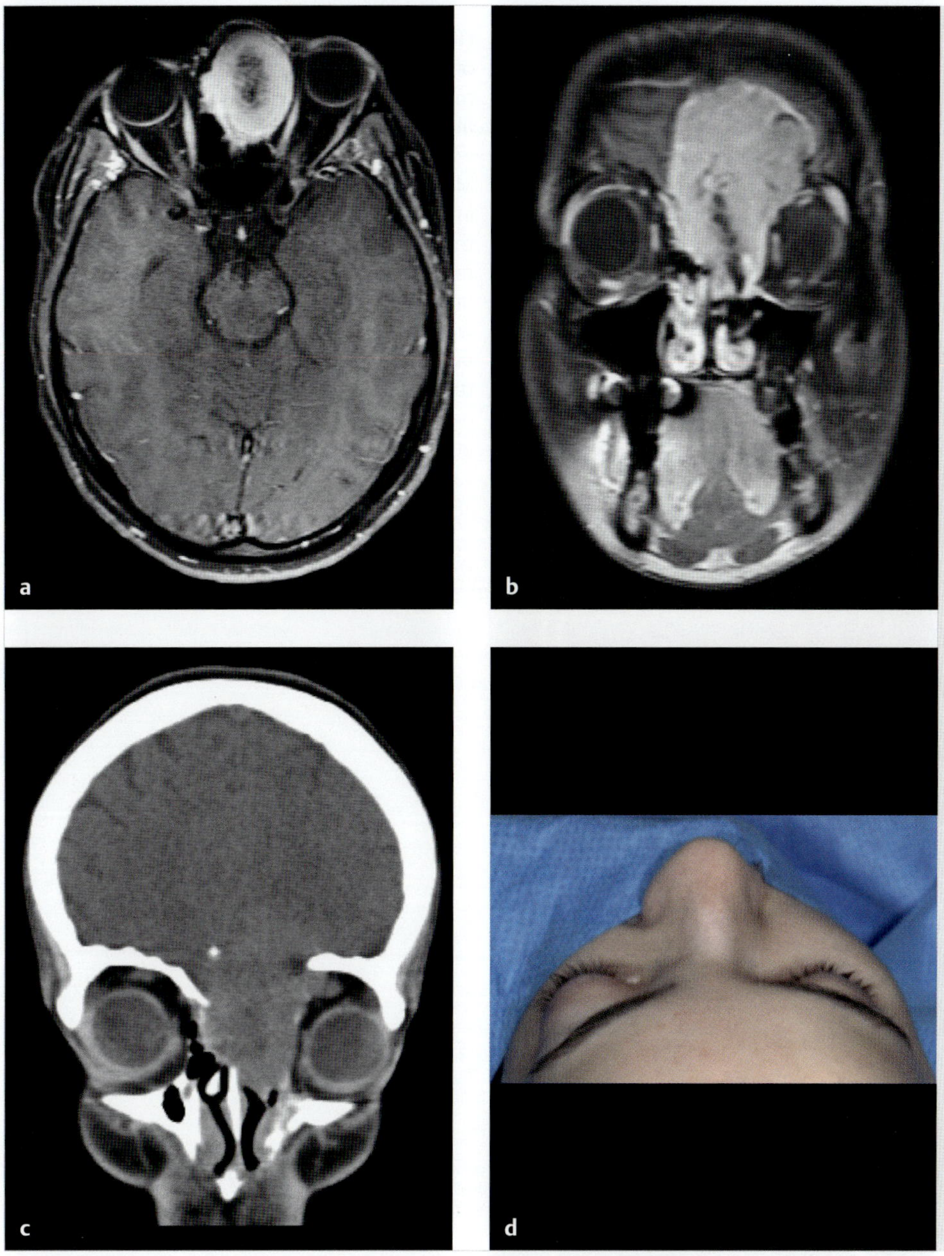

Fig. 12.5 Malignant intranasal, intracranial, and intraorbital tumor. **(a–d)** Malignant tumor of the rhinobase (spindle cell tumor) with osseous destruction and left-sided infiltration of the orbit and infiltration of the periorbita in a 27-year-old woman shown in the contrast enhanced transversal and coronal T1-weighted MRI sequences **(a, b)** and in the coronal reconstruction of the CT scan **(c)**. High-resolution CT imaging for the evaluation of the osseous destruction and planning for reconstruction should be done regularly. Note the left-sided proptosis and left paramedian subcutaneous tumorous swelling of the nasal root **(d)**.

Memorize

The treatment of malignant tumors of the frontal base with involvement of both orbits mostly demands an interdisciplinary treatment plan. Surgical resections and reconstructions can be very extensive and need special care to avoid complications.

12.4 Gliomas of the Optic Nerves and the Intracranial Optic Pathways

Gliomas of the optic nerves and the intracranial optic pathways are rare tumors and especially appear in childhood and adolescence. They represent approximately 2 to 7% of all intracranial tumors in childhood, but a higher percentage in children under 5 years of age, with up to 65%.[18,19,20] They are often associated with neurofibromatosis type I (NF I).[21,22,23,24] They correspond histologically to pilocytic astrocytomas (WHO grade I), rarely to pilomyxoid astrocytomas (WHO grade II). High-grade tumors are extremely rare.[20,25] They can grow purely unilaterally into the orbit or can develop retro-orbitally. They can also occur bilaterally and can be localized in the optic canal. These tumors initially grow slowly and are mostly asymptomatic, whereas gliomas of the optic chiasm can reach large sizes and extend to the hypothalamus or grow there primarily. These young patients usually become symptomatic with visual impairment. In infants and very young children these symptoms are mostly diagnosed at an advanced age. The affected children are amblyopic and the symptoms are recognized later after the appearance of strabismus or nystagmus. Endocrinological disturbances can occur in cases of intracranial growth in the hypothalamus and the manifestation of occlusive hydrocephalus can arise due to the development of giant tumors.[26] Treatment depends on various factors; visual function, the grade of proptosis, and intracranial tumor extension represent important criteria for the different treatment modalities. If the localization of the glioma is limited to the optic nerve and the visual acuity is functionally disturbed, resection is possible via a combined extradural and intradural approach with resection of the optic nerve retrobulbarly and anterior to the

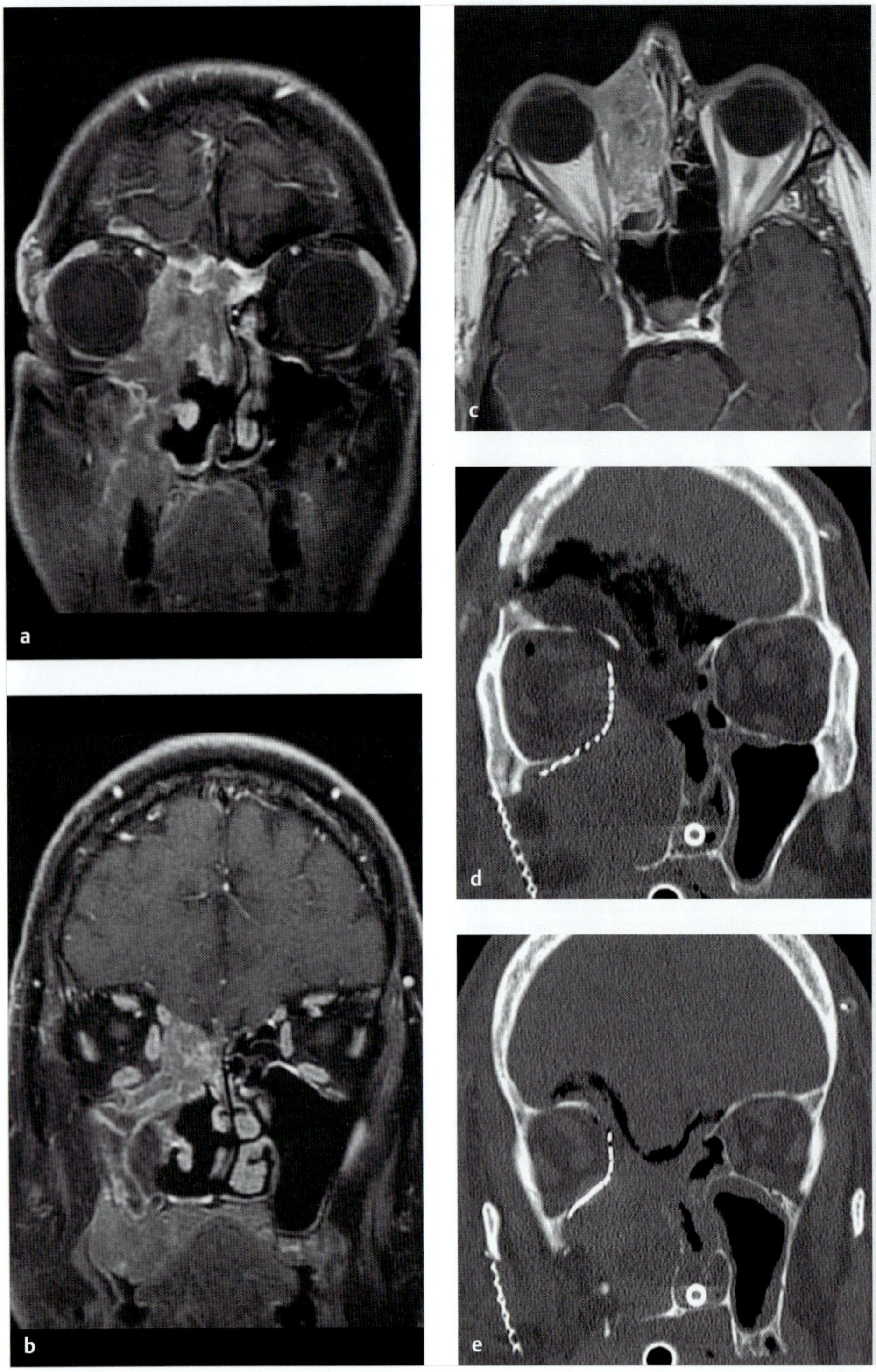

Fig. 12.6 Rhinobasal carcinoma with infiltration of the orbit and reconstruction with allogenic material. **(a–e)** Rhinobasal carcinoma with infiltration of the basal dura, the medial orbital wall, and the periorbita. The contrast-enhanced MRI sequences show infiltration of the periorbita in the coronal and transversal slices **(a–c)**, while the ocular muscles are not involved **(b)**. The resection of such tumors should always be undertaken by an interdisciplinary team, here with neurosurgeons and ENT surgeons. The postoperative CT scan shows the extension of tumor resection. Reconstruction of the medial orbital wall was performed with an intraoperatively adapted titanium mesh **(d, e)**.

optic chiasm. A "wait and see" strategy is preferred in patients with intact visual function with respective clinical, ophthalmologic, and radiological follow-up studies. In cases with distinct proptosis with local symptoms, surgical resection must be evaluated and discussed if there is intact vision. Progressive gliomas of the optic chiasm are treated with radiosurgery, possibly after microsurgical tumor debulking. Chemotherapy must be considered in young patients.[26,27,28]

> **Memorize** (M!)
>
> Optic nerve gliomas and gliomas of the optic pathways mainly occur during childhood and are frequently associated with neurofibromatosis type I. They mostly cause late-diagnosed amblyopia and can reach extensive sizes.

12.5 Vascular Malformations

The most common vascular malformations of the orbit are represented **by cavernous malformations** (CMs).[1,29,30] Clinically they are characterized by recurrent intralesional and/or extralesional hemorrhage or by progressive increase in growth. Patients with familial syndromes and genetic alterations have a significant risk for the development of multiple CMs.[31,32] MRI is the diagnostic imaging tool. CMs can be discerned in the T2-weighted sequences with a typical appearance and mixed signal intensity. One can see the classic perilesional hemosiderin ring, which is especially delineated in the special T2*-weighted gradient echo sequences. A high sensitivity for the detection of CMs is seen in susceptibility-weighted MRI sequences.[33] Microsurgical resection is indicated if CMs are clinically symptomatic with single or recurrent

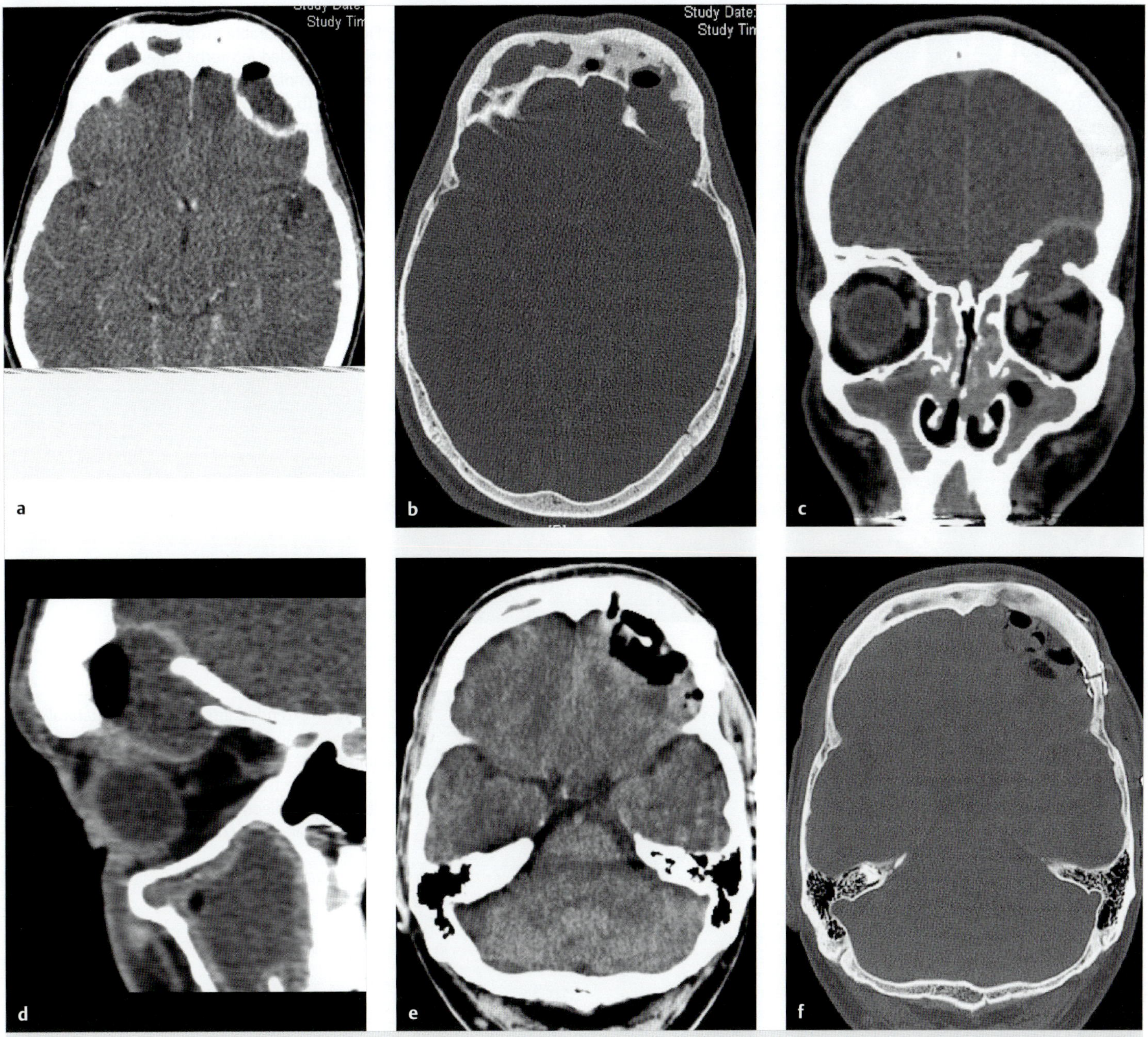

Fig. 12.7 Intracranial und intraorbital abscess. Extensive intracranial abscess (a, b) and intraorbital abscess with compression of the ocular bulb from cranially with pansinusitis (c, d). Postoperative computed tomography after frontal craniotomy and abscess drainage (e, f).

hemorrhages. Asymptomatic lesions can be followed up clinically and radiologically.

Another vascular disease involving the orbit and the ocular bulb is the **carotid–cavernous sinus fistula** (CCF). CCFs commonly appear after traumatic vascular lesions but can also occur spontaneously without any external impact. A pathological short circuit is caused between the arterial vessels of the cavernous sinus, especially the cavernous segment of the internal carotid artery, and the veins of the cavernous sinus. With the increased arterial shunt volume and the resulting venous congestion, characteristic symptoms appear, including pulsating exophthalmos, chemosis, and ciliary injection. Distinct dilatation of the intraorbital veins (ophthalmic vein) and intracranial veins can be seen in the MRI sequences. Conventional digital subtraction angiography (DSA) of the extracranial and intracranial vessels is needed for detailed imaging and localization of the fistula. The treatment of CCF is in the domain of interventional neuroradiology and usually performed by endovascular occlusion of the fistula or the pathological vascular segment.

12.6 Miscellaneous Lesions

There are several more diseases involving the orbital structures, such as hemangiopericytomas, neurofibromas, lymphomas, dermoids, epidermoids, osteomas, mucoceles, infections, and abscesses (▶ Fig. 12.7, ▶ Fig. 12.8, ▶ Fig. 12.9).[1,34,35,36]

12

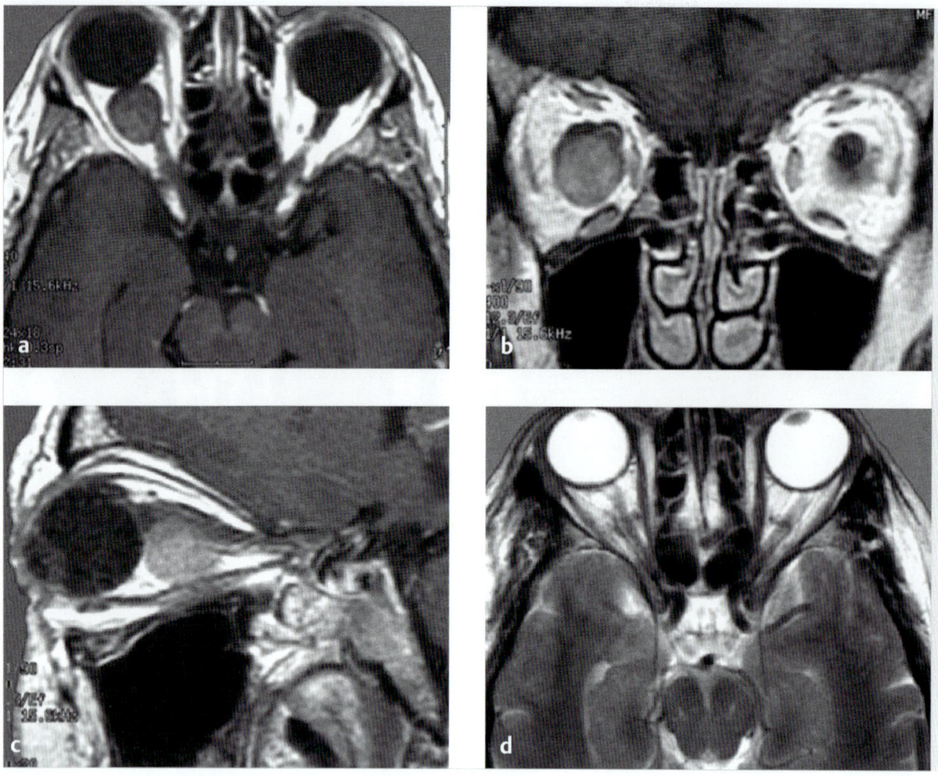

Fig. 12.8 Noticeable proptosis **(a)** in a patient with right-sided intraorbital neurinoma with dislocation of the optic nerve cranially and medially **(b, c)**. Postoperative MRI after fronto-orbital craniotomy and tumor resection **(d)**.

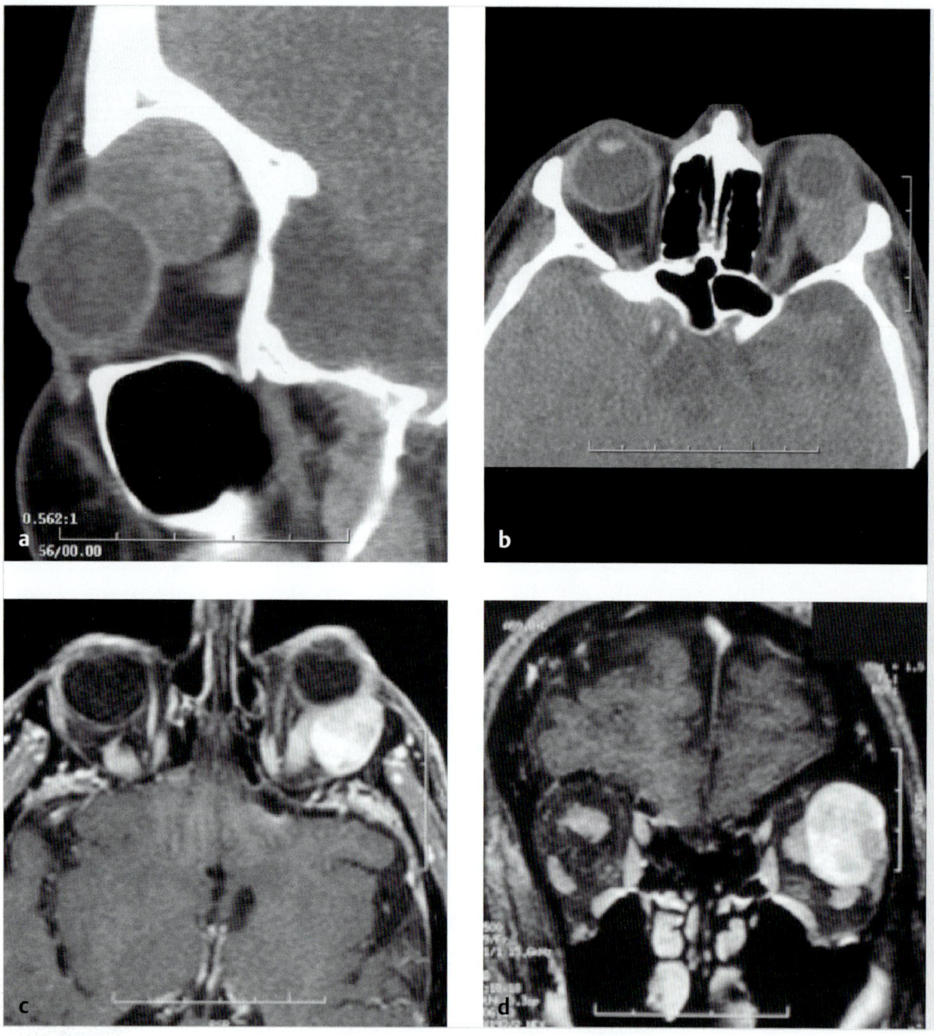

Fig. 12.9 Extended intraorbital craniolateral mass with caudal displacement of the left ocular bulb **(a, b)**. MRI shows the contrast-enhancing tumor in the transversal **(c)** and coronal **(d)** depiction. A pleomorphic adenoma of the lacrimal gland was confirmed histologically.

References

[1] Shields JA, Shields CL, Scartozzi R. Survey of 1264 patients with orbital tumors and simulating lesions: The 2002 Montgomery Lecture, part 1. Ophthalmology. 2004; 111(5):997–1008

[2] Abdel-Aziz KM, Froelich SC, Dagnew E, et al. Large sphenoid wing meningiomas involving the cavernous sinus: conservative surgical strategies for better functional outcomes. Neurosurgery. 2004; 54(6):1375–1383, discussion 1383–1384

[3] Attia M, Patel KS, Kandasamy J, et al. Combined cranionasal surgery for spheno-orbital meningiomas invading the paranasal sinuses, pterygopalatine, and infratemporal fossa. World Neurosurg. 2013; 80(6):e367–e373

[4] Bassiouni H, Asgari S, Sandalcioglu IE, Seifert V, Stolke D, Marquardt G. Anterior clinoidal meningiomas: functional outcome after microsurgical resection in a consecutive series of 106 patients. Clinical article. J Neurosurg. 2009; 111 (5):1078–1090

[5] Louis DN, Ohgaki H, Wiestler OD, et al. The 2007 WHO classification of tumours of the central nervous system. Acta Neuropathol. 2007; 114(2):97–109

[6] Bassiouni H, Asgari S, Stolke D. Tuberculum sellae meningiomas: functional outcome in a consecutive series treated microsurgically. Surg Neurol. 2006; 66(1):37–44, discussion 44–45

[7] Bonnal J, Thibaut A, Brotchi J, Born J. Invading meningiomas of the sphenoid ridge. J Neurosurg. 1980; 53(5):587–599

[8] Miller NR. Primary tumours of the optic nerve and its sheath. Eye (Lond). 2004; 18(11):1026–1037

[9] Sandalcioglu IE, Gasser T, Mohr C, Stolke D, Wiedemayer H. Spheno-orbital meningiomas: interdisciplinary surgical approach, resectability and long-term results. J Craniomaxillofac Surg. 2005; 33(4):260–266

[10] Turbin RE, Pokorny K. Diagnosis and treatment of orbital optic nerve sheath meningioma. Cancer Contr. 2004; 11(5):334–341

[11] Mirone G, Chibbaro S, Schiabello L, Tola S, George B. En plaque sphenoid wing meningiomas: recurrence factors and surgical strategy in a series of 71 patients. Neurosurgery. 2009; 65(6) Suppl:100–108, discussion 108–109

[12] Schick U, Bleyen J, Bani A, Hassler W. Management of meningiomas en plaque of the sphenoid wing. J Neurosurg. 2006; 104(2):208–214

[13] Al-Mefty O, Smith RR. Surgery of tumors invading the cavernous sinus. Surg Neurol. 1988; 30(5):370–381

[14] Mariniello G, Bonavolontà G, Tranfa F, Maiuri F. Management of the optic canal invasion and visual outcome in spheno-orbital meningiomas. Clin Neurol Neurosurg. 2013; 115(9):1615–1620

[15] Herr MW, Gray ST, Erman AB, Curry WT, Deschler DG, Lin DT. Orbital preservation in patients with esthesioneuroblastoma. J Neurol Surg B Skull Base. 2013; 74(3):142–145

[16] Jimbo H, Kamata S, Miura K, et al. Operative management of skull base malignant tumors arising from the nasal cavity and paranasal sinus: recent strategies used in 25 cases. Neurol Med Chir (Tokyo). 2010; 50(1):20–26, discussion 26

[17] Hoffmann TK, El Hindy N, Müller OM, et al. Vascularised local and free flaps in anterior skull base reconstruction. Eur Arch Otorhinolaryngol. 2013; 270(3): 899–907

[18] Schick U, Hassler W. Pediatric tumors of the orbit and optic pathway. Pediatr Neurosurg. 2003; 38(3):113–121

[19] Campagna M, Opocher E, Viscardi E, et al. Optic pathway glioma: long-term visual outcome in children without neurofibromatosis type-1. Pediatr Blood Cancer. 2010; 55(6):1083–1088

[20] Fernandez C, Figarella-Branger D, Girard N, et al. Pilocytic astrocytomas in children: prognostic factors–a retrospective study of 80 cases. Neurosurgery. 2003; 53(3):544–553, discussion 554–555

[21] Nicolin G, Parkin P, Mabbott D, et al. Natural history and outcome of optic pathway gliomas in children. Pediatr Blood Cancer. 2009; 53(7):1231–1237

[22] Chan MY, Foong AP, Heisey DM, Harkness W, Hayward R, Michalski A. Potential prognostic factors of relapse-free survival in childhood optic pathway glioma: a multivariate analysis. Pediatr Neurosurg. 1998; 29(1):23–28

[23] Fouladi M, Wallace D, Langston JW, et al. Survival and functional outcome of children with hypothalamic/chiasmatic tumors. Cancer. 2003; 97(4):1084–1092

[24] Grill J, Laithier V, Rodriguez D, Raquin MA, Pierre-Kahn A, Kalifa C. When do children with optic pathway tumours need treatment? An oncological perspective in 106 patients treated in a single centre. Eur J Pediatr. 2000; 159(9): 692–696

[25] Chikai K, Ohnishi A, Kato T, et al. Clinico-pathological features of pilomyxoid astrocytoma of the optic pathway. Acta Neuropathol. 2004; 108(2):109–114

[26] Silva MM, Goldman S, Keating G, Marymont MA, Kalapurakal J, Tomita T. Optic pathway hypothalamic gliomas in children under three years of age: the role of chemotherapy. Pediatr Neurosurg. 2000; 33(3):151–158

[27] Goodden J, Pizer B, Pettorini B, et al. The role of surgery in optic pathway/ hypothalamic gliomas in children. J Neurosurg Pediatr. 2014; 13(1):1–12

[28] Sawamura Y, Kamada K, Kamoshima Y, et al. Role of surgery for optic pathway/hypothalamic astrocytomas in children. Neuro-oncol. 2008; 10(5):725–733

[29] Günalp I, Gündüz K. Vascular tumors of the orbit. Doc Ophthalmol. 1995; 89 (4):337–345

[30] Schick U, Dott U, Hassler W. Surgical treatment of orbital cavernomas. Surg Neurol. 2003; 60(3):234–244, discussion 244

[31] Siegel AM, Bertalanffy H, Dichgans JJ, et al. [Familial cavernous malformations of the central nervous system. A clinical and genetic study of 15 German families]. [Article in German]. Nervenarzt. 2005; 76(2):175–180

[32] Sürücü O, Sure U, Gaetzner S, et al. Clinical impact of CCM mutation detection in familial cavernous angioma. Childs Nerv Syst. 2006; 22(11):1461–1464

[33] Dammann P, Wrede KH, Maderwald S, et al. The venous angioarchitecture of sporadic cerebral cavernous malformations: a susceptibility weighted imaging study at 7 T MRI. J Neurol Neurosurg Psychiatry. 2013; 84(2):194–200

[34] Schick U, Lermen O, Unsöld R, Hassler W. Treatment of primary orbital lymphomas. Eur J Haematol. 2004; 72(3):186–192

[35] Lim JH, Sardesai MG, Ferreira M, Jr, Moe KS. Transorbital neuroendoscopic management of sinogenic complications involving the frontal sinus, orbit, and anterior cranial fossa. J Neurol Surg B Skull Base. 2012; 73(6):394–400

[36] Duvoisin B, Zanella FE, Sievers KW. Imaging of the normal and pathological orbit. Eur Radiol. 1998; 8(2):175–188

Chapter 13

Intraconal Orbital Tumors

13

13 Intraconal Orbital Tumors

Michael L. Hinni, Devyani Lal, and Karel De Leeuw

13.1 Introduction

Management of intraconal orbital tumors presents several challenges. The intraorbital anatomy can be quite difficult to negotiate, especially in the intraconal segment. Several blood vessels in this area are end-arteries and injury to these can lead to visual field deficits and blindness.

The intraconal orbit can be afflicted with many orbital inflammatory and neoplastic conditions. In many situations, biopsy of these lesions is not feasible due to concern about injuring neurovascular structures, and diagnosis and management must rely on radiographic imaging. Several low-grade tumors in the orbit can be managed by attentive observation, whereas many inflammatory conditions such as inflammatory pseudotumor and Graves's ophthalmopathy may require urgent medical and surgical management. When the orbit becomes involved with a malignant neoplasm, a careful evaluation of the therapeutic modality to be utilized and the extent of resection and exenteration must be determined with careful consideration.

13.2 Anatomy

The bony orbit is a pyramidal structure comprising seven bones. The bony framework is lined by orbital periosteum. Within the bony orbital framework exists the globe, and the contents occupy two additional compartments, the intraconal and extraconal regions. The extraconal compartment is separated from the intraconal compartments by a fascial sheath known as Tenon's capsule. Within the cone are found the extraocular muscles, the optic nerve, the ciliary ganglion, numerous small blood vessels, and small branches of the first and second divisions of the trigeminal nerve. The globe is held firmly in the anterior orbit by the medial and lateral canthal ligaments (for details see Chapter 1).[1]

13

Entering and/or exiting the bony orbit are numerous structures, most of which pass through either the inferior or the superior orbital fissure (see ▶ Fig. 13.1).

Although covered by a tendinous sheath, the superior and inferior orbital fissures provide a potential pathway for spread of tumors via neural and vascular pathways into the pterygomaxillary space, infratemporal fossa, cavernous sinus or cranial cavity. The lamina papyracea (ethmoid bone), the lacrimal bone, and even the maxillary bone can often be quite thin, and may not provide a robust barrier to the spread of malignant disease. Based on lymphatic drainage, the intraparotid, facial, and/or submandibular level-1 neck lymph nodes as well as the retropharyngeal lymph nodes are the first echelons of lymphatic drainage, and may be involved with metastasis.

13.3 Evaluation/Diagnosis

As seen already in other chapters, when presented with an orbital mass the treating clinician must first decide whether the mass is an infectious or inflammatory condition, or whether it represents a true neoplasm. This determination can generally be made with an astute elicitation of history from patients, caregivers, or parents, thorough examination (vital signs, a complete head and neck examination, visual acuity, and ophthalmologic examinations), and laboratory testing(white blood cell count, red cell count, and sedimentation rate) and imaging. Several imaging modalities may have complementary roles and these may include ultrasound, computerized tomography (CT scan) and magnetic resonance imaging (MRI) (see Chapter 4). These tests enable the clinician to differentiate the infectious or inflammatory conditions from true neoplasms. If an intraconal neoplasm is suspected, the next step is to make a histopathologic diagnosis. When possible, fine needle aspiration can be very helpful and minimizes the risk of seeding tumor. Fine needle aspiration is particularly useful for tumors in the lateral orbit involving the lacrimal gland, as well as tumors generally located in the anterior orbit. Tumors more posterior in the orbit or those that may involve the optic nerve might be best suited by a direct surgical biopsy. The clinician is encouraged to develop a careful differential diagnosis so that any incision on the face or on the eyelids is made with consideration of the need for subsequent surgical management. Possible approaches besides fine needle aspiration can include transconjunctival, subciliary, brow, direct access through the oral cavity and the buccal gingival sulcus, or—as in the case of many medially placed and posteriorly placed lesions—transnasal endoscopic approaches. The latter approaches are particularly appealing when the lamina papyracea or intrasinus contents will

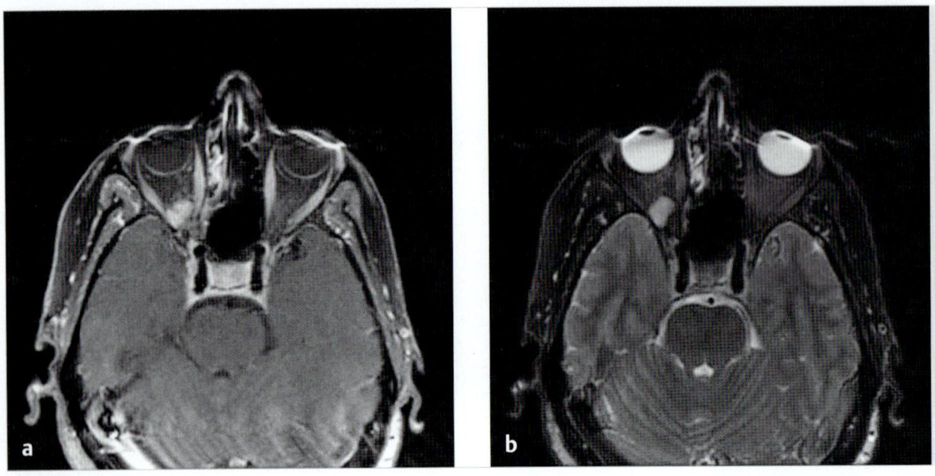

Fig. 13.1 On MRI, hemangiomas of the orbit have a classic heterogeneous appearance with areas of gadolinium enhancement and flow voids within the tumor **(a)**. These tumors are also inherently bright on T2-weighted images **(b)**.

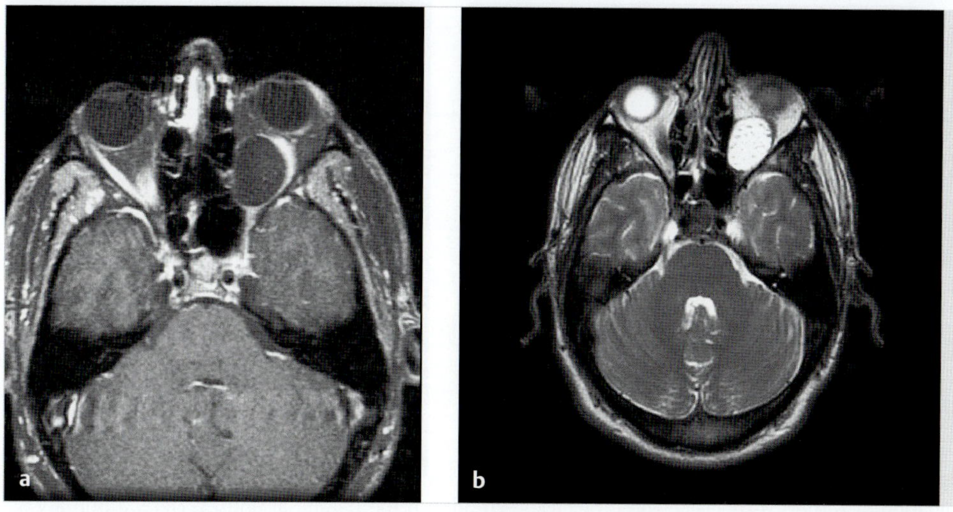

Fig. 13.2 Nonneoplastic masses, such as dermoid cysts, can also be mistaken for a tumor. This figure illustrates the MRI appearance of dermoid cysts. These appear dark on T1 images and do not enhance with gadolinium **(a)**. They appear to be brilliantly bright on T2-weighted MRI images **(b)**.

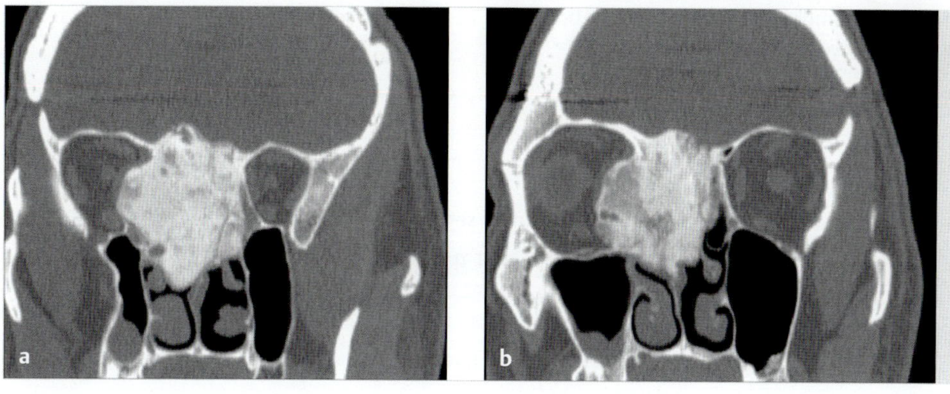

Fig. 13.3 Ossifying fibroma shows a characteristic, sharply demarcated, expansile mass covered by a thick shell of bone; the tumor mass appears to be multiloculated and is of varying density on CT **(a, b)**.

be a component of the overall definitive surgical approach. However, several tumors may be located in areas where a biopsy may pose a serious risk of loss of vision. In such cases, radiological imaging can be very useful in narrowing down the diagnosis.

Often, several tumors such as orbital hemangioma have classic pathognomic features (▶ Fig. 13.1) and a biopsy may be bypassed in favor of close and watchful observation with repeat imaging. In addition, a nonneoplastic mass such as orbital dermoid also has a classic appearance (▶ Fig. 13.2) that can be observed without biopsy. Orbital involvement by lymphoma is not unusual in patients with systemic leukemia-lymphoma and often these may not require additional biopsy in known disease history. Bony tumors such as ossifying fibroma (▶ Fig. 13.3) and osteoma have a classic appearance on CT. In several infiltrative lesions close to the orbital apex, the optic nerve, and the optic canal, the history may be suspicious for orbital pseudo tumor, and response to a trial of systemic glucocorticosteroids can often be diagnostic as well as therapeutic. IgG_4-related disease is another newly described inflammatory entity mediated by plasma cells that can afflict the orbit, lacrimal gland, and paranasal sinuses and present as a mass. Biopsy can be avoided if other afflicted areas are available for safer sampling, and these lesions also tend to respond to immunosuppressant and corticosteroid therapy.

Orbital tumors are generally evaluated radiographically by CT scanning, either with or without contrast (or preferably both). Images should be available and studied in all three planes (coronal, sagittal, and axial planes) to map the tumor and obtain a three-dimensional understanding of the lesion and surrounding pertinent anatomy The MRI scan is critical in refining the diagnosis and assessing soft tissue invasion of tumors, and must be performed for almost all complex orbital pathology for diagnostic or management purposes (▶ Fig. 13.4) (see Chapter 4). In the case of carcinomas, particularly the high-grade ones, as well as sarcomas and other mesenchymal tumors, body-wide staging with total body PET/CT scanning may be important.

In general, patients with intraconal orbital tumors should be evaluated from the beginning by a multidisciplinary team of experts including ophthalmologists specializing in orbital surgery, otolaryngologists with special training in head and neck surgery, and specialists in endoscopic skull base surgery, medical oncology, radiation oncology, pathology, and neuroradiology.

13.4 Classification of Tumors

Classification of orbital and orbit-related tumors is complicated. In general, orbital lesions can be grouped into inflammatory, primary, and secondary or metastatic. Several authors subclassify true neoplasms (either primary or secondary) into intracoronal or extracoronal on the basis of the anatomical location. The reader is referred to ▶ Table 13.1, ▶ Table 13.2, and ▶ Table 13.3 for lists of common inflammatory conditions (▶ Table 13.1), benign primary tumors (▶ Table 13.2), and primary and secondary malignant tumors (▶ Table 13.3) that involve the orbit. These tables are not comprehensive, as several rarer tumors can affect the orbit, but they provide a reference framework for the treating physician to begin with.

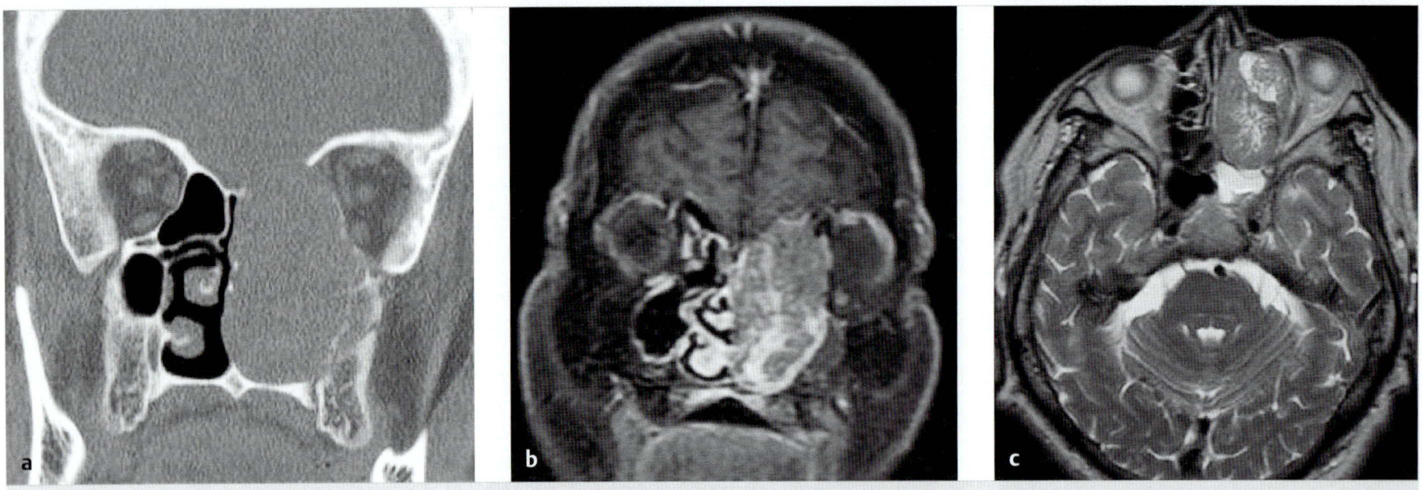

Fig. 13.4 CT and MRI are complementary in evaluation of tumors, especially when they also extend into the paranasal sinuses. Here, a primary sinonasal adenocarcinoma extending into the orbit is shown. The CT scan shows the extent of tumor and bony destruction **(a)**. On MRI, The T1 sequence with contrast shows the tumor as an enhancing mass, whereas retained fluid in the sinuses is dark **(b)**. The T2-weighted sequence shows the retained sinonasal secretions to be bright, whereas the tumor itself does not appear bright **(c)**. T2-weighted sequences differentiate tumor from secretions. Secretions appear dark on T1 and bright on T2-weighted sequences.

Table 13.1 Malignant primary tumors of the orbit

Primary orbital tumors (malignant)	Localization
Vascular tumors	
• Hemangiopericytoma	Entire orbit
• Angiosarcoma	
• Kaposi's sarcoma	
Neurogenic tumors	
• Malignant schwannoma	Can appear in the entire orbit and periorbita
• Esthesioneuroblastoma	Medial and cranial orbit
• Neuroblastoma	Entire orbit
• Optic nerve glioma	Posterior orbit/orbital apex
• Retinoblastoma	Medial or posterior orbit
• Malignant melanoma	Intraocular/retinal
• Malignant meningioma	Can appear in the entire orbit and periorbita
Salivary gland-/Lacrimal gland tumors	
• Adenoid cystic carcinoma	Lateral and superior orbit
• Adenocarcinoma, not otherwise specified	Lateral and superior orbit
• Carcinoma ex pleomorphic adenoma	Lateral and superior orbit
• Mucoepidermoid carcinoma	Lateral and superior orbit
Lymphatic tumors	
• Malignant lymphoma	Can appear in the entire orbit and periorbita
Mesenchymal tumors	
• Rhabdomyosarcoma	Can appear in the entire orbit
• Leiomyosarcoma	Can appear in the entire orbit and periorbita
• Fibrosarcoma	
• Osteosarcoma	
• Chondrosarcoma	

Table 13.2 Malignant secondary tumors of the orbit

Secondary malignant tumors	Localization
Sinonasal tumors	Medial and inferior or posterior orbit
Nasopharyngeal carcinoma	Posterior and medial orbit
Malignant skin tumors	
• Basal cell carcinoma	Anterior orbit, eyelid
• Squamous cell carcinoma	
• Malignant melanoma	
• Merkel cell carcinoma	
• Sweat gland carcinoma	
• Microcystic adnexal carcinoma	
Secondary malignant orbital tumors (metastases)	
Carcinoma	
• Breast	Posterior orbit/extraocular muscles
• Lung	
• Prostate	
• Gastrointestinal tract	
• Kidney	
Malignant melanoma	Can appear in the entire orbit and periorbita
Malignant lymphoma	Can appear in the entire orbit and periorbita

Table 13.3 Nontumorous–pseudotumorous pathology and benign tumors of the orbit

Pathology	Localization
Orbital complication of an acute sinusitis (orbital cellulitis)	Medial orbit/eyelids
Paranasal sinus mucocele	Medial/superior orbit
Orbital pseudotumor	In most cases in only one compartment, occasionally diffuse occurrence
Grave's ophthalmopathy	Enlargement of extraocular muscles
Invasive fungal infection (e.g., aspergillosis)	Medial/inferior orbit
Primary orbital tumors (benign)	
Vascular lesions	
• Orbital varicose veins	Superior orbit
• Vascular malformations	Can appear in the entire orbit
• Hemangioma	Preferentially anterior in the orbit, in the skin, or in the eyelid
• Arteriovenous shunts	Retrobulbar
Neurogenic tumors	
• Neurofibroma	Superior orbit/upper lid
• Schwannoma	Originates preferentially from the infraorbital or supraorbital nerves
• Meningioma	Sphenoid wing or posterior orbit
Salivary gland/lacrimal gland tumors	
• Pleomorphic- or monomorphic adenoma	Lateral superior orbit
Lymphatic tumors	Preferentially subconjunctival or upper lid

13.5 Orbital Neoplasia

13.5.1 Benign Lesions

While this chapter will focus primarily on malignant neoplasms of the orbit, occasionally the clinician is faced with a benign lesion. Lacrimal gland tumors are quite uncommon, representing as few as 2% of all the neoplasms identified in the orbit.[2,3] Approximately half of the lacrimal gland masses represent inflammatory lesions, cystic lesions, or lymphatic lesions, and are generally benign. Approximately half of lacrimal gland masses or tumors are true neoplasms and are split generally evenly between benign mixed tumors (pleomorphic adenoma) or carcinomas, with adenoid cystic being most common and mucoepidermoid carcinomas being less common. Carcinoma ex pleomorphic adenoma is more common in the lacrimal gland than it is in other salivary type glands. Pleomorphic adenomas in this gland can be resected through a lateral orbital approach; however, in the experience of the authors, even benign tumors of the lacrimal gland tend to be more fibrotic and more difficult to operate on than their counterparts in traditional salivary gland tissue.

Lymphatic malformations and true hemangiomas (which are true neoplasms) are most common in the pediatric age group, and they are often treated with intermittent doses of antibiotics and steroids, beta blockers, and more recently beculizimab in conjunction with the judicious use of surgery. In a recent review from 2011 on the use of propranolol for infantile hemangioma, 58.8% of 85 cases were treated with a dose of 2 mg/kg per day. Improvement or complete resolution of the lesion was noted in 96%, with recurrences in only one-fifth of cases.[4] In another study, of 42 patients with cavernous hemangiomas of the orbit, all treated surgically, 83% achieved good visual function.[5] In general, localized benign orbital lesions can and probably should be safely removed, with vascular neoplasms perhaps being the one exception where a trial of medication is indicated, particularly for obvious hemangiomas or those vascular anomalies that are microscopically and radiographically microcystic.

13.5.2 Primary Malignant Tumors

Malignant Vascular Tumors

Malignant vascular tumors within the orbit include hemangiopericytomas, angiosarcomas, and Kaposi's sarcomas (this last lesion is included here rather than with the mesenchymal tumors). As a rule, vascular malignant tumors within the orbit are rare with angiosarcoma in the orbit as a primary neoplasm is extremely rare.[6] Few if any centers have more than simple case reports to share on the subject. The treatment of malignant vascular tumors within the orbit has included surgery with complete resection whenever possible, as well as with adjuvant radiotherapy. As these lesions develop nests of malignant cells running along blood vessels, often outside the palpable boundary of the neoplasm, obtaining negative margins can sometimes be challenging. Careful preoperative counseling with approval for enucleation or orbital exoneration when necessary is an important part of the preoperative evaluation. It must be borne in mind that while the orbit may be preserved, loss of bony support can often present additional changes to functional vision due to enophthalmos, diplopia, and loss of the upper and lower eyelids. In addition, adjuvant radiotherapy also carries significant risk of injuring the lens, the optic nerve, and the retina, which can cause intractable treatment pain and/or blindness. This is one of several critical reasons why thorough multidisciplinary input and planning agreement upon therapeutic plan must precede initiation of treatment. All of the oncologic specialties involved must be "on the same page."

Neogenic Tumors

Retinoblastoma

Retinoblastoma is a neuroendocrine tumor and the most common orbital tumor in children, often being evident before 1 year of age.[7] Although most cases are sporadic, as many as 40% are genetic via an autosomal dominant gene that predisposes the patient to additional primary tumors such as sarcomas. It has been demonstrated that small tumors (those that are confined the retina) have a more favorable prognosis than larger tumors that extend outside the orbit or involve the optic nerve. Unfortunately, many patients do not present until metastasis or direct brain extension occurs. Some authors have proposed avoiding the use of fine needle aspiration to make the diagnosis in the case of retinoblastoma due to the fear of seeding the tumor within the orbital fat. The offending gene mutation is reported to be at the 13q14 locus of the chromosome, with possession of one normal gene copy offering protection.[7] Histologically, three distinct patterns have been described. The first pattern is completely undifferentiated with extensive necrosis and a high mitotic rate. This subtype has the worst prognosis. The second type, containing "Homer–Wright rosettes" (cuboidal cells arranged around a central lumen), and a third type containing "fleurettes" (where the retinoblasts are arranged in an organized pattern reminiscent of the "fleur-de-lis") are both considered to offer a better prognosis.[7] This malignancy is often devastating due to the age of onset and the common need for multimodal therapy, including definitive or adjuvant radiotherapy, which can inhibit craniofacial growth and induce second malignancies despite curative treatment of the retinoblastoma. It is hoped that, with the increasing availability of proton beam therapy, the morbidity associated with treating young children with orbital retinoblastoma can be reduced.

Rhabdomyosarcoma

Rhabdomyosarcoma is overall the most common orbital malignancy, with most cases occurring in children less than 10 years of age, though it can be relatively common up to 20 years of age.[8,9] It is the most common sarcoma that occurs in the head and neck region; according to the Intragroup Rhabdomyosarcoma Study (IRS), the head and neck was the location of over one-third of all cases, with most of those occurring in the orbit.[10] Rhabdomyosarcoma also occurs in the middle ear and mastoid region, nasal cavity, nasopharynx, paranasal sinuses, and occasionally the infratemporal fossa. The differential diagnosis may include hemangiomas, neurofibromas, and optic nerve gliomas as well as more common inflammatory conditions. Growth can be rapid, with the appearance of proptosis with or without visual loss over one or two days.[8] Fine needle aspiration can generally make the diagnosis, often with the assistance of ultrasound. CT and MRI in combination are recommended to assist with staging and treatment planning. Several histological subtypes have been described for rhabdomyosarcoma including embryonal, botryoid (a variant of embryonal), alveolar, and pleomorphic. Most orbital tumors (95%) belong to the embryonal/botryoid variant, with the remainder of the orbital tumors being of the alveolar type. The embryonal variant tends to be better differentiated but occasionally presents in a poorly differentiated pattern with very few rhabdomyoblasts. Cells are often spindle-shaped or fusiform with an elongated nucleus and tapered ends. Mitoses are common. The botryoid ("bag of grapes") variant is common in small children under 5 years of age and typically presents with grapelike structures associated with hollowed areas such as the nasal cavity, and may be mucosa-covered. The botryoid variant carries the best prognosis.

Alveolar rhabdomyosarcomas are usually found in slightly older children, such as teenagers or young adults. Histologically, tumor cells are arranged in an alveolar pattern centrally attached to a fibrous septum. Often special stains to identify myogenesis within the cytoplasm are necessary or even critical for making the diagnosis. The pleomorphic variant is the least common and is almost always a disease of the extremities in adults. Light microscopy can usually demonstrate striated muscle differentiation, and the diagnosis can be assisted by positive stains for desmoid muscle–specific actin and myoglobin.[11,12] It is noteworthy that S100 and cytokeratin stains are occasionally positive in some rhabdomyosarcomas. The alveolar rhabdomyosarcoma has been linked to a chromosomal rearrangement t(2;13)(q35; q14),[13,14] While embryonal rhabdomyosarcomas may be linked to the loss of heterozygosity on chromosome 11, carefully identifying the histological subtype has prognostic significance, with the botryoid variant doing better than the embryonal variant, which has a better prognosis than the alveolar variety. The 5-year overall survival ranging between 20 and 83% is dependent upon the respective group.

Treatment is generally initiated with concurrent radiation and chemotherapy. While prompt surgery is not necessarily wrong, aggressive tumors may recur before adjuvant radiotherapy and chemotherapy can be initiated. Surgery is therefore generally reserved for a salvage role or when there is residual tumor following chemoradiotherapy.

Optic Nerve Glioma

The optic nerve glioma is essentially an astrocytoma of cranial nerve II. The ascending cell is the fibrillary astrocyte that exists in the oligodendroglioma supporting fascia that exits the brain with the optic nerve.[9] These lesions represent only about 2% of orbital tumors, often occurring in patients with neurofibromatosis.[3] Only about 20% are purely intraorbital with most extending up to or involving the optic chiasm.[2,9] The lesion tends to grow slowly and run a fairly benign course in children and young adults. The lesion often attains considerable size before total visual loss is evident. In very young children, however, or in mature adults, the optic nerve glioma can be a fairly aggressive lesion, demonstrating rapid growth and progressive loss of vision. The diagnosis can often be made radiographically due to the homogeneous fusiform dilatation evident of the optic nerve on CT scan. Slowly progressive proptosis with gradual loss of vision is the key presenting symptom. The tumor is not considered to be particularly chemosensitive or radiosensitive and the treatment approach is generally surgical through a frontal orbital craniotomy (see Chapter 12).

Less common lesions including malignant schwannomas and non–optic nerve neuroblastomas. These often involve sensory nerves within the superior orbital fissure and can be quite aggressive, commonly extending intracranially. These lesions often initially present with distant metastases. Postoperative radiotherapy is all but universally indicated in this setting for these uncommon aggressive tumors.

Meningiomas

Meningiomas within the orbit account for approximately 5% of orbital tumors.[15] Generally considered benign, meningiomas in the orbit can involve the optic nerve or can directly spread from an intracranial meningoma through the superior orbital fissure (▶ Fig. 13.5). It is occasionally difficult to know whether the tumor began intracranially and grew downwards. Most have a benign course and are occasionally recognized incidentally and can simply be monitored. Occasionally, however, an intraorbital meningioma can be aggressive, requiring combined transorbital and transcranial approaches for complete excision (see Chapter 12).

Lymphomas and Leukemias

Both primary orbital lymphomas and leukemic infiltrates within the orbital contents occur. Unfortunately, fine needle aspiration can be of limited value in sorting out the diagnosis as this test

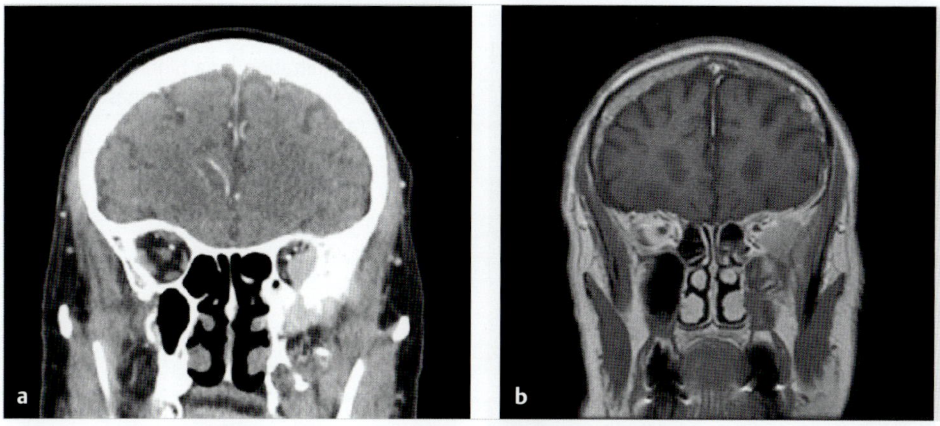

Fig. 13.5 A left sphenoid wing meningioma (high grade) is shown as appearing on CT **(a)** and T-1 with gadolinium contrast on MRI **(b)**. These masses infiltrate into the orbit, showing bony, meningeal, and soft-tissue infiltration.

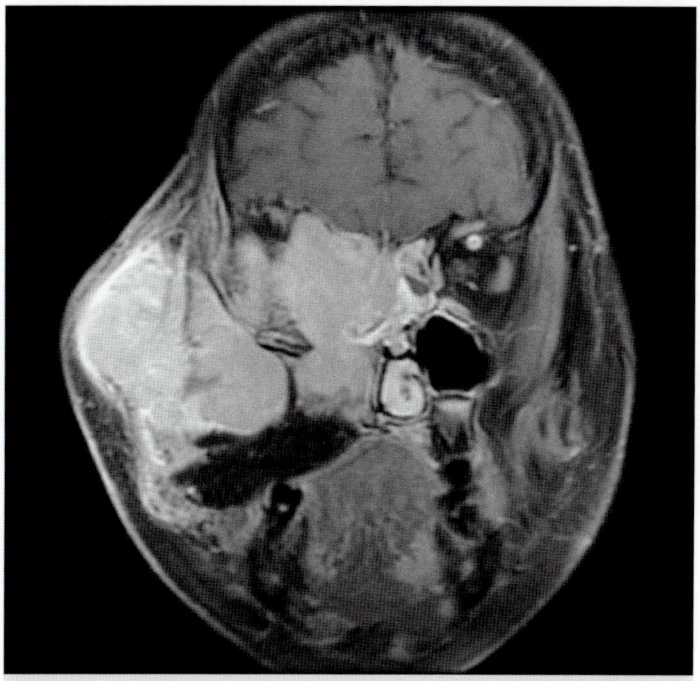

Fig. 13.6 A recurrent and high-grade osteosarcoma shows diffuse and extensive infiltration of several bones around the orbit and also infiltrates into the orbit, soft tissue of the cheek, and the nasal cavity.

may simply suggest a lymphoid process. Non-Hodgkin's lymphomas are more common and can present in the orbit bilaterally.[16] While orbital lymphomas may have a fairly benign course they can be aggressive and are generally treated like stage 1 lymphomas elsewhere. The role of surgery is essentially to confirm the diagnosis. Surgery may be necessary in rare circumstances to remove residual disease refractory to nonsurgical therapy.

Leukemic infiltrates are usually associated with known leukemia and can often simply be observed.

Osteogenic Sarcoma

This rare, aggressive malignancy may involve any of the seven bones that make up the orbit (▶ Fig. 13.6). Onset is often rapid with a quick progression of proptosis. Often a thorough history will reveal that there was previous radiation such as for a retinoblastoma. It is more common in males. CT often reveals the classic sunburst pattern. In the absence of distant metastatic disease, complete surgical resection is recommended, usually to be followed by radiotherapy and chemotherapy.[7]

Mesenchymal Chondrosarcoma

Mesenchymal chondrosarcoma is more deadly. This is primarily a disease of teenagers and young adults and in the orbit is more commonly seen in females. This tumor is highly malignant with rapid growth, regional spread, and distant disease. Historically these tumors have been surgically removed with attempts made to clear all surgical margins. Radiotherapy is reserved for histologically close or positive margins. Other very rare malignant mesenchymal tumors that can occur in the orbit are fibrosarcomas and angiosarcomas.

13.6 Secondary Orbital Tumors

Secondary orbital tumors are more common than primary ones in the adult patient.[9] The various types are dominated by skin cancers. However, direct extension from the paranasal sinuses, nasal cavity, and nasopharynx is seen with some frequency in the adult head and neck cancer practice. Direct extension from minor salivary gland cancers evolving in the nasal cavity or lacrimal sac are also encountered infrequently.[17]

13

13.6.1 Esthesioneuroblastoma

The esthesioneuroblastoma or olfactory neuroblastoma is a malignancy from the basal cells of the olfactory neuroepithelium. Because of the lesion's origin, the cribriform plate is invariably involved. The lesion often herniates into the nose in a highly vascular polypoid mass, causing obstruction and sometimes bleeding. Intracranial extension is also common as is direct invasion of the ethmoid and sphenoid sinus. As many as three-quarters of patients can experience orbital symptoms. Orbital involvement with direct invasion is evident in more than half of these cases[18] (▶ Fig. 13.7).

From a histopathologic standpoint, the tumor is made up of small, round cells that occasionally form rosettes or pseudorosettes. This is a neuroendocrine lesion and is positive for synaptophysin and/or chromogranin on immunohistochemistry. The tumors may be positive for cytokeratin as well as the S100 stain. The differential diagnosis includes other small cell neuroendocrine malignancies including metastatic ones. The full gamut of sinonasal carcinomas including sinonasal undifferentiated carcinomas, squamous cell carcinoma, less commonly lymphomas, and melanomas must be considered. A complete differential diagnosis also includes hemangiopericytoma, plasmacytoma, and sarcomas. Treatment is universally complete tumor removal through

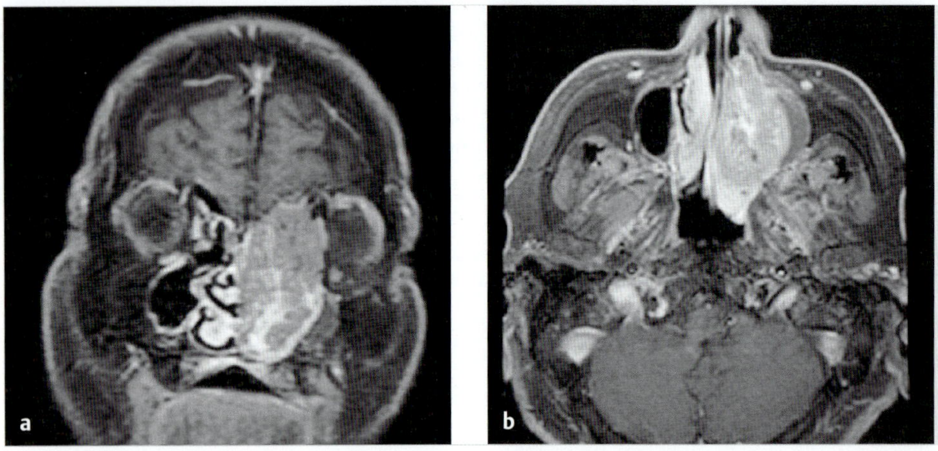

Fig. 13.7 MRI (T1 with contrast sequences) shows orbital infiltration by a high-grade neuroendocrine carcinoma of the paranasal sinuses on coronal **(a)** and axial **(b)** images.

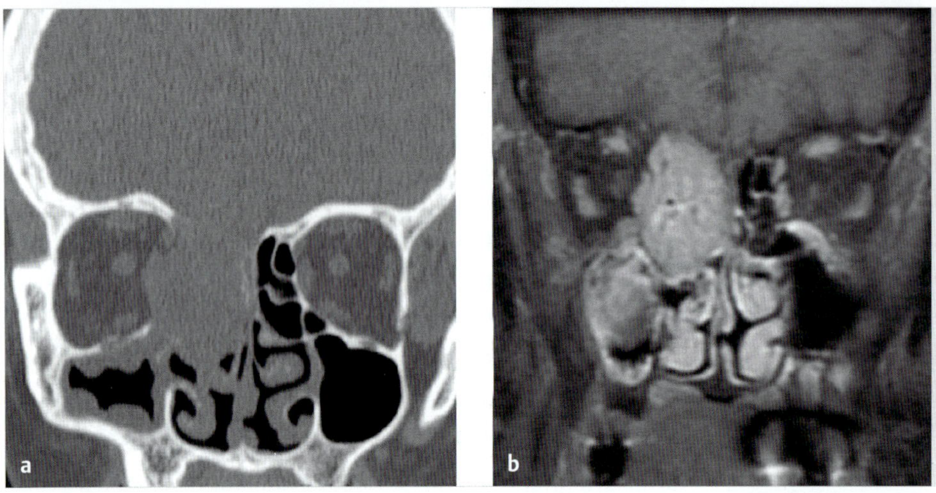

Fig. 13.8 Renal cell carcinoma metastatic to the nose, ethmoid sinus, and adjacent orbit. The CT scan **(a)** shows the area of bony involvement. The MRI (T1 with contrast) image shows the hypervascular nature of the tumor with multiple flow voids and areas of contrast uptake **(b)**.

whatever approach is necessary (endoscopic, transfacial, combined craniofacial resection, or unfortunately perhaps even orbital exoneration). While generally not evident at presentation, regional lymphadenopathy occurs in upward of 50% of patients, with the positive nodes sometimes appearing more than a year later. When they occur, regional metastases are best treated by neck dissection with adjuvant radiotherapy.[19,20]

13

13.6.2 Nasopharyngeal Carcinoma

Nasopharyngeal carcinoma (NPC) has been classified by the World Health Organization into two main groups: type 1 represents traditional squamous cell carcinomas based on their squamous differentiation on light microscopy; type 2 includes the former nonkeratinizing carcinoma and the undifferentiated carcinoma (or lymphoepithelioma). These latter two were found—after the initial classification was created—to have significant overlap. Today most clinicians simply designate these as squamous cancers or as undifferentiated cancers. The less common squamous cell carcinomas have a weak relationship to the Epstein–Barr virus (EBV), but EBV is strongly associated with poorly differentiated carcinomas. Positivity for EBV antigens helps to distinguish nasopharyngeal undifferentiated carcinoma from the less common lymphomas. The Epstein-Barr early antigen, as well as the viral capsid antigen (VCA) can be very helpful during follow-up in screening patients for evidence of recurrence.[21]

Nasopharyngeal carcinomas can track along the surface of the anterior cranial fossa and directly involve the orbit or extend through the superior orbital fissure. More commonly they erode laterally through the sphenoid wing and into the orbit posteriorly. Slightly more anteriorly, the lamina papyracea is not a robust barrier and the medial orbit can often be involved as well.

Transfacial, endoscopic transoral, combined transfacial and transcranial, and even transnasal endoscopic approaches have been described to surgically address nasopharyngeal carcinoma. More commonly, concurrent chemoradiotherapy is employed. Both approaches can have quite high morbidity should orbital involvement be present at presentation.

13.6.3 Metastatic Tumors

Metastatic cancers arising hematogenously are rare in the orbit and represent as few as 1% of tumors in the orbit.[9] Most commonly a metastatic tumor of the orbit derives from breast (50%). Less commonly metastases from cancers of the lung, prostate, gastrointestinal tract, and kidney also occur (▶ Fig. 13.8).[22] Interestingly, intraocular metastases outnumber orbital metastases. Neuroblastoma from an adrenal gland site can occasionally metastasize to the orbit in children. In one series, metastatic neuroblastoma was second only to rhabdomyosarcoma in an evaluation of the incidence of orbital neoplasms.[9] Understandably, orbital neuroblastoma generally involves additional metastases and sadly treatment is often palliative only.

13.7 Surgical Approaches to the Orbit

The cardinal principle in approaching the orbit surgically does not differ from that for other regions of human anatomy.

Essentially, one must select an approach that affords the best exposure so that one has the optimum opportunity at the initial operation to remove all the disease and preserve functioning orbital contents. There are several basic approaches that can be utilized for accessing orbital tumors, including anterior, medial, superior, lateral, and inferior approaches. In addition, many orbital tumors involving the medial inferior posterior or even the superior orbit can now be successfully approached and removed via transnasal endoscopic techniques (see Chapter 18).

The medial approach to the intraconal orbit is afforded through the classic **lateral rhinotomy** incision. Through this access the medial canthal tendon can be released and the globe and uninvolved orbital contents lateralized. The ethmoid sinus and lacrimal fossa can be nicely exposed through his approach, affording reasonable visibility from the medial aspect of the orbit to the orbital apex. This approach can also be combined with an anterior approach for additional exposure. Both extracoronal and intracoronal tumors can be successfully visualized and addressed with this approach. It is important that the medial canthal tendon be repaired at closure to prevent telecanthus. In general, the lateral rhinotomy incision (if appropriately placed) heals well without significant sequelae. The pyriform aperture and frontal nasal buttress as well as portions of the superior and inferior orbit can be removed en bloc with this approach and replaced with miniplates following tumor removal. This can significantly enhance exposure of the skull base and posterior orbit.

The superior approach, lateral approach, and transnasal approach to the orbit are detailed in Chapter 18.

13.8 Conclusion

Orbital tumors present the clinician with a host of challenges. Perhaps nowhere else are the consequences of the disease and its selective treatment more serious or potentially morbid. A careful understanding of the precise histopathologic diagnosis and careful preoperative imaging is important. Further, a designated team of experts should be assembled, including head and neck surgeons, endoscopic rhinologists, ophthalmologists with skills in both orbital and oculoplastic surgery, neuroradiologists, pathologists, radiation oncologists, medical oncologists, and others including social services. They should all bring their talents to bear on the group of patients stricken with these challenging diseases. The very best results will be achieved with careful forethought from such a multidisciplinary team and the precise execution of planned treatment. Long-term follow-up will be necessary depending on the specific disease.

References

[1] Garrity JA, Henderson JW, Cameron JD, Eds. Henderson's Orbital Tumors. 4th ed. rev. Philadelphia, PA: Lippincott Williams & Wilkins; 2007

[2] Holds JB. Orbital tumors. In: Bailey BJ,ed. Head and Neck Surgery—Otolaryngology. Philadelphia, PA: JB Lippincott; 1993:1110–1124

[3] Janecka I, Housepian E, Trokel S, Rankow R, Jones I, Jakobiec F. Surgical management of malignant tumors of the lacrimal gland. Am J Surg. 1984; 148 (4):539–541

[4] Spiteri Cornish K, Reddy AR. The use of propranolol in the management of periocular capillary haemangioma–a systematic review. Eye (Lond). 2011; 25 (10):1277–1283

[5] Yang M, Yan J. Long term surgical outcomes of orbital cavernous haemangiomas (low-flow venous malformations) as performed in a tertiary eye hospital in China. J Craniomaxillofac Surg. 2014; 42(7):1491–1496

[6] Kansy K, Juergens P, Krol Z, et al. Odontogenic myxoma: diagnostic and therapeutic challenges in paediatric and adult patients–a case series and review of the literature. J Craniomaxillofac Surg. 2012; 40(3):271–276

[7] Waldstein G, Keyser R, Stocker JT. The eye. In: Stocker JT, Dehner LP, eds. Pediatric Pathology. Philadelphia, PA: JB Lippincott; 1992;463–489

[8] Levine MR, Larson DW. Orbital tumors. In: Podos SM, Yanoff M, eds. Textbook of Ophthalmolgy. Vol 4. New York, NY: Gower Medical; 1991

[9] Henderson JW. Orbital Tumors. 3rd ed. New York, NY: Raven Press; 1994

[10] Maurer HM, Gehan EA, Beltangady M, et al. The Intergroup Rhabdomyosarcoma Study-II. Cancer. 1993; 71(5):1904–1922

[11] Parham DM, Webber B, Holt H, Williams WK, Maurer H. Immunohistochemical study of childhood rhabdomyosarcomas and related neoplasms. Results of an Intergroup Rhabdomyosarcoma study project. Cancer. 1991; 67(12):3072–3080

[12] Dickman PS, Triche TJ. Extraosseous Ewing's sarcoma versus primitive rhabdomyosarcoma: diagnostic criteria and clinical correlation. Hum Pathol. 1986; 17(9):881–893

[13] Whang-Peng J, Knutsen T, Theil K, Horowitz ME, Triche T. Cytogenetic studies in subgroups of rhabdomyosarcoma. Genes Chromosomes Cancer. 1992; 5(4): 299–310

[14] Douglass EC, Shapiro DN, Valentine M, et al. Alveolar rhabdomyosarcoma with the t(2;13): cytogenetic findings and clinicopathologic correlations. Med Pediatr Oncol. 1993; 21(2):83–87

[15] Janecke IP, Sekhar LN. Meningiomas: head and neck oncological perspectives. In Fisch U, ed. Neurological Surgery of the Ear and the Skull Base. Berkeley, CA: Kugler & Ghedini; 1989:139

[16] Medeiros LJ, Harmon DC, Linggood RM, Harris NL. Immunohistologic features predict clinical behavior of orbital and conjunctival lymphoid infiltrates. Blood. 1989; 74(6):2121–2129

[17] Howard GR, Nerad JA, Carter KD, Whitaker DC. Clinical characteristics associated with orbital invasion of cutaneous basal cell and squamous cell tumors of the eyelid. Am J Ophthalmol. 1992; 113(2):123–133

[18] Rakes SM, Yeatts RP, Campbell RJ. Ophthalmic manifestations of esthesioneuroblastoma. Ophthalmology. 1985; 92(12):1749–1753

[19] Kennerdell JS, Maroon JC, Malton ML. Surgical approaches to orbital tumors. Clin Plast Surg. 1988; 15(2):273–282

[20] Patel SG, Singh B, Stambuk HE, et al. Craniofacial surgery for esthesioneuroblastoma: report of an international collaborative study. J Neurol Surg B Skull Base. 2012; 73(3):208–220

[21] Neel HB, III, Pearson GR, Weiland LH, et al. Anti-EBV serologic tests for nasopharyngeal carcinoma. Laryngoscope. 1980; 90(12):1981–1990

[22] Shields JA, Shields CL. Rhabdomyosarcoma of the orbit. Int Ophthalmol Clin. 1993; 33(3):203–210

Chapter 14

Radiotherapy of Orbital Diseases

14

14 Radiotherapy of Orbital Diseases

H. Christiansen and R. M. Hermann

14.1 Introduction

All malignant tumors of the human body can also afflict the orbital structures. Treatment is mostly in line with the principles of treatment in other localizations. Thus, for example, basaliomas are surgically resected. Equally effective radiotherapy of these lesions is only carried out as a therapeutic alternative to mutilating operations, after incomplete resections, or in accordance with the patient's expressed wish.

First a brief overview of the various radiation techniques routinely used is given. In the following only entities are discussed that exhibit special features in the area of the orbit, in occurrence, or in treatment. The radiotherapeutic possibilities are dealt within the context of overarching treatment concepts and alternative therapeutic options.

14.2 Technique

14.2.1 Percutaneous Radiotherapy (External Beam Radiotherapy)

Linear accelerators are used in the main to produce ultrahard photon or electron radiation for percutaneous radiation (external beam radiotherapy, EBRT) Occasionally, X-ray tubes are also used as a source for very soft photon beams (e.g., in the postoperative radiation of pterygium, see Chapter 14.4.4).

Operating Principle and Use of the Linear Accelerator

High-frequency microwave beam is fed into a vacuum pipe ("waveguide") and an electron beam is guided onto it. The electrons absorb energy from this and reach a much higher energy than is achievable through direct acceleration between anode and cathode in the classic X-ray tube. This electron beam is then bundled via magnets and directed onto a target of dense material (tungsten), where it is decelerated. The resulting bremsstrahlung is the therapeutically usable photon radiation. This can penetrate the human body easily and is therefore particularly well suited for the radiation of deep-lying structures (▶ Fig. 14.1).

The electron radiation can also be guided directly onto a diffusion foil and then used in treatment. The advantage of this radiation is a prompt build-up of the dose in the body, although it penetrates only a few centimeters in depth. Thus "fast electrons" are ideal for treat target structures close to the body's surface.

> **Memorize** M!
>
> High-energy electron and photon beams can be produced with linear accelerators. Electron beams are suitable for the treatment of tumors close to the body's surface, while photons are good for penetration to depth.

The dose distribution is planned in advance when using therapeutic irradiation so as to ensure sufficient coverage of the target structures while being able to ensure sufficient care is taken of the surrounding normal tissue (so called "organs at risk").

The simplest form of radiation planning is so-called **2D planning**. In this the requisite dose is estimated from the field geometry, the depth of the structure to be irradiated, and the dose prescribed on the basis of sample measurements made previously on an anatomical model. Anatomical characteristics (e.g., influence of bones on the distribution of the dose) are not taken into account here.

3D conformal planning requires planning computed tomography. Through this the electron densities as well as the target structures and organs at risk can be determined individually for the patient. The planning system contains many stored sample measurements with the help of which the computer then calculates a very precise dosage estimate according to specification. In doing this the most accurate systems simulate the irradiation by considering individual photon paths (so-called **Monte Carlo simulation**).

In classical 3D-planning the radiotherapy physicist specifies not only the direction of the beam and the geometry of the radiation fields to the radiotherapy planning system and then checks the dose distribution in the target structures in order to adjust the field configuration after that if needed. In contrast, with **intensity-modulated radiotherapy (IMRT)** the dose desired is specified to the planning computer in terms of the target volume and the maximum tolerated exposure of the organs at risk (so-called *constraints*) (▶ Fig. 14.2, Video 14.1). With the assistance of iterative algorithms the computer optimizes the field configuration independently. In doing this, differently shaped fields are irradiated from one gantry angle so that the intensity of the field is modulated (hence the name) in order to reach the planning target. These plans become so complex that they cannot be checked for plausibility with simple software algorithms. The irradiation of such a plan on a dummy for measurement purposes and comparison between what is measured and the dose calculated is the optimum way to verify such planning before the plan is implemented on a patient.

Imagery-guided radiotherapy (IGRT) requires imagery at the linear accelerator (or at the patient positioning table). Modern equipment uses the high megavoltage photon radiation for imaging. However, these energies are associated with high losses in image quality as this radiation has very poor contrast (only a little radiation is absorbed e.g., in the bone). This is why many accelerators are equipped with a normal X-ray tube as well. Alternatively, X-ray tubes can be directly installed in the radiotherapy bunker that aim at defined angles onto the axis of rotation of the accelerator (the so called "isocenter"). The corresponding image converters are mounted on the other side of the patient table. This way, the anatomy of the patient can be made visible before radiotherapy and, if necessary, corrected by adjustment of the treatment table position.

Ideally, the current position of the tumor is represented by radiopaque markers (e.g., small spirals of gold) and monitored closely during the radiotherapy procedure. The patient can then be adjusted for the respective position of the tumor by automatic movement of the treatment table. This process is designated as **image guided radiotherapy (IGRT)**.

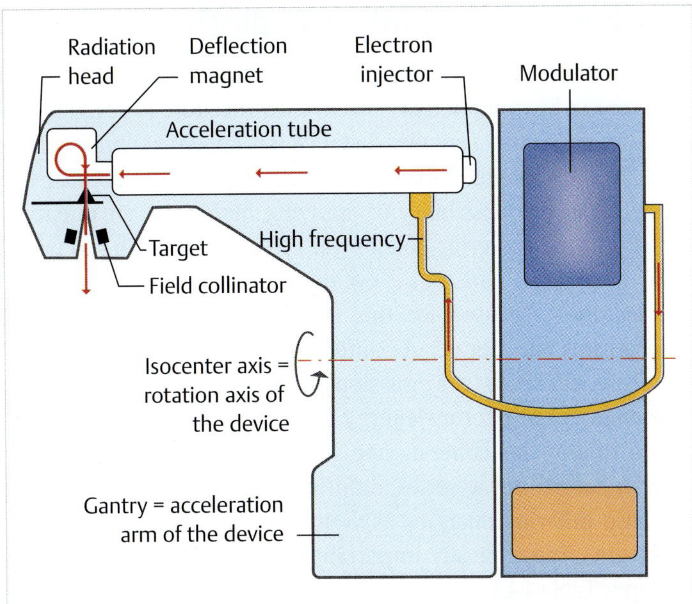

Fig. 14.1 Structure of a linear accelerator. A high-frequency microwave is guided into a high-vacuum tube (called a "waveguide") into which an electron beam is then injected. The electrons are thereby accelerated to high energies, bundled with steering magnets, and fired onto a dense material (e.g., tungsten). This is where the therapeutically useful bremsstrahlung arises as "photon radiation."

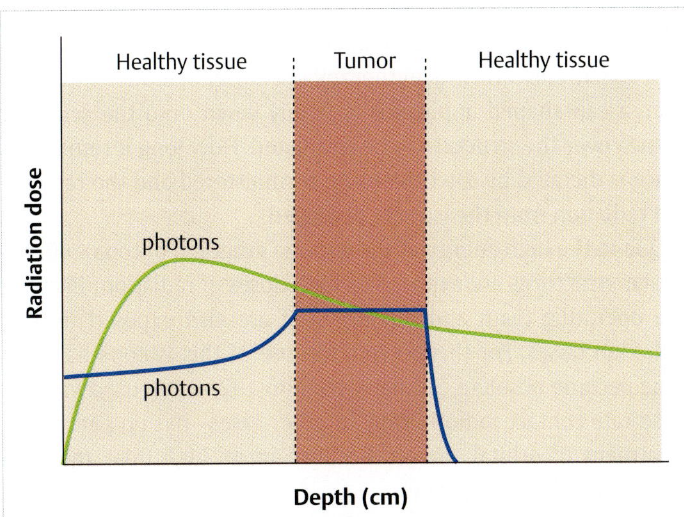

Fig. 14.3 Comparison of the energy transmission (linear energy transfer) of photons and of protons. On the horizontal axis the depth (cm) of the surface in a water dummy is given, the vertical axis represents the dose. Tumor tissue, with normal tissue on either side of it, is assumed at a defined depth.
The photons striking the surface of the water only build up their full energy dose in layers lying somewhat deeper (so-called forward scattering) and then penetrate all further tissue equally. The protons exhibit a different characteristic: on the way to the tumor they ionize the surroundings to only a limited extent, and then virtually the whole of the energy is delivered in the tumor; hardly any radiation penetrates behind the tumor. The diameter of the tumor is covered by using protons with different energies whose Bragg peaks then overlap.

A further example is respiration-gated radiotherapy of a lung carcinoma. In this the respiratory cycle of patients is monitored and the irradiation is administered only in a relatively central position.

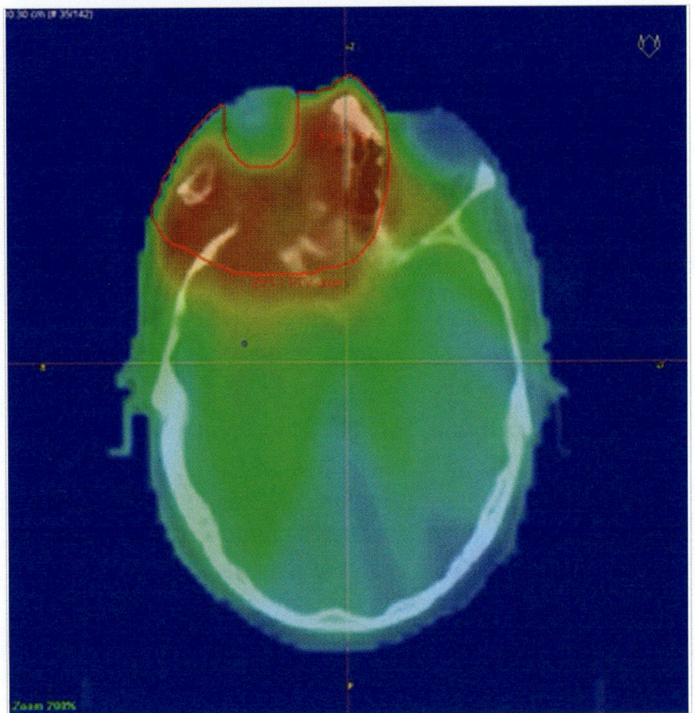

Fig. 14.2 Intensity-modulated irradiation of a carcinoma of the right upper jaw, with extensive destruction of the midfacial bones. The high doses (brown/red) attenuate rapidly in the area of the orbit (green/blue) and this minimizes the side effects of irradiation on the ocular structures.

Proton and Heavy Ion Radiation (Particle Radiation)

Photons and electrons are classified as " sparsely ionizing" radiation. In contrast, protons and "heavy" ions (e.g., helium or carbon ions) lose their energy to a lesser extent during most of their trajectory and then transfer most of it in almost the very last part, the so-called "Bragg peak" (▶ Fig. 14.3). The position of the Bragg peak depends on the acceleration energy and thus can be determined very precisely. Beyond the Bragg peak only a very minimal radiation survives in the tissue.

As a result of this physical feature, the entire radiotherapy dose required can be deposited in the region of the tumor from one or two irradiation directions. In many cases, therefore, the "crossfire technique" needed for classic 3D-conformal radiotherapy with photons, with its correspondingly higher radiation exposure of neighboring tissue, is not required.

As a result of the high release of energy release in one place in the tissue (linear energy transfer, LET), heavy ion irradiation is biologically more effective than photon irradiation. The relative biological effectiveness (RBE) compares the number of biological effects that are triggered by different types of radiation. Sparsely ionizing photon radiation is rated as 1. Compared with this, proton beams have an RBE of 1.1, helium ions 1.3.[1] As this increases biological effectiveness has an effect not only on the tumor cells but on normal tissue as well, the dose of the heavy ion radiation must be adjusted accordingly. For this, the **cobalt gray equivalent (CGE)** is a useful concept that also enables comparison with the results of treatment with conventional photon radiation.

Protons are generated from water through hydrolysis and accelerated by a cyclotron to 2/3 of the speed of light. Upon reaching the appropriate speed, the beam is further modulated from its circular path via beam lines, which are formed by electromagnets, and directed to a gantry in the treatment room. Individually prepared compensators can be used to cover the tumor. Alternatively, the equipment can also be fitted with pencil beam scanning. In this the tumor region is "scanned" with the proton beams and thus the treatment session consists of many "single shots." Although the application of radiation is thereby extended in time, this does mean that no individual collimators have to be produced and disposed of after use (radioactive waste).

A disadvantage of this technique is the extremely high technical effort and thus financial cost necessary for the creation of these types of radiation. For this reason proton radiation is at present only available in a few places.

A further disadvantage is low energy transfer of the particles on their way to the Bragg peak. As the tumor must be covered in its entire depth, particles with the requisite energy differences must be fired into this area and already on the way to the tumor volume the energy emissions overlap. When irradiating tumors in the fundus of the eye, there is therefore significant radiogenic exposure in the anterior parts of the eye. This is why ~35% of patients later develop neovascular glaucomas after proton radiotherapy of uveal melanomas.[1]

In summary, so far it has only been clinically demonstrated for a few entities and situations that radiotherapy with particles provides a clinical advantage in the sense of higher tumor control and/or fewer side effects. Among those entities are, for example, the adenoid cystic carcinomas as well as chondrosarcomas of the base of the skull (evaluation of the German Society for Radiooncology at http://www.degro.org/dav/html/download/pdf/Protonen_Stellungnahme_010808.pdf). The aim of the radiooncological research in the abovementioned centers is to examine further indications in clinical studies and to evaluate treatment results.

> **Memorize** M!
>
> The physical characteristic of proton and heavy-ion irradiation consists in the release of a large part of the energy at a certain point (the so-called Bragg peak). This means that the radiation dose can be applied very precisely. The increased biological effectiveness in comparison with photon irradiation must be taken into account when prescribing the dose.
>
> A disadvantage is the high cost of production so that this form of treatment is only available in a few centers.
>
> Thus far, a clinical advantage for proton irradiation compared with photon radiation has been shown for only a few entities.

14

Brachytherapy: Contact Radiotherapy

With distance between the radioactive source and the target structure to be irradiated of > 10 cm the procedure is described as "teletherapy"; with a smaller distance it is known as "brachytherapy." The advantage of contact radiotherapy in the area of the orbit lies in the possibility of applying high doses of radiation directly in the posterior pole of the eye without having to penetrate the anterior parts of the eye or other areas of the orbit. Various isotopes are used for this that emit radiation by natural mechanisms of decay. A differentiation is made clinically between beta decay (the emission of electrons) and gamma decay (the emission of photons/energy quanta). Alpha emitters do not play a role in this context. One should take account of the fact that, in natural decay series, differing types of decay often occur and also differing energies as well (the so-called natural decay spectrum). The clinically important characteristics are summarized in ▶ Table 14.1.[2]

In general, two different forms of contact radiotherapy in the area of the orbit can be differentiated: episcleral and intraocular brachytherapy. In this, **intraocular brachytherapy** for the selective radiotherapy of the macula (epimacular brachytherapy) after vitrectomy with strontium-applicators is so far still classed as experimental (see Chapter 14.4.5). In contrast, the epibulbar application of strontium-applicators of ~1 cm diameter in the treatment of pterygia is well established (see Chapter 14.4.4). For this, the applicator is held manually directly over the area to be irradiated or is moved slowly in circling movements. With highly active sources, this procedure takes only a few minutes.

In classic episceral brachytherapy during an operative intervention, a cap-shaped applicator is firmly sewn onto the sclera or cornea over the structure to be irradiated. How long it remains in place is dictated by the dose to be administered and the range of the radiation from the isotope deployed.

Due to the high energy of the gamma emission of cobalt 60, the ocular structures are exposed to high doses of radiation; likewise the operating team and nursing staff are also exposed to high radiation doses. For this reason, the use of this isotope has over time become obsolete. Similarly iridium 192—often used for high dose rate contact radiotherapy in other cases—has no part in the treatment of orbital tumors because to its high dose rate and comparatively high energy.

Iodine 125 and palladium 103 are characterized by the emission of gamma radiation with much lower energies. Because of this the surrounding ocular structures can be relatively well protected with gold shields as the rear applicator wall.

Table 14.1 Radionuclides used for ocular brachytherapy

Isotope	Clinically relevant radiation	Energy (mean or spectrum) (MeV)	HLP	HVLD in water (mm)
Iodine 125 (^{125}I)	gamma	0.022–0.031 0.035	60 days	20
Palladium 103 (^{103}Pd)	gamma	0.021	17 days	15
Cobalt 60 (^{60}Co)	gamma	1.17–1.33	5.26 years	108
Iridium 192 (^{192}Ir)	gamma	0.38	74 days	63
Ruthenium 106 (^{106}Ru)	beta	2.07–3.54	1 year	24
Strontium 90/yttrium 90 ($^{90}Sr/^{90}Y$)	beta	^{90}Sr 0.546 ^{90}Y 2.28	28 years 64 hours	1.5

Abbreviations: HLP: half-life period HVLD: half-value layer density.

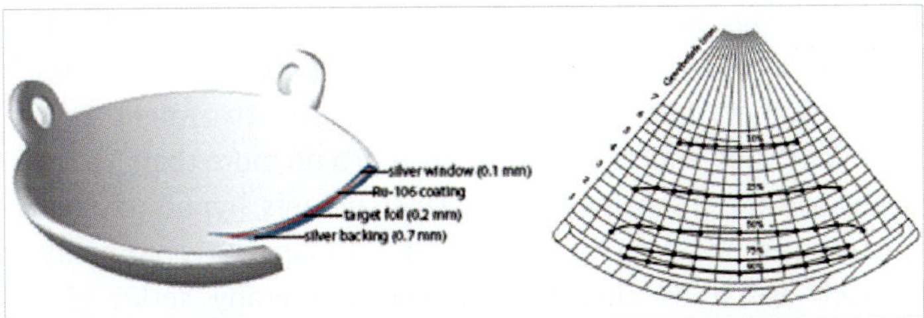

Fig. 14.4 Structure of a ruthenium 106 applicator of the Bebig Company and the depth distribution of a CCA applicator. *Left*: the rear of the applicator is screened with 0.7 mm silver, while the 0.1 mm-thick silver foil on the inside allows through the beta radiation used in treatment. *Right*: the emitter is fixed externally to the sclera; at a distance of 0.5 mm 90% of the dose is measured, at 1 mm 75%, at 2 mm more than 50%, and at 4 mm 25% can still be measured. With the kind permission of Eckert & Ziegler BEBIG, Berlin.

This works even better with the beta radiation of ruthenium 106 (▶ Fig. 14.4). All of the radiation is absorbed by the 0.7-mm silver posterior shielding, while a 0.1-mm thin silver foil on the concave side screens out only the low-energy electrons (0.039 MeV) and lets the high-energy electrons at 3.54 MeV exit almost unhindered. The dose gradient is even steeper than with iodine 125 or palladium 103, at a distance of 7 mm from the applicator the dose is reduced to 1/10 of the starting dose. Thus neighboring ocular structures can be well protected. A disadvantage is the unavoidably high dose at the sclera with a tumor apex of > 6 mm in order to still maintain a sufficient dose in the areas of the tumor lying farthest from the applicator. For this reason, the use of this isotope should remain limited to tumors < 5 mm in height (+ 1 mm sclera) (▶ Fig. 14.4, ▶ Fig. 14.5).

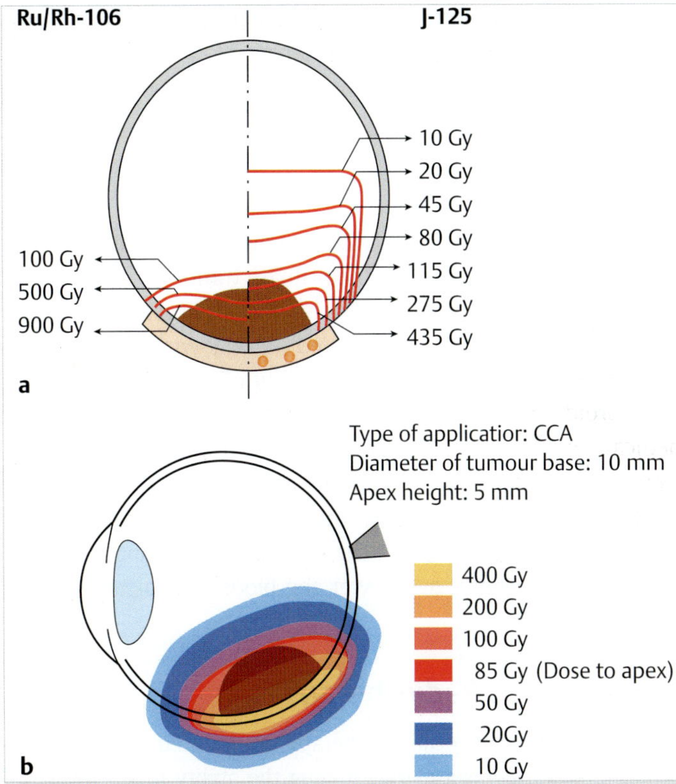

Fig. 14.5 Comparison of depth–dose curves between a ruthenium 106 and a iodine 125 applicator on the model of an eye. The clearly steeper dose gradient from the ruthenium 106 is striking. This gives the advantage of lower exposure of the unaffected ocular structures. However, with the irradiation of tumor cells lying > 6 mm from the applicator, very high doses are necessarily required at the sclera. With the kind permission of Eckert & Ziegler BEBIG, Berlin.

Memorize M!

In brachytherapy a natural emitter is placed directly onto the lesion to be treated or the overlying sclera. Episcleral brachytherapy is well established, for example, with iodine 125 and ruthenium 106. As the beta radiation of the ruthenium does not reach as far as the γ gamma radiation of the iodine, ruthenium can only be used to treat tumors at an apical distance of up to 6 mm from the emitter. Tumors up to 10 mm can be treated with iodine applicators; but the surrounding ocular structures will be subject to greater exposure.

14.3 Radiotherapy of Malignant Neoplasias of the Orbit

14.3.1 Metastases in the Area of the Orbit

In principle, any malignant neoplasia of the human body can form metastases in all structures of the orbit. In the course of this the symptoms depend on the particular localization of the metastasis. When the eye muscles are afflicted this is often associated with exophthalmos, pain, and diplopia. Occasionally, however, enophthalmos can also be observed (in particular with cirrhotic adenocarcinomas) if constricting, scarlike infiltrations arise.

Due to the blood flow characteristics and, also probably, due to interactions between surface antigens of the tumor cells with vascular endothelia, most of the secondary metastases are located in the area of the uvea.[3] It is estimated that up to 10% of patients suffering from advanced tumor stages develop metastases in the uvea (literature overview[4]); of these, however, ~90% remain asymptomatic and, for that reason, are not detected without ophthalmological examinations.[5]

The most frequent originating tumors for uveal metastases are ~80% breast carcinomas in women and the same for bronchial carcinomas in men.[6] The average survival time after diagnosis of such metastases is ~9 months,[7] although the prognosis can differ hugely depending on the primary tumor, previous treatments, and the response of the disease to systemic therapies.

Choroid Metastases

Almost 90% of uveal metastases affect the choroid; metastases rarely occur in the iris, and are even rarer in the ciliary body.[3,8,9] In the area of the choroid most of the metastases are localized between the macula and the equator.[9]

In up to 50% of choroid metastases they are synchronous or associated with cerebral metastases occurring in the later course of the disease.[6] Multiple choroid metastases are seen in up to 30% of patients.[6] In almost 50% of patients (in particular with breast cancer), bilateral affliction is seen, with half of those afflicted not experiencing any symptoms.[3]

The symptoms are dependent on the localization of the metastases. Patients afflicted notice a worsening of their sight or

14

blurred vision; less often they report floaters, photopsia, or scotomas.[3] If it is untreated, there is a danger of complete blindness and a painful, treatment-refractory glaucoma that ultimately will make enucleation unavoidable.

Therapy

Treatment depends on the localization of the metastasis, its size, and the treatment options for the primary tumor.

Small metastases without acute risk to sight in systemically still responsive tumors can be monitored initially within the context of systemic therapies, as the probability of a remission is high. The choroid lies outside the blood–vitreal barrier so that systemic medicaments can flow freely. Very good remission rates have been described for systemic administration of the VEGF-antibody bevacizumab.[10] Astonishingly, intravitreal injections are also effective, probably because of the very high local concentrations, which can sufficiently overpower the blood–vitreal barrier in a reverse direction.

Percutaneous Radiotherapy

Prompt induction of localized therapy is indicated with progression of choroid metastases threatening the ability to see by growing into the macula, subretinal fluid accumulation, or bleeding into the vitreous humor. The aim of such treatment is local control.

In this situation external beam radiotherapy with photons (EBRT) plays a very important role. It is available everywhere, effective, and cheap. The total and single doses of EBRT published since the 1970s vary between 5 × 5 Gy and 25 × 2 Gy (overview[4]). Due to variations in irradiation techniques and in the dosages, and the nonstandardized definition of the end point of sight improvement, direct comparison of the study results is difficult. Local control of the tumor was reported in 70 to 90% of patients and stabilization or improvement of the sight in > 70%.

In the only prospective phase II study a total dose of 40 Gy with 2 Gy single dose in 65 afflicted eyes (50 patients) was examined with regard to effectiveness and toxicity.[5] The median survival was 7 months. Sonographically, 17% of the tumors exhibited no change as a result of the radiotherapy, 39% a full remission, the others a partial remission. With regard to clinical end points, 85% profited from the therapy: a significant improvement in sight was experienced by 36%, a stabilization by 50% of patients. None of the initially asymptomatic patients experienced a deterioration in their sight. In the further course of the disease, metastases recurred in 14% of the eyes. Half of the patients developed temporary skin erythemas or conjunctivitis during treatment. Severe radiogenic side effects were described in a no more than 5%.

Because of the sensitivity of ocular structures, hypofractionated treatment schedules (e.g., 5 × 5 Gy) are no longer recommended. Instead, as far as clinically possible, a therapy series giving 5 × 2 Gy up to 40 Gy should be followed in accordance with the findings mentioned above.

In clinical practice a dosage of 10 × 3 Gy has also proved to be effective, in particular when concurrent brain metastases are identified and the choroid metastases are to be treated at the same time with whole-brain radiotherapy by widening the radiation fields. Based on radiobiological formulae, comparable effectiveness can be assumed with regard to not only the normal tissue but also the tumor cells. At 10 × 3 Gy, assuming an α/β quotient of 3 for late-reacting normal tissues, the biologically effective dose is 100 Gy_3 in comparison to 93.3 Gy_3 with a fractionation of 20 × 2 Gy. For tumor cells a distinctly higher α/β quotient (~9) is postulated, the biologically effective dose at 20 × 2 Gy is calculated at 84.3 Gy_9 and 93.3 Gy_9 at 10 × 3 Gy. No allowance has been made here for the acceleration of the therapy at 10 in comparison to 20 fractions and the thus additionally increased biological effectiveness.

Technique

The EBRT takes place with the patient in a supine position, with the head fixed in a mask positioning system.

The eye structures afflicted, including the orbital optic nerve, are mapped as the CTV (clinical target volume) in the planning CT. The safety margins for the definition of the PTV (planning target volume) only have to cover unsafe positioning of the mask (depending on the system used) and, where necessary, the movement of the eye(s).

If it is anatomically possible, the lenses should be protected. For this, lateral-opposing fields offer good options. The central radiation plane is placed ventrally behind the lenses to avoid divergence of the beam paths in this direction (▶ Fig. 14.6).

If the metastasis lies in the iris area, the lens cannot be protected by conventional means. Here irradiation with several field angles ("wedge") is generally unavoidable.

If affliction is unilateral, it is justified not only to irradiate with laterally opposing fields with inclusion of the contralateral ocular

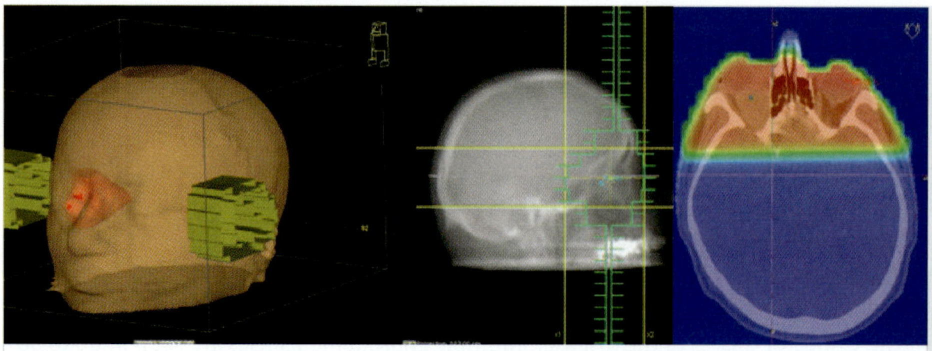

Fig. 14.6 Radiotherapy of an extensive orbital metastasis, right, with lateral opposing fields. This means both orbits are covered with the same radiation dose homogeneously. Protecting the lenses does not make clinical sense in this example because of the extent of the metastases and therefore has not been attempted. On the left side of the illustration, the angle and the configuration of both fields are shown schematically; in the center the field aperture is shown in yellow and the configuration of the multileaf collimator (MLC) from the line of sight of the accelerator onto a digitally produced radiograph is shown in green. On the right, the dose distribution is shown in a transversal layer as an example, where the reddish-brown colors correspond to the prescribed dose.

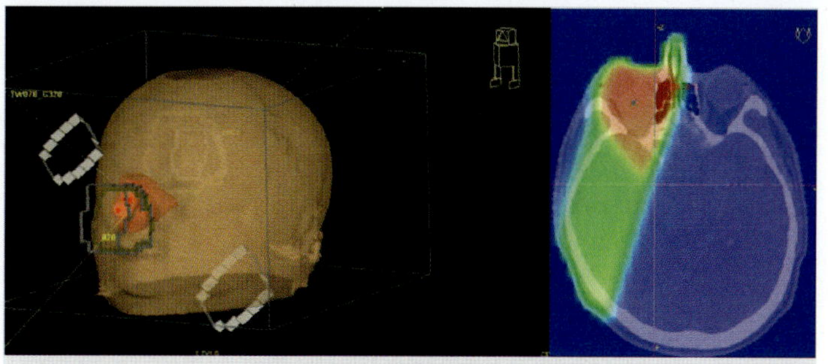

Fig. 14.7 Irradiation of an extensive orbital metastasis, right, unilateral. The aim of this technique is comprehensive protection of the contralateral orbit.
On the left side of the illustration the entry angle and the configuration of the three fields are shown schematically. On the right side, the dose distribution is depicted in a transversal layer as an example, where the reddish-brown colors correspond to the prescribed dose. In comparison to ▶ Fig. 14.6, the temporal right brain is more exposed, but the contralateral orbit has now been taken out of the irradiation fields.

fundus (due to the synchronous contralateral metastases found in up to 50% of cases) but also to irradiate unilaterally only on the side afflicted (▶ Fig. 14.7). Through the unilateral irradiation only 50 to 70% of the dose will be applied in the area of the contralateral eye.[5] In the above-mentioned prospective study, with this procedure no contralateral choroid metastases recurred. The authors postulated that this dose had effectively prevented the occurrence of contralateral metastases.[11] However, the low number of cases ($n = 35$ with unilateral occurrence) must be taken into account. Furthermore, so far there have been no further clinical data on dose–effect relationships, either for the elective or for the therapeutic, scenario.

Memorize M!

EBRT is suitable for treating choroidal metastases with 10 × 3 Gy or 20 × 2 Gy. With this regimen, sight can be improved in 85% of patients or at least stabilized. If the affliction is unilateral both the ipsilateral and the contralateral orbit can be treated. With cerebral metastases the choroid together with the whole cerebrum is irradiated.

Other Radiotherapy Techniques

An alternative to percutaneous irradiation with photons is provided by protons or heavy ions. With this technique very high single doses can be used saving time vis-à-vis EBRT. Furthermore, the eyeball can be sufficiently immobilized through a "light point" technique, so that operative interventions (as in brachytherapy) are not necessary.[12] As there have so far not been any prospective randomized studies comparing it with EBRT, the effectiveness and toxicity of this irradiation technique in comparison with EBRT cannot be assessed. However, the production of these beams is extremely time-consuming, equating to cost-intensive, and thus only possible in a few centers. In the highly palliative situation of the treatment of uveal metastases, the use of this method is mostly not justified.

Alternatively, the deployment of brachytherapy in smaller patient series for the treatment of a single, well-defined choroid metastasis has also been reported.[13] The technique of episcleral treatment is described under "Technical Procedure in Episcleral Brachytherapy" in Chapter 14.3.3. This does, however, require the operative attachment (and subsequent removal) of an appropriate applicator episclerally on the metastasis. The theoretical advantage vis-à-vis EBRT is the shorter treatment duration and the more precise coverage of the metastasis. As an effective dose, in the largest series a dose of ~68 Gy at the tumor apex and 236 Gy at the base of the tumor metastasis have been reported.[14]

Clinical advantages of this more costly therapy over EBRT on a group of patients suffering from an advanced malignant disease have not yet been substantiated. However, the possibility of re-irradiation by brachytherapy is undisputed in the event of a recurrence or renewed progression after EBRT has been given.

Metastases and Tumors of the Eyelid

Systemically far advanced tumors rarely metastasize in the eyelids. Their frequency is assessed at < 1% of malignant changes in the eyelids. These lesions grow in a diffusely infiltrating manner as well as locally,[15] so that operative resections can be very complex due to the reconstruction required. As a therapeutic alternative, palliative EBRT can be offered. In a series of seven patients with eyelid metastases, local control with EBRT was reported in four patients.[15]

Basaliomas or squamous epithelial carcinomas of the skin can likewise occur in the eyelid area. Here EBRT represents an alternative treatment of equal value to operative procedures, with excellent local control rates.

Therapeutically, either kilovolt-photon irradiation or electron irradiation is used. In order to achieve maximum effect with electron irradiation, a layer of material isodense to water is placed onto the region affected (e.g., a silicone cushion 1 cm in diameter). The radiation builds up in this layer (forward scattering, see ▶ Fig. 14.2) so that 100% of the prescribed dose covers the area of the tumor at skin level. To protect the ocular structures (sclera, lens, retina), before each radiotherapy session a calotte of dense material (gold, lead) is placed onto the sclera under the eyelids after a local anesthetic has been given. Thus these organs at risk (except for the lacrimal gland) can be protected effectively despite the administration of higher doses of radiation.

Technically kilovolt-photon irradiation (if still available) is the easier to use. It is characterized by a smaller half shadow than electron irradiation[16] in the area of the field margin. This must be taken account of in the field definition in order to avoid underdosing in the tumor. Also in favor of the use of kilovolt irradiation is the fact that it can be blocked more easily: eye calottes with lead 2 mm thick with a 0.1-mm gold coating are found to be sufficient for 250 kV (▶ Fig. 14.8).[16] For electron irradiation the calottes used must be measured in advance and adjusted appropriately for the energies used as regards the density of the material and the diameter of the calotte. Lead calottes are impractical due to the thickness required at, for example, an electron energy of 9 MeV. Calottes of tungsten or gold have proved to be significantly better suited.[17] The calottes should be coated additionally with 2 mm of acrylic[17] to reduce any backscattering that would give additional exposure to the inside of the eyelids.[17]

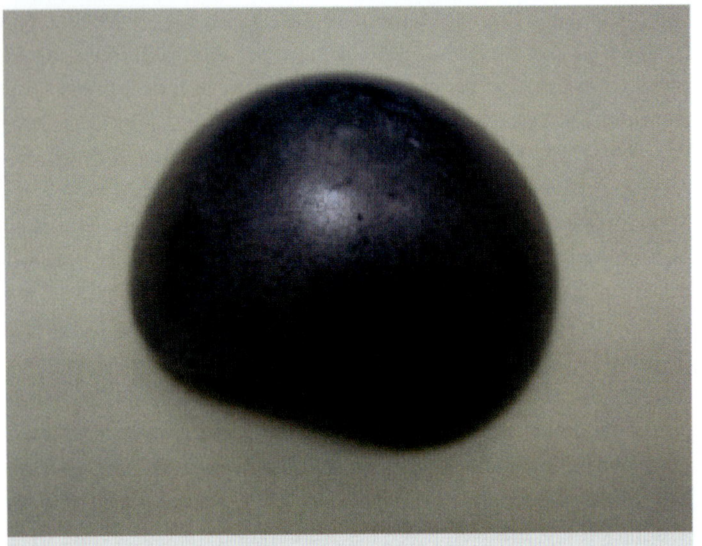

Fig. 14.8 Example of an eye calotte.

> **Memorize**
>
> With metastases and tumors of the eyelid, EBRT with kilovolt-photon irradiation or with electron irradiation is well suited for achieving local control as an alternative to operative interventions. Eye calottes are placed on the sclera before each administration of radiation to protect unaffected ocular structures.

14.3.2 Orbit Lymphomas

Primary intraocular lymphomas (PIOL) are rare. They belong to the group of extranodal non-Hodgkin's lymphomas and are mostly derived from the B cell line. T cell lymphomas in this location are a rarity in Europe.

The retina, the vitreous humor, and the optic nerve can be afflicted.[18] In 80% of cases there is CNS involvement within 2 years of diagnosis (so-called oculocerebral lymphoma); in ~20% of primary CNS lymphomas the eye becomes infiltrated in the course of the disease.[19] In this respect, PIOL constitutes one entity of the primary CNS lymphomas (PCSNL). These are mostly diffuse large B-cell lymphomas and accordingly highly malignant lymphomas.

14

The primary lymphomas of the uvea have to be distinguished from these. These are mostly differentiated as low-malignant B cell lymphomas (extranodal marginal zone lymphomas).[18]

With secondary involvement of the orbit within the context of an extraocular lymphoma growth, mostly the uvea or the adnexa are affected.

Due to the radiosensitivity of lymphoma cells, although radiotherapy is associated with high remission rates, it is only for low-malignant lymphomas with long-term tumor control. This is why therapeutically highly malignant lymphomas must be differentiated from low-malignant (indolent) ones.

> **Memorize**
>
> For the treatment of orbit lymphomas it is imperative to differentiate them into low-malignant lymphomas, curable by radiotherapy, and highly malignant ones, curable by chemotherapy.

> Low-malignant lymphomas mostly afflict the uvea and the orbit adnexa; highly malignant ones afflict the retina, the vitreous humor, and the optic nerve. Of highly malignant lymphomas in the orbit, 80% manifest themselves in the CNS as well over the further course of the disease.

Treatment of Highly Malignant Lymphomas

So far, due to the rarity of the disease, there is no standard procedure. In principle, the condition should be treated locally as long as the disease is restricted to the eye and systemically if the CNS is primarily involved.[20]

The polychemotherapy generally deployed for highly malignant lymphoma according to the CHOP protocol (cyclophosphamide, vincristine, doxorubicin, prednisolone) is largely ineffective for eye and CNS involvement as it scarcely overcomes respectively the blood–eye or blood–brain barriers.[20]

With the involvement of an eye only, either intravitral methotrexate (MTX) or rituximab is applied or the orbit is irradiated with 30 to 35 Gy.[20] Here it is postulated that the generous covering of both orbits by use of laterally opposing fields without protection of the lenses could be associated with a lower recurrence rate than the strict unilateral irradiation of the afflicted orbit with wedged fields or technical omission of orbital structures (e.g., of the lens), even if there is no prospectively randomized corroboration of this assumption.[21] As so far the superiority of no one treatment modality has been demonstrated, treatment can be according to the patient's wishes and adjusted for any previous treatments.

When both eyes are afflicted simultaneously, bilateral local therapy can be combined with systemic treatment.

> **Memorize**
>
> Highly malignant lymphomas that are localized only to the eyes are treated locally. For this EBRT and also intravitreal MTX or rituximab can be deployed.

With simultaneous CNS involvement the therapy is orientated on the treatment of PCNSL, where necessary combined with local therapy to compensate for the limited penetration of the chemotherapy and antibodies into the eye chambers.

With PCNSL, the whole cerebrum is treated by radiotherapy (WBRT). After WBRT with 40 Gy and 20 Gy additional boost doses in the regions afflicted, 5-year survival rates of between 10 and 30% are achieved, and ~60% after a combination of ~45 Gy WBRT with high-dose MTX.[22] However, with combination therapy there is a raised risk for chronic neuronal toxicity. This shows itself on the one hand in a reduction of the neurocognitive capabilities, in particular of the executive functions (alertness, learning and reproducing new information) as well as of psychomotor coordination.[23] On the other hand, ~30% of patients develop therapy-associated leukoencephalopathy and brain atrophy after combination therapy, which is associated with dementia, ataxia, and incontinence and can have a lethal progression in one-third of patients.[24]

For this reason in phase II studies—at least in patients with complete remission after MTX induction—the dose of the WBRT is successively reduced to 30.6 Gy and 23.4 Gy.[25] In this way the neurotoxicity is indeed distinctly reduced, but in younger patients the oncologic therapy results seemed also to become compromised. Good long-term results have been published for a dose reduction of the WBRT to 23.4 Gy after complete remission with polychemotherapy (MTX, procarbazine, vincristine) including administering rituximab with cytarabine as consolidation.[26] The 3-year survival rate was 87%, in contrast with only 40% in patients who did not exhibit complete remission for the induction therapy and who were irradiated with 45 Gy.

Only one prospective randomized phase III study (G-PCNSL-SG) examined the value of WBRT. In this it was shown that WBRT up to 45 Gy with 1.5 Gy single dose after high-dose MTX or high-dose MTX and ifosfamide significantly improved progression-free survival in some subgroups but not the overall survival of patients.[27] However, a definitive evaluation of the results is not possible as the study was calculated to have a power of 60%, thus being not big enough to substantiate the noninferiority of the chemotherapy alone arm.[25]

Nevertheless, in current German therapy studies, when there is complete remission on chemotherapy the cerebrum is not subject to further irradiation. The focus of therapy is on polychemotherapy, with high-dose MTX as a fixed component, flanked by araC, thiotepa, and alkylating agents. With this regimen, 8-year survival rates of 50% are achievable for those under 65 years of age.[28] In addition, rituximab is currently given in the protocols. Although this is poor at penetrating the CNS, nevertheless it is apparently relatively effective in low concentrations in the CNS.

The value of high-dose chemotherapy with autologous stem cell transplantation has still not been definitively established and is being investigated in various randomized studies.[24]

The value of whole-brain radiation with optional boost for the regions afflicted with primary or secondary therapy failure after system therapy is undisputed. In this a whole-brain dose of 36 Gy and a single dose of 1.5 Gy should not be exceeded due to the otherwise distinctly raised risk of neurological late toxicity.[29] In patients who are unable to receive chemotherapy, higher overall doses are applied in line with the results described above. When the eyes are affected, the orbits are included in the radiotherapy volume via laterally opposing fields.

Memorize M!

Highly malignant oculocerebral lymphomas are treated like CNS lymphomas. Here polychemotherapy plays the primary role. In current therapy studies, consolidating irradiation of the CNS still plays a role only in incomplete remission of the lymphomas after chemotherapy. In this, the radiation dose planning must avoid the occurrence of a radiogenic leukoencephalopathy, which proves fatal in 30% of those afflicted.

In patients who for reasons of comorbidity cannot receive chemotherapy, or with recurrences after polychemotherapy, the value of whole- brain radiotherapy is undisputed.

Therapy of Low-Malignant Lymphomas

The role of radiotherapy in these entities is considerably better defined.

Traditionally, indolent lymphomas of all localizations were treated locally with radiation doses between 24 Gy and more than 40 Gy. This reliably gives local control with very high cure rates for MALT lymphomas of the orbit.[30] A SEER analysis on 1111 patients with low-malignant orbit lymphomas who were treated from 1998 to 2010 showed that over the further course none of the patients receiving radiotherapy died as a result of lymphoma, whilst 11.5%[31] of the patients who did not receive radiotherapy died.

The equivalence of 24 Gy and 36 Gy dosage in diverse lymphoma localizations was demonstrated in a randomized prospective study.[32] Various series reported good and long-lasting remission rates after a dose de-escalation to 2 × 2 Gy. This concept too was compared prospectively in a randomized study in diverse localizations with 12 × 2 Gy.[33] However, significantly lower rates of complete remission (44% at 2 × 2 Gy; 60% at 12 × 2 Gy) were reported and a lower local progression-free survival.

In contrast to the experiences with indolent lymphomas of other localizations, a retrospective series has been published with outstanding results after low-dose radiotherapy in the area of the orbit. This can be attributed to the generally lower tumor burden in the orbit area and its earlier diagnosis with visible or early clinical symptomatic disease in contrast to lymphoma occurring in other locations. Fasola et al report on 20 patients with 27 lymphomas manifesting in the area of the orbit adnexa, which were irradiated with 2 × 2 Gy.[34] After a median follow-up of over 2 years, a complete remission was seen in 85% of the lymphomas treated, a partial remission in 11%. Only one patient experienced an intraorbital recurrence outside the radiotherapy fields. No acute side effects were reported by 80% of the patients; in 20% there were mild, self-limiting toxicities such as periorbital edema, dry eyes, or conjunctivitis. Chronic toxicities did not occur. Although these are retrospective data on a patient group with only 2 years of follow-up monitoring, in several respects these results are normative for radiotherapy of indolent lymphomas of the orbit, as they enable a very gentle treatment option:

1. Higher doses of radiation are associated with higher risks for acute and chronic toxicities; thus over 50% reported acute complications with doses between 19 and 48 Gy[35]; for details see Chapter 14.5. Even with a local progression after 2 × 2 Gy of previous exposure, re-irradiation is possible with few complications.
2. Additionally, the target volume definition has been disputed: after selective radiotherapy of the afflicted orbit region, in up to 30% of the patients a recurrence was reported outside the radiation volume, so that initial irradiation of the whole orbit has been considered.[36] Fractionation of 2 × 2 Gy enables partial orbit irradiation since if there is recurrence there can be unproblematic re-irradiation even with fields that overlap previously irradiated structures. On the other hand, a complete orbit irradiation can also be carried out on a primary fractionation schedule with 2 × 2 Gy with minimal toxicity.
3. Partial orbit irradiation with low-dose radiation does, however, require close follow-up. In so doing, the contralateral orbit is also to be examined as even in this area recurrences have occasionally been described.[34]

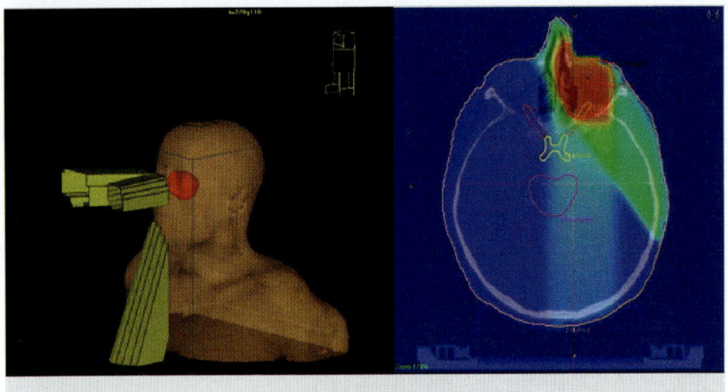

Fig. 14.9 Dose distribution of an irradiation for a low-malignant orbital lymphoma, left. Through the use of three different beam angles, in which one enters cranially via the skull calotte, very good coverage of the target volume is achieved with a sharp dose decay into the surrounding, unaffected structures. The intended dose can be identified as a reddish-brown colors in the transversal section (*right*) and low radiation doses as green/blue colors.

> **Memorize**
>
> Low-malignant MALT lymphomas of the orbit are curable by EBRT with low doses of radiation (2 × 2 Gy or 12 × 2 Gy). It has not been established whether the whole of the afflicted parts of the orbit have to be treated. With the extremely low radiation doses, treatment of only the afflicted part can be strongly justified.

Technique

The patient is placed in an individually prepared thermoplastic mask. The GTV (gross tumor volume) is determined by the clinical considerations and the imagery. The CTV embraces either the GTV including the afflicted ocular structure (lacrimal gland or conjunctiva), or else the whole orbit (see discussion above). In principle, tumors lying on the surface should be treated with electrons using bolus material (silicone cushion) in order to guarantee an optimal dose build up effect. Volumes lying deeper (e.g., lacrimal gland) are treated with photons after 3D planning (▶ Fig. 14.9).

Whenever appropriate and possible, the lens should be protected with a calotte (see Chapter 14.3.1).

14.3.3 Uveal Melanomas

The treatment of uveal melanomas has changed fundamentally since the 1980s. Whereas enucleation previously represented the mainstay of treatment, since then—whenever technically possible and desired by the patient—the focus has been on procedures that preserve the eye.

Radiotherapy can control uveal melanomas oncologically and at the same time preserve the sight as well as the eyeball.[2] However, the radiation doses required are above the tolerance doses of the retina, the optic nerve, lenses, eyelids, and lacrimal gland. For this reason, correspondingly adjusted techniques or radiation planning are necessary. The necessary dose distributions can be achieved via episcleral brachytherapy, irradiation with protons/heavy ions, or via radiosurgical techniques. Internationally, brachytherapy is the most frequently used.

Value of Radiotherapy: COMS Studies

The value of radiotherapy was investigated to derive guidance from long-term, prospective, randomized studies by the COMS group.[37] This data is very significant because uveal melanoma is a rare disease[38] with an estimated 1,400 new cases reported per year in the United States. In 1986 three multicenter prospective studies were started at the initiative of the National Eye Institute, into which ~2,500 patients with unilateral choroidal melanomas were recruited.

The melanomas were divided into three categories[39]:

- Small melanomas: 1.5 to 2.4 mm tumor height, diameter 5 to 16 mm.
- Medium-sized melanomas: 2.5 to 10 mm tumor height, diameter ≤ 16 mm (since November, 1990).
- Large melanomas: > 10 mm tumor height, diameter > 16 mm.

Small Melanomas

Patients with small tumors on the criteria above were offered the chance of being included in a prospective monitoring study. With these patients there was the risk of a misdiagnosis by confusion with a benign nevus, so the closely monitored growth process would ultimately provide information about the nature of the tumor. Initially 188 tumors were monitored, of which ~10%, 20%, or 30% were progressing after 1, 2, or 5 years.[40] Although most patients were not treated, only 1% of the patients had died from melanoma within 5 years.

Conclusion

Small uveal melanomas with tumor heights under 2.4 mm and diameters less than 16 mm can often be differentiated from benign nevi only through the long-term growth process. Within 5 years only 30% exhibit progression.

Medium-sized Melanomas

Patients with medium-sized melanomas on the criteria above (no localization peripapillarly or in the ciliary body, cM0) were randomized between episcleral brachytherapy with an iodine 125 applicator or primary enucleation. Over a 12-year period a total of 1,317 patients were treated.[41] The 5-year survival rates did not differ significantly, being 81% after enucleation and 82% after brachytherapy, nor did the tumor-specific survival rates. Long-term data with 10- and 12-year survival rates exhibited no significant differences.[42] Almost half of the patients in the study were still alive after 12 years free of disease. Negative prognostic factors were tumor diameter > 11 mm and age > 60 years.

The organ-preserving procedure exhibited good oncological effectiveness. In the first 5 years after brachytherapy only ~12.5% of the patients underwent enucleation: 10% for tumor progression (mainly in the first 3 years of primary treatment), 2.5% due to other causes (pain, loss of sight).[43] In 2% of the patients, although a recurrence was documented, enucleation was not done. A recurrence was defined here as an increase in the height of the tumor by 15% in ultrasound or growth of 250 µm in photographs in two consecutive examinations. Age > 50 years, tumor height > 5 mm, and tumor growth up to the fovea were correlated with the frequency of recurrence.

The mortality of patients after a secondary enucleation might be increased (risk ratio 1.5). After adjustment for other risk factors, however, this finding just failed statistical significance at $p = 0.08$ and did not affect the survival rates of the whole group (see above). For this reason, brachytherapy can be regarded as a safe alternative in this patient group.

With regard to radiogenic side effects, 532 patients without cataracts before brachytherapy were monitored in follow-up examinations.[44] The first cataract developed a median 2.5 years after primary therapy; the first operation became necessary after a median 3.5 years (with no defined criteria preset for the indication for the operation). After 5 years cataracts had developed in 83% of the affected eyes, but only 12% had to be operated on because of this. After a lens dose of ≥ 24 Gy, 18% of the patients were operated on; after < 12 Gy this was only 4%. Sight improved in most patients after cataract operations or stabilized. Cataract surgery was effective despite the tumor treatment.

Functional limitation in the sense of a substantial loss of sight after brachytherapy was experienced by only 17% of patients after 1 year, by 33% after 2 years, and by > 40% after 3 years.[45] The risk was associated with diabetes mellitus, tumor height [≤ 5 mm vs. > 5–7.5 vs. > 7.6], distance between tumor and macula, and tumor-associated detachment of the retina (in particular when the macula was involved). The tumor height was directly correlated with the radiation dose required; likewise, the proximity of the tumor to critical structures also determined the dose applied there. Surprisingly, however, they all the patients lost visual acuity, even those with good sight before therapy: approximately 2 lines per year after treatment, to a greater extent in patients with risk factors.[45]

The implications of these findings for the quality of life have been examined in an accompanying study on 209 patients at 6 months and then annually after the treatment.[46] Both after brachytherapy and also after enucleation, a significant rise in difficulties was experienced in activities that require visual guidance. The differences in visual function (night-time driving, peripheral vision) between the treatment groups were significantly in favor of brachytherapy, at least during the first 2 years, even if to only a limited extent. After 3 to 5 years, however, the differences leveled out. At the same time, anxious patients suffered more from anxiety symptoms after brachytherapy than did anxious patients after enucleation.

Overall it was demonstrated that enucleation and iodine 125 brachytherapy are equally effective in melanomas with medium-sized tumors regarding survival and tumor control. Although the eye-preserving procedure did favor some functional parameters during the first 2 years after treatment, these differences in functionality and quality of life leveled out in the long-term. In this respect treatment can be selected according to the personal preferences of the individual patient.

M!

Memorize

In medium-sized melanomas of tumor height < 10 mm and diameter ≤ 16 mm, episcleral brachytherapy with eye preservation and enucleation exhibit the same results oncologically. The minimal and only temporary nature of the advantage demonstrable with regard to the quality of life after eye-preserving treatment is surprising. Even in the event of a favorable localization, an evident sight loss is exhibited in the course of the follow-up care.

Brachytherapy is not indicated with extrascleral growth, a major encroachment on the ciliary body, ring melanomas, and a peripapillary localization.

After a thorough consultation on the treatment options, each patient must make a decision based on his or her own preferences; in particular, anxious patients seem to benefit more from enucleation than from brachytherapy.

Likewise, an important consideration is the sight of the contralateral eye and the individual wishes of the patient.

Primary enucleation is indicated for large tumors, which involve > 40% of the intraocular volume, for a primary blind and painful eye and for neovascular glaucomas.[47]

Large Melanomas

The third study attempted to improve the results of therapy for locally advanced uveal melanomas. In this the effectiveness of neoadjuvant hypofractionated EBRT of the afflicted orbit with 5 × 4 Gy was compared with enucleation alone. The rationale was the fear of triggering tumor cell dissemination through the enucleation and thus worsening the prognosis. Neoadjuvant irradiation preoperatively inactivates the tumor cells and tumor vessels are thrombosed. In total, 1,003 patients with a tumor of height ≥ 2 mm and diameter > 16 mm, or with a tumor height of over 10 mm, were randomized. With the neoadjuvant irradiation the rate of postoperative and late complications was not increased[48]; there were no significant differences in the 5- and 10-year survival rates between the two therapy arms (5-year survival rate 62% for EBRT + enucleation vs. 57% for enucleation).[49,50] Nor was the tumor-specific survival improved, but the prior irradiation did significantly reduce the rate of histologically confirmed local recurrences from 5 to 0.[48] Given this minimal effect, neoadjuvant irradiation prior to a planned enucleation for uveal melanomas no longer has a part to play.

M!

Memorize

Neoadjuvant EBRT before enucleation with large uveal melanomas exhibits no benefits with regard to the occurrence of metastases.

Technical Procedure in Episcleral Brachytherapy

For treatment planning purposes, the basal maximum tumor diameter and tumor height must be measured precisely using ultrasonography.[2] Additionally, a fundus diagram has to be produced showing the tumor boundaries relative to the optic nerve, the papilla, the equator, the ora serrata, and the lens. The exact distance between the edge of the tumor and the macula as well as the papilla must be known.

Iodine 125

The advantage of using iodine 125 seeds is the individually plannable dose distribution and the full coverage even of relatively high tumors up to 10 mm. However, the use of such a system

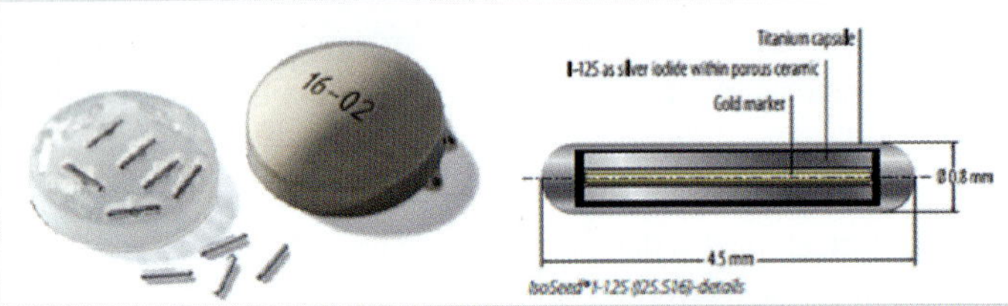

Fig. 14.10 Basic construction of an applicator with iodine 125 seeds and schematic construction of one such seed. Following the previously derived plan, the seeds are inserted in a Silastic capsule, which is then taken inserted into the applicator. With the kind permission of Eckert & Ziegler BEBIG, Berlin.

does require appropriate experience with the handling and planning as well as an expensive dosimetric measuring station in order to be able to verify the calculated dose distributions.[47] The geometric information is transferred into a computer planning system designed for this task, which enables the calculation of dose distributions.

The procedure most used with iodine 125 was published in the COMS studies mentioned above.[43] The dose was prescribed for a point 5 mm from the inner sclera with an apical height of < 5 mm. For tumor heights ≥ 5 mm the dose is prescribed to the tumor apex. A dosage of 85 Gy was administered with a dose rate between 0.42 and 1.05 Gy/h. Thus the 85 Gy isodose covered the dosing points and the whole tumor. The planning system used must meet the TG-43 recommendations[51] in regard to various effects such as back-scatter with a gold shield or anisotropy, as otherwise up to 30% less dose is actually applied than planned.[2]

As lower dose rates can be associated with less control of the tumor, a minimum of 0.6 Gy/h is recommended[2] and for this reason the hospital stay is between 3 and 7 days. The size of the applicator selected is such that the base of the tumor encompassing all pigmented areas is irradiated with an excess margin of 2 to 3 mm. Circular diameters of standard iodine 125 applicators are 12, 14, 16, 18, and 20 mm. The seeds are inserted individually into the applicator using a Silastic capsule and held there (► Fig. 14.10). Specially shaped applicators with gaps can reduce the dose exposure of the optic nerve when it is reached by the tumor or enable optimized dose distributions.

14

First of all a pre-plan is calculated. If an asymmetric seed distribution or the use of seeds with varying activity be determined here, then an exact seed distribution in preparing the applicator and, during surgery, precise orientation and placement of the applicator are essential. After receipt of the seeds ordered according to the calculated plan, a definitive plan is produced based on the actual activity measured, and the applicator is then loaded. The inside is covered with a concave spacer (e.g., contact lens) and then the applicator is ideally sterilized with gas.

Memorize M!

In episcleral brachytherapy with iodine 125 seeds the dose distribution can be adjusted individually to the requirements of the tumor's extent and geometry by distributing the individual seeds correspondingly in the applicator casing; a corresponding planning system and a measuring station are required for this. Tumors up to an apical height of 10 mm can be sufficiently covered.

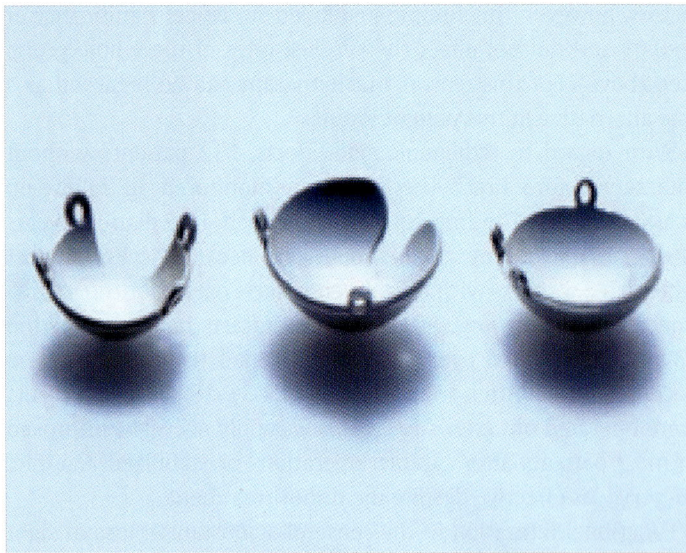

Fig. 14.11 Various forms of ruthenium 106 applicators. With the kind permission of Eckert & Ziegler BEBIG, Berlin.

Ruthenium 106

Because of its distinctly steeper dose gradients, ruthenium 106 was introduced by Lommatzsch into the treatment of uveal melanomas.[52] In contrast to the procedure described above, ruthenium 106 applicators are delivered ready-to-use in different sizes by the manufacturer (Bebig, Berlin, Germany). The three standard sizes administer doses at diameters of 13.5, 15.8, and 18 mm (CCA, CCD, CCB) (► Fig. 14.11). Further shapes with notches to protect the optic nerve are available. The geometry of the dose distribution is essentially pre-set. Although it is desirable to make an individual plan using a planning system, it is not mandatory as the radiation exposure of the critical structures can be estimated based on the depth–dose distributions and using the geometry of the eye.

At the tip of the tumor a dose of 100 to 150 Gy is aimed at, whilst the dose at the sclera is between 700 and 1500 Gy (overview[53]). These terms of reference only apply with tumor heights of up to ~5 mm (included in the calculation is an additional 1 mm for the thickness of the sclera) so that this form of treatment is only indicated for small to medium-sized melanomas.

Memorize M!

In episcleral brachytherapy with ruthenium 106, prefabricated applicators are used with known dose distributions. Tumors with an apical height of 5 mm (+ 1 mm sclera) can be treated with this procedure because of the sharp decay of the dose. At the tip of the tumor the aim is for between 100 and 150 Gy.

Administration and Radiation Protection

With the patient under a general anesthetic the applicator is placed in position by the ophthalmologist. With transillumination the boundaries of the anterior localized tumors on the sclera/cornea are marked with dye; with posteriorly located tumors a point light source or ultrasound is used. Overlying eye muscles have to be removed if necessary. Dummy applicators are used so that the seam can be positioned accurately before the radiating applicator is used.

The soft photon radiation of the iodine 125 applicators can be blocked by lead aprons without any problem in the operating room. However, when the applicators are being loaded with the seeds they do have to be handled manually.

From the radiation protection aspect, the high-energy beta radiation of ruthenium 106 is more problematic. Although this radiation has a short range in water, in the air it can penetrate up to 15 m. When the particles collides with dense materials (e.g., metal), bremsstrahlung results for which the lead aprons can be insufficient. For this reason the applicators should be stored for as long as possible behind layers of silicone, which absorbs the electrons. During the operation the surgeon's hand is exposed to ~2 to 6 mSv.[54]

During the time the radiation sources are in place, patients in Germany are treated as in-patients for reasons of radiation protection, while internationally some are treated as outpatients.

The removal of the applicator can often be conducted under local anesthetic. The exact time of the removal is documented, the dose actually delivered checked, and if necessary recalculated (if in place for longer than planned, e.g., because of shortage of operating room capacity). In this procedure one must guarantee that all iodine seeds are removed and none are unintentionally left behind in the patient or in the operating room.

Combination of Brachytherapy with Transpupillary Thermotherapy

Because of the restrictions on brachytherapy with ruthenium 106 described in Chapter 14.2.1. and Chapter 14.3.3, underdosing can occur in the apex area of melanomas with an apical height > 5 mm. These areas or remnants of tumors, which can remain clinically after brachytherapy, can be destroyed by heating selectively to 45 to 65°C with an infrared laser of wavelength 810 nm (transpupillary thermotherapy, TTT).

The problem-free combination of both therapy modalities was demonstrated in a large series of 425 consecutive patients with tumors of a medial apex height of 4.2 mm.[55] After ruthenium 106 irradiation with apex doses of < 100 Gy at 23% and > 200 Gy at 26%, nearly 90% of the patients were treated with TTT 2 months after radiation, and—where necessary—again after 6 months. As well as an excellent local control rate, no specific TTT complications were reported.

The retrospective comparison of two patient groups, of which 70 patients were treated only with ruthenium 106 and 63 were treated with ruthenium 106 + TTT, suggests a higher local control and eyeball preservation after combination therapy, but without raising the complication rate.[56]

Radiation with Protons/Helium Ions

Radiotherapy with protons lends itself to uveal melanomas due to the physical characteristics of the depth–dose distribution. Experience has been collected on this therapy for some 30 years.

A disadvantage is the high cost, not only of the construction of the cyclotrons but also of the preparation of the patients. Intraoperatively, the tumor boundaries have to be marked with tantalum clips sewn onto the sclera. For irradiation purposes it is sufficient to immobilize the patient with the normal means. A dose of 50 to 70 CGE (cobalt Gray equivalent) is applied in 4 to 5 fractions.

In a randomized study a dose de-escalation of 70 CGE to 50 CGE in 5 fractions (applied over 7 days) was tested.[57] Patients ($n = 188$) with a tumor height of < 5 mm and localization in the proximity of the papilla or the macula were randomized. The oncological effectiveness was not restricted by the dose reduction, however, nor was the sight improved (5 years post therapy ~55% at least 20/200). The field of vision was only significantly better after 50 CGE. From this a dose of 50 CGE can be justified in this situation.

The therapy series published so far suggest a very good local tumor control. Despite high patient numbers these are, nevertheless, the experiences of individual institutions with differing inclusion criteria and ways of representing results. So far there is only one randomized study that compares irradiation with helium ions and conventional brachytherapy.[58] In this, 86 patients were treated with helium ions (70 CGE) and 98 with iodine 125 brachytherapy. The tumors measured < 10 mm in apical height and < 15 mm in maximum diameter. After brachytherapy, significantly more local recurrences were reported with consequent enucleations. However, there were more neovascular glaucomas after helium ion irradiation. There was no difference in overall survival between the two groups.

The disadvantages of proton radiation have to be considered: Despite the good dose distribution the beams do hit the anterior eye. This region, which is generally protected in brachytherapy, is exposed to radiation—only a little but nevertheless biologically active. Thus, keratites, loss of eyelashes, cataracts, and sicca syndrome can be observed.[58] One problem in particular is the occurrence of neovascular glaucomas in up to 35% of the patients in individual series.[1] Almost 30% of patients whose tumors were not situated in the proximity of the papilla or macula experience a distinct loss of sight within 2 years of radiation; after 10 years 65% of the patients have become blind.[59]

In this respect proton radiation has so far not been proven with sufficient evidence. Furthermore, the indication for it is still completely unclear. A review accordingly concludes that "currently, there is too little evidence to make informed decisions on which treatment should be preferred"[60]. Theoretically, proton radiation can provide benefits in tumors close to the macula or the papilla or in the area of the ciliary body and the iris. However, this will only be accepted if the tumors are not accessible to brachytherapy.

M!

Memorize

In principle, proton radiotherapy with 50 CGE can be used with good local control rates. A problem is the high rate of neovascular glaucomas in some therapy series (~30%) with this procedure and the evident sight loss even with favorably localized tumors. Due to the lack of randomized studies, the importance of this type of radiation cannot be defined with certainty at the current time.

Hypofractionated Stereotactic Photon Radiotherapy

Photons of 6 MV energy can provide a therapeutic alternative for posteriorly localized melanomas. A mandatory requirement, however, is either immobilization of the eye or online-tracking of the eye position in order to avoid fatally misdirected irradiation.

In the largest series to date, 212 patients were treated who, with a tumor height of > 7 mm or with a juxtapapillary or juxtamacular tumor position, were not suitable for a ruthenium 106 brachytherapy.[61] The tumor volume delineated in the MRT was expanded with 2 mm safety margins; this volume should be covered by 80% isodose. For this, 10 to 12 microcollimated radiation directions were used; 24 patients were irradiated with 5 × 14 Gy, 158 with 5 × 12 Gy, and 30 with5 × 10 Gy within 7 days.

The 5-year total survival was 85%; local tumor control was 96% after 5 years (definition of recurrence: 2 × 25% size increase) and 93% after 10 years. After 5 years 18% of the eyes that had received radiation were enucleated, above all due to neovascular glaucoma, and more rarely due to recurrence. The sight deteriorated clearly: prior to therapy 83% had sight of > 0.1, after 1.5 years 43% still had, after 3 years 20%, and after 5 years only 9%. One must, though, consider the unfavorable tumor position in the proximity of critical structures as a selection criterion for this therapy. Within the first 5 years, 33% of the patients did not develop retinopathies, 39% had no optic nerve neuropathies, and 75% no glaucomas.[62] Tumor control was not dependent on the overall dose, but the sight deteriorated at 10 Gy and 12 Gy single dose significantly more slower than with 14 Gy.

In this respect the results are similar to those of the therapy series with proton irradiation. However, with the latter, tumor localization on the iris and the ciliary body can be covered; this is mostly not possible with stereotactic photon irradiation.

When comparing treatment results between stereotactic photon irradiation, proton irradiation, and brachytherapy with ruthenium 106, distinctly different regression dynamics have to be differentiated: After radiation with ruthenium, melanomas very quickly reduce in size, with often only a scar remaining. In contrast with this, the reduction of tumors after stereotaxy and proton irradiation is clearly slower, and often wave-shaped as well.[61,63]

Memorize M!

Stereotactic photon irradiation with high single doses is possible. As there have so far not been any randomized studies, the importance of this therapy has not been defined.

Adjuvant EBRT for Extrascleral Tumor Spread

When the melanoma invades over the eye into the bordering soft tissue, adjuvant EBRT of the orbit with up to 60 Gy is recommended after enucleation as prophylaxis against recurrence, in particular after R1-resection.[2] This recommendation is based above all on fundamental considerations and on an older therapy series, but not on randomized data. After enucleation, 17 patients received further irradiation of the orbit with a median dose of up to 50 Gy (35–60 Gy) in 22 fractions.[1,3,6,10,15,18,19,20,23,30,34,38,41,57,58,61,62,63,64,65,66,67,68,69,70,71,72,73] In the further course there was an orbital recurrence in only one patient after 60 Gy of normofractionated radiation. Despite the high risk of developing systemic metastases, achieving local control in the orbit does seem to influence the prognosis favorably: in an historical group the 5-year survival rate of patients with extrascleral growth without adjuvant radiotherapy was reduced from 34 to 11% by the appearance of local recurrence.[74]

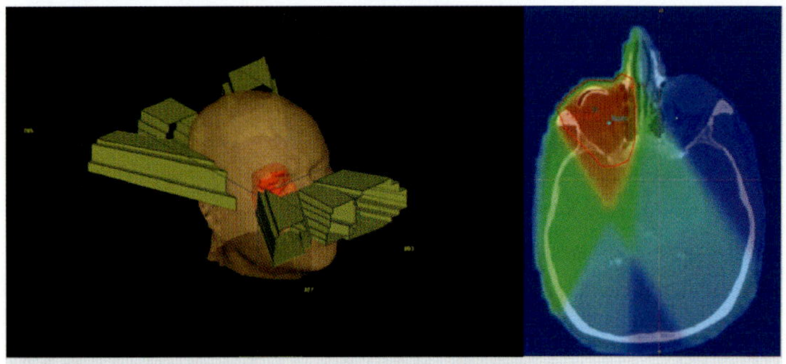

Fig. 14.12 Adjuvant radiation of a T4 melanoma after enucleation of the right eyeball. By selecting three different gantry angles for the radiation, a homogeneous coverage of the entire affected orbit is achieved, with the osseous boundaries included within the target volume. Surrounding structures can be sufficiently protected.

After an orbital exenteration, adjuvant radiotherapy only makes sense after a R1/R2-resection (▸ Fig. 14.12).[75]

14.3.4 Retinoblastoma

It is estimated that about 750 children a year in the US develop retinoblastoma. The tumor genesis is very well known and is attributed to the hereditary or acquired loss of the tumor suppressor gene *RB1*.[76] In 40% a bilateral, multiple tumor growth (in hereditary form) is found. The children concerned are very young when the disease develops; the median age is approximately 12 months.

Tumors develop in the retina and tend to grow into the optic nerve. Dissemination in CSF can take place via the chiasma. Hematogenous metastases are also possible (although rare).[76]

Therapy is based on the extent of the disease. The indications for enucleation, for laser therapy, and for cryotherapy and TTT are discussed in Chapter 13.

By bringing chemotherapy forward, tumors are first of all put into remission ("chemoreduction") to make them better accessible for the focal therapy. In current protocols, vincristine, etoposide, carboplatin, and cyclophosphamide are used for this.[77] Selective administration paths (intravitreal, periocular, or the administration of superselective melphalan into the ophthalmic artery) are distinctly less toxic and mutagenic.[77]

Ionizing radiation provides important therapy options, but does require a high degree of specialized expertise. Due to the high risk of radiogenically induced tumors (in particular of osteosarcomas) in these patients, who are particularly susceptible, the volume exposed should be kept to the minimum possible. Furthermore, the known maximum tolerance doses for orbital structures and also the growing midfacial bones represent a problem as, when there is a unilateral premature termination to growth, massive asymmetries arise in the middle of the face. For this reason one must take care to ensure a symmetrical dose distribution in both halves of the middle of the face. Due to these special requirements, radiotherapy of these patients should only be undertaken in centers with special expertise.

With localized, unifocal, or oligofocal tumors without involvement of the vitreous humor and with an apical tumor height between 2 and 4 mm, episcleral brachytherapy with ruthenium 106 is ideal.[77] However, this therapy is not suitable for tumors that are situated close to the papilla or macula because of the unavoidable destruction of the retina in the area being treated.

EBRT offers the possibility of preserving the organ and the chance of cure with bilateral, multifocal tumors, or with locally advanced growth with vitreous humor involvement, or with localization on the posterior pole of the eyeball.[76] The technique used today was described for the first time by Schipper.[78] Children are treated under anesthetic, the lenses fixed with vacuum lenses. The radiation takes place via highly collimated opposing temporal fields. In order to avoid beam divergence, the anterior field boundary is the central beam. An add-on collimator is placed as close as possible to the eye in order to minimize the "half shadow," the region of dose build-up in the area of the field boundary. Avoidance of underdosing in the anterior area of the eye is decisive with regard to recurrence.[76]

Normofractionated doses with a total dose of 50 Gy are administered. Under this treatment the occurrence of radiogenic side effects and complications such as cataract development and retinopathy is relatively rare. The main side effect is the disruption to mid-facial development, the other main risk in radiotherapy on children with hereditary retinoblastomas is the induction of a second tumor, ~23% within 25 years (in contrast with 6% for non-hereditary retinoblastoma).[79]

Other radiotherapy techniques, such as stereotactic treatment, can indeed apply precise, high doses in a small area but, in so doing, expose large volumes to low doses and the correspondingly high mutagenic risks. The use of an IMRT (intensity-modulated radiotherapy) technique for a unilateral tumor is the subject of controversy as the radiation dose in the bony orbit is supposed to be easy to calculate.[80] However, prospective proof of clinical benefits vis-à-vis the classic procedure described above is lacking.

Proton irradiation can offer theoretical advantages, but in Germany has been reserved until now for isolated cases only.[76] In a retrospective series from Boston, MA, however, significantly fewer secondary tumors developed in the proton-irradiated field in a comparison between 55 patients treated with protons and 31 irradiated with photons (0 vs. 14%), though this was with varying median follow-up monitoring periods (7 vs. 13 years), with younger patients in the photon group, and with a photon irradiation technique that exposes distinctly more volume than the "Schipper technique" described above.[81]

Memorize M!

Retinoblastomas can be destroyed with ionizing radiation. The young ages of the patients and their particular susceptibility to radiogenic tumor induction are problematic. For this reason the volumes exposed to radiation are to be kept as low as possible. For unilateral, small tumors still restricted in growth, brachytherapy with ruthenium 106 is ideally suited. For bilateral and multifocal tumors, or with locally advanced growth with involvement of the vitreous body or with localization at the posterior pole of the eye, EBRT can offer a cure while preserving the eyeball and the sight. With the assistance of a highly collimated, laterally opposing technique ("Schipper technique") an equal exposure of the midfacial bones can be guaranteed with sharp dose gradients ventrally and dorsally.

The treatment of these tumors is reserved for specialist centers.

14.4 Radiotherapy of Benign Diseases of the Orbit

14.4.1 Optic Nerve Meningiomas

Approximately 1 to 2% of all meningiomas arise in the nerve sheath of the optic nerve. Progressive loss of sight can occur through local growth with consecutive compression of the nerve fibers or of the blood vessels supplying the nerve. Displacement can cause proptosis, pain, or motility disturbances.[82] Furthermore, other neurological disturbances can be triggered by growth per continuitatem into the brain.

Due to the localization, operative therapies can be associated with a high rate of blinding. This underpins the importance of conservative therapies, in particular that of radiotherapy. As the optic nerve reacts relatively sensitively to high single doses (see Chapter 14.5.8), conventionally fractionated EBRT with 28 to 31 × 1.8 Gy is recommended.

As a result, the sight can be preserved in over 90% of patients, as has been demonstrated in various therapy series.[83,84] Regression of the tumor occurs—if at all—only very slowly, while the sight can improve distinctly after treatment.[82]

Here it makes sense to use highly conformal stereotactic treatment techniques in order to minimize the exposure of other ocular structures and thus to improve the functional long-term results. The tumor can be delineated by the MRI and is expanded for planning purposes with safety margins of 5 mm, which are to be covered by 95% of the dose prescribed (► Fig. 14.13).

Memorize M!

With optic nerve meningiomas, normofractionated EBRT causes the growth to be inhibited. Through this the sight is preserved in 90% of those afflicted.

14.4.2 Idiopathic Inflammation of the Orbit

The historic term "pseudotumor orbitae" covered a whole range of diverse diseases; it should no longer be used because of its lack

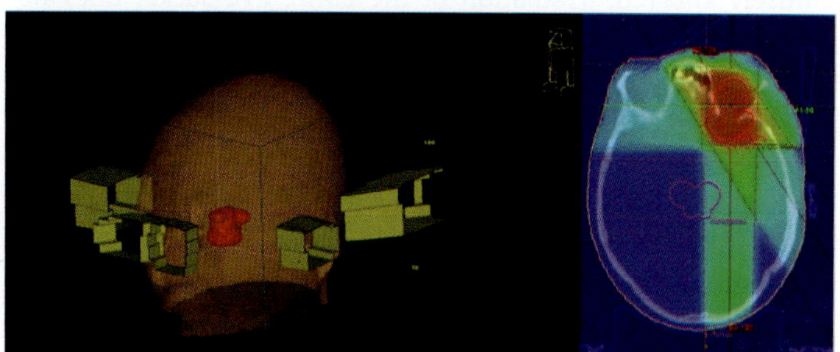

Fig. 14.13 Dose distribution of an irradiation with extensive left-side optic nerve sheath meningioma. By selecting different beam angles, a homogeneous coverage of the target volume is achieved and surrounding structures, such as the contralateral eye, can be amply protected. The high-dose areas can be identified as reddish-brownish colors in the transversal section (*right*) and low radiation doses as green/blue colors.

of rigor and because of the development of standard histopathological classifications in the meantime.[85] Instead, all acute or chronic inflammation of orbital structures without identifiable local or systemic cause is classified as "idiopathic inflammation of the orbit"[86]. The most frequent manifestation is the swelling of the lacrimal gland, followed by the eye musculature, and the orbital fat. It is a matter of debate whether the diagnosis has to be corroborated by the histopathological demonstration of benign lymphoplasmacytic infiltrates and sclerosis and the exclusion of other etiologies.[87]

Oral corticosteroids form the backbone of the treatment due to their immunosuppressive and anti-inflammatory action with response rates of between 30 and 80%.[88]

For patients, who do not respond sufficiently well to this treatment, who suffer relapses after dose reduction or tapering, or for whom steroids are contraindicated, EBRT offers an effective treatment option.

In a therapy series with 20 patients (26 irradiated orbits), the alleviation of symptoms was achieved in 85% after 27 Gy (25.2–30.6 Gy); in 45% of patients it was possible to completely taper off cortisone.[89] In another series, similar therapy results were demonstrated in 16 patients after a dose of 20 Gy (14–30 Gy) with symptom alleviation in over 80% and over 50% of patients no longer requiring cortisone treatment.[90] Interestingly, the patients with bilateral disease responded to the radiation significantly better in both therapy series than did patients with unilateral disease, so that a distinct, apparently more radiation-sensitive entity is postulated in these patients.[89]

The optimally effective radiation dose has not yet been found. Because of the inflammatory cause of the disease, low immunomodulatory radiation doses would also have to demonstrate effectiveness. In a retrospective series with 22 patients, no difference was found in the treatment results after 20 Gy vs. 40 Gy.[91] An older patient series reports response with as little as 16 Gy.[92] So far, however, there are still no therapy studies that have examined the lower doses or alternative fractionating schedules with 10 or 20 × 1 Gy weekly, such as in endocrine orbitopathy (see Chapter 7.4.2).

The tumor volume (GTV) to be delineated in the imagery is to be treated here as the target volume, with ample safety margins for the subclinical invasion of surrounding structures, mobility, and accuracy of reproducibility. As long as the orbit has not been diffusely affected, irradiation of the entire eye socket does not appear to be necessary.[93] For superficially situated processes, there are electron treatments that include lens shielding; for processes lying deeper in the orbit there are 3D conformal or IMRT planned photon irradiation.

> **Memorize**
>
> With idiopathic inflammation of the orbit, EBRT with ~20 Gy can effect a remission in the majority of patients if the steroid treatment is not successful or is contraindicated.

14.4.3 Choroidal Hemangiomas

Arising from the blood vessels of the choroid, hemangiomas develop as slowly growing vascular tumors. Differentiation is made between the diffuse growth type, which appears in childhood (in half of the patients with an encephalofacial angiomatosis [Sturge–Weber syndrome]), and a solitary, local growth, which manifests between the 30th and 50th years of life. The position and size determine the symptoms because the overlying retina can be damaged by the underlying vascular growth (loss of photoreceptors, cystic degeneration, gliosis).[94] Mostly a reduction of visual acuity occurs through exudative retinal detachments, cystic macula edemas, subretinal fibroses, or, rarely, neovascular glaucomas.

The aim of treatment is the reabsorption of subretinal fluid accumulations and of a macula edema to preserve or improve visual acuity.[94] The treatment strategy is based on symptoms and localization and size of the tumor. Asymptomatic hemangiomas are monitored, treatment is not necessary.[94]

The results with regard to long-term preservation of sight are most favorable for an extrafoveal tumor location, limited for a parafoveal location, and poorest for a subfoveal location.[95]

Symptomatic defined hemangiomas with exudative retinal detachment have for the most part been treated with laser photocoagulation. In this, subretinal fluid accumulations are resorbed, but later recurrences are frequent.[94] Repeat treatment can then lead to the loss of visual fields.[71] For this reason, after a maximum of two failed laser treatments an alternative treatment option should be chosen.

Transpupillary thermotherapy stimulates the resorption of subretinal fluid, but can lead to secondary changes to the photoreceptors, so it should not be used for subfoveal tumors.[94]

The advantage of photodynamic treatment (PDT) vis-à-vis the above-mentioned therapeutic modalities resides in its selective effect on vascular endothelial cells, so that it is also suitable for subfoveal tumors. In a prospective study on 31 patients with circumscribed hemangiomas, Boixadera et al show good effectiveness of PDT with verteporfin 6 mg/m^2 and 689-nm laser light, with administration of 50 J/cm^2.[64] Only one application was required in 80% of patients; in 14% two treatments at an interval of 3 months. Under the treatment, visual acuity increased significantly, and macula edemas and retinal detachments reduced in size. The diameters of the hemangiomas halves during treatment.

Radiotherapy

When there has been unsatisfactory response to previous therapies or with subfoveal localization or with extensive subretinal collection of fluid, radiotherapy provides therapeutic alternatives. With this treatment vascular proliferations can be stopped, blood vessels thrombosed, and tumors brought into partial remission at least. Subretinal fluid is resorbed, the risk of retinal detachments is reduced, and often the sight improves again. Different forms of radiotherapy are possible as discussed below.

Episcleral Brachytherapy

Various isotopes have been used with good results. The largest patient group was treated with cobalt 60 applicators (dose in the apex 40–60 Gy),[96] but other isotopes have been used as well (ruthenium 106, iodine 125, palladium 103) (though with distinctly smaller patient numbers). All tumors were brought into regression, the subretinal fluid was resorbed, and sight was preserved or improved in the majority of patients (overview[97]). Currently a dose of 20 Gy at the apex is regarded as sufficient.[97]

The general disadvantage of episceral brachytherapy is the necessity of two operative interventions—for the application and for the removal of the isotopes. As a further restriction, it has been considered up until now that this form of therapy could only be administered on circumscribed hemangiomas. With ones that are growing diffusely, the tumor is often so spread out that it cannot be completely covered by the applicators. However, this restriction is at present being questioned it as a result of a case series of 5 patients.[98] In this series, iodine 125 applicators were only placed on the largest tumor diameters and 35 Gy was dosed at the apex. There was no requirement for complete tumor coverage. Nevertheless, the tumor reduced in all patients and only in one patient did the sight deteriorate. Therapy-associated complications were not recorded.

Proton Irradiation

Zografos et al reported therapy results in 53 patients (54 eyes), in 48 of which tumor grew in a circumscribed manner.[99] The tumor height of the circumscribed hemangiomas was 3.3 mm on average and the maximum diameter was 9.5 mm on average. For localization of the tumors tantalum clips were sewn onto the sclera. Doses between 4 × 4.1 Gy (16.4 Gy) and 4 × 6.8 Gy (27.2 Gy) were applied on consecutive days. Although the tumors reduced down to scar level, all patients after 27.2 Gy ($n = 4$) went on to develop neuropathies of the optic nerve with consecutive losses of visual acuity. With the low doses of radiation, these changes did not occur. It was therefore concluded that a total dose between 16.4 Gy and 18.2 Gy proton radiation is safe and effective in this context.

Another case series with 17 patients confirms the safety of low total doses when protons are used.[70] Here 4 × 5 CGE were applied without it leading to complications considered worth reporting.

Only one study examined case series that were treated either with conventional photon irradiation ($n = 19$, between 16 and 30 Gy) or with proton irradiation ($n = 25$, mostly 20 CGE).[100] The groups were unequally divided with reference to tumor height and follow-up. More retinopathies seem to have appeared after proton irradiation, where they were self-limiting in half of the patients. In one patient a severe neuritis occurred after proton irradiation. Hardly any advantage was demonstrated for proton treatment in terms of the functional results.

Given the current state of knowledge, no general recommendation for proton treatment can be made from methodological considerations as so far no benefits have been demonstrated over other radiotherapies. Benefits for the treatment of children with Sturge–Weber syndrome are at any rate plausible due to the more precise dose application.[101]

EBRT

For **diffuse hemangiomas** with extensive retinal detachment, EBRT represents an effective therapy option. In 15 patients an improvement in sight after 10 × 2 Gy was demonstrated in ~45% with a follow-up period of 5 years.[102] The patients who did not benefit had clinically non-controllable secondary glaucomas in the foreground. A highly conformal technique was used with vacuum-affixed eye lenses, which are used elsewhere for the treatment of patients with retinoblastoma (see Chapter 14.3.4).

Normofractionated irradiation with 10 × 2 Gy is also effective in **circumscribed hemangiomas**. In 36 patients thus treated, after 5 years there was a reattachment of the retina in over 60%; sight was improved in 40%, stable in 40%, and had deteriorated in 20%.[102] Similar results were also reported in another series with 8 patients after 20–24 Gy, and in fact in this group there was improvement in the sight of all patients.[103]

Technically a dorsally angled lateral treatment field can be used with photons. Due to the angling, the lens of the opposite side is not radiogenically exposed. By placing the central beam plane directly behind the lenses, beam divergence into the ipsilateral lens can be avoided. With cooperative patients who can look straight ahead without moving during planning and therapy, there is no need to immobilize the eye during the radiotherapy. As an aid, a point light source can be placed in a corresponding position over the radiation mask.

Stereotactic radiation with high single doses has also been reported in small case series. The "gamma knife" was used among other tools. In 7 patients the tumor for the single irradiation was covered by the 10 Gy isodose (or at least the most prominent part of the tumor).[104] The results on tumor reduction and sight improvement were indeed very promising, but there is a lack of prospective studies which would define the importance of this therapy option in comparison with other treatment possibilities. However, the planning and administration of the radiation dose are relatively time consuming, involving temporary paralysis of the eye musculature and immobilization in a stereotactic treatment context.

The treatment of **young children with Sturge–Weber syndrome** and diffuse hemangiomas, often with almost complete retinal detachment, is problematic. The treatment of choice for these children is proton treatment in specialized centers, as in this way the radiogenic exposure of the surrounding tissue, in particular of the still-growing orbital bone structures, can be kept as low as possible. Currently, a fractionation of 10 × 2 CGE instead of the conventional 4 × 3.75 CGE is recommended.[101] Alternatively, as mentioned above, episcleral brachytherapy can also be also considered despite the diffuse growth.[98]

> **Memorize** (M!)
>
> For localized hemangiomas after unsatisfactory response to photodynamic treatment or with a critical localization, radiotherapy is promising for tumor regression and resorption of subretinal fluid. With localized tumors good results are reported after episcleral brachytherapy (20 Gy at the apex) or after EBRT with 10 × 2 Gy. Diffuse hemangiomas are a domain of EBRT. Alternatively, children can be also treated in a center for proton radiation.

14.4.4 Pterygium

Treatment is indicated only if the sight is threatened with growth in the direction of the pupil or for reasons of subjective cosmetic impairment. The treatment of choice is surgical resection, for which various procedures are used, but up to 70% of patients can experience recurrence after the operation.

The probability of regression is distinctly reduced by postoperative contact irradiation. Strontium 90 applicators with a diameter of 1 cm (±0.2 cm), which due to the low energy beta radiation have a therapeutic range of only 1 mm and thus protect the orbital structures, have proved effective.

In a prospective, randomized, double-blind study the effectiveness of 1 × 25 Gy within 24 hours postoperatively was demonstrated.[105] Of 42 eyes with placebo radiation during a median follow-up monitoring of 18 months, 67% developed a recurrence after a primary resection in contrast to 7% of 44 eyes after radiation. Severe side effects were not observed.

In retrospective series of several thousand patients the effectiveness of various fractionation schemes (1 × 22 [-30] Gy, 2 × 10 Gy, 3 × 8 [-10] Gy, 4 × 7 [-9] Gy, 6 × 5 [-10] Gy, 4 × 12 Gy, 8 × 3 Gy), in part in weekly, in part in daily fractionation] was examined. There were recurrence rates of between 2% and 20%.[106] Severe damage to the sclera was only reported after single irradiations over 20 Gy in ~5% of the patients; in this regard the hypofractionated schemes commend themselves.

In terms of the success of the treatment, there were negative prognostic factors in a large Japanese series with 1,320 lesions and 30 Gy within 48 hours postoperatively or with 35 Gy at intervals over 48 hours; patients were male, age < 40 years, treated for recurrence and irradiated within 2 hours postoperatively.[107] Acute, temporary side effects occurred in 15% of patients (conjunctivitis, pain, sight impairment, photophobia, tear production).

As an alternative to the strontium source, very soft (20 kV) X-rays can be used. Here perioperative application (preoperatively 1 × 7 Gy; postoperatively 4 × 5 Gy every second day) appears more effective with surgery for a recurrence than postoperative radiation with 4 × 5 Gy.[108]

Even primary irradiation (without surgical resection) of a pterygium can be successful, although its importance has not yet been proven prospectively.[106]

> **Memorize**
>
> Brachytherapy with strontium 90 applicators lowers the risk of recurrence after resection of a pterygium to under 20%. The treatment should be applied in several individual fractions so as to prevent damage to the sclera.

14

14.4.5 Age-Related Macular Degeneration

Within the context of age-related macular degeneration (AMD), the sight can be threatened either by atrophy of the pigment epithelium or through neovascularization of the choroid underneath the pigment epithelium (so-called exudative or "wet" AMD). Serum lipids and proteins can leak out via the new vascular formations, which leads to swelling of the retina. Bleeding can also occur. Ultimately, scarring processes start to destroy the architecture of the retina, restricting vision.[69]

These aberrant vascular sproutings consist of particularly radiation-sensitive, rapidly proliferating endothelial cells. They thus represent a promising target for radiotherapy (overview[109]).

Initial prospective experiences with EBRT of the rear third of the eye were reported by Chakravarthy et al in 19 patients who received either 5 × 2 Gy or 5 × 3 Gy.[65] After 1 year, sight was preserved or improved in 63% of the patients treated, and in 77% regression of the choroidal neovascular membrane was demonstrated. These results led to many randomized phase III studies that examined the value of EBRT. The results of 14 studies with over 1,200 evaluable patients were analyzed in summary form in a Cochrane review.[69] Thirteen of the studies used EBRT (2 × 8 Gy, 1 × 7.5 Gy, 4 × 6 Gy, 4 × 4.5 Gy, 4 × 4 Gy, 5 × 4 Gy, 4 × 2 Gy, 6 × 2 Gy, 7 × 2 Gy, 10 × 2 Gy); one used episcleral brachytherapy (12.6 Gy). In 9 studies the control groups received no treatment, in 3 studies they received a placebo irradiation, and in one study they received a very low radiation dose. The loss in sight after 1 or 2 years was reduced marginally by the radiotherapy (risk ratio 0.75 [0.55–1.03], 0.9 [0.74–1.10]); only the occurrence of a very obvious sight loss (≥ 6 lines) within 2 years was clearly statistically diminished (risk ratio 0.41 [0.18–0.94]. The total dose given had no influence on the results (≤ 14 Gy vs. > 14 Gy). On the whole the studies with placebo irradiation in the control group exhibited distinctly less effect than those with monitoring alone in these study arms. From this the authors concluded that so far there is no convincing evidence in favor of EBRT as an effective treatment for wet AMD.

Similarly, so far there is no convincing evidence for the effectiveness of episcleral brachytherapy.[110]

> **Memorize**
>
> EBRT or brachytherapy of the rear third of the eye has no significant influence on the clinical course of wet AMD.

The introduction of intravitreal injections of antibodies against VEGF (e.g., ranibizumab) represented a decisive therapeutic advance in the treatment of AMD. Through combination with ionizing radiation in various application forms it was attempted to reduce the frequency of the intraocular injections needed. In vitro and in vivo studies exhibited tumor biological synergistic effects between both forms of therapy.[111]

Promising data are available for further development of conventional EBRT. In a stand-alone system (IRay) microcollimated, highly focused radiation beams are produced with an energy of only 100 kV, which are used for stereotactic single irradiation. Three radiation beams are sent into the eye via the lower pars plana and cross each other in the macula in an area of ~0.5 cm. The application of 24 Gy lasts 5 minutes; the optic nerve is exposed to ~1.3 Gy, the lens to only 0.17 Gy.[72] These doses are classified as harmless. Because the radiation is relatively soft, the brain is effectively shielded by the cranial bone. The eye position is continually monitored during irradiation by means of a contact lens with low suction; if there is deviation from the planned position, the irradiation procedure is halted automatically.

Jackson et al examined the effectiveness of such single irradiation delivered in this way (16 Gy vs. 24 Gy vs. placebo irradiation) in combination with ranibizumab as needed in 230 patients after at least 3 injections.[112] The primary end point was the number of the ranibizumab injections required within 52 weeks. Changes in sight and the size of the neovascularizations were also assessed.

After irradiation with 16 Gy or 24 Gy, a median of 2 ranibizumab injections was significantly lower than the 3.5 after placebo irradiation. All other end points did not differ to any significant extent, with sight well preserved on the whole. There were no side effects from the radiotherapy. Thus, through the radiotherapy, it was possible to significantly reduce the requirement for ranibizumab in the first year after treatment. However, at the time of writing, it is not yet possible to assess the value of stereotactic radiotherapy over the long-term course of this combination therapy.

M!

Memorize

There is promising data on single radiotherapy of the macula with 16 Gy or 24 Gy of highly collimated 100 kV radiation (IRay) with reference to the reduction in the frequency of intravitreal injections of VEGF antibodies in wet AMD. It remains to be seen whether this system can be established in clinical routine.

Another form of application of this combination therapy is a surgical procedure, **intraocular (epimacular) brachytherapy (EMBT)**. In this, an afterloading system is used with a strontium source. In the context of a posterior vitrectomy, a 19-gauge applicator is manually placed directly over the region to be treated on the retina in the area of the macula; then the strontium 90 emitter is moved from its shielded parking position into the specially formed apex. A dose of 24 Gy is then applied within ~3 minutes. The optic nerve and lens are also effectively protected. Due to the sharp drop in dose (10% at 100 µm), precise positioning of the source during the irradiation process is essential, otherwise there is a risk of significant under- or overdosing. As the applicator is held by hand during the treatment, suboptimal dose distributions can result. In addition, the retina is exposed to more dose than the actual target, the choroid.

Dugel et al randomized 494 previously untreated patients 2:1 between 2 ranibizumab injections with subsequent EMBT followed by ranibizumab only if required, and only ranibizumab treatment (3 injections at monthly intervals; then a fixed schedule of another injection every 3 months).[66] With EMBT it was possible to preserve the sight after 2 years in only 77% of the patients; in the injections-only group in contrast the figure was 90%. Thus the EMBT failed the "not inferior" criterion. Instead, sight deteriorated after EMBT in comparison with an improvement in the injection-only group. Furthermore, complications arose in 54% of the patients after EMBT, which were mostly connected with vitrectomy (e.g., cataract formation independently of radiogenic dose exposure). Despite the possible precision of the radiotherapy applied, EMBT in this clinical situation is not sufficiently effective and is encumbered with unavoidable operative trauma.

A further prospective randomized study is currently investigating the value of EMBT in reducing the injection frequency within the context of a PRN protocol in patients previously treated (Merlot study). Results are not yet available.

M!

Memorize

Intraocular (epimacular) brachytherapy for wet AMD cannot be recommended within the current state of knowledge.

In comparison with EMBT, the conceptual advantage of percutaneous stereotactic single radiotherapy (IRay) as previously described employed in combination with VEGF antibodies appears evident from the avoidance of any surgical trauma and from the exact positioning of the radiation dose by means of robot-guided eye position tracking, with which the quality of the dose distribution is reproducible and controllable.

Due to the precise dose delivery at the Bragg peak, the use of protons seems to make sense. Although in initial series administration of 14 CGE as single radiotherapy demonstrated more effectiveness than 8 CGE, almost 50% of treatments were associated with unacceptable risks of retinopathy within 30 months. In subsequent studies it was possible to reduce the retinopathy rate to almost 10% by fractionating the dose application (2 × 12 CGE).[109]

Ultimately, the significance of proton therapy is minimal due to its sparse availability. A randomized study (PBAMD2) is recruiting at present in order to clarify its value in combination with VEGF antibody treatment.

14.5 Radiogenic Side Effects and Toxicities in the Orbit Area

Radiogenic side effects in orbit radiotherapy range from transient irritation right through to blinding. This depends on the total dose and the single dose that strike the structure being irradiated. In general, normofractionated radiotherapy (daily doses between 1.5 and 2 Gy) has to be distinguished from hypofractionated radiotherapy (higher single doses, right through to the extreme of radiosurgery [= single irradiation]).

Here a difference is maintained between acute side effects appearing during the radiotherapy series and within the first 3 months, and chronic toxicities that manifest themselves with a chronically advancing progress only months and years after the conclusion of the therapy. Of course, chronification of acute normal tissue reactions can also happen with very high doses.

In the following the side effects are listed according to organ. The breakdown of the radiogenic side effects is based on the current CTC (Common Terminology Criteria) categorization: the respective current recommendations are available at http://ctep.cancer.gov/protocolDevelopment/electronic_applications/ctc.htm.

In summary, in the last few decades the rate of severe side effects has been statistically reduced by the increased deployment of modern methods of high-precision irradiation also in clinical routine (e.g., 3D conformal radiotherapy, IMRT, IGRT). Nevertheless, high doses of radiation must be applied to sensitive areas.

As well as the purely physically aspect of doses applied to high-risk organs, biological aspects also play a role, such as the individual's radiosensitivity, so that, despite the technical innovations high-precision radiotherapy, the individual risk continues to be a factor in the development of severe side effects.

14.5.1 Eyelid

The cutis of the eyelids reacts essentially like the cutis in other parts of the human body. The changes due to radiotherapy are dependent on the reactions of the basal cells of the epidermis and of the endothelial cells in the supplying capillaries.

Under **normofractionated radiotherapy**, from the third week of radiotherapy an increasing basal cell depletion is evident, while the mitosis rate of the basal cells clearly rises subsequently.[113] Increasing perivascular infiltration by inflammatory cells and dilatation of the papillary vessels are clinically visible as edema and erythema at ~30 Gy. Hyperpigmentation occurs from ~45 Gy and moist epitheliolysis is possible from ~50 Gy.

In the longer term, after doses of ~40 Gy a rarefaction of the papillary vessels occurs with a simultaneous increase in the diameter of the vessels. With total doses of 50 to 60 Gy these processes can manifest themselves as telangiectasias; the poor supply to the epidermis then leads to atrophy from total doses > 60 Gy.[113] Once there is a failure to achieve a critical number of supplying papillary vessels—even years after a course of radiotherapy—secondary necrosis can occur. Today it is very rare that chronic scarring occurs after a secondary wound healing. This can, however, prevent the eyelid from closing due to the development of entropion or ectropion. With cobalt-era treatments such findings were distinctly more frequent due to the unavoidably higher skin dose than with modern linear accelerators.

With **higher single doses** these changes are observed with low cumulative overall doses.

The eyelashes fall out from doses of 20 Gy normofractionated radiotherapy. An irreversible loss can be expected from doses over 40 Gy.[114] This can be a consequence of irritation of the conjunctiva and the cornea. However, when the eyelashes grow back after radiation the growth direction can be inwards (trichiasis) with associated painful irritation of the eye.

> **Memorize** (M!)
>
> Skin erythema is to be expected from an ongoing, normofractionated radiotherapy from a skin dose of ~30 Gy, hyperpigmentation from ~45 Gy, and moist epitheliolysis from ~50 Gy.
>
> Chronic side effects can occur in the form of telangiectasias from ~50 Gy even years afterwards. The development of skin atrophy is possible from ~60 Gy.

14.5.2 Tear Ducts

Xerophthalmia can result from damage to the meibomian glands and the lacrimal gland. Chronic dryness of the eyes can lead to vascularization of the cornea and opacifications, which in turn affect the sight.

A sigmoid dose–effect curve is assumed for the development of xerophthalmia after normofractionated radiotherapy, with minimal risk for doses under 30 Gy, a sharp rise over 40 Gy, and an almost 100% risk at 57 Gy.[114] With 30 to 45 Gy, the symptom occurs within 4 to 11 years after the conclusion of the radiotherapy; with 57 Gy as early as within the first year.

Radiation doses > 65 Gy often lead to scarring and stenosis of the tear ducts.[114]

> **Memorize** (M!)
>
> The risk of chronic dryness of the eye after normofractionated radiotherapy clearly increases with doses from ~40 Gy. The higher the dose delivered, the earlier the manifestation of the xerophthalmia.

14.5.3 Conjunctiva

Acute conjunctivitis with reddening and pain occurs in nearly half of patients after 27 Gy dose.[35] Super infections with bacteria or viruses are possible here.

With radiation doses over 50 Gy, the risk clearly increases for the development of chronic conjunctivitis.[114] Histologically, squamous cell epithelial metaplasias are observed. With > 60 Gy, scarring is possible with adhesions between conjunctiva and eyelid or eyeball.

The dose at the conjunctiva can be effectively reduced by patients in whom only one part of the orbit has to be treated by opening their eyes as wide as possible while the radiotherapy is in progress.

> **Memorize** (M!)
>
> Transient irritation of the conjunctiva can occur even with low doses of radiation. Chronic conjunctivitis is observed from > 50 to 60 Gy; this can cause metaplasias and scarring.

14.5.4 Cornea

In general, the cornea is regarded as radiotherapy-resistant; this is why doses up to ~1,000 Gy are administered in episcleral brachytherapy.

Normofractionated radiotherapy doses from 30 Gy can trigger transient epithelial erosion and 40 to 50 Gy doses can also trigger (sometimes chronic) edemas, with the sight being affected depending on the localization.[114] Ulcers of the cornea are observed with > 60 Gy, but also with single treatments with 20 Gy.

The cornea can also be damaged in a secondary development as a consequence of a radiogenic keratitis sicca.

To avoid high doses on the cornea, the dose build-up effect on surfaces can be exploited. Also, gold calottes can be used that are placed under the eyelids before each irradiation (see Chapter 14.3.1). These can provide marked shielding from low-energy photons or electron radiotherapy.

> **Memorize** (M!)
>
> The cornea is radiation-resistant; chronic side effects are anticipated only from doses of > 50 Gy of normofractionated radiotherapy. With brachytherapy with ruthenium 106 the sclera withstands "single doses" of ~1,000 Gy. Secondary damage to the cornea is possible with xerophthalmia.

14.5.5 Iris

The iris is regarded as relatively radiation-resistant. Normofractionated radiotherapy doses > 70 Gy (hypofractionated 30–40 Gy) can lead to persistent iritis.[114]

Neovascular glaucomas as a consequence of neovascularization after ischemia and fibrosis in the Schlemm's canals are very frequently observed; presumably additional risk factors such as age, diabetes mellitus, retinal detachments, or vitreous humor bleeds play a role in combination with the radiation. With proton irradiation for uveal melanomas, the percentage of lens-penetrating radiation almost equates to the rate of neovascular glaucomas appearing at a later date.[1]

To avoid such complications it is important to spare the anterior chamber of the eye as far as possible.[81] Intensive follow-up by an ophthalmologist is usually indispensable to identify and treat neovascularization early. In this respect, intravitral injection of bevacizumab seems to be effective.[114] In the event of secondary glaucomas occurring with iridocorneal angle closure, these must be treated surgically with trabeculectomy.

M!

Memorize

Persistent iritis after normofractionated radiography is observed only with doses > 70 Gy. One feared complication of radiogenic exposure of the anterior part of the eye is the occurrence of neovascular glaucoma as a consequence of neovascularization and fibrosis of the Schlemm's canals.

14.5.6 Lens

Acute reactions of the lens to radiotherapy do not occur. However, the lens does react with great sensitivity to low radiation doses with the slow development of a cataract.[114] Cells in the germinative zone die and this is followed by increased mitosis in surviving cells, resulting in gradual opacification so that patients suffer from an increasing loss of sight and limited-contrast vision. Phacolytic glaucomas are possible.

A cataract can occur even after a single dose of 2 Gy. With dose between 2.5 and 6.5 Gy a cataract develops after a latency period of 8 years in 33% of irradiated patients; with dose between 6.5 and 11.5 Gy the latency period halves to 4 years, while the percentage of patients affected doubles to 66%.[115]

The sensitivity of the lens in childhood is expected to be even greater: a 50% risk is assumed after 1 Gy.[114] Experiences in whole-body radiotherapy prove that a higher single dose is associated with a raised risk in comparison with fractionated, lower single doses.

For avoidance of cataracts, gold calottes should be used (wherever it is appropriate to use them) to shield low energy photon radiation or electron radiation (see Chapter 14.3.1). The physical-technical options are fairly limited, however, as the lens is reactive to even low doses of radiation. The recommendation often given in the literature for the use of modern planning and radiotherapy techniques such as IMRT is meaningless in this regard: it is precisely IMRT that deposits low doses of radiation in large areas of the body that are not used as beam paths in conventional techniques.

The method of choice with a significant cataract is lens surgery, with success rates as high as in the normal population.[114]

M!

Memorize

A contract can arise after only 2 Gy of exposure. With 6 Gy, one-third of patients irradiated develop a cataract within 8 years. In the decision on therapy, the risk of developing cataracts is no longer relevant as lens surgery delivers excellent functional results.

14.5.7 Retina

The retina is part of the CNS. Acute reactions to radiation are not known; the retina reacts to radiotherapy like late-reacting normal tissue. Slow-progressing microangiopathic changes are at the forefront. Clinically, microaneurysms, telangiectasia, and exudates are observed as signs of retinopathy.[114] Retinal detachments, bleeds into the vitreous humor, and macular edemas can occur to complicate matters. With macular involvement in these changes, a massive loss of sight is possible.

The latency period between radiotherapy and the occurrence of the first changes lies between 0.5 and 3 years but occasionally they can occur significantly later. The latency period diminishes with the size of the dose applied. The threshold dose for the development of retinopathy is considered to be 30 to 35 Gy,[114] although occasionally such changes have also been reported after distinctly lower doses (then, however, there is nearly always a connection with comorbidity such as diabetes or arterial hypertension). Between 30 and 50 Gy the risk rises sharply: as the TD 5/5 45–50 Gy are taken, already with 55 Gy the TD is 50/5.[68] Higher daily single doses are associated with a significant rise in the risk, while hyperfractionated radiotherapy (twice daily 1.1–1.2 Gy) significantly reduces the risk.[116] One should note that simultaneous chemotherapy can increase the risk for the development of retinal changes.

To avoid retinopathy, fractionated radiotherapy—and where necessary hyperfractionated radiotherapy—should be administered (to the extent it makes sense in terms of the tumor biology), or only the smallest possible area of the retina (sparing the macula as far as possible) should be exposed to high doses of radiation.

Therapeutically, few interventions are proven effective; laser treatment is used for the reduction of macula edemas; and intravitreal VEGF antibodies appear to open up new therapeutic alternatives.[114]

M!

Memorize

Retinopathy (often reversible) can appear from ~30 Gy dose. In patients with diabetes and arterial hypertension, however, distinctly lower threshold doses are possible. The risk can be significantly lowered by delivering hyperfractionated radiotherapy.

14.5.8 Optic Nerve

Radiogenic optic nerve neuropathy is rare but, because of the lack of treatment options, it is serious for the patient afflicted when it occurs. It is characterized by a painless loss of sight or visual field. Damage anterior of the chiasma afflict the ipsilateral eye; damage in the proximity of the chiasma can involve both optic nerves (in the sense of a bitemporal hemianopsia with injury of the intersecting fibers). Correspondingly, damage to the chiasma can lead to complete blindness. Pathophysiologically, disruption of the blood supply to the optic nerve concerned is assumed.[117]

With normofractionated radiotherapy and exposure of the entire optic nerve, a 5% risk of sight loss (< 20/100) is reported within 5 years with a total dose of 50 Gy, and a risk of 50% with 65 Gy.[68] However, in various series no optic nerve damage has been observed when the maximum dose in the area of the nerves is limited to < 56 Gy and in the chiasma to < 54 Gy.[117] For this reason the TD5/5 is currently assumed for 55–60 Gy, with a distinct rise in doses > 60 Gy.

An exception seems to be the radiotherapy of pituitary tumors as there complications have been repeatedly reported at as little as 46 Gy with 1.8 Gy single dose. Neuropathy also appeared in these patients within the first year after radiotherapy, not within the first 3 years as in the other groups.[117]

The risk is further dependent on the dose of the individual fraction, with a distinct rise with daily doses > 1.9 Gy. A hyperfractionation (twice daily 1.2 Gy) seems particularly safe with regard to the avoidance of optic nerve neuropathy.[117]

With stereotactic single radiotherapy, a maximum dose < 8 Gy in the optic nerve seems to be safe. Maximum doses between 8 and 12 Gy are associated with a risk clearly under 10%.[117]

These results with photon radiotherapy are in the main also valid for proton radiotherapy (where the CGE equivalent dose is generally stated).

Memorize

Neuropathy of the optic nerve is extremely rare with a dose < 56 Gy in the optic nerve and < 54 Gy in the chiasma. A 5% risk for occurrence within 5 years after normofractionated radiotherapy is proposed between 55 and 60 Gy. With single radiotherapy, doses < 8 Gy are probably safe, while single doses between 8 and 12 Gy are associated with a 10% risk.

14.5.9 Radiogenic Tumor Induction

In addition to the deterministic side effects of a radiotherapy, which are the consequences of radiotherapy that do not occur below a threshold dose, there are also stochastic effects. These concerns mutations for which there is no safe threshold dose (▶ Table 14.2). A photon can trigger a mutation, which in turn leads to tumor induction many years later. The higher the radiation dose, the higher the probability of such an event occurring; on the other hand, the higher also is the chance that the mutated cell is killed by the radiotherapy.

The carcinogenic risk in irradiating benign changes such as endocrinal orbitopathy is discussed in detail in Chapter 7.4.2.

Only sparse data are available on the irradiation of malignant changes. It is certain that patients with hereditary retinoblastoma are particularly prone to radiogenic tumor induction (see Chapter 14.3.4). In one therapy series the rate for second tumors was 23% within 25 years of the therapy.[79]

Patients with sporadically occurring malignant tumors are clearly less prone to the risk of tumor induction. The best data on estimating the associated risk with a full-dose EBRT are available for breast cancer treatment. Here, for almost 11,000 patients with a follow-up monitoring period of over 20 years, it was demonstrated that the risk of a radiation-induced tumor is ~1% per decade after conclusion of the therapy.[67] The transferability of this risk for the therapy of nonhereditary tumors in the orbit area is evident.

Memorize

The risk of a radiogenic tumor induction in the radiotherapy of sporadically appearing, not genetically caused tumors is roughly 1% per decade of life after the conclusion of the radiotherapy.

For children with retinoblastomas, due to the particular sensitivity of these patients to ionizing radiation, the risk lies distinctly higher, up to 30% within 25 years.

The risks are plainly smaller for the radiation of benign lesions due to the lower radiation doses.

Table 14.2 Summary of tolerance doses for acute and chronic side effects in radiotherapy of the orbit. The doses stated correspond to median threshold doses. In isolated cases the occurrence of side effects with distinctly lower cumulative doses is possible in patients who are particularly sensitive to radiation. A regular clinic visit by the patients during ongoing radiotherapy and after conclusion of the treatment is obligatory for this reason. All dose details relate to normofractionated radiotherapy protocols

Tissue	Acute side effects	Chronic side effects[a]
Epidermis	Edema/erythema 30 Gy	Telangiectasias 50–60 Gy
	Hyperpigmentation 45 Gy	Atrophy > 60 Gy
	Moist epitheliolysis 50 Gy	
Tear glands		Xerophthalmia > 40 Gy 100% 57 Gy inside 1 year
		> 65 Gy stenoses of the tear ducts
Conjunctiva	Conjunctivitis > 27 Gy in 50% of patients	> 50 Gy conjunctivitis with metaplasias > 60 Gy scarring
Cornea		> 60 Gy ulceration possible
		Secondary damage with xerophthalmia
Iris		> 70 Gy iritis
Lens		Cataract possible at 2 Gy 6 Gy 30% cataract in 8 years TD5/5 10 Gy TD 50/5 18 Gy
Retina		Retinopathy TD5/5 45–50 Gy TD50/5 55 Gy
Optic nerve		Neuropathy TD 5/5 55–60 Gy > 60 Gy 20% risk

[a]TD5/5: tolerance dose in which one effect occurred in 5% of the patients within 5 years. TD50/5: tolerance dose in which one effect occurred in 50% of the patients within 5 years.

References

[1] Daftari IK, Char DH, Verhey LJ. Anterior segment sparing to reduce charged particle radiotherapy complications in uveal melanoma. Int J Radiat Oncol Biol Phys. 1997; 39(5):997–1010

[2] Nag S, Quivey JM, Earle JD, Followill D, Fontanesi J, Finger PT, American Brachytherapy Society. The American Brachytherapy Society recommendations for brachytherapy of uveal melanomas. Int J Radiat Oncol Biol Phys. 2003; 56 (2):544–555

[3] Demirci H, Shields CL, Chao AN, Shields JA. Uveal metastasis from breast cancer in 264 patients. Am J Ophthalmol. 2003; 136(2):264–271

[4] Wiegel T, Bornfeld N, Kreusel KM. Inzidenz und Therapie von Aderhautmetastasen. Onkologe. 1999; 5(9):813–818

[5] Wiegel T, Bottke D, Kreusel KM, German Cancer Society. External beam radiotherapy of choroidal metastases–final results of a prospective study of the German Cancer Society (ARO 95–08). Radiother Oncol. 2002; 64(1):13–18

[6] Giuliari GP, Sadaka A. Uveal metastatic disease: current and new treatment options (review). Oncol Rep. 2012; 27(3):603–607

[7] Rudoler SB, Corn BW, Shields CL. External beam irradiation for choroid metastases: identification of factors predisposing to long-term sequelae. Int J Radiat Oncol Biol Phys. 1997; 38(2):251–256

[8] Shah SU, Mashayekhi A, Shields CL. Uveal metastasis from lung cancer: clinical features, treatment, and outcome in 194 patients. Ophthalmology. 2014; 121(1):352–357

[9] Shields CL, Shields JA, Gross NE, Schwartz GP, Lally SE. Survey of 520 eyes with uveal metastases. Ophthalmology. 1997; 104(8):1265–1276
[10] Chen CJ, McCoy AN, Brahmer J, Handa JT. Emerging treatments for choroidal metastases. Surv Ophthalmol. 2011; 56(6):511–521
[11] Wiegel T, Kreusel KM, Schmidt S, Bornfeld N, Foerster MH, Hinkelbein W. Radiotherapy of unilateral choroidal metastasis: unilateral irradiation or bilateral irradiation for sterilization of suspected contralateral disease? Radiother Oncol. 1999; 53(2):139–141
[12] Tsina EK, Lane AM, Zacks DN, Munzenrider JE, Collier JM, Gragoudas ES. Treatment of metastatic tumors of the choroid with proton beam irradiation. Ophthalmology. 2005; 112(2):337–343
[13] Kanthan GL, Jayamohan J, Yip D, Conway RM. Management of metastatic carcinoma of the uveal tract: an evidence-based analysis. Clin Experiment Ophthalmol. 2007; 35(6):553–565
[14] Shields CL, Shields JA, De Potter P. Plaque radiotherapy for the management of uveal metastasis. Arch Ophthalmol. 1997; 115(2):203–209
[15] Bianciotto C, Demirci H, Shields CL, Eagle RC, Jr, Shields JA. Metastatic tumors to the eyelid: report of 20 cases and review of the literature. Arch Ophthalmol. 2009; 127(8):999–1005
[16] Amdur RJ, Kalbaugh KJ, Ewald LM. Radiation therapy for skin cancer near the eye: kilovoltage x-rays versus electrons. Int J Radiat Oncol Biol Phys. 1992; 23 (4):769–779
[17] Shiu AS, Tung SS, Gastorf RJ, Hogstrom KR, Morrison WH, Peters LJ. Dosimetric evaluation of lead and tungsten eye shields in electron beam treatment. Int J Radiat Oncol Biol Phys. 1996; 35(3):599–604
[18] Coupland SE, Heimann H. Primäres intraokuläres Lymphom. [Primary intraocular lymphoma]. Ophthalmologe. 2004; 101(1):87–98
[19] Davis JL. Intraocular lymphoma: a clinical perspective. Eye (Lond). 2013; 27 (2):153–162
[20] Chan CC, Sen HN. Current concepts in diagnosing and managing primary vitreoretinal (intraocular) lymphoma. Discov Med. 2013; 15(81):93–100
[21] Rajagopal R, Harbour JW. Diagnostic testing and treatment choices in primary vitreoretinal lymphoma. Retina. 2011; 31(3):435–440
[22] Illerhaus G, Finke J, Korfel A. Therapie von primären zerebralen Lymphomen. [Treatment of primary cerebral lymphomas]. Onkologe. 2011; 17(4):308–317
[23] Correa DD, Maron L, Harder H. Cognitive functions in primary central nervous system lymphoma: literature review and assessment guidelines. Ann Oncol. 2007; 18(7):1145–1151
[24] Korfel A, Schlegel U. Primäre Zentralnervensystemlymphome. [Primary central nervous system lymphomas]. Der Onkologe. 2014; 20(1):75–86
[25] Nayak L, Batchelor TT. Recent advances in treatment of primary central nervous system lymphoma. Curr Treat Options Oncol. 2013; 14(4):539–552
[26] Morris PG, Correa DD, Yahalom J. Rituximab, methotrexate, procarbazine, and vincristine followed by consolidation reduced-dose whole-brain radiotherapy and cytarabine in newly diagnosed primary CNS lymphoma: final results and long-term outcome. J Clin Oncol. 2013; 31(31):3971–3979
[27] Thiel E, Korfel A, Martus P. High-dose methotrexate with or without whole brain radiotherapy for primary CNS lymphoma (G-PCNSL-SG-1): a phase 3, randomised, non-inferiority trial. Lancet Oncol. 2010; 11(11):1036–1047
[28] Juergens A, Pels H, Rogowski S. Long-term survival with favorable cognitive outcome after chemotherapy in primary central nervous system lymphoma. Ann Neurol. 2010; 67(2):182–189
[29] Hottinger AF, DeAngelis LM, Yahalom J, Abrey LE. Salvage whole brain radiotherapy for recurrent or refractory primary CNS lymphoma. Neurology. 2007; 69(11):1178–1182
[30] Harada K, Murakami N, Kitaguchi M. Localized ocular adnexal mucosa-associated lymphoid tissue lymphoma treated with radiation therapy: a long-term outcome in 86 patients with 104 treated eyes. Int J Radiat Oncol Biol Phys. 2014; 88(3):650–654
[31] Olszewski AJ, Desai A. Radiation therapy administration and survival in stage I/II extranodal marginal zone B-cell lymphoma of mucosa-associated lymphoid tissue. Int J Radiat Oncol Biol Phys. 2014; 88(3):642–649
[32] Lowry L, Smith P, Qian W. Reduced dose radiotherapy for local control in non-Hodgkin lymphoma: a randomised phase III trial. Radiother Oncol. 2011; 100(1):86–92
[33] Hoskin P, Kirkwood A, Popova B. FoRT: a phase 3 multi-center prospective randomized trial of low dose radiation therapy for follicular and marginal zone lymphoma. (abstract). Int J Radiat Oncol Biol Phys. 2013; 85(1):22
[34] Fasola CE, Jones JC, Huang DD. Le QT, Hoppe RT, Donaldson SS. Low-dose radiation therapy (2 Gy × 2) in the treatment of orbial lymphoma. Int J Radiat Oncol Biol Phys. 2013; 86(5):930–935
[35] Stafford SL, Kozelsky TF, Garrity JA. Orbital lymphoma: radiotherapy outcome and complications. Radiother Oncol. 2001; 59(2):139–144
[36] Pfeffer MR, Rabin T, Tsvang L, Goffman J, Rosen N, Symon Z. Orbital lymphoma: is it necessary to treat the entire orbit? Int J Radiat Oncol Biol Phys. 2004; 60(2):527–530
[37] Hawkins BS. Collaborative ocular melanoma study randomized trial of I-125 brachytherapy. Clin Trials. 2011; 8(5):661–673
[38] Egan KM, Seddon JM, Glynn RJ, Gragoudas ES, Albert DM. Epidemiologic aspects of uveal melanoma. Surv Ophthalmol. 1988; 32(4):239–251
[39] Margo CE. The Collaborative Ocular Melanoma Study: an overview. Cancer Contr. 2004; 11(5):304–309
[40] The Collaborative Ocular Melanoma Study Group. Factors predictive of growth and treatment of small choroidal melanoma: COMS Report No. 5. Arch Ophthalmol. 1997; 115(12):1537–1544
[41] Diener-West M, Earle JD, Fine SL, Collaborative Ocular Melanoma Study Group. The COMS randomized trial of iodine 125 brachytherapy for choroidal melanoma, III: initial mortality findings. COMS Report No. 18. Arch Ophthalmol. 2001; 119(7):969–982
[42] Collaborative Ocular Melanoma Study Group. The COMS randomized trial of iodine 125 brachytherapy for choroidal melanoma: V. Twelve-year mortality rates and prognostic factors: COMS report No. 28. Arch Ophthalmol. 2006; 124(12):1684–1693
[43] Jampol LM, Moy CS, Murray TG, Collaborative Ocular Melanoma Study Group (COMS Group). The COMS randomized trial of iodine 125 brachytherapy for choroidal melanoma: IV. Local treatment failure and enucleation in the first 5 years after brachytherapy. COMS report no. 19. Ophthalmology. 2002; 109 (12):2197–2206
[44] Collaborative Ocular Melanoma Study Group. Incidence of cataract and outcomes after cataract surgery in the first 5 years after iodine 125 brachytherapy in the Collaborative Ocular Melanoma Study: COMS Report No. 27. Ophthalmology. 2007; 114(7):1363–1371
[45] Melia BM, Abramson DH, Albert DM, Collaborative Ocular Melanoma Study Group. Collaborative ocular melanoma study (COMS) randomized trial of I-125 brachytherapy for medium choroidal melanoma. I. Visual acuity after 3 years COMS report no. 16. Ophthalmology. 2001; 108(2):348–366
[46] Melia M, Moy CS, Reynolds SM, Collaborative Ocular Melanoma Study-Quality of Life Study Group. Quality of life after iodine 125 brachytherapy vs enucleation for choroidal melanoma. COMS QOLS report no. 3. Arch Ophthalmol. 2006; 124:226–238
[47] Ray SK, Bhatnagar R, Hartsell WF, Desai GR, American Association of Physicists in Medicine. Review of eye plaque dosimetry based on AAPM Task Group 43 recommendations. Int J Radiat Oncol Biol Phys. 1998; 41(3):701–706
[48] The Collaborative Ocular Melanoma Study (COMS) randomized trial of pre-enucleation radiation of large choroidal melanoma III: local complications and observations following enucleation COMS report no. 11. Am J Ophthalmol. 1998; 126(3):362–372
[49] Hawkins BS, Collaborative Ocular Melanoma Study Group. The Collaborative Ocular Melanoma Study (COMS) randomized trial of pre-enucleation radiation of large choroidal melanoma: IV. Ten-year mortality findings and prognostic factors. COMS report number 24. Am J Ophthalmol. 2004; 138(6): 936–951
[50] The Collaborative Ocular Melanoma Study (COMS) randomized trial of pre-enucleation radiation of large choroidal melanoma II: initial mortality findings. COMS report no. 10. Am J Ophthalmol. 1998; 125(6):779–796
[51] Nath R, Anderson LL, Luxton G, Weaver KA, Williamson JF, Meigooni AS, American Association of Physicists in Medicine. Dosimetry of interstitial brachytherapy sources: recommendations of the AAPM Radiation Therapy Committee Task Group No. 43. Med Phys. 1995; 22(2):209–234
[52] Lommatzsch PK, Werschnik C, Schuster E. Long-term follow-up of Ru-106/Rh-106 brachytherapy for posterior uveal melanoma. Graefes Arch Clin Exp Ophthalmol. 2000; 238(2):129–137
[53] Hermann RM, Pradier O, Lauritzen K, Ott M, Schmidberger H, Hess CF. Does escalation of the apical dose change treatment outcome in β-radiation of posterior choroidal melanomas with 106Ru plaques? Int J Radiat Oncol Biol Phys. 2002; 52(5):1360–1366

[54] Laube T, Flühs D, Kessler C, Bornfeld N. Determination of surgeon's absorbed dose in iodine 125 and ruthenium 106 ophthalmic plaque surgery. Ophthalmology. 2000; 107(2):366–368, discussion 368–369
[55] Verschueren KMS, Creutzberg CL, Schalij-Delfos NE. Long-term outcomes of eye-conserving treatment with Ruthenium(106) brachytherapy for choroidal melanoma. Radiother Oncol. 2010; 95(3):332–338
[56] Yarovoy AA, Magaramov DA, Bulgakova ES. The comparison of ruthenium brachytherapy and simultaneous transpupillary thermotherapy of choroidal melanoma with brachytherapy alone. Brachytherapy. 2012; 11(3):224–229
[57] Gragoudas ES, Lane AM, Regan S. A randomized controlled trial of varying radiation doses in the treatment of choroidal melanoma. Arch Ophthalmol. 2000; 118(6):773–778
[58] Char DH, Quivey JM, Castro JR, Kroll S, Phillips T. Helium ions versus iodine 125 brachytherapy in the management of uveal melanoma. A prospective, randomized, dynamically balanced trial. Ophthalmology. 1993; 100(10): 1547–1554
[59] Linstadt D, Castro J, Char D. Long-term results of helium ion irradiation of uveal melanoma. Int J Radiat Oncol Biol Phys. 1990; 19(3):613–618
[60] Bekkering GE, Rutjes AWS, Vlassov VV. The effectiveness and safety of proton radiation therapy for indications of the eye : a systematic review. Strahlenther Onkol. 2009; 185(4):211–221
[61] Dunavoelgyi R, Dieckmann K, Gleiss A. Local tumor control, visual acuity, and survival after hypofractionated stereotactic photon radiotherapy of choroidal melanoma in 212 patients treated between 1997 and 2007. Int J Radiat Oncol Biol Phys. 2011; 81(1):199–205
[62] Dunavoelgyi R, Dieckmann K, Gleiss A. Radiogenic side effects after hypofractionated stereotactic photon radiotherapy of choroidal melanoma in 212 patients treated between 1997 and 2007. Int J Radiat Oncol Biol Phys. 2012; 83 (1):121–128
[63] Georgopoulos M, Zehetmayer M, Ruhswurm I. Tumour regression of uveal melanoma after ruthenium-106 brachytherapy or stereotactic radiotherapy with gamma knife or linear accelerator. Ophthalmologica. 2003; 217(5):315–319
[64] Boixadera A, García-Arumí J, Martínez-Castillo V. Prospective clinical trial evaluating the efficacy of photodynamic therapy for symptomatic circumscribed choroidal hemangioma. Ophthalmology. 2009; 116(1):100–105.e1
[65] Chakravarthy U, Houston RF, Archer DB. Treatment of age-related subfoveal neovascular membranes by teletherapy: a pilot study. Br J Ophthalmol. 1993; 77(5):265–273
[66] Dugel PU, Bebchuk JD, Nau J, CABERNET Study Group. Epimacular brachytherapy for neovascular age-related macular degeneration: a randomized, controlled trial (CABERNET). Ophthalmology. 2013; 120(2):317–327
[67] Darby S, McGale P, Correa C, Early Breast Cancer Trialists' Collaborative Group (EBCTCG). Effect of radiotherapy after breast-conserving surgery on 10-year recurrence and 15-year breast cancer death: meta-analysis of individual patient data for 10,801 women in 17 randomised trials. Lancet. 2011; 378 (9804):1707–1716
[68] Emami B, Lyman J, Brown A. Tolerance of normal tissue to therapeutic irradiation. Int J Radiat Oncol Biol Phys. 1991; 21(1):109–122
[69] Evans JR, Sivagnanavel V, Chong V. Radiotherapy for neovascular age-related macular degeneration. Cochrane Database Syst Rev. 2010(5):CD004004
[70] Frau E, Rumen F, Noel G, Delacroix S, Habrand JL, Offret H. Low-dose proton beam therapy for circumscribed choroidal hemangiomas. Arch Ophthalmol. 2004; 122(10):1471–1475
[71] Gündüz K. Transpupillary thermotherapy in the management of circumscribed choroidal hemangioma. Surv Ophthalmol. 2004; 49(3):316–327
[72] Hanlon J, Firpo M, Chell E, Moshfeghi DM, Bolch WE. Stereotactic radiosurgery for AMD: a Monte Carlo-based assessment of patient-specific tissue doses. Invest Ophthalmol Vis Sci. 2011; 52(5):2334–2342
[73] Hykin PG, McCartney AC, Plowman PN, Hungerford JL. Postenucleation orbital radiotherapy for the treatment of malignant melanoma of the choroid with extrascleral extension. Br J Ophthalmol. 1990; 74(1):36–39
[74] Starr HJ, Zimmermann LE. Extrascleral extension and orbital recurrence of malignant melanomas of the choroid and ciliary body. Int Ophthalmol Clin. 1962; 2(2):369–384
[75] Robertson DM. Changing concepts in the management of choroidal melanoma. Am J Ophthalmol. 2003; 136(1):161–170
[76] Sauerwein W, Stannard CE. Auge und Orbita. In: Bamberg M, Molls M, Sack H, eds. Radioonkologie. Vol. 2. 2nd ed. Munich, Germany: W. Zuckschwerdt; 2009:304–310
[77] Temming P, Lohmann D, Bornfeld N, Sauerwein W, Goericke SL, Eggert A. Current concepts for diagnosis and treatment of retinoblastoma in Germany: aiming for safe tumor control and vision preservation. Klin Padiatr. 2012; 224(6):339–347
[78] Schipper J. An accurate and simple method for megavoltage radiation therapy of retinoblastoma. Radiother Oncol. 1983; 1(1):31–41
[79] Sauerwein W, Zehetmayer M. Strahlentherapie intraokularer Tumoren. [Radiotherapy of intraocular tumors]. Onkologe. 1999; 5(9):781–791
[80] Reisner ML, Viégas CM, Grazziotin RZ. Retinoblastoma–comparative analysis of external radiotherapy techniques, including an IMRT technique. Int J Radiat Oncol Biol Phys. 2007; 67(3):933–941
[81] Sethi RV, Shih HA, Yeap BY. Second nonocular tumors among survivors of retinoblastoma treated with contemporary photon and proton radiotherapy. Cancer. 2014; 120(1):126–133
[82] Pacelli R, Cella L, Conson M. Fractionated stereotactic radiation therapy for orbital optic nerve sheath meningioma - a single institution experience and a short review of the literature. J Radiat Res (Tokyo). 2011; 52(1):82–87
[83] Baumert BG, Villà S, Studer G. Early improvements in vision after fractionated stereotactic radiotherapy for primary optic nerve sheath meningioma. Radiother Oncol. 2004; 72(2):169–174
[84] Turbin RE, Thompson CR, Kennerdell JS, Cockerham KP, Kupersmith MJ. A long-term visual outcome comparison in patients with optic nerve sheath meningioma managed with observation, surgery, radiotherapy, or surgery and radiotherapy. Ophthalmology. 2002; 109(5):890–899, discussion 899–900
[85] Rootman J. Why "orbital pseudotumour" is no longer a useful concept. Br J Ophthalmol. 1998; 82(4):339–340
[86] Mombaerts I, Goldschmeding R, Schlingemann RO, Koornneef L. What is orbital pseudotumor? Surv Ophthalmol. 1996; 41(1):66–78
[87] Matthiesen C, Bogardus C, Thompson S. In Reply to Dr. Mombaerts. Int J Radiat Oncol Biol Phys. 2011; 81:901–902
[88] Mombaerts I, Schlingemann RO, Goldschmeding R, Koornneef L. Are systemic corticosteroids useful in the management of orbital pseudotumors? Ophthalmology. 1996; 103(3):521–528
[89] Prabhu RS, Kandula S, Liebman L. Association of clinical response and long-term outcome among patients with biopsied orbital pseudotumor receiving modern radiation therapy. Int J Radiat Oncol Biol Phys. 2013; 85(3):643–649
[90] Matthiesen C, Bogardus C, Jr, Thompson JS. The efficacy of radiotherapy in the treatment of orbital pseudotumor. Int J Radiat Oncol Biol Phys. 2011; 79 (5):1496–1502
[91] Lee JH, Kim Y-S, Yang SW. Radiotherapy with or without surgery for patients with idiopathic sclerosing orbital inflammation refractory or intolerant to steroid therapy. Int J Radiat Oncol Biol Phys. 2012; 84(1):52–58
[92] Sergott RC, Glaser JS, Charyulu K. Radiotherapy for idiopathic inflammatory orbital pseudotumor. Indications and results. Arch Ophthalmol. 1981; 99(5): 853–856
[93] Prabhu RS, Kandula S, Crocker I. In reply to Marks. Int J Radiat Oncol Biol Phys. 2013; 86(5):808–809
[94] Mashayekhi A, Shields CL. Circumscribed choroidal hemangioma. Curr Opin Ophthalmol. 2003; 14(3):142–149
[95] Shields CL, Honavar SG, Shields JA, Cater J, Demirci H. Circumscribed choroidal hemangioma: clinical manifestations and factors predictive of visual outcome in 200 consecutive cases. Ophthalmology. 2001; 108(12):2237–2248
[96] Zografos L, Bercher L, Chamot L, Gailloud C, Raimondi S, Egger E. Cobalt-60 treatment of choroidal hemangiomas. Am J Ophthalmol. 1996; 121(2):190–199
[97] López-Caballero C, Saornil MA, De Frutos J. High-dose iodine-125 episcleral brachytherapy for circumscribed choroidal haemangioma. Br J Ophthalmol. 2010; 94(4):470–473
[98] Arepalli S, Shields CL, Kaliki S, Emrich J, Komarnicky L, Shields JA. Diffuse choroidal hemangioma management with plaque radiotherapy in 5 cases. Ophthalmology. 2013; 120(11):2358–2359, 2359.e1–2359.e2
[99] Zografos L, Egger E, Bercher L, Chamot L, Munkel G. Proton beam irradiation of choroidal hemangiomas. Am J Ophthalmol. 1998; 126(2):261–268
[100] Höcht S, Wachtlin J, Bechrakis NE. Proton or photon irradiation for hemangiomas of the choroid? A retrospective comparison. Int J Radiat Oncol Biol Phys. 2006; 66(2):345–351
[101] Yonekawa Y, MacDonald SM, Shildkrot Y, Mukai S. Standard fractionation low-dose proton radiotherapy for diffuse choroidal hemangiomas in pediatric Sturge-Weber syndrome. J AAPOS. 2013; 17(3):318–322

[102] Schilling H, Sauerwein W, Lommatzsch A. Long-term results after low dose ocular irradiation for choroidal haemangiomas. Br J Ophthalmol. 1997; 81 (4):267–273

[103] Ritland JS, Eide N, Tausjø J. External beam irradiation therapy for choroidal haemangiomas. Visual and anatomical results after a dose of 20 to 25 Gy. Acta Ophthalmol Scand. 2001; 79(2):184–186

[104] Kim YT, Kang SW, Lee JI. Gamma knife radiosurgery for choroidal hemangioma. Int J Radiat Oncol Biol Phys. 2011; 81(5):1399–1404

[105] Jürgenliemk-Schulz IM, Hartman LJ, Roesink JM. Prevention of pterygium recurrence by postoperative single-dose beta-irradiation: a prospective randomized clinical double-blind trial. Int J Radiat Oncol Biol Phys. 2004; 59 (4):1138–1147

[106] Ali AM, Thariat J, Bensadoun RJ. The role of radiotherapy in the treatment of pterygium: a review of the literature including more than 6000 treated lesions. Cancer Radiother. 2011; 15(2):140–147

[107] Isohashi F, Inoue T, Xing S, Eren CB, Ozeki S, Inoue T. Postoperative irradiation for pterygium: retrospective analysis of 1,253 patients from the Osaka University Hospital. Strahlenther Onkol. 2006; 182(8):437–442

[108] Willner J, Flentje M, Lieb W. Soft X-ray therapy of recurrent pterygium–an alternative to 90Sr eye applicators. Strahlenther Onkol. 2001; 177(8):404–409

[109] Kishan AU, Modjtahedi BS, Morse LS, Lee P. Radiation therapy for neovascular age-related macular degeneration. Int J Radiat Oncol Biol Phys. 2013; 85(3): 583–597

[110] Jaakkola A, Heikkonen J, Tommila P, Laatikainen L, Immonen I. Strontium plaque irradiation of subfoveal neovascular membranes in age-related macular degeneration. Graefes Arch Clin Exp Ophthalmol. 1998; 236(1):24–30

[111] Timke C, Zieher H, Roth A. Combination of vascular endothelial growth factor receptor/platelet-derived growth factor receptor inhibition markedly improves radiation tumor therapy. Clin Cancer Res. 2008; 14(7):2210–2219

[112] Jackson TL, Chakravarthy U, Kaiser PK, INTREPID Study Group. Stereotactic radiotherapy for neovascular age-related macular degeneration: 52-week safety and efficacy results of the INTREPID study. Ophthalmology. 2013; 120 (9):1893–1900

[113] Adamietz IA. Strahlendermatitis: Prophylaxe und Behandlung. [Radiodermatitis: Prevention and treatment]. Onkologe. 2011; 17:61–74

[114] Jeganathan VSE, Wirth A, MacManus MP. Ocular risks from orbital and periorbital radiation therapy: a critical review. Int J Radiat Oncol Biol Phys. 2011; 79(3):650–659

[115] Merriam GR, Focht EF. The effects of ionizing radiations on the eye. Radiat Ther Oncol. 1972; 6:346–385

[116] Parsons JT, Bova FJ, Fitzgerald CR, Mendenhall WM, Million RR. Radiation retinopathy after external-beam irradiation: analysis of time-dose factors. Int J Radiat Oncol Biol Phys. 1994; 30(4):765–773

[117] Mayo C, Martel MK, Marks LB, Flickinger J, Nam J, Kirkpatrick J. Radiation dose-volume effects of optic nerves and chiasm. Int J Radiat Oncol Biol Phys. 2010; 76(3) Suppl:S28–S35

Chapter 15

Surgery of the Lacrimal Drainage System

15

15 Surgery of the Lacrimal Drainage System

15.1 Anatomy, Clinical Evaluation, and Treatment of Common Lacrimal Drainage Disorders

M. A. Varde and B. Wiechens

15.1.1 Anatomical Considerations

The **tear film** is important for the integrity of the ocular surface and thus for sight. It consists of three parts: *mucin*, *water*, and *lipid*, which are produced by the lacrimal gland, the lids, and the outer surface of the eye respectively. The tears are evenly distributed by the blink mechanism.

The tears are eliminated through evaporation and drainage via the **excretory system**. It consists of the *puncta*, *canaliculi*, *lacrimal sac*, and the *nasolacrimal duct*. The latter terminates in the inferior meatus of the nose (Chapter 1)[1,2,3,4,5] (▶ Fig. 15.1).

15.1.2 Examination of the Lacrimal Pathway

Tearing can be caused by **hyperlacrimation** or **epiphora**. The former describes an *excess production of tears* due to neuronal effects or disorders of the lacrimal gland as well as reflex secretion in ocular surface disorders or evaporative dry eye syndrome.[4]

The accumulation of tears due to **insufficient drainage** is referred to as *epiphora*. The elimination of tears via the excretory system is dependent not only on the *patency of the system* but also on the *position of the lid* and an *intact lacrimal pump*.

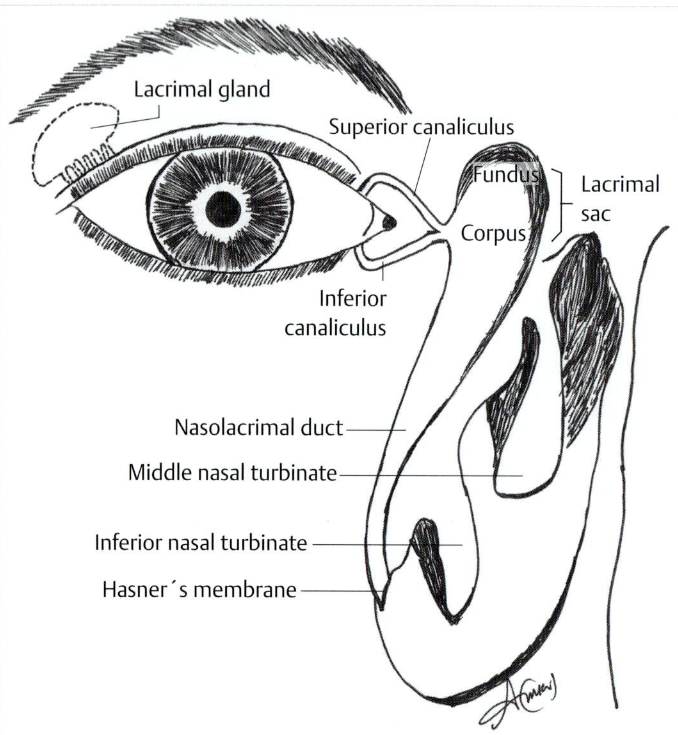

Fig. 15.1 Anatomy of the excretory tear duct system.

The lacrimal pump describes the different parts of the pretarsal orbicularis oculi muscle, which forms loops around the canaliculi and lacrimal sac and actively influences the tear flow by contraction. If constant tearing occurs due to malposition of the eyelid (retraction, ectropion) or reduced orbicularis oculi muscle tone, it is referred to as **functional epiphora**.

A **blockage of the lacrimal drainage system** can be classified by the anatomical localization and the degree of stenosis (absolute or relative). The clinically relevant anatomical localizations of lacrimal duct stenoses along with their recommended treatment options are summarized in ▶ Table 15.1.

The examination of a patient with epiphora is described in detail in the remainder of Chapter 15.1.2.

Evaluation of the Eyelids

The clinical examination starts with the *inspection of the eyelids and of the periocular region* (see Chapter 3.1). Significant **lid laxity** can be diagnosed by the *"snapback test"*: the lower lid is pulled downward with a finger and its repositioning is observed. If this happens spontaneously and rapidly, there is no laxity. A significant laxity is present if repositioning is delayed, if it requires blinking, or if there is no apposition to the eyeball at all. In the *"distraction test"* the eyelid is held between thumb and index finger, and drawn away from the eyeball. The distance between the eyeball and the eyelid is then measured. Significant laxity of the eyelid can be assumed when this is 10 mm or more.

Evaluation of the Lacrimal Excretory System

Dye Disappearance Test (DDT)

Fluorescein (a yellow dye that fluoresces green under blue light) is instilled into the conjunctival sac. After 5 minutes a blue light is used to examine whether the dye has been eliminated. If there is no dye detectable, a problem with lacrimal drainage is unlikely. This test is particularly useful in children, since diagnostic syringing usually cannot be done.

Table 15.1 Localization of lacrimal stenoses and possible surgical treatment options

Localization	Surgical treatment
Lacrimal punctum	Punctoplasty
Proximal canaliculus	Canalicular endoscopy Trephination CDCR (conjunctivodacryocystorhinostomy)
Distal canaliculus	Canalicular endoscopy Trephination DCR (dacryocystorhinostomy)
Common canalicular duct	Canalicular endoscopy DCR (dacryocystorhinostomy)
Nasolacrimal duct	Probing, lacrimal duct intubation Balloon dilation Canalicular endoscopy DCR (dacryocystorhinostomy) (Endonasal surgery)

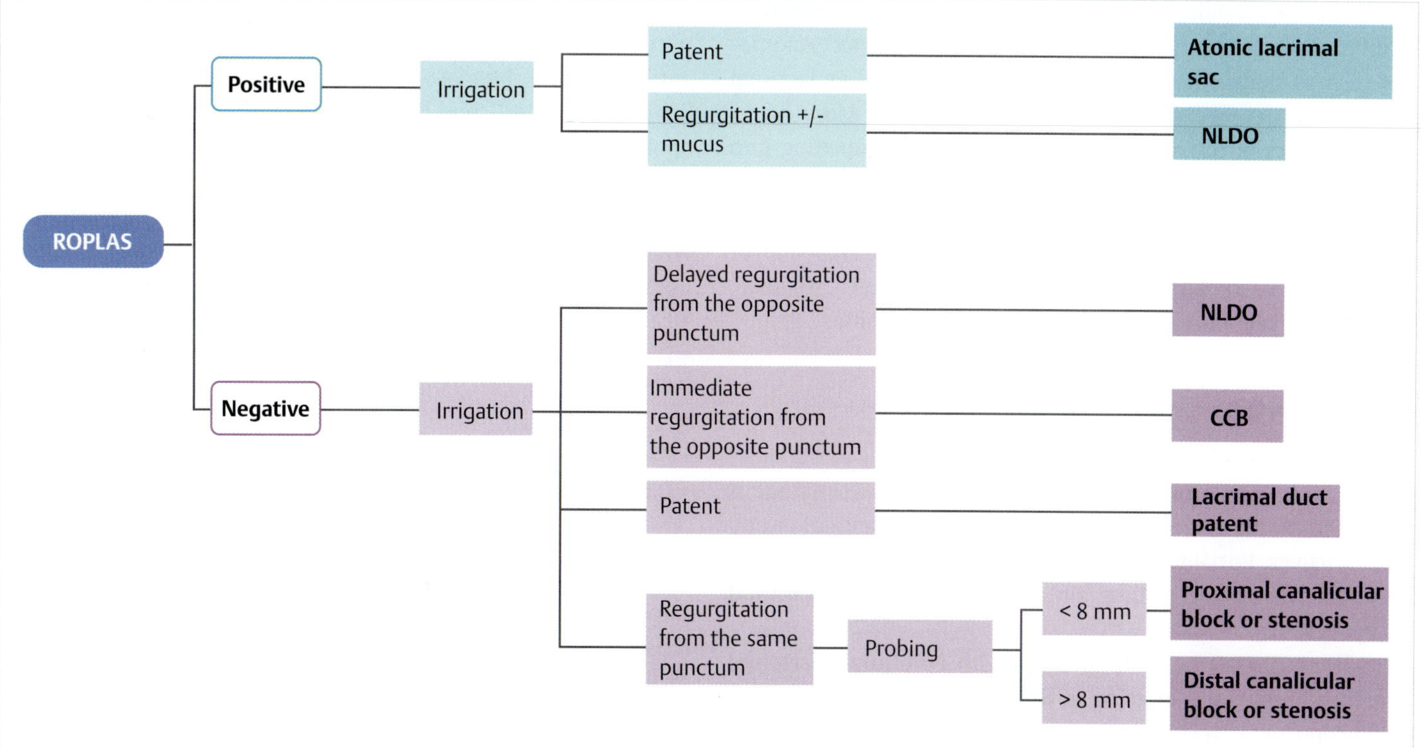

Fig. 15.2 Flowchart for the clinical diagnosis of lacrimal duct stenosis. NLDO, nasolacrimal duct stenosis; CCB, common canalicular block; ROPLAS, regurgitation on pressure over the lacrimal sack.

Jones Test

This test is rarely used due to its low sensitivity and specificity. Basically the DDT is carries out, but the investigator then attempts to detect fluorescein in the nose with a swab (Jones I). If the test is negative, the lacrimal ducts are flushed with saline (Jones II). A relative nasolacrimal duct obstruction (NLDO) is indicated when fluorescein is detected. If no dye can be detected, this either means an absolute or a canalicular stenosis, as there is no accumulation of fluorescein in the lacrimal sac.

ROPLAS Test

ROPLAS is an initialism for "regurgitation on pressure over the lacrimal sac". It describes the expression of mucous or mucopurulent material via the canaliculi upon retrograde compression of the lacrimal sac. If secretions are accumulated in the lacrimal sac due to NLDO or atonic sac, the test is positive. It is helpful for children with lacrimal duct stenosis and when contemplating the indications for a dacryocystorhinostomy (DCR).

Diagnostic Probing

The canaliculus is probed using a Bowman's probe with the lid held under lateral traction. A "soft stop" is an elastic resistance and indicates canalicular stenosis (the localization of the block can then be measured and the canaliculus on the opposite side likewise probed) or common canalicular stenosis. A "hard stop" is an indication of the patency of the canalicular system into the lacrimal sac. The probe is stopped by the bone of the lacrimal sac fossa.

Diagnostic Syringing

Syringing is performed through either the upper or the lower lacrimal punctum. The end point of the examination is whether the saline or water that is used reaches the patient's pharynx. The patient will confirm patency, perhaps swallow or cough. The examiner should also pay attention to the pressure required for flushing. A 5-mL syringe with a blunt, short lacrimal duct cannula is best suited for this procedure. The lacrimal ducts are patent if 100% of the liquid flushed goes through. A patency with increased pressure or partial regurgitation occurs with partial (or relative) stenosis. A reflux of fluid via the same lacrimal punctum is an indicator of a canalicular stenosis. The immediate regurgitation of clear liquid via the opposite punctum occurs with common canalicular block (CCB), the delayed regurgitation, sometimes associated with mucoid flakes or pus, is indicative of NLDO. Sometimes, dilatation of the sac can be seen on syringing in these cases (▶ Fig. 15.2).

Imaging

Imaging of the lacrimal system by means of **dacryocystography** (DCG) was first described in 1909 by Ewing. A water-soluble or iodized, oily contrast medium is instilled into the lacrimal ducts via the canaliculus with a lacrimal cannula or a catheter and radiography (**digital subtraction DCG**), CT (**CT-DCG**) or MRI (**MR-DCG**) are carried out. This is helpful especially in posttraumatic stenoses, as with CT-DCG in particular the surrounding bony structures can be visualized.[4]

15

15.1.3 Congenital NLDO

Epidemiology and Pathogenesis

Symptomatic **congenital nasolacrimal duct obstructions** (CNLDO) affect some 2 to 12% of newborns.[6,7] The incidence is even reported as high as 20%, with the majority of cases developing spontaneous remission[8] and are therefore often not being presented for consultation. In children with **Down syndrome** a significantly higher incidence of 22 to 35%[9,10] is reported. Anomalies such as punctum or canalicular atresias as well as lacrimal sac fistulas are rare causes of infantile epiphora. More often, CNLDO occurs in the area of Hasner's valve at the opening into the inferior nasal meatus due to an incomplete canalization of the nasolacrimal duct. These "simple" stenoses are mostly membranous and unilateral. Other "complex" variants are bony or canalicular obstructions,[11] as well as lacrimal duct stenoses, which are linked with dysmorphia or Down's syndrome.

Clinical Signs

An accumulation of amniotic fluid in the lacrimal sac of the newborn is termed an **amniontocele**. Draining of the lacrimal sac is prevented by the obstruction in the area of the Rosenmüller and Hasner valves. Initially, the content is sterile, but can develop an infection over course of time and then lead to **acute neonatal dacryocystitis**.

However, CNLDO typically presents with **epiphora**, **increased tear film height**, and **matting of the eyelashes** through mucous or mucopurulent secretion. The symptoms often appear within the first 4 weeks of life.[12] Spontaneous remission during the first year of life is reported in 90 to 97% of cases.[8,12]

Treatment

For an **amniontocele, massaging** the sac in a downward direction can be tried. Due to hydrostatic pressure this can lead to drainage of the sac contents into the inferior nasal meatus. If this is unsuccessful, prompt **probing of the lacrimal duct** is recommended in order to avoid neonatal dacryocystitis.

Neonatal dacryocystitis is an **emergency** and must be treated with intravenous administration of antibiotics in order to avert progression into orbital cellulitis or sepsis. An abscess should be punctured with a small cannula and the fluid obtained should be sent for microbiological analysis including an antibiogram. During this procedure, antibiotics can also be injected directly into the abscess. Therapeutic probing of the lacrimal duct should be done a few days after the acute infection subsides. If this treatment is unsuccessful, a **dacryocystorhinostomy** should be carried out where necessary a few days later.[13]

In the more common chronic course of CNLDO there is controversy with regard to the **timing for an intervention**. Therapeutic lacrimal duct probing during the first year of life leads to remission in up to 96% of cases.[13] Some authors report that the rate of spontaneous canalization decreases with increasing age of the child.[14] This is probably because, after the first year of life, persistent lacrimal duct stenoses are **complex stenoses** in most cases. Most authors recommend surgical intervention, primarily as **probing**, at the age of 1 year and before then conservative treatment with **Crigler's massage** and, if needed, topical antibiotics.[15,16]

There has been increasing discussion whether an earlier surgical intervention from the age of 6 months can be recommended. One argument in favor of this is the potential of congenital lacrimal duct stenoses to be **amblyogenic**.[17] The prevalence of amblyopia and anisometropia in children with CNLDO seems to be significantly higher than in children who are unaffected.[18] However, this hypothesis has not been confirmed to date. A further reason for early intervention is the parents' wishes. Although conservative measures are possible and effective, the purulent discharge, the necessity for repeated treatment with antibiotics, and the massage do have an impact on the quality of life of parents and child.[19] Furthermore, the probability of developing acute dacryocystitis increases with the duration of the stenosis and reduces the success of probing.[20]

Irrespective of the timing of intervention, the question of which surgical procedure should be performed is also increasingly under discussion. Treatment options are:

- Lacrimal duct probing.
- Lacrimal duct probing with silicone intubation (mono- or bicanalicular).
- Balloon dilation.
- Lacrimal endoscopy.
- Dacryocystorhinostomy.

Lacrimal Duct Probing

Depending on the age of the child, **probing** can be conducted mostly under **analgosedation**; general anesthesia is not necessary. Many authors in the United States and United Kingdom conduct this procedure as an "office procedure" without sedation,[21] but this can however only be done in children under 1 year of age.

First the puncta and canaliculi are examined and the upper punctum is carefully dilated with a Nettleship probe, and the lacrimal passage is irrigated with a cannula. Probing of the lacrimal duct can either be done with the long, slightly curved lacrimal cannula or with the Bowman probe (sizes 0 to 0000). The probing should be done primarily via the upper canaliculus to avoid injury to the lower canaliculus. It is assumed that due to gravity the majority of tears will flow out via the lower punctum, although varying results are reported on this in the literature. It is advisable to stand at the patient's head end. The probe is pushed first into the ampulla and then into the horizontal part with the lid under lateral traction. Attention is paid to identifying obstructions. Once the periosteum is reached, the direction of the probe is changed downward, laterally and posteriorly, following the course of the nasolacrimal duct. The instrument normally slides on its own with the use of soft pressure in the appropriate direction. After passage through the nasolacrimal duct, the bend in the instrument is directed medially, and the resistance in the area of the Hasner valve is overcome with gentle pressure in order to exit into the inferior nasal meatus (▶ Fig. 15.3). Using force can easily result in a wrong passage. When this is suspected, the probe can be withdrawn and a new attempt made to push forward. The patency of the lacrimal system can either be confirmed directly by irrigation (the patient in analgosedation swallows spontaneously; in general anesthesia flushing can be performed using fluorescein solution and can be detected in the nose as in the Jones test) or by means of nasal endoscopy. The examination of the nose has the advantage that the surgery can be combined, if necessary, with a **medialization of the inferior nasal concha**, should the latter obstruct the ostium. To achieve this, a periosteal elevator is pushed under the concha and the concha is infractured medially. Postoperative medication with oxymetazoline nose drops and eye drops and antibiotic eye drops (e.g., azithromycin, kanamycin) for a week is recommended.[13] The parents should be informed about the possibility of minor bleeding from the nose or the puncta. This often occurs

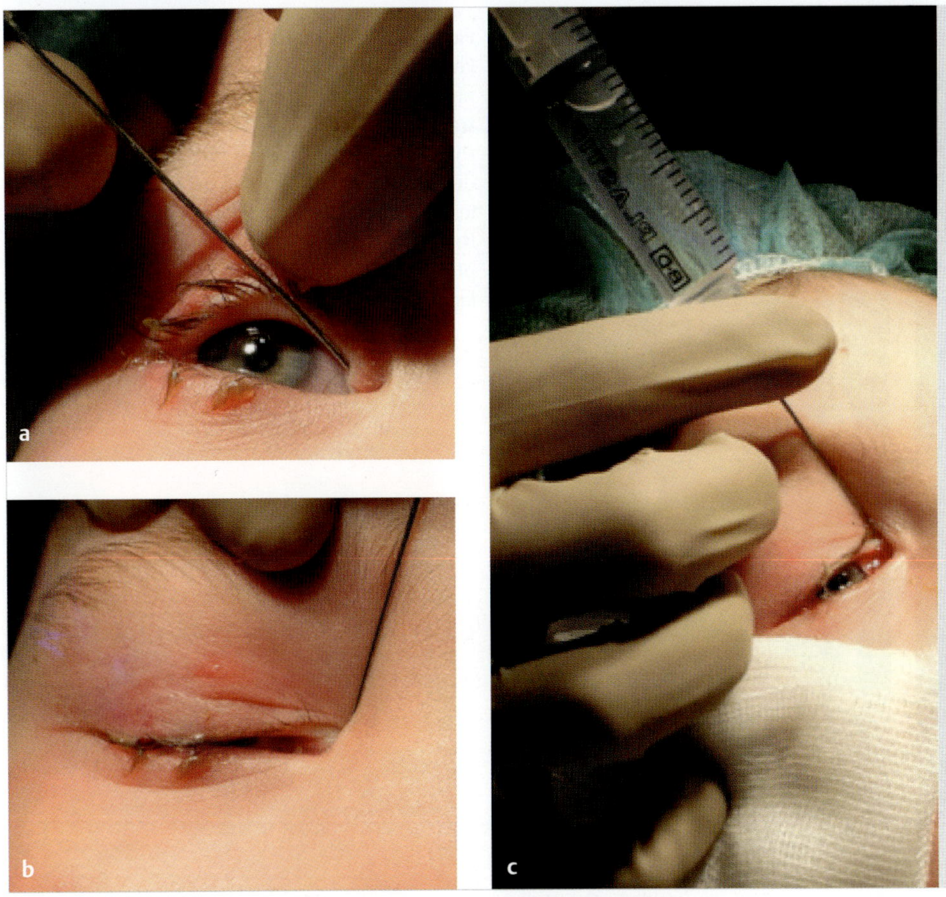

Fig. 15.3 Therapeutic probing and syringing of the lacrimal system. (a) Probe insertion into the upper canaliculus under constant lateral traction of the eyelid. (b) After contact with the periosteum, the probe's direction is turned toward the first premolar tooth. (c) Syringing of the lacrimal system. Successful recanalization is confirmed by observing the swallowing reflex under sedation, alternatively direct view with the endoscope.

intraoperatively and postoperatively and is usually harmless. In the initial period after the intervention, an early treatment of any possible rhinitis with decongestant nasal drops is recommended to prevent further obstruction. Lacrimal probing can be repeated if necessary.

The success rate of lacrimal duct probing in the first 4 years of life for CNLDO is reported to be 70 to 92%.[22,23] A more recent study found no statistically significant differences in the success rate of the primary probing related to the age of the children.[19]

Probing and Silicone Intubation

The **intubation of the lacrimal passage with a silicone tube** is done in recurrences following previous probing or in complicated lacrimal stenoses. It is more physiological and significantly less invasive than DCR. General anesthesia is recommended for the intubation.

After the probing, a silicone stent is inserted into the lacrimal passage. Mono- and bicanalicular silicone intubation systems are available for this; the success rate is independent of the type of intubation.[24] We use **bicanalicular intubation** with the rigid Jünemann probe (▶ Fig. 15.4). The probe, loaded with a 4–0 polypropylene thread, is inserted into the nasolacrimal duct and the metal probe is removed after retrieval of the thread in the nose. The suture remains as a splint for the silicone tube. The hollow tube is placed onto the punctual end of the suture and drawn into the nose. The procedure is repeated via the opposite punctum and the tube is knotted in the nose. **Monocanalicular intubation** likewise is done with a rigid system. The advantages of this method are the protection of the other canaliculus during the surgery, the avoidance of punctal erosion by a tight tube, as well as the simplicity of removal of the device in children. The disadvantage is the relatively traumatic retrieval of the probe from the nose. To date there are also flexible monocanalicular intubation systems available, which have an olive-shaped end of the metal probe and are recovered from the inferior meatus with a special hook (Crawford method). If necessary, the tube can be fixed with a nonresorbable thread to the nasal mucous membrane to avoid premature dislocation. It is recommended to leave the intubation in place for at least 4 weeks. In general a tube removal is recommended after 6 months.[25] With a normal dye disappearance test it can be removed earlier to avoid complications.

The success rate of primary silicone intubation with CNLDO before the fourth year of life is reported as 89 to 94%.[24,25] Here too there is evidence of a higher success rate in younger children.[25]

Balloon Dilation

Balloon dilation was introduced in the 1990s.[26,27] For this procedure an inflatable balloon made of polyurethane on a semiflexible catheter is introduced into the nasolacrimal duct, inflated to 8 to 9 atmospheres (depending on manufacturer) and left for 90 seconds. The catheter is then removed. The effect is due to the dilatation of the duct and the Hasner valve.[28] The success rate is 79 to 96%.[26,29,30]

General anesthesia is required for balloon dilation. A disadvantage of the procedure is the additional cost. Balloon dilation is mainly used in cases where probing has been unsuccessful.

Complications

Intraoperative complications of CNLDO surgery are **epistaxis, injury to the nasal mucous membrane** and the inferior nasal concha, as well as to the **canaliculi**. Some authors recommend packing the nose with 4% cocaine or oxymetazoline to minimize

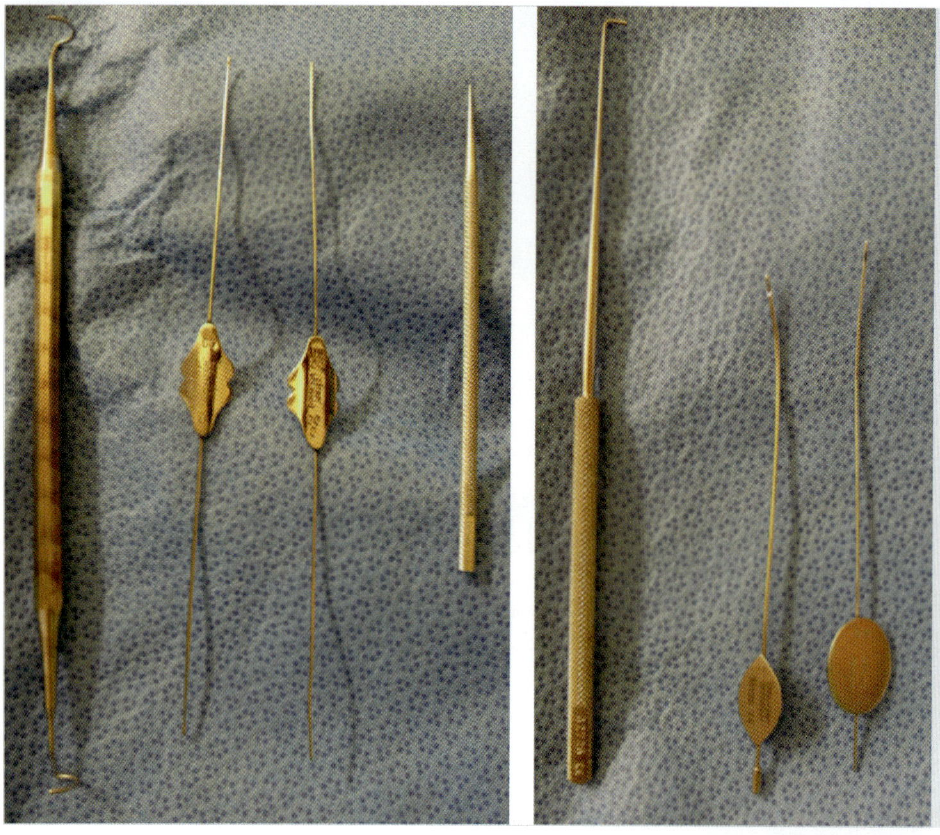

Fig. 15.4 Instruments for lacrimal probing. From left to right: Pigtail probe (for retrograde finding of a lacerated canaliculus via the contralateral punctum), Bowman probe (for probing the lacrimal system, sizes 00000), Nettleship dilator (to dilate the punctum prior to probe insertion), hook (to locate the polypropylene thread in the inferior nasal meatus), Jünemann probes (1.0 mm and 0.8 mm in diameter for lacrimal intubation).

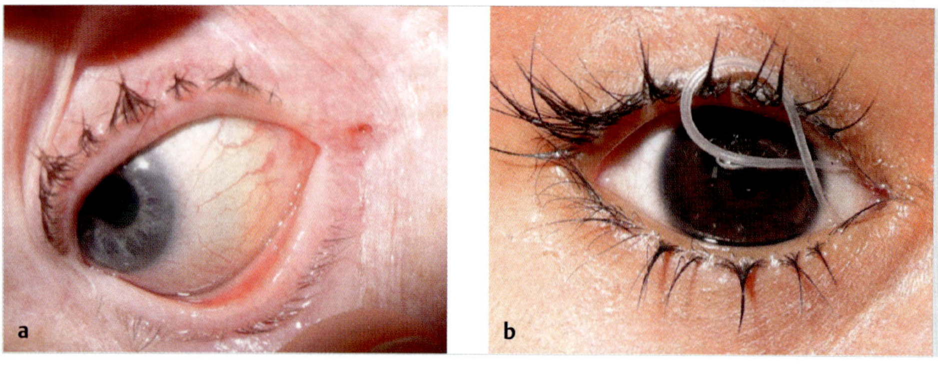

Fig. 15.5 Complications of silastic tubing. **(a)** Complete erosion of the canaliculi with consecutive symblepharon and migration of the bicanalicular intubation into the lacrimal sac. **(b)** "Spaghetti-syndrome": dislocation of the tube. (Image courtesy of Dr. B. Mukherjee, Sankara Nethralaya Eye Hospital, Chennai, India.)

intraoperative bleeding and for a planned nasal endoscopy.[31] The use of Jünemann or Ritleng probes or the flexible Crawford probe for lacrimal intubation, along with careful probing, helps in minimizing of these complications. Bleeding is mostly self-limiting and requires additional nasal packing or coagulation only in rare cases. A **false passage** can be avoided by using the correct probing technique.

Bicanalicular intubation bears the risk of **slitting of the puncta** through erosion as a result of knotting the tube ends too tightly in the nose. With facial growth in children the intubation becomes tight and this causes the tube to cut in. These patients need regular follow-up and, if necessary, early tube removal. Intraoperatively, care should be taken not to knot the tube too tightly. A further complication is **migration of the tube** (▶ Fig. 15.5a) into the medial canthal area. This can occur either with monocanalicular intubation or with complete canalicular erosion. Particularly in children, silicone can lead to granuloma **formation** in the area of the puncta or in the nasolacrimal duct. This is one reason for possible re-stenosis even after DCR. **Dislocation of the silicone tube** (▶ Fig. 15.5b), for example, after rubbing in the medial canthus, can necessitate early removal of the tube and thus endanger the success of the treatment. A loop in the medial canthus, if untreated, can lead to corneal epithelial defects and ulcers.

Prognosis and Recommendation for Treatment

The **overall prognosis** for congenital lacrimal stenoses is very good,[7] with remission in 90% of cases. For atresias the prognosis is significantly poorer and dependent on the success of surgical reconstruction; however, data on this are not currently available. Simple congenital NLDO has the best prognosis with a spontaneous remission of up to 100% in the first year of life. Probing, silicone intubation, and balloon dilation likewise show very good results. Due to the high rate of spontaneous remission when the clinical course of the disease is uncomplicated, the general recommendation is to postpone surgical intervention until the child is 1 year old and instead perform Crigler massage.[20,32]

After the first year of life probing is recommended as a primary intervention. Primary silicone intubation can be considered in case of narrow lacrimal passage or canalicular strictures.

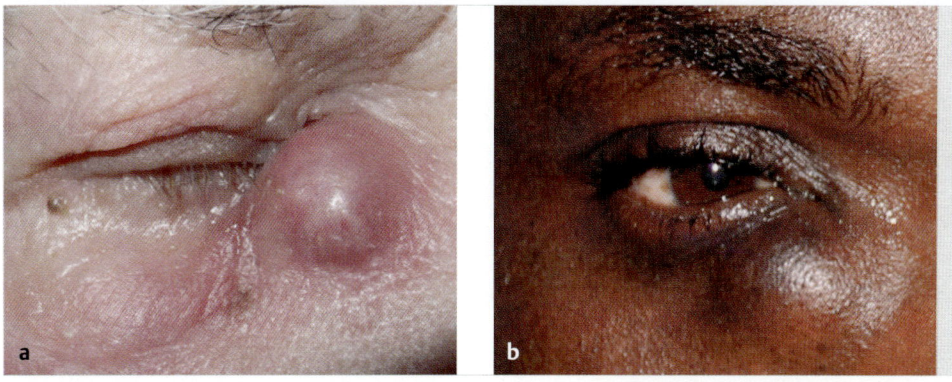

Fig. 15.6 Acute and chronic dacryocystitis. **(a)** Acute dacryocystitis with abscess formation. **(b)** Chronic dacryocystitis with mucocele formation. (Image courtesy of Dr. F. Ngounou, Presbyterian Eye Service, Acha-Bafoussam, Cameroon.)

There may be recurrence despite successful probing and postoperative decongestant measures. Repetition of probing with or without intubation and, if necessary, medialization of the inferior nasal concha is recommended. In our view, balloon dilation can be tried as next choice to avoid a DCR.

With tight NLDs, bilateral stenoses, Down's syndrome, craniofacial dysmorphias, or following acute dacryocystitis, **primary lacrimal duct intubation** should be considered with the primary procedure because in these cases probing alone generally delivers poorer results.[20]

In bony stenosis, repeated re-stenosis, or recurrent dacryocystitis, a **dacryocystorhinostomy** has to be done. As an alternative, from the age of 2 years **endoscopic lacrimal duct surgery** is a newer, more physiological surgical approach.

15.1.4 Acquired Lacrimal Stenoses

Etiology and Pathogenesis

Acquired lacrimal stenoses do not occur only in childhood but can also occur also in adults. The prevalence of symptomatic acquired stenoses is reported in a US cohort study as ~30 per 100,000 inhabitants.[33] Primary or secondary causes for this are **inflammation, infection, neoplasia, trauma**, or **mechanical causes**. In the following paragraph only the most common causes are addressed.

Punctal and canalicular stenoses often occur secondarily to involutional ectropion or chronic blepharitis. Stenosis can also occur in scarring conjunctival diseases, chronic topical treatment (e.g., for glaucoma), following epidemic keratoconjunctivitis and due to chemotherapy (especially breast cancer treated with docetaxel), acid burns, or trauma.[34]

Primary **nasolacrimal duct stenosis** (NLDO) mostly occurs in middle-aged women with an incidence of 20 per 100,000 inhabitants. The primary acquired NLDO is often described as PANDO ("primary acquired nasolacrimal duct obstruction"). Women have a narrower nasolacrimal duct than do men.[35] Postmenopausal hormonal factors appear to cause an alteration in the mucous membrane, which in turn causes the stenosis or occlusion.[36] Secondary NLDO mostly arises in intranasal pathologies (polyps, scarring, tumors) or granulomatous inflammations (sarcoidosis, Wegener's disease), or posttraumatically following mid-face fractures.[37]

Clinical Signs

In most patients canalicular stenoses lead to **epiphora**. NLDO often presents with matting of lashes and mucous or mucopurulent **discharge**. Complications of NLDO include **acute dacryocystitis** (possibly with empyema formation), which may lead to orbital cellulitis or sepsis if left untreated (▶ Fig. 15.6a). Old and immunosuppressed patients are especially at risk.

NLDO in combination with common canalicular block produces an accumulation of trapped mucous in the dilated lacrimal sac, which is termed **mucocele**. An indolent, well-circumscribed swelling without signs of acute inflammation can be seen in the medial canthal angle inferior to the medial canthal tendon (MCT) (▶ Fig. 15.6b).

Treatment

If possible, treatment of secondary stenosis is primarily treatment of the cause (immunosuppressive therapy for granulomatous diseases, reduction of topical glaucoma treatment, and treatment of canaliculitis).

Acute dacryocystitis needs immediate treatment with intravenous antibiotics and, in case of abscess formation, with incision and drainage. This can be carried out with short topical anesthesia (local cold spray) or under general anesthesia. As with most abscesses, it is mandatory to ensure healing from the base of the wound (local application of antibiotic tablets or a tamponade into the abscess cavity). Once healed, **dacryocystorhinostomy** (DCR) should be carried out as soon as possible in order to avert a recurrence.

Punctal and canalicular stenoses can, if necessary, be treated by **slitting** ("punctal snip" operation) or by **trephination and silicone intubation**.

With distal and common canalicular stenoses as well as NLDO, **dacryocystorhinostomy** is a possible therapeutic option.

External Dacryocystorhinostomy (External DCR)

Addeo Toti first described the DCR procedure in 1904. The principle of the surgery is to create a **direct connection between the lacrimal sac and the nasal cavity**, thus enabling lacrimal drainage into the nose, bypassing the nasolacrimal duct. Most authors report a success rate of 90 to 95%. Revision surgery can be done in case of failure.

Indications for external DCR are PANDO, secondary NLDO, persistent CNLDO, mucocele, and chronic dacryocystitis. It can also be indicated in incomplete NLDO or common canalicular block (CCB), or for treatment of functional epiphora in facial nerve palsy (see Chapter 16). The **contraindication** for external DCR is acute dacryocystitis.

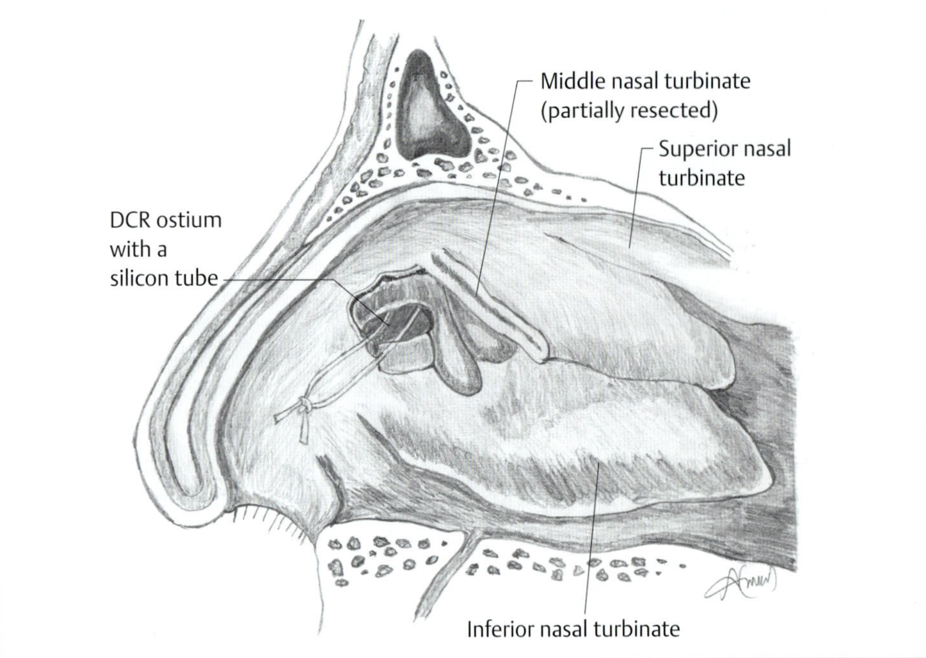

Fig. 15.7 Intranasal localization of the lacrimal sac ostium following dacryocystorhinostomy with silicone tube intubation.

15

▶ **Steps of an External DCR.** The surgery is often performed with general anesthesia, but can also be done under local anesthesia (infraorbital and supratrochlear nerve block, local infiltration of the incision site) with sedation. At the beginning of the surgery, a nasal pack with Moffet's solution is inserted into the nose near the location of the ostium at the insertion of the middle turbinate. Moffet's solution contains epinephrine, cocaine, and bicarbonate as local vasoconstrictors and anesthetics.[31]

The site of the incision is infiltrated with a local anesthetic containing epinephrine 1:200,000. The **incision** is made approximately 3 mm medial to the medial canthus, protecting the angular vein with a slightly bowed course of 10 to 12 mm length. A blunt pair of scissors is now inserted horizontally and the periosteum of the lateral nasal wall is exposed via blunt dissection. Only in some cases is it necessary to separate the anterior part of the MCT for a better view. The **periosteum** can be incised with a scalpel or directly reflected laterally with an elevator, taking the lacrimal sac with it. Now the anterior lacrimal crest and the lacrimal sac fossa are visualized. The **ostium** is initiated inside the fossa with the periosteum elevator. Once the ostium has been initiated, it is extended anteriorly with a bone punch (Kerrison, Citelli), posteriorly by removing the anterior ethmoidal cells, superiorly to about 2 mm above the medial canthus (here the MCT can be a good guide), and inferiorly up to the edge of the bony nasolacrimal canal.[38] The expansion of the ostium superiorly should be done carefully, avoiding the injury of the cribriform plate with consequent **liquorrhea**. A frequently occurring anatomical variant of the ethmoidal cells are the so-called **agger nasi cells**, part of the ethmoid displaced anteriorly between lacrimal sac fossa and nasal cavity. The agger nasi cells can cause pneumatization of the lacrimal bone and the lacrimal process of the maxillary bone. In these cases, during osteotomy a cavity lined with a thin mucosa is encountered, and only after breaking through a second bone is the nasal mucosa seen. In case of doubt, the nose can be probed with a curved artery forceps. The **nasal mucosa** is now infiltrated with local anesthetic and epinephrine and the **lacrimal sac** is tented with a Bowman probe and incised lengthwise. It is important to incise the sac along its entire length as otherwise, although the ostium might be patent, a "**sump syndrome**" (accumulation of secretion in the residual lacrimal sac) can occur. Further incisions are made to fashion anterior and posterior mucous membrane and lacrimal sac flaps. The posterior ones can be excised or anastomosed. If a posterior mucous membrane anastomosis is planned, this is the next step. Thereafter **bicanalicular intubation** can be done with a silicone tube. The tube is introduced into the nose via the ostium and knotted. It is important to ensure that the ends of the mucous membranes that form the anastomosis are adequately apposed and do not collapse into the ostium. The wound is closed in two layers (orbicularis and skin). A **nasal packing** is normally done at the end of the procedure. Postoperatively, topical antibiotics and nasal decongestants are given. The nasal pack is removed on the first or second postoperative day, the skin sutures after a week. The intubation remains in place for 6 weeks to 3 months in most cases; in complicated cases (revision surgery, following dacryocystitis, traumatic NLDO) it can be left for a longer time (▶ Fig. 15.7).

There are numerous variations of the technique described above. The success rate is roughly 80 to 99%.[39] This is more dependent on the experience of the surgeon than on the variation. The use of anterior vs. anterior and posterior mucosal flaps for anastomosis seems to have no influence on the success of the surgery,[40] nor does the intraoperative use of 5-fluoruracil.[41] In some studies, intraoperative use of **mitomycin C** has shown positive effects on keeping the ostium patent and is, where necessary, a possible **adjuvant therapy**, namely in revision DCRs.[42,43] According to a meta-analysis, **silicone intubation** seems to have no influence on the patency of a primary DCR.[44]

Conjunctivodacryocystorhinostomy (CDCR)

CDCR is the creation of a **connection from the conjunctival sac into the nasal cavity** through an external DCR, thereby circumventing the canalicular system. The main indication is **proximal bicanalicular stenosis**. A glass tube (Lester–Jones or Putterman tube) or silicone tube is inserted into the conjunctival sac, exiting in the nasal cavity. The method has a high complication and

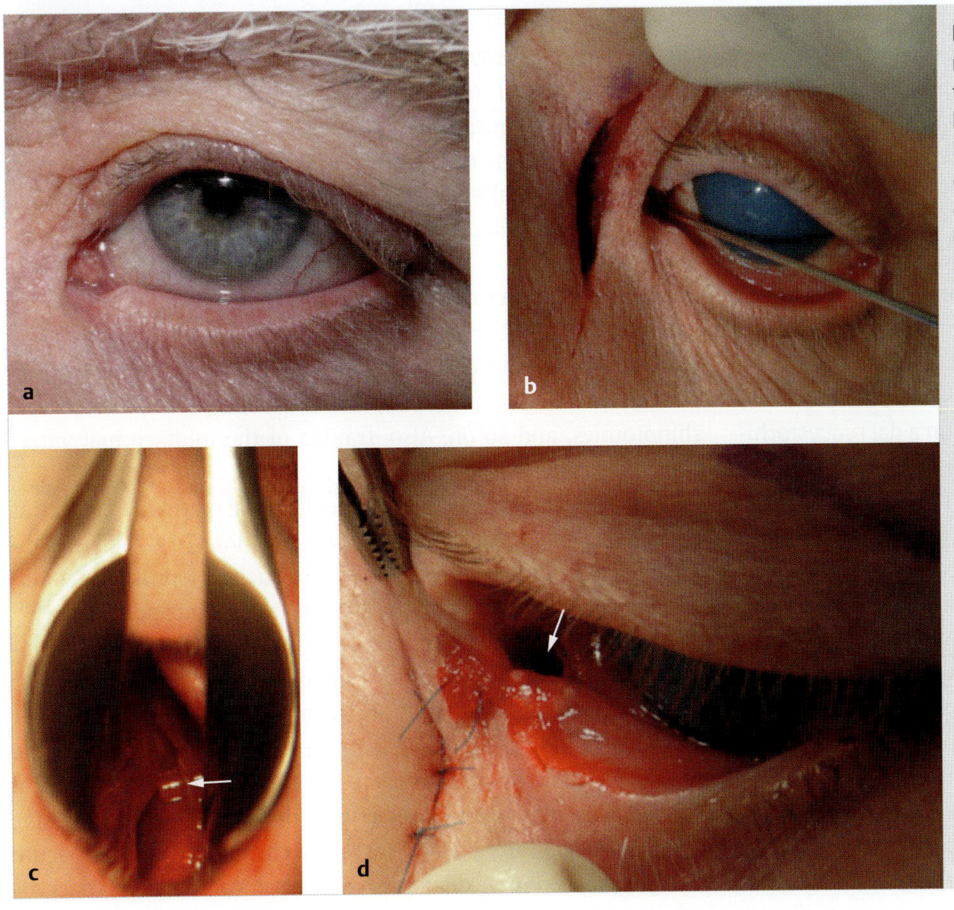

Fig. 15.8 A patient with a posttraumatic bicanalicular stenosis and telecanthus formation following multiple surgical procedures on the lacrimal duct system. Intraoperative picture of a Lester Jones tube (LJT) placement through the dacryocystorhinostomy ostium into the nose. (In collaboration with Dr. L. Bauer, Department of Otorhinolaryngology, Head and Neck Surgery, Nordstadt Clinic, Hannover, Germany.) **(a)** Preoperative clinical view. **(b)** Probing of a placeholder into the nasal cavity. **(c)** Position of the LJT anterior to the attachment of the middle nasal concha without contact with the nasal septum (*arrow*, distal edge of the LJT). **(d)** Tube position in the medial canthus (*arrow*, proximal edge of the LJT).

failure rate and is very intensive in postoperative care for the patient. The surgery is therefore limited to rare indications (▶ Fig. 15.8).

Transcanalicular Endoscopy

Dacryoendoscopy was introduced in the 1990s. Diagnostic endoscopes are flexible and have an external diameter of approximately 0.5 mm; they can have a resolution as high as 6000 pixels. A therapeutic lacrimal endoscope is rigid with two or three working channels and has an external diameter of 0.8 to 1.1 mm. The therapeutic options are briefly described here.

Short canalicular or other stenoses can be opened with a diode laser (**laser dacryoplasty**). So far the reported success rate is up to 81%.[45] A further option is the dilation of stenoses with a microdrill (**microdrill dacryoplasty**).

A pilot study, published in 2012, reports promising results with the **transcanalicular laser DCR**, in which a diode laser is used to create the ostium and a balloon catheter to dilate it[46] (Chapter 15.2).

The advantage of endoscopic lacrimal surgery is the restoration of the original anatomy without disrupting the medial canthus. This method also allows the underlying pathology to be diagnosed by direct visualization. Disadvantages of the procedure so far experienced are increased costs and limited indications.

Complications

A rare complication of **punctoplasty** is an excessive slitting of the puncta. If the opening is too large, the punctum loses its capillary action and a (paradoxical) **functional lacrimal insufficiency** results.

Significant intraoperative complications with **external DCR** are **bleeding, injury to the canaliculi, liquorrhea** due to fracturing of the cribriform plate, and **opening of the periorbita** with the prolapse of orbital fat. With a minor liquorrhea, the site of the fracture can be covered with orbicularis muscle fibers. The patient needs systemic antibiotics. Postoperatively, delayed **bleeding** can occur. In most cases elevated positioning, local cooling, and blood pressure control of the patient are sufficient to stop the bleeding that mostly originates from the nasal mucosa. If necessary, the nose has to be repacked. Nasal endoscopy with visualization of the source and cauterization are rarely necessary. Delayed complications of the external DCR are possible **fistula formation**, mainly in early surgery following acute dacryocystitis or after local radiotherapy, as well as **complications of the silicone intubation** (see above). The most common complication is **failure of the surgery** due to closure of the ostium. Reasons include a small bony ostium, secondary common canalicular stenosis, or scarring inside the nose (septal deviation or spur and hypertrophy of the middle nasal turbinate being predisposing factors). For this reason, nasal endoscopy for preoperative evaluation has to be carried out in all cases before an external DCR. An **epicanthus** in the area of the incision can be corrected with a Z-plasty (Chapter 16).

15.2 Endoscopic Dacryocystorhinostomy

Andreas Neumann, Mauricio López-Chacón, and Manuel Bernal-Sprekelsen

15.2.1 Introduction

Epiphora is the main symptom when problems arise along the pathway drainage of the lacrimal system. Accumulation of tears

15

leads to blurred vision. The differential diagnosis of epiphora is key for a correct indication of a surgical solution. Overproduction of tears can be temporary under certain emotional conditions; irritation or inflammation of the conjunctiva may also increase the tear production, but the assessment is pretty obvious. Alterations of the drainage pathways may be produced by changes of the pumping mechanism or by obstruction of the pathways at different anatomical levels. Thus, one has to distinguish between a proximal stenosis (presaccal) at the lacrimal punctum, at the superior or inferior canaliculus, or at the common canaliculus, and an obstruction of the lacrimal sac itself (saccal stenosis), as well as a distal stenosis (postsaccal) in the nasolacrimal duct.

In cases of a saccal and postsaccal obstruction a dacryocystorhinostomy (DCR) can solve the problem of epiphora or of chronic dacryocystitis. The principles of a DCR consist in a broad opening ("-ostomy") of the lacrimal sac ("dacryocysto-") into the nasal fossa ("-rhino-"). To achieve this, the bone medially to the sac needs to be removed and the sac has to be incised or its medial wall be removed.

The horizontal aspect of the lacrimal pathways (canaliculi) are not reached by an endoscopic approach. Thus, presaccal stenosis is not suitable for solving saccal or postsaccal stenosis. Nonetheless, an endoscopic DCR is not a formal contraindication for a presaccal obstruction. Here, the DCR might facilitate the later insertion of a Lester–Jones tube (a small tube, crystal-like in appearance, overcoming the presaccal stenosis by forming communication between the inferior lacrimal punctum and the inner orifice of the common canaliculus, or inserted at the inner angle of the conjunctiva into the lacrimal sac). Without prior resection of the bony medial wall this could not be achieved.[47]

15.2.2 Etiology of Obstructions of the Lacrimal Pathways

During adulthood, chronic dacryocystitis with acute flare-ups—which may even produce an abscess of the sac—is among the most frequent causes of stenosis. In childhood the failure to open or delayed/insufficient opening of the Hasner valve is a common cause of epiphora. Many newborns suffer from an obstruction of the lacrimal pathways, which later resolves spontaneously during their first months of life. The incidence of these basically membranous stenoses of the nasolacrimal duct is around 25 to 50%[48]; that of incomplete stenosis as much as 50 to 70%.[49] The rate of a spontaneous resolution during the first months of life is of about 85%.[12] Thus, the indication of an endoscopic DCR in newborns is to be approached conservatively. True malformations of the lacrimal pathway in children are usually associated with craniofacial malformations.[50,51] Nevertheless, chronic epiphora, congenital dacryoceles, and posttraumatic or postinflammatory obstructions remain clear indications for a surgical opening of the lacrimal sac. Prior probing of the pathways, which may open a small (membranous) obstruction is indicated, as it may sometimes avoid surgery. As in children general anesthesia or at least sedation is needed, prior consent for a DCR should be obtained in case the probing is not successful. Even in cases of a rare agenesis of the inferior lacrimal punctum, good results can be obtained with a DCR.[52] Because of the high rate of spontaneous resolution in children and the narrow anatomical conditions, it is recommended not to indicate a DCR before the age of 12 months.[51]

Women are more prone to suffer from drainage problems of the lacrimal pathway then are men. A hypothesis to explain this could be the use of cosmetic products over decades, which would induce a chronic unspecific irritation of the lacrimal sac. A histologic study of the medial wall of the lacrimal sac of Arabic women using "kol" as a make-up on the cheeks could find "kol" in the lacrimal sac, surrounded by a chronic unspecific inflammatory reaction.[53]

Lesions of the lacrimal pathways can be produced during surgical procedures of the nose and paranasal sinuses, such as lateral osteotomies during a rhinoplasty, middle meatal antrostomies performed too far anteriorly, Caldwell–Luc procedures, lateral rhinotomies, and so on. Also, trauma of the midface may interrupt the pathways.[54]

Other diseases may involve the lacrimal pathways: such as allergies, chronic rhinosinusitis, viral infections (e.g., herpes simplex[55]), or more rare specific infections such as leprosy, sarcoidosis, tuberculosis, Wegener disease, or rhinosporidiosis.[56,57] Finally, tumors infiltrating the area, radiotherapy, and chemotherapy with 5-FU[58] may induce stenosis.

A facial palsy is a frequent functional cause of epiphora.

A typical indication for DCR in those situations in which the drainage pathways are obstructed at the level of the sac (saccal stenosis) or along the nasolacrimal duct (postsaccal stenosis). These situations are given in cases of a chronic or recurrent acute dacryocystitis, when dilatation of the sac can be seen (dacryocele) or when a stone formation (dacryolythiasis) can be proven radiologically.

> **Memorize** M!
>
> Stenosis of the lacrimal pathways in adults is usually due to chronic dacryocystitis; in children there is delayed opening of the Hasner valve or a malformation is present. A wait-and-see policy is advised in children.

15.2.3 Preoperative Diagnosis

All potential causes of obstruction should be excluded. An interdisciplinary approach (Ophthalmology and ENT) is recommended.

The duration of epiphora and clinical history, particularly acute recurrent or chronic dacryocystitis, has to be elicited. The latter often leaves a scar at the inner angle of the eye; if there is retention of pus or mucous in the sac, a protrusion may be visible or palpable.

Considering the close anatomical relationships in the nose and paranasal sinuses, it is the task of the rhinologist to exclude potential causes of obstruction by of rhinoscopy, endoscopy, and, if needed, radiologically. Also, there are some anatomical conditions, such as septal deviation, agger nasi cells, chronic rhinosinusitis, or hyperplastic turbinates, that may play a role in the obstruction, or pathologic situations that may induce recurrent stenosis after surgery, such as tumors or previous surgery (Caldwell–Luc, etc.). In around 20% of the DCR there is indication for additional corrections within the nose to reach the lacrimal sac.[59]

During the clinical inspection it has to be checked whether the lacrimal punctum is in contact with the conjunctiva. In patients with facial palsy or with ectropium of the lower lid the secondary lagophthalmos prevents the tears to drain through the inferior lacrimal punctum, producing pseudo epiphora. Overproduction of tears can be assessed with Schirmer's test.

Further exploration aims at the differential diagnosis between presaccal and saccal or postsaccal stenosis. This is key for a correct indication of DCR and to obtain good results thereafter.

Preoperative probing of the superior/inferior canaliculus and the common canaliculus can confirm or rule out a stenosis at this level, allowing differentiation between a presaccal and saccal or a postsaccal stenosis. Simultaneous irrigation with saline solution of fluorescein dye (Jones's test) can be helpful to assess the permeability. The probing can be performed during an ophthalmologic exploration or a radiological assessment (dacryocystography) of the lacrimal system. However, as dacryocystography implies a prior probing of the proximal pathway in order to inject the contrast material, this probing can already confirm or exclude a potential stenosis at precisely this level, rendering the dacryocystography redundant. In our clinical routine, dacryocystography has become obsolete. In any case, a dilated lacrimal sac shown in the dacryocystography has a positive prognostic value on the long-term result after DCR.[60,61] An alternative radiologic approach can be performed when probing with a balloon catheter. Here, a saccal or postsaccal stenosis may be dilated to solve the drainage problems. DCR can then be indicated should the epiphora still persist.[62]

Computed tomography and other imaging techniques are indicated for revision DCR, for example, after midface trauma, or when there is a suspicion of tumor but usually not as routine exploration for epiphora or dacryocystitis.

> **Memorize**
>
> Clinical history, inspection, and exploration together with probing (±irrigation) of the lacrimal pathways are diagnostic keys to assessing the level of obstruction. Further diagnostic tools may be indicated in particular cases. In around 20% of cases additional changes of the nose and/or paranasal sinuses need to be addressed as well (e.g., septal deviation).

15.2.4 Surgical Technique of DCR

Over a century ago, two surgical approaches had been developed in parallel for Ophthalmology and ENT: the external approach of Toti[63] and the endonasal one described West.[64] Recent technological developments have allowed the incorporation of so-called minimally invasive techniques, such as the transcanalicular or endoluminal, the endoscopic, and the balloon dilation procedures.[45,65] The endonasal approach (which should more correctly be called **rhinodacryocystostomy**) offers some advantages:

- Preservation of the whole attachment of the lacrimal system (which preserves the pumping mechanism) and of the trochlea by retaining all structures around the horizontal pathways, including the medial palpebral ligament.
- The possibility of carrying out the surgery even in cases of acute infection of the sac (drainage into an already contaminated nasal cavity; no risk of thrombosis of the vena angularis as no external incision is performed).
- No external scar.

The endonasal approach can be performed under the microscope, as described by Hans Heermann in 1958,[66] or endoscopically.[67,68] Nowadays, endoscopic DCR is being described as the "gold standard" for the treatment of saccal and postsaccal stenosis.[69] The surgical steps are very similar, independently of the optical tools employed (Video 15.1).

Perioperative antibiotics are not needed.[70,71] The fact that anticoagulation therapy can be continued was confirmed by observations of Smith[72,73,74] in 9 patients operated under warfarin and in 40 patients under ASS. The surgical procedure is usually performed under general anesthesia, but can also be done under local.

Neurosurgical cottonoids soaked in topical anesthesia and vasoconstrictor (epinephrine 1:100.000) are kept in the nasal fossa for around 15 minutes to achieve anesthesia of the mucosa at the anterior septum, the lateral nasal wall, and the anterior aspect of the middle turbinate. For interventions under local anesthesia, anesthetics have to be injected into the frontal nerves and the external nasal wall. Additional sedation is recommended, particularly immediately before incising the lacrimal sac, as its full anesthesia is difficult when an acute inflammation or infection is present. Other measures to improve the exposure include the trimming of the head of the middle turbinate or a (mini)septoplasty in cases of a high deviation at the level of the agger nasi.

The lacrimal sac can be localized laterally to the ascending process of the maxillary bone (which corresponds to the agger nasi). This bone can have several millimeter in thickness.

The posterior edge of the ascending process is the so-called "linea maxillaris", right in front of the anterior edge of the uncinate process. Introducing one branch of a bayoneted forceps into the nose while pointing the other branch at the lacrimal puncti helps to identify the area of dissection. If available, probing with small cold-light optical fibers can be helpful to identify the lacrimal sac itself. However, this technique may conduce to errors (see below). The regular anterior removal of the uncinate process, as advocated elsewhere,[75] for a better exposure of the sac is not needed according to our experience.

Two vertical incisions about 1 cm apart through the mucoperiosteum and down to the bone are made on the agger nasi (▶ Fig. 15.9). A Beaver or a Montserrat knife is adequate for the incision. A monopolar Colorado needle can keep the bleeding low. The posterior incision lies on the linea maxillaris, right in front of the uncinate process. Connecting both incisions cranially allows the creation of an inferiorly based flap, which is dissected subperiostially toward the inferior turbinate (▶ Fig. 15.10). The length of the flap is between 1.5 and 2 cm. Following the recommendations of Massegur et al[76] this flap is repositioned at the end of the surgery to cover the exposed lateral nasal wall (see ▶ Fig. 15.18). Sometimes the flap needs to be shortened slightly to avoid closure of the opened sac and the common canaliculus, although in most cases the flap undergoes shrinkage that makes its trimming unnecessary. We formerly resected this flap. However, it was observed preserving it to cover denuded areas effective reduced blood clot crusting, fibrin exudation, and granulation tissue formation, thus shortening the postoperative healing period. Uncovered areas at the lateral nasal wall are more prone to produce ecchymosis in the cheek and emphysema.[53] To obtain a good patency it is important to remove the bone superiorly and to conduct the incision of the lacrimal sac so as to widely expose

15

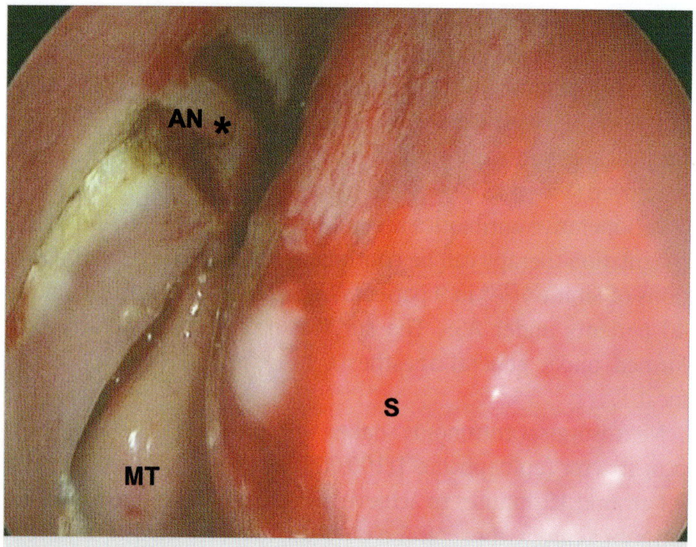

Fig. 15.9 DCR of the right side. Creation of an inferiorly based mucoperiosteal flap of 1 cm width on the ascending process of the maxilla. Cranially, the flap reaches the insertion of the middle turbinate (MT) and is partially resected there (*). S, septum. AN, agger nasi.

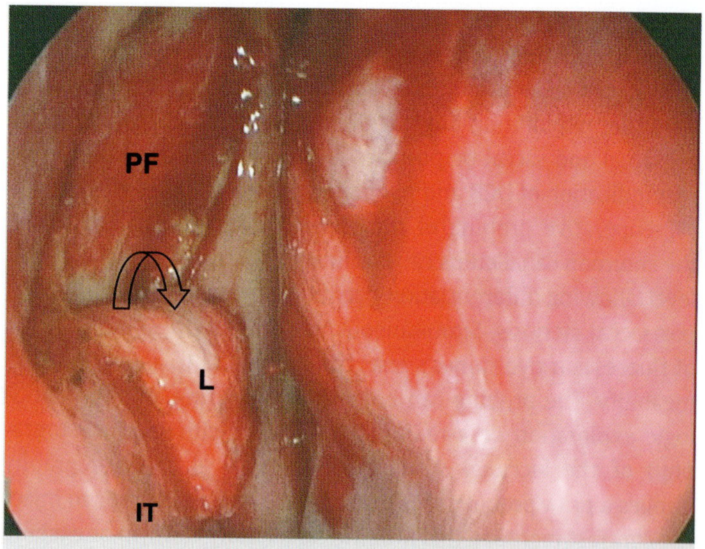

Fig. 15.10 The inferiorly based flap (L) is pushed downwards onto the inferior turbinate (IT). Submucoperiosteal dissection is key to preserving the flap. It also exposes the underlying bone.

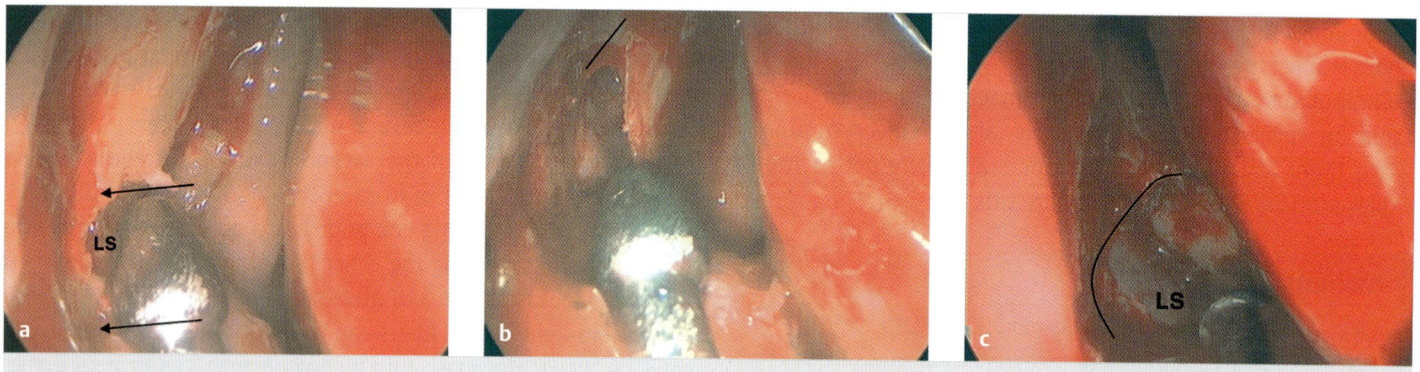

Fig. 15.11 **(a)** The posterior edge of the ascending process of the maxilla (called the "maxillary line") is approached with a 90° Kerrison rongeur to first detach the lacrimal sac (LS). Then, the inferior third is removed anteriorly (*arrows*). **(b)** Next, the ascending process is removed laterally and superiorly with a 45° Kerrison rongeur (*line*). **(c)** Due to leverage forces, the frontal process (FP) gets broken and the sac (LS) is exposed.

15

the common canaliculus. Removing the bone cranially prevents that area acting as a scaffold for potential obliterative scarring.

The ascending process of the maxilla can be resected from the maxillary line anteriorly (▶ Fig. 15.11). The Kerrison rongeurs (90° and 45°) may serve when that bone is thin enough. With the 90° rongeur positioned right behind the maxillary line the bone is resected anteriorly. The 45° rongeur is worked superiorly and as laterally as possible along the ascending process until the superior third of the sac is exposed, which is where the common canaliculus drains (▶ Fig. 15.12). If the ascending process is very thick, prior drilling with a diamond burr allows partial exposure of the sac, which can be then completed with the Kerrison. Care must be taken not to catch the mucoperiosteal flap with the burr. Should there be doubts about the right location of the sac at this stage, then probing through the inferior canaliculus will bulge its mucosa. Soft tissues of the cheek may be exposed if the bone is removed too far anteriorly. One may palpate the cheek from outside to identify the soft tissue.

The thin lacrimal bone lies lateral and posterior to the ascending process of the maxilla. This explains why probing with a small cold-light fiber might disorientate the surgeon when the bony structures are still preserved, as the light would transilluminate through the thin lacrimal bone, which corresponds to the most posterior aspect of the sac, right in front of the orbit.

A bony septation between the sac and the orbit may be missing; thus, opening of the periorbita can occur in 10 to 15% of cases.[53] The use of hammer and chisel has been described by some authors.[77,78,79] These must be employed very carefully, as the chisel has to be directed in the direction of the orbit.

Once the sac has been exposed, its medial wall is incised (▶ Fig. 15.13). It is important to have a helping "third hand" stabilizing the sac from outside by exerting pressure on the inner angle of the eye. This prevents the sac being displaced laterally while it is being incised. The incision can be made with an angled Beaver knife or a phaco knife. Inflamed sacs may have thickened walls that may render the incision incomplete or superficial. We prefer a full resection of the medial wall to enable a large drainage and to allow study of the specimens histopathologically (▶ Fig. 15.14). Such histopathologic study is advised to rule out other diseases, such as aspergilloma, inverted papilloma, granulomatosis, or malignant tumors.[62,80,81] Alternative techniques have been described that preserve the medial aspect of the sac,

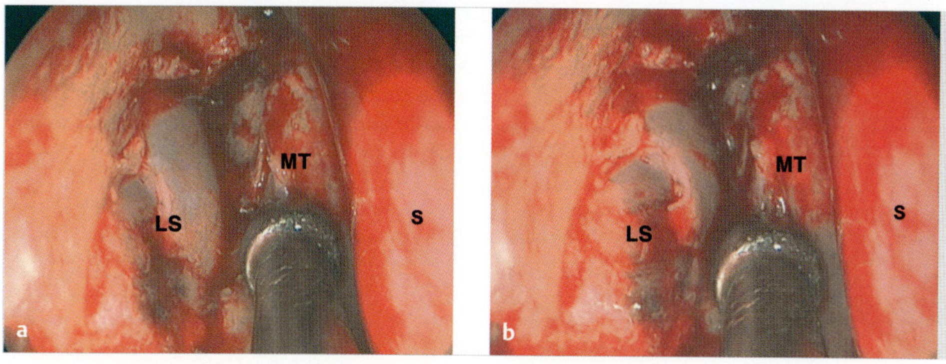

Fig. 15.12 The superior third of the lacrimal sac is exposed, as the common canaliculus drains there. Panel **(a)** shows the exposed sac (LS) right in front of the middle turbinate (MT). **(b)** The lacrimal sac is compressed from outside (at the level of the inner canthal area) in order to avoid a lateralization during its incision. S, septum.

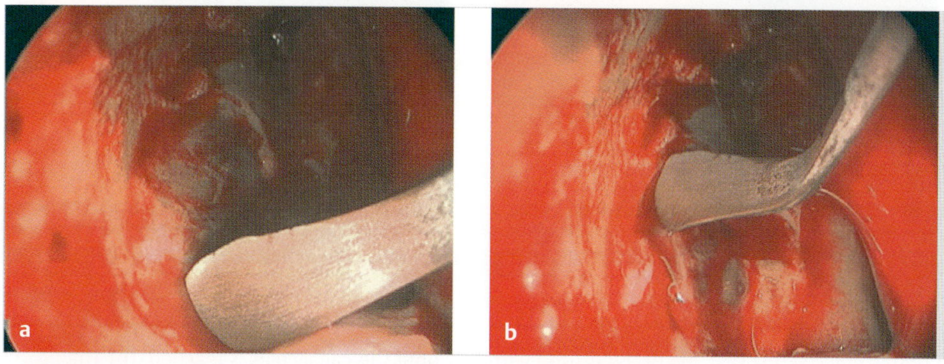

Fig. 15.13 (a, b) The lacrimal sac is incised with an angled phaco-knife from inferiorly to superiorly. Meanwhile, the external pressure has to be maintained on the sac to avoid its lateralization.

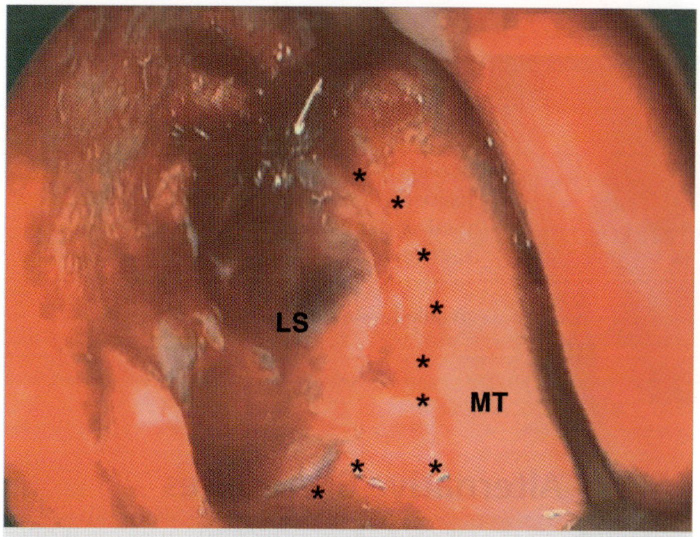

Fig. 15.14 The sac (LS) is now opened like a book (*), its medial aspect toward the middle turbinate (MT). Depending on the surgical technique, the medial aspect of the sac can be resected (our preference) or displaced posteriorly to be adapted with the mucosa of the uncinate process.

creating a flap attached to surrounding mucosa to maintain patency.[76]

Both canaliculi are now probed with a silicone catheter (▶ Fig. 15.15, ▶ Fig. 15.16). Probing must be performed smoothly to avoid a "via falsa." It can be checked endoscopically whether both ends leave the common canaliculus (▶ Fig. 15.17). Probing and leaving the silicone catheter seem to have little influence on the final outcome (see below). However, it facilitates the follow-up and particularly the removal of fibrin exudations and crusts by simply following the silicone and avoiding touching the opened lacrimal sac, as this is painful.

The silicone probes can be fixed on or knotted inside the nose. We prefer to fix them on the nose, as this allows us to conduct the probes toward the septum while avoiding burying them below the mucoperiosteal flap. The silicone probe should not contact the conjunctiva avoiding irritations and subsequent foreign body reaction or lesions of the conjunctiva. Also, it has to leave enough free movement to open the eyelids completely. Knotted or clipped probes can be left in the middle meatus. This is particularly helpful in children,[52] to avoid manipulations.

Sometimes, probing of the smaller superior canaliculus is not possible, particularly in children. In such a situation the silicone probe can be introduced in only the inferior canaliculus. As this may be badly tolerated by children, it has to be evaluated whether probing is needed or can be skipped.

Finally, the mucoperiosteal flap is repositioned covering the previously denuded bone (▶ Fig. 15.18). Usually, packing is not needed. The repositioned mucosal flap can be fixed with resorbable material or a small piece of PVA sponge. A loose application of ointment can be used as well.

DCR in children is demanding and can be challenging due to the narrowness of working simultaneously with an endoscope and a burr. The bone is worked preferably with 1-mm 90° and 45° Kerrison rongeurs. The exposure is similar to that in adults,[76,82] but slightly more anteriorly as described by Veiss-Claus-Güttich.

Memorize

M!

The endoscopic approach is the "gold standard" for DCR. Endoscopic localization of the sac is essential to avoid lesions of the cheek or the orbit.

Surgical principles are essentially resection of the ascending process of the maxilla and of the medial aspect of the lacrimal sac. Wide exposure of the superior third enables the patency of the drainage of the common canaliculus. Prior dissection of a caudally based mucoperiosteal flap allows the covering of denuded areas and eases and shortens the healing process.

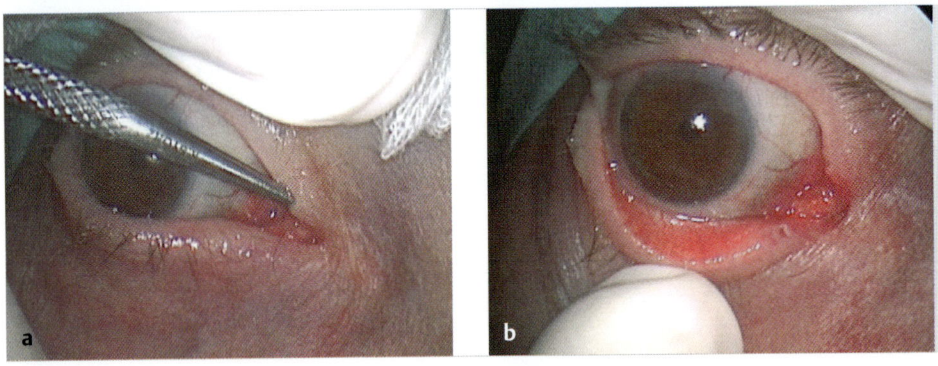

Fig. 15.15 (a, b) Both lacrimal puncti are now dilated with a Castroviejo dilator. The Bowmann probe confirms the permeability of the inferior, superior and common canaliculi. Care has to be taken to avoid damage to the cornea.

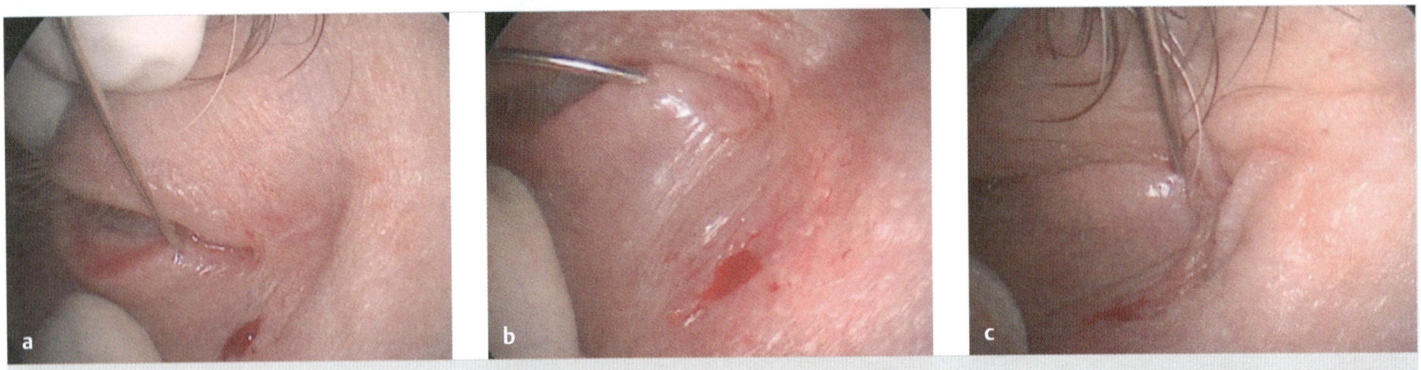

Fig. 15.16 A silicone probe is introduced through both canaliculi. **(a)** First the probe is used vertically until the canaliculus is reached. **(b)** Then the probe goes horizontally into the common canaliculus into the lacrimal sac. **(c)** Next the probe is used vertically again to enter the nasal fossa. Dilation and probing must be performed smoothly to avoid a "via falsa."

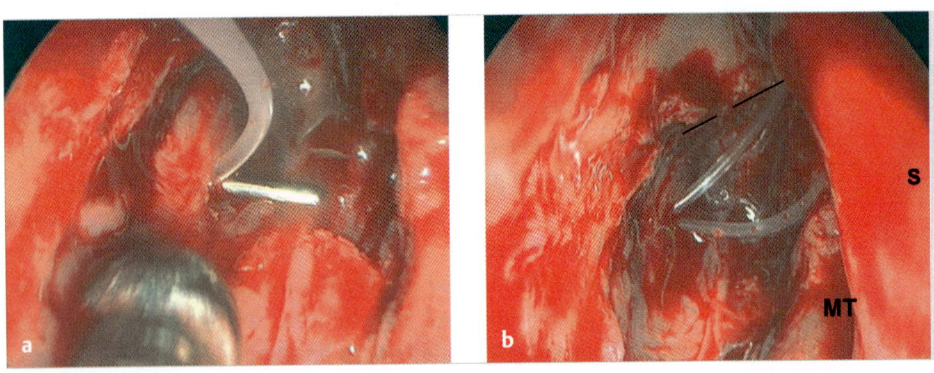

Fig. 15.17 Panel **(a)** shows the horizontal probing of the sac. A Blakesley forceps grasps the probe and pulls it out of the nose. Panel **(b)** displays the level of bone resection superiorly (*black dashed line*) to fully expose the superior third of the sac with its common canaliculus. Note in **(a)** and **(b)** that both ends of the silicone probe leave the common canaliculus. MT, middle turbinate. S, septum.

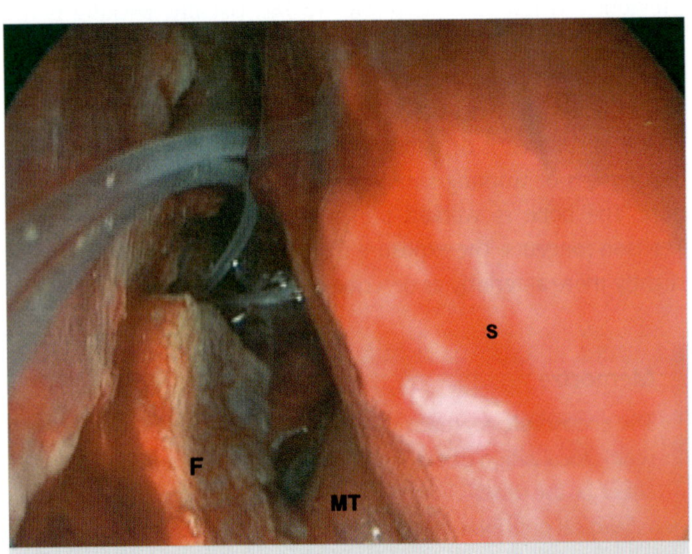

Fig. 15.18 Shows the situation after reposition of the inferiorly based flap (F). Thanks to the initial trimming of the flap cranially, the opening of the sac remains patent. A small resorbable packing keeps the flap onto the lateral wall. Care has to be taken not to leave the silicone probes under the flap. Covering the lateral wall again with mucosa speeds up the healing process and reduces granulation tissue formation. MT, middle turbinate. S, septum.

15.2.5 Alternative Procedures

The availability of very small endoscopes allows transcanalicular, endoluminal surgery (overview in[45]; see Chapter 15.1).

Balloon dilation under radiographic control has been available since 1989.[65] However, in most centers it is not the first choice, even though from the results it seems to achieve rates up to 92%.[83] The results after introduction of a polyurethane stent[84] are rated as bad or very bad.[85,86]

Opening of the sac with different types of **lasers** seems to provide better hemostasis. However, it induces a higher fibroblastic activity and subsequent scarring.[87] The results vary in the literature and are even contradictory. Most authors report a worse patency rate than with nonlaser DCR.[71,87,88,89,90]

The use of **ultrasonic bone aspirators** (Sonsopet) instead of a drill has been reported to show good results.[91]

Local application of Mitomycin C to avoid excessive scarring and re-stenosis has repeatedly been reported without a clear advantage.[71,92] No long-term positive effect on the patency has been observed after intranasal application.[92]

In order to avoid a DCR in **children** it has been recommended to probe and rinse the lacrimal pathway, and to perform an endoscopic intranasal incision of the Hasner valve with rinsing.[93] The advantages are not clear, particularly because a general anesthesia is needed and because it is technically demanding to identify the Hasner valve endoscopically. Additionally, causes beyond the Hasner valve can be overlooked and obliterative scarring after the procedure cannot be excluded. The same applies for the nasolacrimal intubation, with which Aggarwal et al[94] avoided DCR in 25 of 28 children.

15.2.6 Follow-up

Similarly to endoscopic surgery, there is little evidence about the effects of different modalities of follow-up. The following recommendation may be adapted individually:

Vasoconstrictors may be applied during the early days. If pus was found in the sac, eye drops containing antibiotics (e.g., gentamycin) may be prescribed. Some authors basically prescribe eye drops with steroids and antibiotics.

PVA sponge can be left inside for about 6 days, as it keeps the mucosal flap on the lateral wall. When the packing is being removed it has to be rotated to avoid tangential detachment of the flap. On the right side the rotation has to be performed clockwise, on the left counterclockwise. Recent experiences without any packing do not show a worse outcome. As after endoscopic sinus surgery, rinsing with saline solution is recommended.

Fibrin exudations and crusts can be removed once per week, when needed. The silicone probe can then be followed endoscopically up to the common canaliculus, avoiding painful manipulations of the sac itself. Type and frequency of the follow-up are addressed differently by different authors. Rosique López et al[95] did not note any difference in the outcome 24 months after laser-assisted DCR whether they had scheduled a follow-up once or 4 to 6 times within the first 6 months after surgery.

To avoid emphysema, blowing the nose should be avoided for around 10 days. Also, when the patient is sneezing the mouth should be opened to avoid emphysema formation.

15.2.7 Stenting

Varying recommendations have been made for the duration of maintenance of the stenting, from up to 6 months to not at all. If the knotted stent is well tolerated it can be left until the healing process is finalized. Arguments again stenting are formation of granulation tissue, infection,[96] damage to the canaliculi, granulation tissue formation around the common canaliculus, dislocation, discomfort of the patient, cost, and the need for crust removal around the stent and for removal. Randomized controlled studies did not show any advantage for stenting.[97,98,99,100] Also, a meta-analysis of 5 randomized and 4 cohort studies did not show any positive effect of stenting, although it was indicated that a larger prospective study was needed.[44] But it can also be argued that stenting has no negative influence on the outcome. Chong et al[101] did not observe any difference in the formation of granulation tissue with and without a stent. Chan and Selva[102] described a shrinking of the ostium in about 35% 12 months after endonasal DCR, although this did not correlate with a bad outcome.

In our practice we leave the stent in for around 8 to 14 days.

> **Memorize** M!
>
> Postoperative stenting with a silicone probe is handled in various ways. There is no evidence for advantages or disadvantages of stenting.

15.2.8 Complications

Overall, complications after DCR are rare[53] and not threatening. Usually they do not need a specific treatment.

Ecchymosis

Bleeding (as well as emphysema, see below) into the soft tissue of the cheek may occur as the lateral wall of the nose has been partially removed and the resection may have been too far anteriorly. In these cases bleeding can already happen during surgery, specifically because at the anterior aspect of the inflamed sac the arteries are larger. Bleeding into the orbit is possible when additional surgery of the paranasal sinuses has been performed. Small hematomas of the eyelids were described in around 12.5%.[76]

Epistaxis

Epistaxis is rather a complication of surgery at the turbinates and/or the anterior ethmoid. Fayet et al[103] reported small bleeding in 60.6%, moderate bleeding in 27.3%, and severe bleeding in 11.6% of cases when the uncinate process had simultaneously been removed. Dolman et al[104] observed bleeding that needed packing in 5.5%. Other authors report a much lower incidence of severe bleeding, below 1%.[105] The "hammer-and-chisel" technique seems to produce little tendency to bleed.[77]

Treatment of epistaxis is carried out as after endoscopic surgery of the paranasal sinuses.

Lesions of the Orbit

Occasionally, the sac is located more posteriorly, directly in front of the orbit or even without any bony barrier intervening. In such situations incision of the sac may also involve the periorbita: the orbital fat will then protrude. No emphysema need be expected so long as the patient avoids blowing the nose. Prophylactic antibiotics should be prescribed if the sac contains pus. Bleeding into the orbit is a potential risk but has not yet been described in the literature. One case of a temporary diplopia was described after accidental intraoperative touching of the medial rectus muscle.[104]

Synechia

Scarring between the middle turbinate and the lateral nasal wall is observed in around 20% of cases. Fortunately, this is not automatically linked to new epiphora or obstruction of the sinuses and the need to transect synechiae is confined to few cases.

Emphysema

When blowing the nose or when sneezing with the mouth closed, air may enter the soft tissue of the cheek during the first week after surgery. Resorption of the air is rapidly progressive and the emphysema disappears quickly. No specific treatment is needed, but it is better to prevent emphysema.

An increasing number of patients are being fitted with CPAP masks due to obstructive sleep apnea. After DCR this may lead to regurgitation of air bubbles through the lacrimal puncti.[106] This can be prevented with a change from a nasal to a facial mask.

Displacement of the Stent

Silicone stents that have been knotted inside the nose can become displaced when sneezing or blowing the nose, showing through the lacrimal puncti. It is better then to remove the probe, as it is highly probable that the problem will recur. Unknotted silicone stents or those fixed at the dorsum of the nose can also become displaced or may even accidentally be removed by the patient. In any case, it is not necessary to reposition the stent as there are no differences in the outcomes (see above).

Lesion of the Nasal Vestibule

When the drill is being used to remove the ascending process of the maxillary bone, care must be taken not to heat up the skin at the entrance of the nose.

Others

Blowing the nose may produce air bubbles at the lacrimal puncti. It has no consequences at all and shows that the DCR has been successful.

Complications at the punctum, such as granulations or cyst formation, or synechia formation between both lacrimal puncti, are infrequent.[107]

Formation of granulation tissue around the inner ostium of the common canaliculus has been described in 17.5% of cases.[53,107] Topical steroids (nasal spray and eye drops) are indicated, particularly if these granulations become symptomatic. The stent is a potential source of the granulation tissue and thus should be removed.

> **Memorize** M!
>
> Complications after DCR are rare and usually minor. Main complications, such as bleeding, lesions of the orbit, emphysema, and displacement of stents can be avoided with a careful surgical technique and can easily be treated when they occur.

15.2.9 Results

Outcome measures after endoscopic DCR are patency of the lacrimal after probing, rinsing, application of fluorescent dye, or imaging. The patient's subjective impression of having got rid of the epiphora is another criterion.

Functional results after endonasal and external DCR are comparable.[71,88,89,108,109] Only the laser-assisted DCR (instead of the use of a burr) shows a worse outcome in a meta-analysis than an external approach (see above). The rate of long-term patent dacryocystorhinostomies, and the associated very good and good subjective results, is 85 to 95% and above.[60,69,110,111,112] This is also reflected in studies on the quality of postoperative life.[113] Endoscopic endonasal techniques seems to show better results than nonendoscopic approaches, although the results using the binocular microscope seem to match the endoscopic technique.[66,79,114,115]

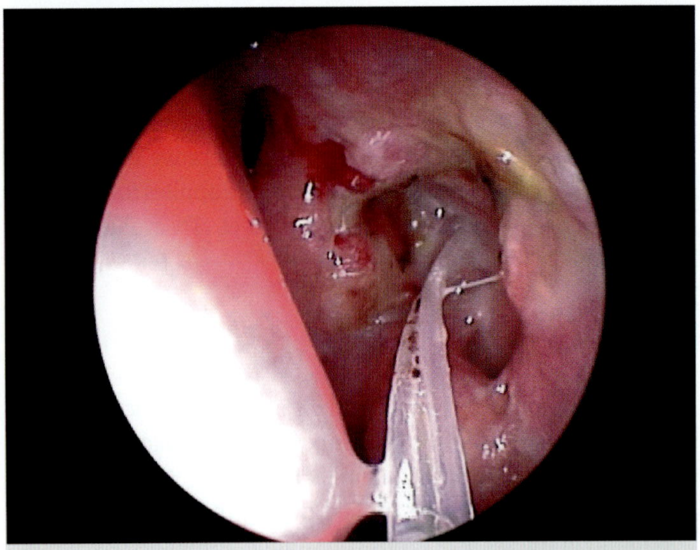

Fig. 15.19 "Lacrimal sump syndrome". The preserved inferior aspect of the opened sac may still produce mucus, which then may block the drainage superiorly. Repeated external massage of the inner canthus with the finger can help to drain mucus accumulation in the remnant sac.

In children the surgical procedure is more demanding because of the narrow spaces. Nevertheless, as in adults, the results show a patency rate above 85%.[51,52,82,116] Only when a craniofacial malformation or a syndromic disease is present does the success rates seem to drop.[117,118]

Recurrent epiphora may be experienced due to retractile scarring or because not enough bone of the ascending process of the maxilla was removed superiorly (around the common canaliculus). The latter may then serve as a scaffold for ingrowing fibroblasts. Insufficient exposure of the lacrimal sac is the most frequent cause of failure after DCR.[119] Also, insufficient resection of the medial wall of the sac or irregular margins may be the basis of an obliterative scarring and re-stenosis. Eye drops containing antibiotics and steroid can be prescribed for 4 to 6 weeks, as well as nasal topical steroids to reduce the tendency to scarring.

True recurrences need to be differentiated from the so-called "lacrimal sump syndrome" (▶ Fig. 15.19)[120]: the common canaliculus can become blocked due to the accumulation of mucous in the inferiorly located remnant sac. Soft external massage of the internal canthus of the eye can help to empty the remnant sac. Revision surgery is not indicated.

In summary, endoscopic endonasal DCR is an effective treatment of saccal and postsaccal stenosis of the lacrimal pathways with few complications.

References

[1] Forrester JV. The Eye: Basic Sciences in Practice. 2nd ed. Edinburgh, Scotland; New York, NY: WB Saunders; 2002

[2] Yazici B, Yazici Z. Frequency of the common canaliculus: a radiological study. Arch Ophthalmol. 2000; 118(10):1381–1385

[3] Hartikainen J, Aho HJ, Seppä H, Grenman R. Lacrimal bone thickness at the lacrimal sac fossa. Ophthalmic Surg Lasers. 1996; 27(8):679–684

[4] Cohen AJ, Brazzo BG, Mercandetti M. The Lacrimal System: Diagnosis, Management, and Surgery. New York, NY: Springer; 2006: xx

[5] Thale A, Paulsen F, Kohla G, Schauer R, Rochels R, Tillmann B. [The efferent lacrimal ducts of the human. Morphological and biochemical studies]. [Article in German]. Ophthalmologe. 2001; 98(1):67–73

[6] Noda S, Hayasaka S, Setogawa T. Congenital nasolacrimal duct obstruction in Japanese infants: its incidence and treatment with massage. J Pediatr Ophthalmol Strabismus. 1991; 28(1):20–22

[7] Bashour M. Congenital anomalies of the nasolacrimal duct. MedScape Reference [Internet]. 2012. Available at: http://emedicine.medscape.com/article/1210252. Accessed Sptemebr 1, 2016

[8] MacEwen CJ, Young JD. Epiphora during the first year of life. Eye (Lond). 1991; 5(Pt 5):596–600

[9] Stephen E, Dickson J, Kindley AD, Scott CC, Charleton PM. Surveillance of vision and ocular disorders in children with Down syndrome. Dev Med Child Neurol. 2007; 49(7):513–515

[10] Fimiani F, Iovine A, Carelli R, Pansini M, Sebastio G, Magli A. Incidence of ocular pathologies in Italian children with Down syndrome. Eur J Ophthalmol. 2007; 17(5):817–822

[11] Kushner BJ. The management of nasolacrimal duct obstruction in children between 18 months and 4 years old. J AAPOS. 1998; 2(1):57–60

[12] Petersen RA, Robb RM. The natural course of congenital obstruction of the nasolacrimal duct. J Pediatr Ophthalmol Strabismus. 1978; 15(4):246–250

[13] Katowitz JA, ed. Pediatric Oculoplastic Surgery. New York, NY: Springer; 2002

[14] Honavar SG, Prakash VE, eds. Outcome of Probing for Congenital Nasolacrimal Duct Obstruction in Older Children. New Orleans, LA: American Academy of Ophthalmology; 1998

[15] Frick KD, Hariharan L, Repka MX, Chandler D, Melia BM, Beck RW, Pediatric Eye Disease Investigator Group (PEDIG). Cost-effectiveness of 2 approaches to managing nasolacrimal duct obstruction in infants: the importance of the spontaneous resolution rate. Arch Ophthalmol. 2011; 129(5):603–609

[16] Hughes RK, Fitzgerald DE. Congenital nasolacrimal duct obstruction—an optometric perspective. J Behav Optom. 2000; 11(4):94–96

[17] Piotrowski JT, Diehl NN, Mohney BG. Neonatal dacryostenosis as a risk factor for anisometropia. Arch Ophthalmol. 2010; 128(9):1166–1169

[18] Ozgur OR, Sayman IB, Oral Y, Akmaz B. Prevalence of amblyopia in children undergoing nasolacrimal duct irrigation and probing. Indian J Ophthalmol. 2013; 61(12):698–700

[19] Repka MX, Chandler DL, Beck RW, et al. Pediatric Eye Disease Investigator Group. Primary treatment of nasolacrimal duct obstruction with probing in children younger than 4 years. Ophthalmology. 2008; 115(3):577–584.e3

[20] Al-Faky YH, Al-Sobaie N, Mousa A, et al. Evaluation of treatment modalities and prognostic factors in children with congenital nasolacrimal duct obstruction. J AAPOS. 2012; 16(1):53–57

[21] Pediatric Eye Disease Investigator Group. A randomized trial comparing the cost-effectiveness of 2 approaches for treating unilateral nasolacrimal duct obstruction. Arch Ophthalmol. 2012; 130(12):1525–1533

[22] Katowitz JA, Welsh MG. Timing of initial probing and irrigation in congenital nasolacrimal duct obstruction. Ophthalmology. 1987; 94(6):698–705

[23] Robb RM. Success rates of nasolacrimal duct probing at time intervals after 1 year of age. Ophthalmology. 1998; 105(7):1307–1309, discussion 1309–1310

[24] Repka MX, Melia BM, Beck RW, et al. Pediatric Eye Disease Investigator Group. Primary treatment of nasolacrimal duct obstruction with nasolacrimal duct intubation in children younger than 4 years of age. J AAPOS. 2008; 12(5):445–450

[25] Prokosch V, Busse H, Thanos S, Eter N, Stupp T. [Impact of age on success rate of lacrimal duct irrigation with silicone tube intubation in connatal lacrimal duct stenosis]. [Article in German]. Klin Monatsbl Augenheilkd. 2013; 230 (10):1020–1024

[26] Becker BB, Berry FD, Koller H. Balloon catheter dilatation for treatment of congenital nasolacrimal duct obstruction. Am J Ophthalmol. 1996; 121(3): 304–309

[27] Hutcheson KA, Drack AV, Lambert SR. Balloon dilatation for treatment of resistant nasolacrimal duct obstruction. J AAPOS. 1997; 1(4):241–244

[28] Lüchtenberg M, Bartel JH, Bink A, Kuhli-Hattenbach C, Berkefeld J. Clinical effectiveness of balloon dacryocystoplasty in circumscribed obstructions of the nasolacrimal duct. Ophthalmologica. 2007; 221(6):434–438

[29] Goldich Y, Barkana Y, Zadok D, et al. Balloon catheter dilatation versus probing as primary treatment for congenital dacryostenosis. Br J Ophthalmol. 2011; 95(5):634–636

[30] Chen PL, Hsiao CH. Balloon dacryocystoplasty as the primary treatment in older children with congenital nasolacrimal duct obstruction. J AAPOS. 2005; 9(6):546–549

[31] Benjamin E, Wong DK, Choa D. 'Moffett's' solution: a review of the evidence and scientific basis for the topical preparation of the nose. Clin Otolaryngol Allied Sci. 2004; 29(6):582–587

[32] Pediatric Eye Disease Investigator Group. Resolution of congenital nasolacrimal duct obstruction with nonsurgical management. Arch Ophthalmol. 2012; 130(6):730–734

[33] Woog JJ. The incidence of symptomatic acquired lacrimal outflow obstruction among residents of Olmsted County, Minnesota, 1976–2000 (an American Ophthalmological Society thesis). Trans Am Ophthalmol Soc. 2007; 105: 649–666

[34] Esmaeli B, Amin S, Valero V, et al. Prospective study of incidence and severity of epiphora and canalicular stenosis in patients with metastatic breast cancer receiving docetaxel. J Clin Oncol. 2006; 24(22):3619–3622

[35] Groessl SA, Sires BS, Lemke BN. An anatomical basis for primary acquired nasolacrimal duct obstruction. Arch Ophthalmol. 1997; 115(1):71–74

[36] CJGe. Obstruction Nasolacrimal Duct. Emedicine [Internet]. 2012. Available from: http://emedicine.medscape.com/article/1210141

[37] Mukherjee B, Dhobekar M. Traumatic nasolacrimal duct obstruction: clinical profile, management, and outcome. Eur J Ophthalmol. 2013; 23(5):615–622

[38] Ali MJ, Naik MN, Honavar SG. External dacryocystorhinostomy: Tips and tricks. Oman J Ophthalmol. 2012; 5(3):191–195

[39] Harish V, Benger RS. Origins of lacrimal surgery, and evolution of dacryocystorhinostomy to the present. Clin Experiment Ophthalmol. 2014; 42(3):284–287

[40] Pandya VB, Lee S, Benger R, et al. The role of mucosal flaps in external dacryocystorhinostomy. Orbit. 2010; 29(6):324–327

[41] Costa MN, Marcondes AM, Sakano E, Kara-José N. Endoscopic study of the intranasal ostium in external dacryocystorhinostomy postoperative. Influence of saline solution and 5-fluorouracil. Clinics (Sao Paulo). 2007; 62(1):41–46

[42] Feng YF, Yu JG, Shi JL, Huang JH, Sun YL, Zhao YE. A meta-analysis of primary external dacryocystorhinostomy with and without mitomycin C. Ophthalmic Epidemiol. 2012; 19(6):364–370

[43] Xue K, Mellington FE, Norris JH. Meta-analysis of the adjunctive use of mitomycin C in primary and revision, external and endonasal dacryocystorhinostomy. Orbit. 2014; 33(4):239–244

[44] Feng YF, Cai JQ, Zhang JY, Han XH. A meta-analysis of primary dacryocystorhinostomy with and without silicone intubation. Can J Ophthalmol. 2011; 46(6):521–527

[45] Amin S, Emmerich KH, Meyer-Rüsenberg HW. [Modern, minimally invasive surgery of the lacrimal duct system]. [Article in German]. HNO. 2013; 61 (12):1053–1059, quiz 1060

[46] Emmerich KH, Ungerechts R, Meyer-Rüsenberg HW. [Transcanalicular microendoscopic laser DCR: technique and results] [Article in German]. Klin Monatsbl Augenheilkd. 2012; 229(1):39–41

[47] Hakin KN, Sullivan TJ, Sharma A, Welham RA. Paediatric dacryocystorhinostomy. Aust N Z J Ophthalmol. 1994; 22(4):231–235

[48] Pau H. Ophthalmologische Aspekte bei Tränenwegsstenosen. Otorhinolaryngol Nova. 1991; 1:221–226

[49] Bernal Sprekelsen M. Afecciones de la vía lagrimal. In: Bernal M, Massegur H, Sprekelsen C, eds. Cirugía Endoscópica Nasosinusal Básica y Avanzada. Gerona, Spain: Gràfiques Alzamora; 2001:223–226

[50] Barnes EA, Abou-Rayyah Y, Rose GE. Pediatric dacryocystorhinostomy for nasolacrimal duct obstruction. Ophthalmology. 2001; 108(9):1562–1564

[51] Struck HG, Weidlich R. Indikation und Prognose der Dakryozystorhinostomie im Kindesalter. Eine klinische Studie 1970–2000. [Indications and prognosis of dacryocystorhinostomy in childhood. A clinical study 1970–2000]. Ophthalmologe. 2001; 98(6):560–563

[52] Bernal-Sprekelsen M, Massegur Solench H, Tomás Barberán M. Paediatric endoscopic sinus surgery (PESS): review of the indications. Rev Laryngol Otol Rhinol (Bord). 2003; 124(3):145–150

[53] Sprekelsen MB, Barberán MT. Endoscopic dacryocystorhinostomy: surgical technique and results. Laryngoscope. 1996; 106(2 Pt 1):187–189

[54] Osguthorpe JD, Hoang G. Nasolacrimal injuries. Evaluation and management. Otolaryngol Clin North Am. 1991; 24(1):59–78

[55] McLean CJ, Rose GE. Postherpetic lacrimal obstruction. Ophthalmology. 2000; 107(3):496–499

[56] Hardwig PW, Bartley GB, Garrity JA. Surgical management of nasolacrimal duct obstruction in patients with Wegener's granulomatosis. Ophthalmology. 1992; 99(1):133–139

[57] Vasquez RJ, Linberg JV, McCormick SA. Histopathology of nasolacrimal duct obstruction compatible with localized sarcoidosis. Ophthal Plast Reconstr Surg. 1988; 4(3):147–151

[58] Prasad S, Kamath GG, Phillips RP. Lacrimal canalicular stenosis associated with systemic 5-fluorouacil therapy. Acta Ophthalmol Scand. 2000; 78(1): 110–113

[59] Nussbaumer M, Schreiber S, Yung MW. Concomitant nasal procedures in endoscopic dacryocystorhinostomy. J Laryngol Otol. 2004; 118(4):267–269

[60] Hosemann WG, Weber RK, Keerl RE, Lund VJ. Minimally Invasive Endonasal Sinus Surgery. Stuttgart: Thieme; 2000:66–69

[61] Stupp T, Spaniol K, Prokosch V, Thanos S, Pavlidis M. Einflussfaktoren auf den langfristigen Erfolg von Tränenwegsoperationen und der prognostische Wert der Dakryozystografie. [Factors influencing the long-term success of lacrimal duct surgery and the prognostic value of dacryocystography]. Klin Monatsbl Augenheilkd. 2010; 227(1):43–46

[62] Herberhold S, Lindner R, Wilhelm K, et al. Dakryozystorhinostomie nach West in der interdisziplinären Behandlung von Tränenwegsstenosen. [Dacryocystorhinostomy as part of the interdisciplinary treatment of lacrimal duct]. HNO. 2013; 61(10):851–858

[63] Toti A. Nuovo metodo conservatore di cura radicale delle suporazioni croniche del sacco lacrimale (dacriocistorinostomia). Clin Mod Firenze.. 1904; 10:385–389

[64] West JM. Die Technik der Eröffnung des Tränensacks von der Nase aus. Arch Laryngol Rhinol. 1913; 27:504–515

[65] Becker BB, Berry FD. Balloon catheter dilatation in lacrimal surgery. Ophthalmic Surg. 1989; 20(3):193–198

[66] Heermann H. Uber endonasale Chirurgie unter Verwendung des binocularen Mikroskopes. Arch Ohren Nasen Kehlkopfheilkd. 1958; 171(2):295–297

[67] McDonogh M, Meiring JH. Endoscopic transnasal dacryocystorhinostomy. J Laryngol Otol. 1989; 103(6):585–587

[68] Rice DH. Endoscopic intranasal dacryocystorhinostomy: a cadaver study. Am J Rhinol. 1998; 2:127–128

[69] Liang J, Lane A. Is postoperative stenting necessary in endoscopic dacryocystorhinostomy? Laryngoscope. 2013; 123(11):2589–2590

[70] Dulku S, Akinmade A, Durrani OM. Postoperative infection rate after dacryocystorhinostomy without the use of systemic antibiotic prophylaxis. Orbit. 2012; 31(1):44–47

[71] Keerl R, Weber R. Dakryozystorhinostomie - heutige Verfahren, Indikationen, Ergebnisse. [Dacryocystorhinostomy—state of the art, indications, results]. Laryngorhinootologie. 2004; 83(1):40–50

[72] Smith W, Merkonidis C, Yung M. Endoscopic dacryocystorhinostomy in patients taking aspirin perioperatively. Am J Otolaryngol. 2006; 27(5): 323–326

[73] Smith W, Merkonidis C, Draper M, Yung M. Endoscopic dacryocystorhinostomy in warfarinized patients. Am J Otolaryngol. 2006; 27(5):327–329

[74] Smithard A, Wynne D, Bingham BJ, Jones NS. Endonasal laser dacryocystorhinostomy: its role in anticoagulated patients. Laryngoscope. 2003; 113(6): 1034–1036

[75] Yang JW, Oh HN. Success rate and complications of endonasal dacryocystorhinostomy with unciformectomy. Graefes Arch Clin Exp Ophthalmol. 2012; 250(10):1509–1513

[76] Massegur H, Trias E, Ademà JM. Endoscopic dacryocystorhinostomy: modified technique. Otolaryngol Head Neck Surg. 2004; 130(1):39–46

[77] Cokkeser Y, Evereklioglu C, Tercan M, Hepsen IF. Hammer-chisel technique in endoscopic dacryocystorhinostomy. Ann Otol Rhinol Laryngol. 2003; 112(5): 444–449

[78] Heermann J. Rhinochirurgische Aspekte bei Tränenwegsstenosen. Otolaryngol Nova. 1991; 1:227–232

[79] Wielgosz R, Hohenhorst W, Fronz T. Die Heermann-Modifikation der intranasalen Mikrochirurgie bei Tränenwegstenosen. Laryngorhinootologie [Eng. abstr.]. 1995; 74(2):112–117

[80] Heindl LM, Treutlein E, Jünemann AG, Kruse FE, Holbach LM. Selektive Tränensackbiopsie bei externer Dakryzystorhinostomie. [Selective lacrimal sac biopsy for external dacryocystorhinostomy: a clinical pathological study]. Ophthalmologe. 2010; 107(12):1139–1144

[81] Raemdonck TY, Van den Broecke CM, Claerhout I, Decock CE. Inverted papilloma arising primarily from the lacrimal sac. Orbit. 2009; 28(2–3):181–184

[82] Komínek P, Cervenka S. Pediatric endonasal dacryocystorhinostomy: a report of 34 cases. Laryngoscope. 2005; 115(10):1800–1803

[83] Silbert DI, Matta NS. Outcomes of 9 mm balloon-assisted endoscopic dacryocystorhinostomy: retrospective review of 97 cases. Orbit. 2010; 29(3):131–134

[84] Song HY, Jin YH, Kim JH, et al. Nonsurgical placement of a nasolacrimal polyurethane stent: long-term effectiveness. Radiology. 1996; 200(3):759–763

[85] Bertelmann E, Rieck P. Polyurethane stents for lacrimal duct stenoses: 5-year results. Graefes Arch Clin Exp Ophthalmol. 2006; 244(6):677–682

[86] Lee JH, Kang MS, Yang JW. Clinicopathologic findings after nasolacrimal polyurethane stent implantations. Korean J Ophthalmol. 2005; 19(4):252–257

[87] Maini S, Raghava N, Youngs R, et al. Endoscopic endonasal laser versus endonasal surgical dacryocystorhinostomy for epiphora due to nasolacrimal duct obstruction: prospective, randomised, controlled trial. J Laryngol Otol. 2007; 121(12):1170–1176

[88] Huang J, Malek J, Chin D, et al. Systematic review and meta-analysis on outcomes for endoscopic versus external dacryocystorhinostomy. Orbit. 2014; 33(2):81–90

[89] Lester SE, Robson AK, Bearn M. Endoscopic 'cold steel' versus laser dacryocystorhinostomy: completing the audit cycle. J Laryngol Otol. 2008; 122(9): 924–927

[90] Moore WM, Bentley CR, Olver JM. Functional and anatomic results after two types of endoscopic endonasal dacryocystorhinostomy: surgical and holmium laser. Ophthalmology. 2002; 109(8):1575–1582

[91] Murchison AP, Pribitkin EA, Rosen MR, Bilyk JR. The ultrasonic bone aspirator in transnasal endoscopic dacryocystorhinostomy. Ophthal Plast Reconstr Surg. 2013; 29(1):25–29

[92] Karkos PD, Leong SC, Sastry A, Assimakopoulos AD, Swift AC. Evidence-based applications of mitomycin C in the nose. Am J Otolaryngol. 2011; 32(5):422–425

[93] Korkmaz H, Korkmaz M, Karakahya RH, Serhatlı M. Endoscopic intranasal surgery for congenital nasolacrimal duct obstruction–a new approach. Int J Pediatr Otorhinolaryngol. 2013; 77(6):918–921

[94] Aggarwal RK, Misson GP, Donaldson I, Willshaw HE. The role of nasolacrimal intubation in the management of childhood epiphora. Eye (Lond). 1993; 7(Pt 6):760–762

[95] Rosique López L, Lajara Blesa J, Rosique Arias M. Usefulness of local postoperative care after laser dacryocystorhinostomy. Acta Otorrinolaringol Esp. 2013; 64(4):279–282

[96] Kim SE, Lee SJ, Lee SY, Yoon JS. Clinical significance of microbial growth on the surfaces of silicone tubes removed from dacryocystorhinostomy patients. Am J Ophthalmol. 2012; 153(2):253–257.e1

[97] Al-Qahtani AS. Primary endoscopic dacryocystorhinostomy with or without silicone tubing: a prospective randomized study. Am J Rhinol Allergy. 2012; 26(4):332–334

[98] Cannon PS, Chan W, Selva D. Incidence of canalicular closure with endonasal dacryocystorhinostomy without intubation in primary nasolacrimal duct obstruction. Ophthalmology. 2013; 120(8):1688–1692

[99] Smirnov G, Tuomilehto H, Teräsvirta M, Nuutinen J, Seppä J. Silicone tubing is not necessary after primary endoscopic dacryocystorhinostomy: a prospective randomized study. Am J Rhinol. 2008; 22(2):214–217

[100] Unlu HH, Gunhan K, Baser EF, Songu M. Long-term results in endoscopic dacryocystorhinostomy: is intubation really required? Otolaryngol Head Neck Surg. 2009; 140(4):589–595

[101] Chong KK, Lai FH, Ho M, Luk A, Wong BW, Young A. Randomized trial on silicone intubation in endoscopic mechanical dacryocystorhinostomy (SEND) for primary nasolacrimal duct obstruction. Ophthalmology. 2013; 120(10): 2139–2145

[102] Chan W, Selva D. Ostium shrinkage after endoscopic dacryocystorhinostomy. Ophthalmology. 2013; 120(8):1693–1696

[103] Fayet B, Racy E, Assouline M. Complications of standardized endonasal dacryocystorhinostomy with unciformectomy. Ophthalmology. 2004; 111(4): 837–845

[104] Dolman PJ. Comparison of external dacryocystorhinostomy with nonlaser endonasal dacryocystorhinostomy. Ophthalmology. 2003; 110(1):78–84

[105] Andrew N, Selva D. Postoperative haemorrhage in powered endoscopic dacryocystorhinostomy. Clin Experiment Ophthalmol. 2014; 42(3):262–265

[106] Cannon PS, Madge SN, Selva D. Air regurgitation in patients on continuous positive airway pressure (CPAP) therapy following dacrocystorhinostomy with or without Lester-Jones tube insertion. Br J Ophthalmol. 2010; 94(7): 891–893

[107] Zílelíoğlu G, Tekeli O, Uğurba SH, Akiner M, Aktürk T, Anadolu Y. Results of endoscopic endonasal non-laser dacryocystorhinostomy. Doc Ophthalmol. 2002; 105(1):57–62

[108] Hii BW, McNab AA, Friebel JD. A comparison of external and endonasal dacryocystorhinostomy in regard to patient satisfaction and cost. Orbit. 2012; 31(2):67–76

[109] Lee DW, Chai CH, Loon SC. Primary external dacryocystorhinostomy versus primary endonasal dacryocystorhinostomy: a review. Clin Experiment Ophthalmol. 2010; 38(4):418–426

[110] de Souza C, Nissar J. Experience with endoscopic dacryocystorhinostomy using four methods. Otolaryngol Head Neck Surg. 2010; 142(3):389–393

[111] Horn IS, Tittmann M, Fischer M, Otto M, Dietz A, Mozet C. Endonasal nasolacrimal duct surgery: a comparative study of two techniques. Eur Arch Otorhinolaryngol. 2014; 271(7):1923–1931

[112] Zenk J, Karatzanis AD, Psychogios G, et al. Long-term results of endonasal dacryocystorhinostomy. Eur Arch Otorhinolaryngol. 2009; 266(11):1733–1738

[113] Jutley G, Karim R, Joharatnam N, Latif S, Lynch T, Olver JM. Patient satisfaction following endoscopic endonasal dacryocystorhinostomy: a quality of life study. Eye (Lond). 2013; 27(9):1084–1089

[114] Dietrich C, Mewes T, Kühnemund M, Hashemi B, Mann WJ, Amedee RG. Long-term follow-up of patients with microscopic endonasal dacryocystorhinostomy. Am J Rhinol. 2003; 17(1):57–61

[115] Velegrakis GA, Prokopakis EP, Panayotaki I, Pagalos AG, Siganos CS, Helidonis ES. Intranasal laser-assisted dacryocystorhinostomy with the use of a surgical microscope. Am J Otolaryngol. 2002; 23(5):272–276

[116] Vanderveen DK, Jones DT, Tan H, Petersen RA. Endoscopic dacryocystorhinostomy in children. J AAPOS. 2001; 5(3):143–147

[117] Al-Nuaimi D, Inkster C, Lobo C. Paediatric powered endonasal dacryocystorhinostomy. Eur Arch Otorhinolaryngol. 2011; 268(12):1823–1828

[118] Jones DT, Fajardo NF, Petersen RA, VanderVeen DK. Pediatric endoscopic dacryocystorhinostomy failures: who and why? Laryngoscope. 2007; 117(2): 323–327

[119] Orhan M, Saylam CY, Midilli R. Intranasal localization of the lacrimal sac. Arch Otolaryngol Head Neck Surg. 2009; 135(8):764–770

[120] Migliori ME. Endoscopic evaluation and management of the lacrimal sump syndrome. Ophthal Plast Reconstr Surg. 1997; 13(4):281–284

Chapter 16

Lid Surgery in Orbital Disorders

16

16 Lid Surgery in Orbital Disorders

M. A. Varde and B. Wiechens

16.1 Anatomy

The anatomy of the eyelids has been discussed in detail in previous chapters. This chapter touches briefly upon the relevant surgical anatomy with reference to lid surgery.

The main functions of the eyelids are to protect the globe and to moisten and clean the ocular surface, thereby maintaining its integrity, as one of the mechanisms that helps keep the cornea transparent. Failure of lid closure (lagophthalmos) or defects in the lids may lead to exposure keratopathy, which may result in visual impairment or loss of sight due to conjunctivalization; or may cause ulceration of the cornea that can escalate to endophthalmitis. Malpositioning of the lids may be the culprit in some unpleasant and nagging symptoms such as epiphora and chronic conjunctivitis. Stability of the lids, their apposition to the globe, and a normal and regular lid closure as in a blink are decisive factors for a normal eyelid function.

From a surgical standpoint, the tarsal plate is suspended laterally and medially by the lateral and medial canthal tendons, respectively. The posterior part of the medial canthal tendon determines the apposition of the lid to the globe. Superiorly, the tarsal plate is suspended by the levator palpebrae superioris muscle to the Whitnall's ligament and superior orbital rim. Inferiorly, the tarsal plate is anchored to the inferior orbital rim by the inferior lid-retractors (capsulopalpebral fascia). The tarsal plates are akin to the skeletal system providing stability to the lids and a smooth apposition to the globe (▶ Fig. 16.1) (see Chapter 1). The levator palpebrae superioris muscle and Müller's muscle open the lids, whereas the orbicularis oculi actively aid in lid closure as does gravity passively to a certain extent.

The eyelid can be divided into posterior and anterior lamellae (▶ Fig. 16.2, ▶ Fig. 16.3); this surgical division is of great significance for the reconstruction of eyelid defects. The tarsus and tarsal conjunctiva constitute the posterior lamella, whereas the anterior lamella is formed by the orbicularis oculi muscle and the eyelid skin. The eyelid skin is characteristically very thin and has little subcutaneous tissue. The blood supply is from a dense network of capillaries that crisscross both in the anterior and the posterior lamellae. This is why in the reconstruction of large defects, a lamella can be replaced by a free graft.

Located at the medial canthal end are the puncta and the tear drainage system. By their normal blink mechanism the eyelids are also responsible for the drainage of tears from the lacus lacrimalis. Malposition of or trauma to the medial aspect of eyelids may result in epiphora.

Lymphatic drainage is mainly by the preauricular and submandibular lymph nodes. The former drains the lateral two-thirds of the upper lid and medial one-third of the lower lid, whereas the latter accounts for the medial one-third of the upper lid and lateral two-thirds of the lower lid. This is of significance during assessment of periocular tumor spread.

16.2 Traumatology

Lid injuries more often than not are associated with injuries to the globe and the periorbita, face, head, and neck regions. In many such patients with polytrauma, stabilizing the more life threatening injuries take precedence over ocular injuries at presentation.

16.2.1 Case History

In evaluating a trauma patient, the importance of eliciting a detailed history of the **sequence of events that led to the traumatic incident** cannot be overemphasized. Hammer-and-chisel injuries are, more often than not, associated with small entry

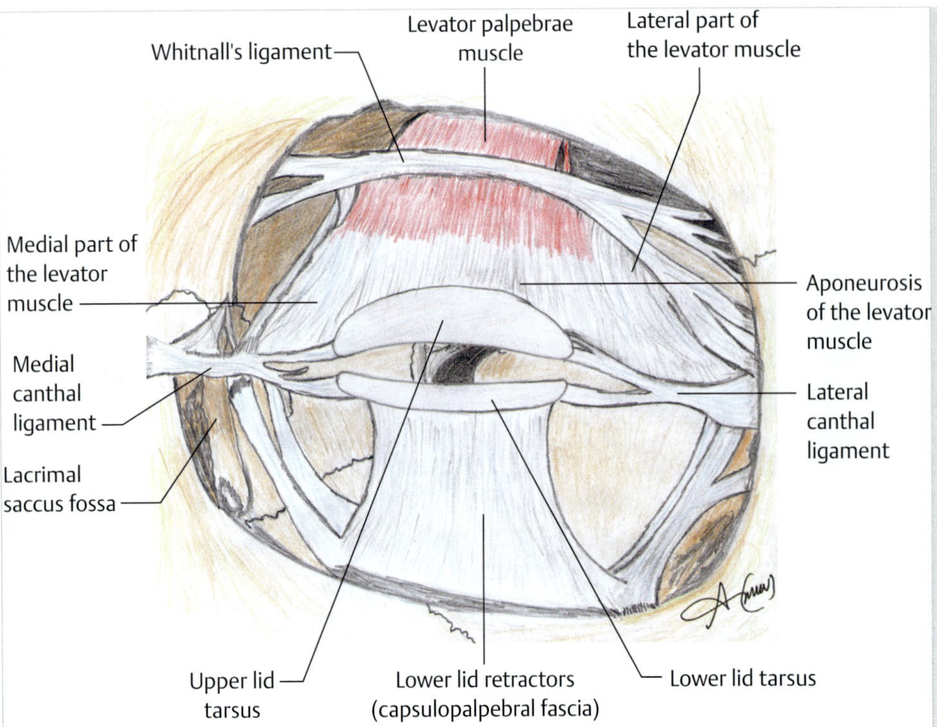

Fig. 16.1 Schematic view of the tarsal plate suspension and stabilization of the lid apparatus.

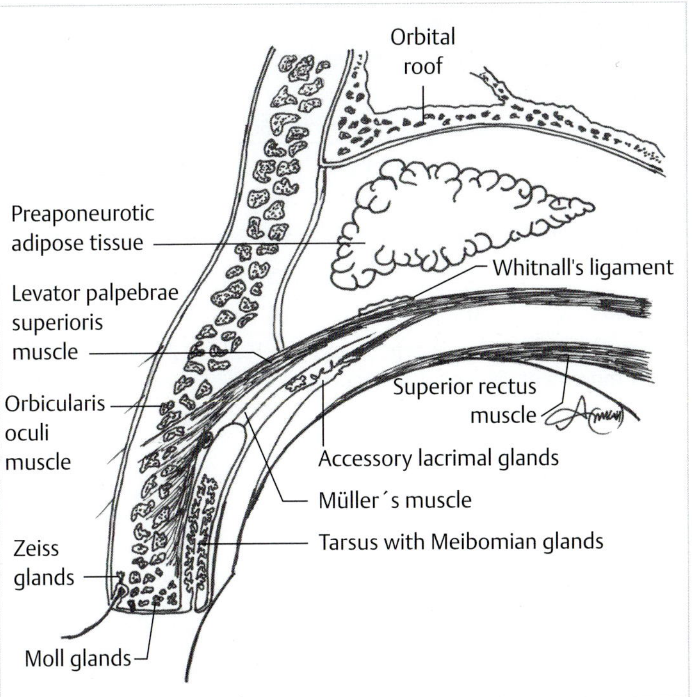

Fig. 16.2 Transverse section through the upper lid.

wounds and intraocular or even intraorbital foreign bodies and in many cases require imaging. It must be remembered to check the adequacy of tetanus immunization in such scenarios.

Bite and claw wounds are often associated with injuries to the lacrimal drainage apparatus and particular attention is required while examining such cases. Canaliculus lacerations have to be suspected in all medial lid injuries, especially when these are associated with a lateral displacement of the lacrimal punctum. Careful probing of the canaliculi and, when necessary, their end-to-end anastamosis during wound repair is pivotal.

16.2.2 Examination

The assessment of ocular and periorbital injuries should be done in four steps:

1. Examination of the eye.
2. Examination of the eyelids and soft tissues.
3. Examination of the orbit.
4. Examination of the face.[1]

The detailed examination of the eye can be hindered by swelling or hematoma of the eyelids; also the visual acuity cannot be determined in unconscious or uncooperative patients. In some cases an examination in the operating theatre under anesthesia may be necessary.

The referring doctor can make a **preliminary assessment of the eye** with the aid of a torch light. If the patient experiences pain when opening the eye, one can place a drop of local anesthetic eye drops (proxymetacaine, tetracaine) into the eye so as to facilitate examination.

First, a rough assessment of visual function should be made. Each eye is examined separately for ability to read fine or large prints, count fingers, or appreciate hand movements at 30 cm distance, and in extreme cases the ability to perceive light.

The next step is to look for a **relative afferent pupillary defect (RAPD)**. Done correctly, this is extremely sensitive in picking up early or mild optic nerve pathology (in this context, traumatic optic neuropathy [TON] or compressive optic neuropathy). As prerequisites, the patient has to fix at a distance target; the examiner must not to get in the way of the patient's line of sight; a fairly bright pointed source of light has to be used; and the examination has to be carried out in a dark or dimly lit room. The pupils are illuminated alternately in quick succession, swinging from one pupil to the other, hence the name **swinging flashlight test**. Normally both the pupils contract equally regardless of which pupil is illuminated, as the direct and consensual pupillary light response are equal due to equal innervation. If illuminating one pupil elicits a dilation of both the pupils, which contract again if the fellow pupil is illuminated in turn, a relative afferent pupil defect in the first eye is to be suspected, for example, in severe globe trauma or traumatic optic neuropathy. RAPD also has prognostic significance and correlates negatively with visual prognosis after trauma.[2] One method for the assessment of visual prognosis after ocular trauma is the so-called **Ocular Trauma Score (OTS)**.[3] Details are depicted in ▶ Table 16.1 and ▶ Table 16.2. This is of significance when discussing visual prognosis with the patient and/or relatives.

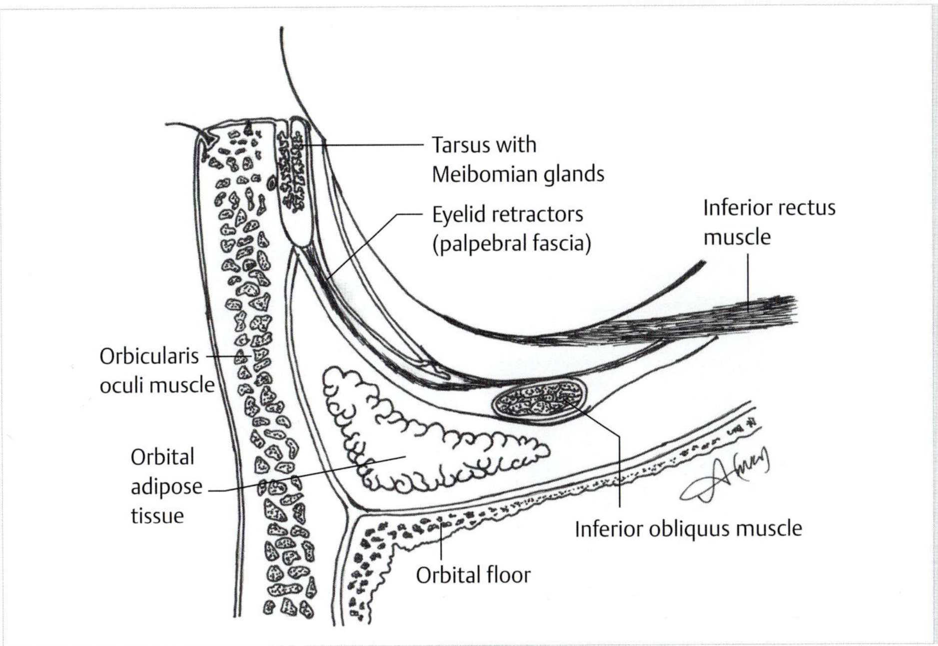

Fig. 16.3 Transverse section through the lower lid.

Table 16.1 Ocular Trauma Score[3]; assessment of the cumulative visual prognosis after ocular trauma

Variable	Points
Vision	
• NPL, loss of the globe	60
• PL, HM	70
• 6/600 to 6/120	80
• 6/60 to 6/15	90
• ≥6/12	100
Globe rupture	-23
Endophthalmitis	-17
Penetrating injury	-14
Retinal detachment	-11
RAPD	-10

Abbreviations: NPL, no perception of light. PL, light perception. HM, hand movement. RAPD, relative afferent pupillary defect.

Table 16.2 Ocular Trauma Score

Points	OTS group	NPL	PL/HM	CF		
				6/60	6/60–6/15	≥6/12
0–44	I	74%	15%	7%	3%	1%
45–65	II	27%	26%	18%	15%	15%
66–80	III	2%	11%	15%	31%	41%
81–91	IV	1%	2%	3%	22%	73%
92–100	V	0%	1%	1%	5%	94%

Abbreviations: NPL, no perception of light. PL, light perception. HM, hand movement. CF, count fingers.

Loss of pupillary shape, blood in the anterior chamber that partially or totally occludes further details, or prolapse of intraocular contents (▶ Fig. 16.4) are an indication of **penetrating globe trauma** through an injury to the cornea or sclera.

If no injury to the eye is apparent, the **intraocular pressure (IOP)** can be carefully assessed by the finger tension method through the closed lid. Lower IOP than in the fellow eye can indicate a concealed globe rupture; a raised IOP can indicate a secondary glaucoma.

Initially, the points assigned in ▶ Table 16.1 are summed. The total gives the score for the OTS group. Using ▶ Table 16.2, the final vision to be anticipated can be roughly assessed. For example, with a **globe contusion** and an initial vision of 6/10 and no further complication, in 94% cases a final vision of at least more than 6/12 can be expected. On the other hand, with a globe rupture, with initial vision of NPL and positive RAPD, 74% cases can end in permanent blindness, but in 11% cases orientation vision may be the end result. This also applies in cases of globe-saving surgeries independent of the initial vision.

When **examining the lids**, attention should be paid to possible malpositioning (traumatic ptosis with disinsertion of the levator aponeurosis) or loss of the angulation in the lateral and/or medial aspect (indicates an avulsion of the lateral/medial or both suspensory ligaments). Measuring the levator function can be helpful as well.

A prolapse of orbital fat tissue indicates a defect in the orbital septum and possibly an injury to deeper-lying structures. Repair entails careful exposure, with understanding of the anatomy so as to restore viable tissues in their anatomically correct location.

Examination of the orbit is dealt in detail in Chapter 3 and Chapter 8.

A superinfected wound needs a course of systemic antibiotics, oral or intravenous according to the severity of the infection.

16.2.3 Diagnostic Measures

The primary imaging modalities when an intraorbital or intraocular foreign body is suspected are conventional radiography, computed tomography (CT), and ultrasound. Magnetic resonance imaging (MRI) should not be used under any circumstances in which a metallic foreign body is suspected. Not only is CT scan (ideally spiral-CT) the most sensitive method for pin-pointing a foreign body but it is also very specific in localizing it and hence should be the method of choice when a foreign body is suspected (▶ Fig. 16.5). Additionally, bony structures are well discernible and fractures better localized.

If the globe is intact, sonography (specifically B-mode) should also be used because intraocular foreign bodies can be clearly defined and their exact location better pin-pointed by the B-mode scan.

16

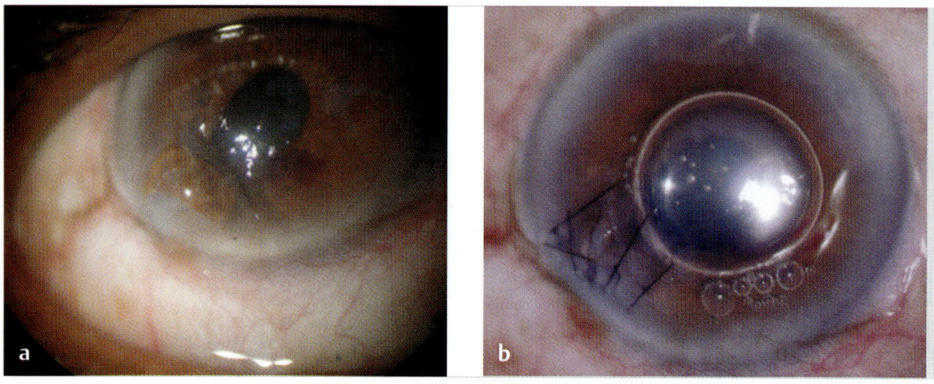

Fig. 16.4 Wound management of a corneal injury. **(a)** Penetrating corneal injury with deformity of the pupil and iris prolapse through the wound. **(b)** Wound repair with placement of corneal sutures. At the end of the operation, an air bubble is placed in the anterior chamber. (Courtesy of Sankara Nethralaya Eye Hospital, Chennai, India.)

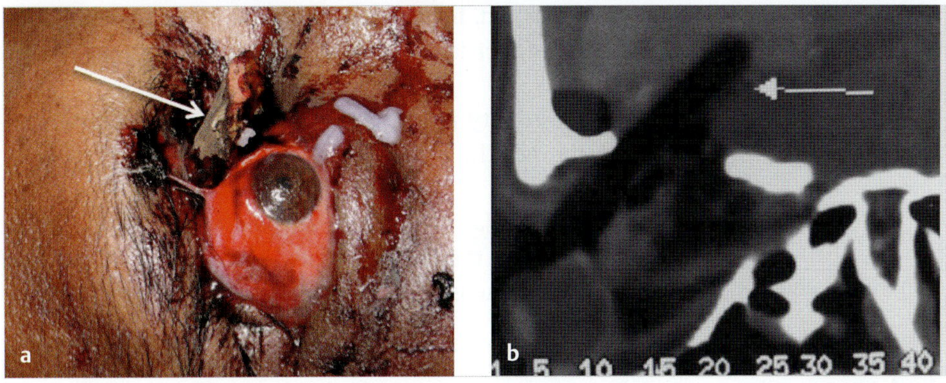

Fig. 16.5 Impalement lesion. **(a)** A patient who had had a road accident causing a penetrating injury with impaled foreign body (*arrow*). Avulsio bulbi. **(b)** CT scan of the same patient shows a large foreign body (corresponding to the density of air) penetrating through an orbital roof fracture into the frontal lobe of the brain. (Courtesy of Sankara Nethralaya Eye Hospital, Chennai, India.)

16.2.4 Surgical Treatment of Lid Injuries

Lateral Canthotomy and Inferior Cantholysis

Before elaborating on the specific surgical protocols of various aspects of lid injuries, a brief note on the method of relieving acute increase in intraorbital pressure (e.g., intraorbital hemorrhage) is worthwhile. **Lateral canthotomy**, alone or in severe cases along with an **inferior cantholysis**, is a quick and easy means of relieving acute increase in intraorbital pressure. These procedures act by decompressing the orbit anteriorly.

The indication, as described above, is sudden and rapid increase in intraorbital pressure that causes compressive optic neuropathy and vision loss. These procedures can be carried out in an emergency setting at the bedside. After local infiltration anesthesia with lidocaine 2% with epinephrine 1:200,000 and topical proparacaine eye drops, a hemostat is applied horizontally on the lateral canthus into the lateral orbital rim. After a couple of minutes, the hemostat is removed and the lateral canthus is incised horizontally up to the lateral orbital rim (lateral canthotomy) with straight scissors. Now the lateral aspect of the lower lid is held with toothed forceps and the inferior band of the lateral canthal tendon of the lower lid is incised along with the lateral insertion of the orbital septum (inferior cantholysis). The wound is left open to decompress the orbit and can be re-sutured at a later date.

Basic Concepts in the Management of Eyelid Trauma

Lid injuries are sometimes associated with **globe injuries.**[4] A globe injury naturally takes precedence over a lid injury. Surgery in cases of globe perforation is generally carried out under general anesthesia as periocular infiltration with a local anesthetic can lead to a rise in orbital pressure, which can lead to a prolapse or loss of intraocular tissues.

Periocular hematomas are, as a rule, treated conservatively with measures to reduce the swelling such as cold compresses and NSAIDs in case of pain. Only when encapsulation and liquefaction of the hematoma has taken place should this be surgically removed in order to avert superinfection (▶ Fig. 16.6).

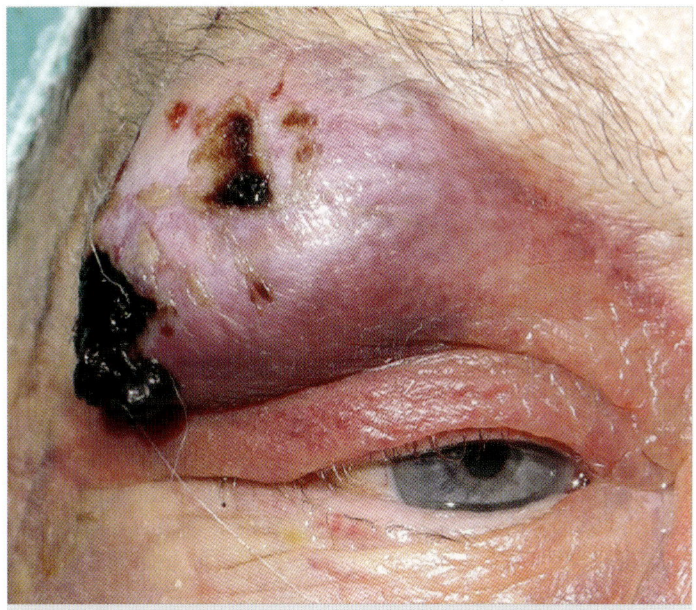

Fig. 16.6 An elderly woman who had fallen on her face 5 days previously, with encapsulated liquefied hematoma of the superolateral orbital rim. A bony fracture was excluded by CT scans. The hematoma was drained.

When inspecting the wound the **extent** and **location** of the wound, involvement of the **lid margins** and **tarsus**, injury to the **canthal tendons** and to the **tear ducts** and potential **loss of tissue**, **contamination**, or **foreign bodies** are important considerations. Most lid injuries can be treated under local anesthetic in cooperative patients. Regional anesthesia is indicated with extensive injuries. On the upper lid the frontolacrimal block anesthetizes the entire lid apart from the medial part. The supratrochlear block anesthetizes the medial aspect of upper lid. The lower lid can be anesthetized with the infraorbital block. Additionally, local infiltration with lidocaine 2% or mixed with bupivacaine 0.5% plus epinephrine 1:200,000 up to 1:100,000 is used when needed. First, a thorough wound cleansing is done with normal saline, or where needed with diluted povidone iodine solution, and inspected for foreign bodies. All foreign bodies are to be carefully removed as they can lead to chronic infections, inflammations, or toxic reactions. The wound should be irrigated continuously under pressure[5] using an irrigating cannula. Due to the excellent blood supply, débridement of devitalized tissue is rarely necessary as these often heal excellently. For this reason only confirmed necrotic tissue should be debrided. The surgical correction of eyelid trauma should not only restore the integrity and protective functions of the lids but also, to the extent possible, deliver a cosmetically acceptable result. For this the following components of the eyelids have to be reconstructed:

- Anterior lamella (skin and orbicularis).
- Posterior lamella (tarsus and conjunctiva).
- Canthal tendons.
- Canaliculi.
- Levator complex.[1]

The canthal tendons, the lacrimal drainage apparatus, and the levator are treated first.

Surgical Correction of the Canthal Tendons Tears

When operating on the canthal tendons it is important that the **directional vector of the canthal tendons** pull inwards so that the lids lie apposed to the convexity of the globe. The **lateral canthal tendon** is sutured to the periosteum of the lateral orbital rim with a nonresorbable 5–0 suture (e.g., 5–0 polypropylene). When the canthal tendon is lost, it can be replaced by a **periosteal flap** from the lateral orbital rim.

The **medial canthal tendon** consists mainly of two parts that circumscribe the lacrimal sac. The posterior part, which is attached to the posterior lacrimal crest, is responsible for the stability and directional vector of the medial canthus. The canthal tendons must be re-attached by suturing them onto the periosteum of the **posterior lacrimal crest** so as to achieve an apposition of the lid to the globe. If the periosteum is not intact, then a **T**-shaped **titanium plate** is sutured posteriorly to the **nasal bone** in order to achieve a posterior vector. Where fractures are more extensive, multiple plates and possibly even **transnasal wiring** may be necessary.[6]

Surgical Correction of Lacrimal Pathway Injuries

With injuries to the lacrimal pathway, reconstruction is necessary with silicone intubation. First, the lacrimal puncta is identified and then carefully dilated with a Nettleship dilator. Under the microscope or a loupe, the medial end of the severed canaliculus can be identified as a white ring. If this cannot be done, then it is possible to inject air into the opposite canaliculus, when it is intact. Once the lacerated end is found, it is intubated with a silicone tube. For this purpose the Mini Monoka (FCI Ophthalmics) is particularly suitable; this is a short tube that can be simply inserted into the canaliculus and that coils itself up in the lacrimal sac, (▶ Fig. 16.7). It sits firmly in the punctum due to a knob at the proximal end. **Intubation all the way into the nose** (see Chapter 15.1) under local anesthesia is very unpleasant for the patient.

Another possibility is **ring intubation using a pigtail probe**. However, the healthy canaliculus must likewise be probed for this.

The pericanalicular tissues are adapted with 60 absorbable sutures and finally the skin is adapted directly taking care that there is not much tension, lest cheese-wiring and wound dehiscence may occur.

Surgical Correction of Injuries to the Levator

A **traumatic ptosis** points to a laceration of the levator palpebrae superioris muscle. In such cases, the torn ends of the muscle need to be identified and sutured with 6–0 absorbable sutures or the distal end of the muscle is sutured to the tarsal plate. The **orbital septum** is generally not sutured.

Surgical Correction of Lid Margin Tears

Blunt traumas can surprisingly result in considerable injuries to the lid margins and the tarsus. Often, the full extent of the injury is not visible upon casual examination and is only determined upon closer examination, sometimes under local anesthesia (▶ Fig. 16.8).

There are several methods of treating lid margin tears. The principle behind all of them is end-to-end adaptation of the posterior edge of the lid margin, meibomian gland orifices, gray line, and eyelash line in an anatomically correct way. In the author's (M. A. Varde) own experience the adaptation of the edges of the eyelid with an oblique absorbable suture is simpler than suturing with silk and produces reproducibly good results (▶ Fig. 16.9). Here the eversion of the edges of the wound is important as they

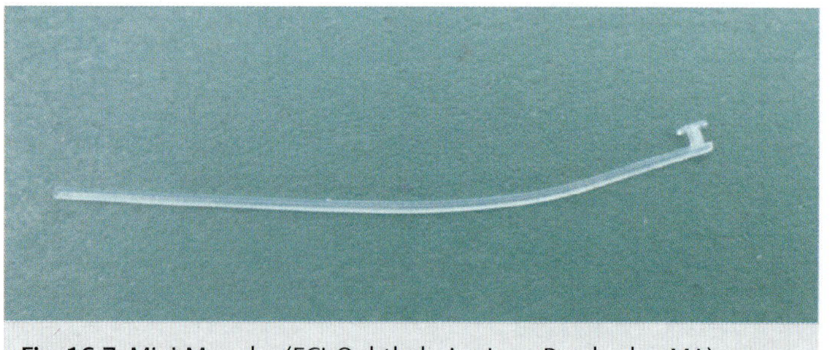

Fig. 16.7 Mini Monoka (FCI Ophthalmics Inc., Pembroke, MA).

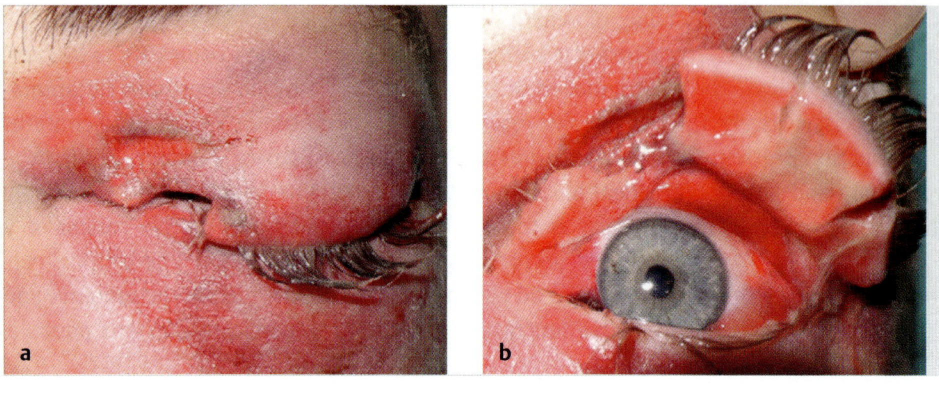

Fig. 16.8 Injury of the medial eyelid margin and the tarsus. **(a)** A patient with blunt trauma of the eyelid edge. **(b)** The extent of the injury becomes obvious only after everting the eyelid.

16

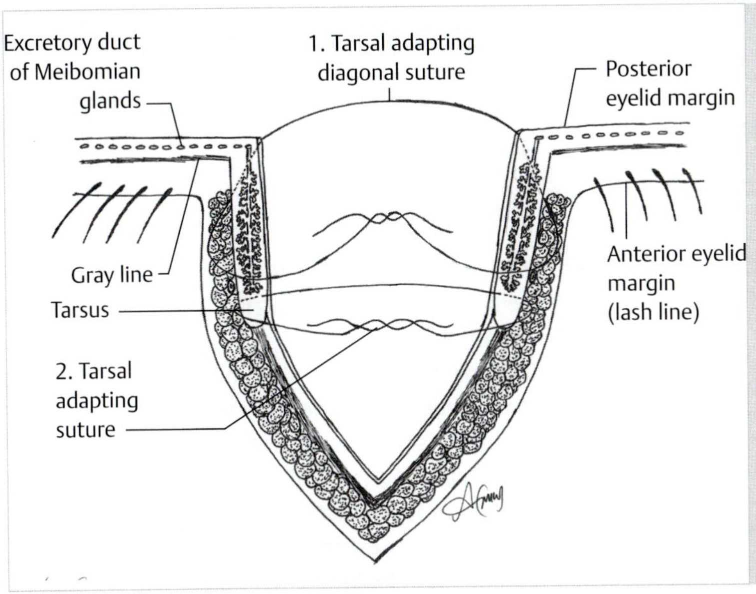

Fig. 16.9 Primary closure of the eyelid margin (here lower lid). The first 6–0 absorbable suture-bite (e.g., Vicryl) is taken from the side of the orbicularis muscle from one cut end, passing diagonally in a supero-posterior direction, within the tarsus, so that the needle emerges from the posterior edge of the upper cut end. The needle is then guided diagonally from the posterior edge of the upper cut end of the other side, antero-inferiorly, so as to emerge at the corresponding point on the opposite edge of the wound. Another suture at the lower end of the tarsus (shown) is placed along with a suture at the eyelash line (not shown). Since this suture is placed at the outer surface, it can be cut short as it does not come in contact with the cornea. The skin is closed above this suture using 6–0 or 7–0 nonabsorbable sutures. The eyelid margin sutures (absorbable) are deeper and hidden, so that the superficial skin sutures can be removed early.

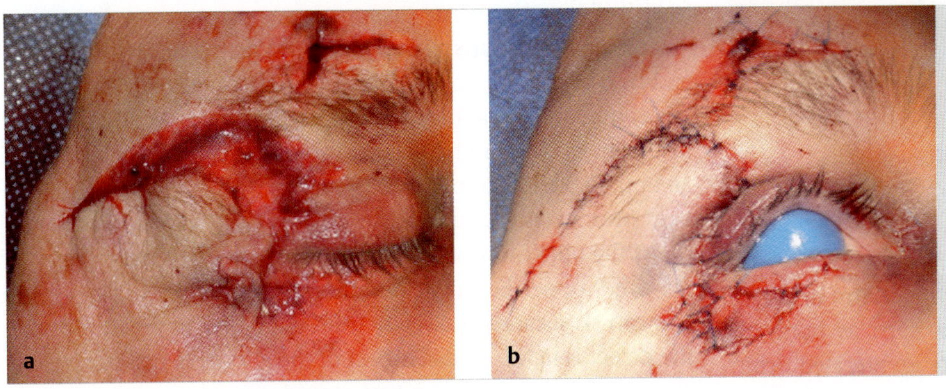

Fig. 16.10 Wound management of a contused laceration. **(a)** Contused laceration involving the lateral upper and lower lid and the eyebrow. **(b)** Favorable postoperative result following repositioning and apposition of the anatomical landmarks.

draw inward due to the contraction of the wound and can thus result in a groove. In some instances there is only a small lid margin defect and, upon everting the tarsus, a tarsal fracture running its entire height is revealed so that the wound needs to be extended superiorly for it to be sutured with 6–0 absorbable sutures. Partial thickness sutures are placed anteriorly through the tarsal plate and knotted on the anterior surface so that the tarsal conjunctiva is free of irregularities. Full-thickness sutures on the upper lid are to be avoided as they will produce painful corneal erosions and in some cases lead to corneal ulcers.

Skin Suture

Skin wounds are sutured according to the general principles of wound closure. The orientations of the wound margins have to be recognized and adapted accordingly. Eyelid wounds often gape significantly due to the forces exerted by the facial musculature and give the impression that tissue has been lost. The angles and corners in the course of the wound aid in orientation as well as, for example, the course of the eyebrow hair (▸ Fig. 16.10). It is important to never involve the septum in the layered wound closure as it can lead to the retraction of the eyelid.

16.3 Reconstruction of Eyelid Defects

When reconstructing the lids after significant tissue loss due to trauma or after excision of lid tumors, some rules of lid reconstruction must be observed. Due to the peculiarities of the lid architecture it is prudent to make the most of the residual lid tissue before harvesting grafts.[7] Differentiating the **anterior** (skin and orbicularis oculi muscle) from the **posterior** (tarsus and conjunctiva) **lid lamella** is mandatory. Each has to be reconstructed separately in order to ensure the stability and functionality of the eyelids. The anterior lamella can be reconstructed with either *local flaps* or *free skin grafts*, and the posterior lamella either with **free tarsoconjuctival grafts, tarsoconjuctival pedicle grafts, or free grafts from the hard palate or nasal septum**. In order to ensure a satisfactory blood supply and thereby their survival, **two free grafts must never be laid on top of each other**. At least one has to be vascularized (▸ Fig. 16.11).[8] The various methods of local flaps and free grafts will be discussed in depth in the following sections.

16

16.3.1 Reconstruction of Defects of the Anterior Lamella of the Periorbital Region

Moderate to large defects of the anterior lamella can be reconstructed with either **free full-thickness** or **split-thickness skin grafts** or with **local flaps**.

Free split-thickness skin grafts (STSGs) consist of the epidermis and a variable percentage of the underlying dermis. The remaining dermis at the donor site regenerates the skin and heals the defect with scar formation. The graft can be harvested with a dermatome in a pre-defined thickness (0.25–0.4 mm)[9] or a

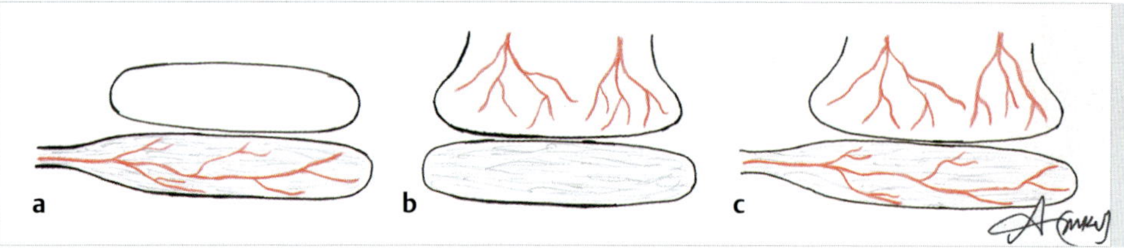

Fig. 16.11 Reconstruction of both lamellae in cases of eyelid defects. Either the anterior **(a)**, or posterior **(b)**, or both lamellae **(c)** must be vascularised.[19]

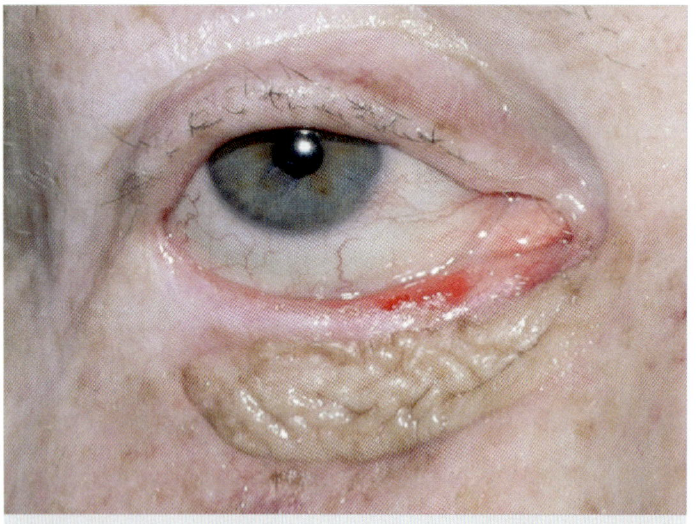

Fig. 16.12 Scarred contraction of a preauricular harvested free skin graft.

Humby knife from the medial aspect of the upper arm or thigh. Indications for STSG are fairly large defects such as burns of the periocular area or the need to cover an exenterated orbit. STSGs tend to contract more than full-thickness skin grafts. This can lead to a shrinkage of up to 40 to 50% of the graft.[8] For this reason if possible, full-thickness skin grafts are used in lid reconstructions.

Free full-thickness skin grafts (FTSGs) consist of epidermis and dermis. For lid reconstruction they should be thin and matched in texture and color to the recipient location. The most suitable donor sites are again the **lids** themselves (e.g. as upper lid blepharoplasty), **retroauricular or preauricular skin grafts**, as well as skin from the **clavicle, the medial aspect of the upper arm** or in children from the **groin**. In male babies the foreskin can also be used as a donor site. Free skin grafts, especially fairly large ones, tend to contract more than local flaps (▶ Fig. 16.12). The contraction of the graft is approximately 10%.[8]

16

Local flaps in oculoplasty are mostly **randomized flaps**. In contrast to **axial flaps** they do not have any defined blood supply from an artery and vein but are supplied from the capillary bed of several collaterals. The ratio of the base of the flap to the length should be planned so that the risk of necrosis is minimized. Normally, for random flaps the ratio is 1:3. In the face, due to the exceptionally good blood supply, even longer flaps are possible as long as no traction is exerted on the base.[10]

Advancement flaps, transposition flaps, and **rotation flaps** are possible for reconstruction. The periorbital region can be principally divided into upper lid, lower lid, and medial and lateral canthal regions. Each of these regions has its own texture. During reconstruction, particular attention is to be paid to the direction of the flap and the alignment of the skin tension lines in order to avert late postoperative lid malpositions or disfiguring scars as a result of wound contraction.

Local flaps are taken from the areas with excess skin. The upper eyelid, the glabellar region, the preauricular region, and the cheek are prime examples.

Advancement flaps are skin or skin-muscle flaps that are drawn in **the same direction** as the incisions. This is why they should always be in the skin tension lines. In the lower lid it is important that the flap is horizontally oriented so that inferior traction and ectropion or lid retraction is avoided. As in lower lid blepharoplasty, one can best estimate the actual excess amount of skin when the patient is looking upward. For the lower lid, a transposition flap from the upper lid is ideal since the vector of force is directed upward.

Transposition flaps place the flap at an angle to the incision and thus alter its direction. The upper lid of most elderly patients has enough redundant skin to compensate for a horizontal defect in the lower lid. Flap harvesting is according to the principles of an upper lid blepharoplasty. This has to be discussed with the patient prior to the reconstruction, as it is possible that an asymmetry of the upper lids will result and a cosmetic blepharoplasty of the other upper lid might become necessary. In most cases, the flap can be sutured in directly from the upper to the lower lid. If the defect is in the medial aspect of the lower lid, options include an advancement flap, or a two-staged procedure with a Pedicle graft, leaving the pedicle in place until vascularization (~2½ to 3 weeks, stage one) followed by a second stage with flap division. It is also possible to place the partially deepithelialized flap into the medial defect underneath the lateral lower lid skin in a single-stage operation (▶ Fig. 16.13). Another method of transposition from the upper lid is the **"bucket handle"** technique, in which the skin muscle flap has a medial and a lateral pedicle (▶ Fig. 16.14). If a transposition flap from the upper lid is not possible, a nasolabial flap is a good alternative, however, this skin is somewhat thicker and less elastic. The skin is somewhat thicker and less elastic. The resulting defect can either be covered primarily or covered with a free graft.

Rotation flaps rotate around a center in order to close a defect. An example of this is the **Mustardé cheek rotation** to treat vertically extensive defects of the lower lid[8] (▶ Fig. 16.15).

16.3.2 Reconstruction of Full-Thickness Defects of the Lower Lid

Smaller defects can be closed **directly** depending on the patient's lid laxity. In older patients, this can be possible for defects of up to one-third of the lid. In younger patients with less lid laxity, this is only possible with very small defects. Too great a tension should be avoided as it causes wound dehiscence. Irregular defects are excised **pentagonally** and sutured so as to maintain a continuous row of eyelashes. In a pentagonal excision it is important to cut the tarsus perpendicularly over its entire height (▶ Fig. 16.9). As the tarsal plate is rather stiff, suturing an oblique defect of the tarsus will result in a notch.

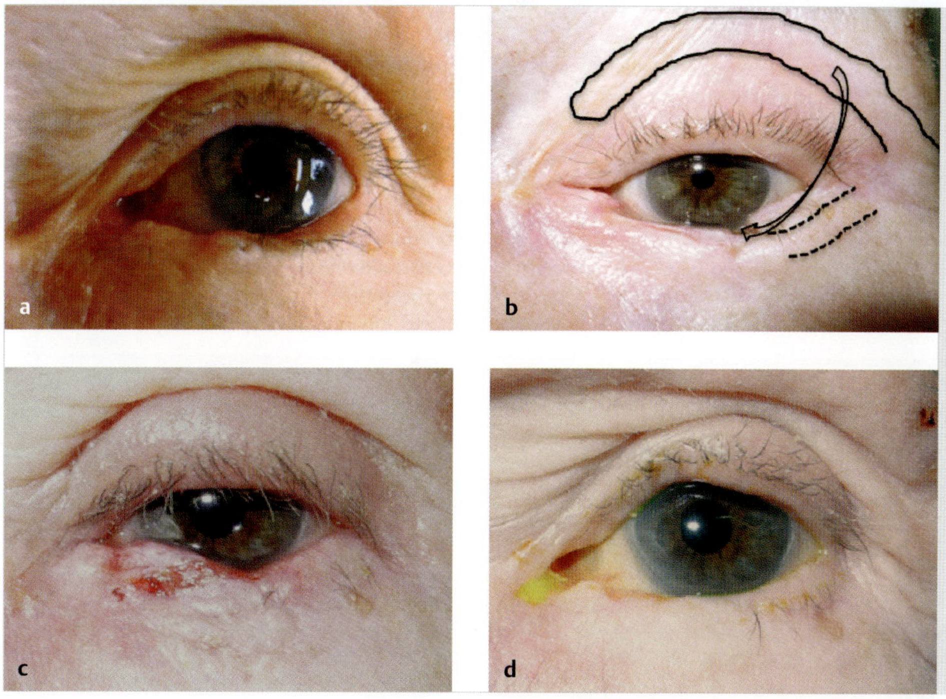

Fig. 16.13 Basal cell carcinoma (BCC) of the lower lid. **(a)** Clinical picture of a female patient with a BCC of the medial aspect of the lower lid. **(b)** After completing an R0 resection, reconstruction of the lower lid is carried out. Steps include probing of the lacrimal duct system; free tarsoconjunctival graft; and a partially deepithelialized, laterally pedicled skin-muscle flap from the upper lid, which is tunneled underneath the lateral aspect of the lower lid (*dotted line*). **(c)** This photo shows the patient 1 week post-op. **(d)** This photo shows 3 months post-op result: discrete deformity of the upper lid contour due to harvesting the tarsoconjunctival transplant, and slight eversion of the lower puctum. Apart from this the lower lid correction showed a cosmetically and functionally satisfying result.

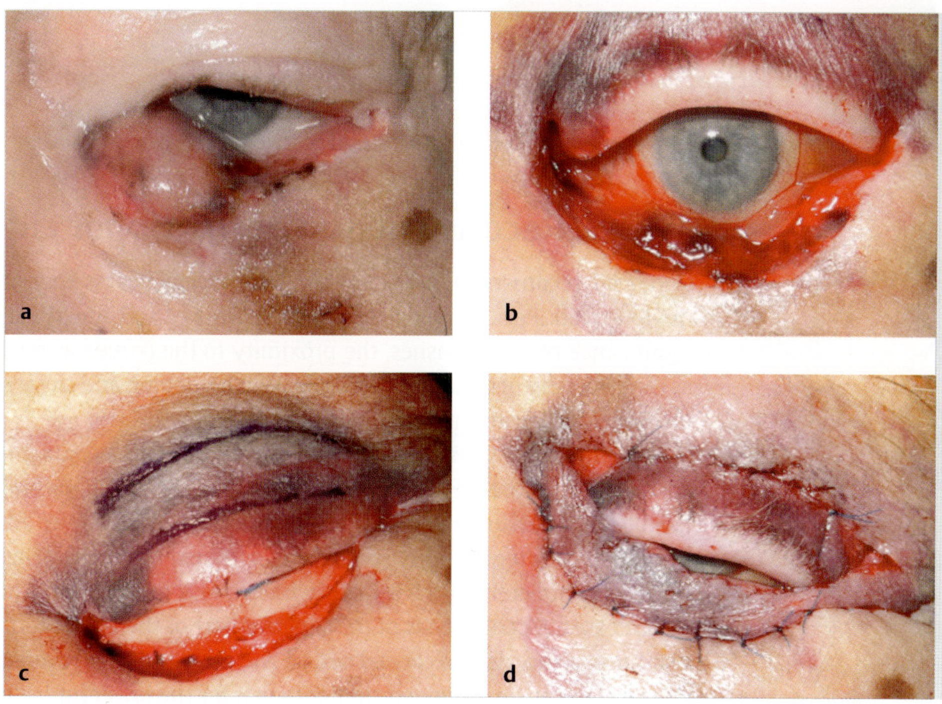

Fig. 16.14 Nodular malignant melanoma of the lower lid. **(a)** Clinical picture of a patient with a nodular malignant melanoma that arose from a lentigo maligna. **(b)** The entire lower lid along with the bulbar conjunctiva in this area has been resected to achieve an R0 resection. **(c)** Free tarsoconjunctival grafts from both upper lids along with a "bucket handle" flap, which is a pedicled skin–muscle flap harvested from the upper lid (marked with a line), were used for lower lid reconstruction. **(d)** Result of the "bucket handle" technique. To reconstruct the conjunctival defect an amniotic membrane transplant was also used.

With full-thickness defects that cannot be primarily closed by a lid margin suture, a little more mobility can be achieved by cutting the lateral canthal tendon (LCT) (**cantholysis**) (Chapter 6). The lateral part of the lid is held with a pair of forceps and pulled in a medial direction in order to be able to palpate the LCT, then the inferior part is cut. The lid is felt to give way and it can then be pulled a little more in order to close the defect.

Further methods for mobilizing the lid are **detaching the septum** and the **Tenzel flap**[11] (► Fig. 16.16, ► Fig. 16.17).

In lid reconstruction care should be taken that the horizontal tension is neither too great (risk of wound dehiscence) nor too little (risk of lid malposition due to laxity, similar to a lax tennis net). Due to gravity and the alignment of the facial muscles, the chance for the lower lid to develop retraction or ectropion is particularly high. Therefore, lateral canthal fixation to the periosteum of the lateral orbital rim or to the LCT of the upper lid is important. Absorbable or nonabsorbable sutures can be used.

If the horizontal defect is too large for a direct closure, both lamellae of the lower lid have to be replaced. The best replacement for the posterior lamella is the posterior lamella of the upper lid either as a **free** or **pedunculated** (*Hughes Surgery*[12,13]) **tarsoconjunctival graft**. If this is not an option or the defect is too large, a posterior lamellar graft can be obtained from the **nasal septum** or the **hard palate**.

Free grafts of the posterior lamella have to be covered with **local flaps** (vascularized anterior lamella), which are fashioned according to the localization and extent of the defect. A pedunculated tarsoconjunctival graft can be covered with a free skin graft or a flap (► Fig. 16.18, ► Fig. 16.19).

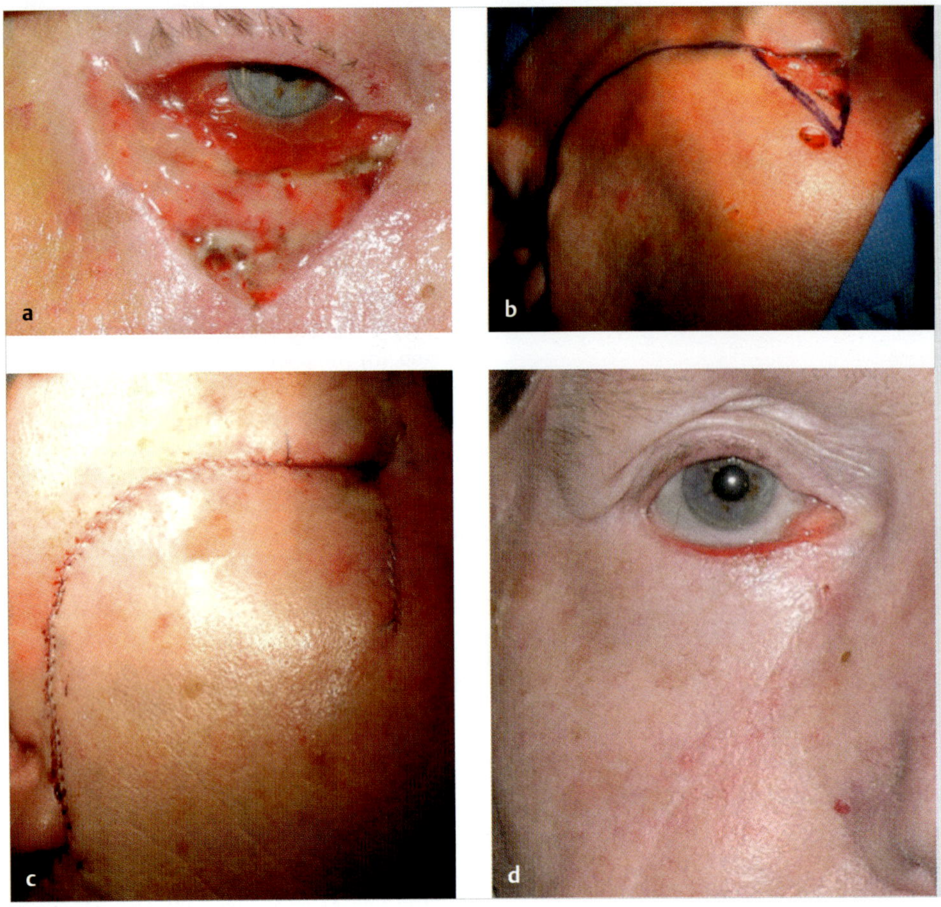

Fig. 16.15 Cheek rotation flap according to Mustarde to reconstruct the anterior lamella of a vertically extended lower lid defect. **(a)** This clinical view shows the defect extension after an R0 resection has been completed. **(b)** Planning of reconstruction procedure. The flap is marked on the skin. **(c)** The patient directly after the procedure. (The posterior lamella has been reconstructed using free tarsoconjunctival grafts harvested from the upper lids). **(d)** The result 6 months postoperatively, with slight ectropion.

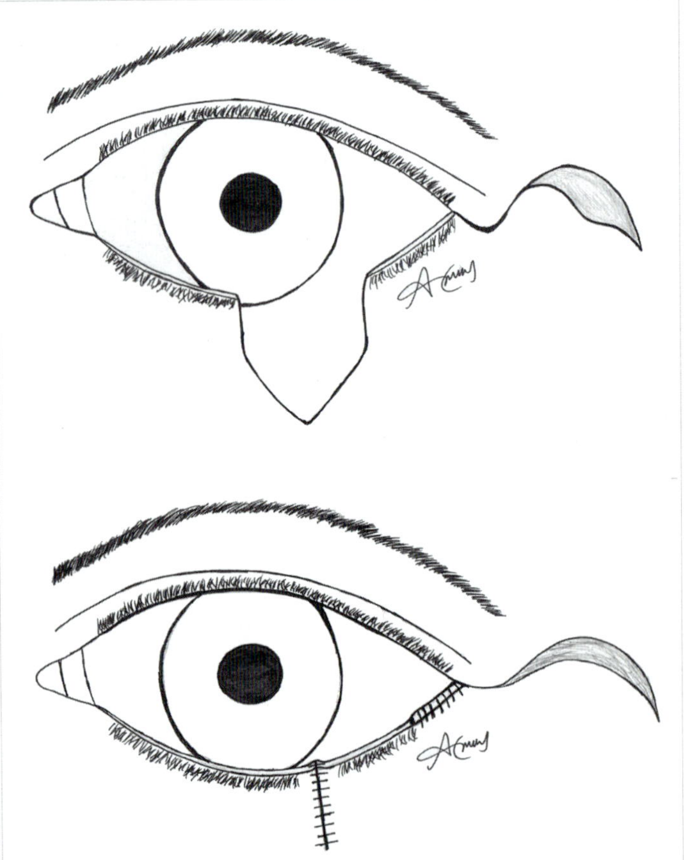

Fig. 16.16 Principle of a Tenzel procedure for reconstruction of penetrating lower lid defects. First a lateral canthotomy and inferior cantholysis is performed, followed by a cut through the septal insertion for mobilizing the residual lateral lower lid medially. A skin-muscle flap is then created in an upward-curved pattern. The procedure is completed by closing the pentagonal defect, reconstructing the lateral canthus with flap fixation at the lateral canthal ligament.

16.3.3 Reconstruction of the Upper Lid

Upper lid reconstruction follows the same principles as that of the lower lid. Peculiarities here are the cosmetic and functional significance of the eyelashes, the proximity to the cornea as well as the necessity of dynamic movement when opening and closing the lid by the levator muscle.

Smaller full-thickness defects can be converted into a pentagon and primarily closed. Here, one should take note of the shape and height of the tarsus, which is different from that of the lower lid. Upper lid shortening often results in a transient **ptosis**. This reverses completely in most cases within a few months even in severe cases. A **cantholysis** of the superior part of the lateral canthal tendon can also be carried out on the upper lid or a **reverse Tenzel flap** can be fashioned similar to that for the lower lid.

The tarsus of the upper lid is ~8 mm high centrally, so that 4 mm is available for the reconstruction of neighboring defects in the sense of a "sliding flap" (**transposition flap** in the same lid (▶ Fig. 16.20).

The anterior lamella can be taken from the upper lid itself by shifting skin from an upper lid blepharoplasty as a **"bucket handle" flap** (▶ Fig. 16.21), from the sides as an **advancement flap**, or from a **free graft**.

A further option for reconstruction of medium-sized upper lid defects is the **switch flap** reconstruction from the lower lid. In this two-stage procedure, a part of the lower lid is turned upward in order to replace anterior and posterior lamella through a pedicled graft. After 2½ weeks the pedicle is cut and the lids are restored.[8] An advantage of the procedure is the reconstruction of a genuine lid edge with continuous lash line (▶ Fig. 16.22).

Another procedure which restores the lash line is the **Hübner tarsomarginal graft** (tarsus with lid margin).[14] Depending on

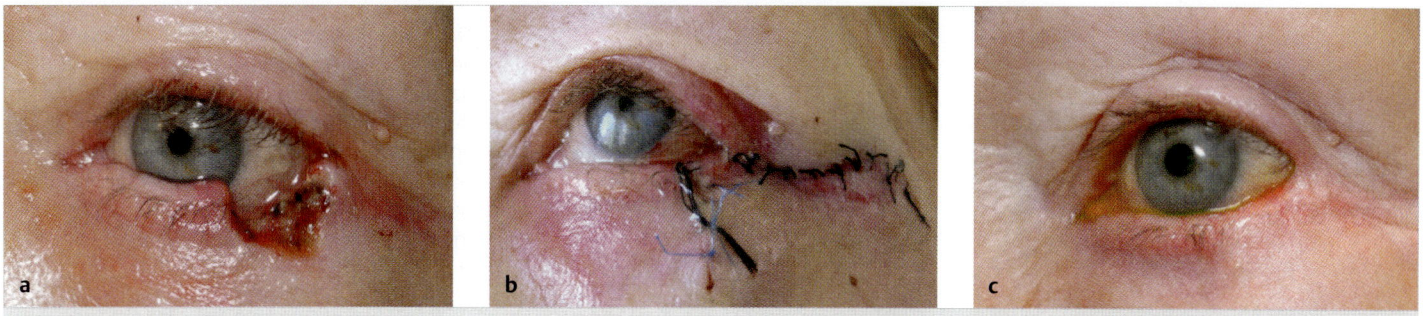

Fig. 16.17 Tenzel plasty. **(a)** A defect in the lateral thirds of the lower lid rim following resection of a basal cell carcinoma. **(b)** Reconstruction of the defect using a Tenzel flap. **(c)** The patient presents 6 weeks postoperatively with a slight rounding of the lateral canthus, but the eyelid position is acceptable.

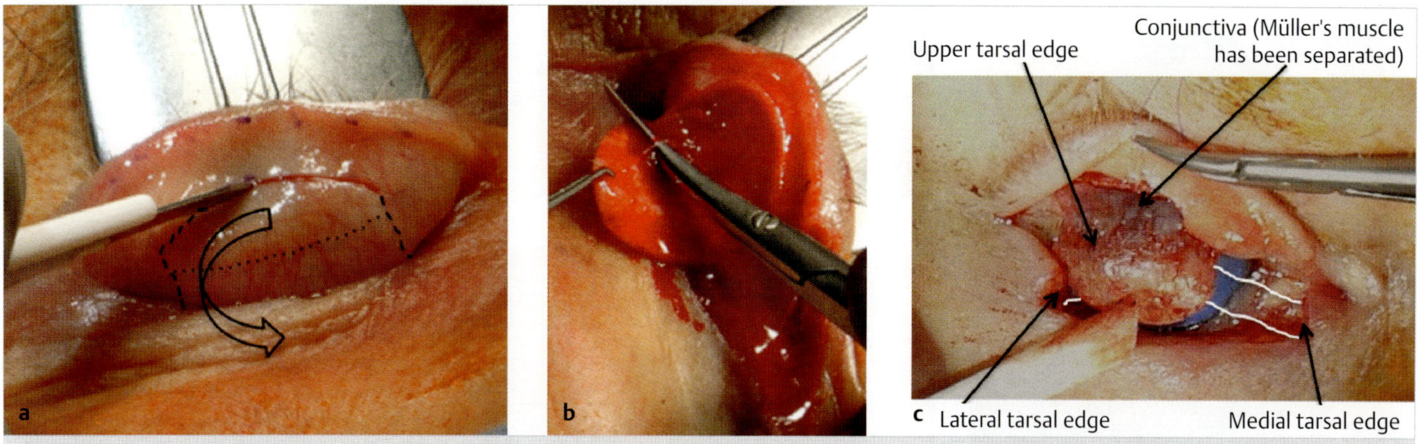

Fig. 16.18 Principle of the Hughes technique. **(a)** The upper lid is everted using a lid scoop and the required horizontal transplant extent is marked with a surgical pen. Distally 4 mm of the tarsus is spared (dotted line, upper tarsal rim; dashed line, incisions). **(b)** The pedicled tarsoconjunctival graft is separated from the orbicularis muscle. Müller's muscle is dissected carefully. **(c)** The pedicled tarsoconjunctival graft is sutured inferiorly into the lower lid defect as a posterior lamella (white lines delineate the edge of the eyelid sutures).

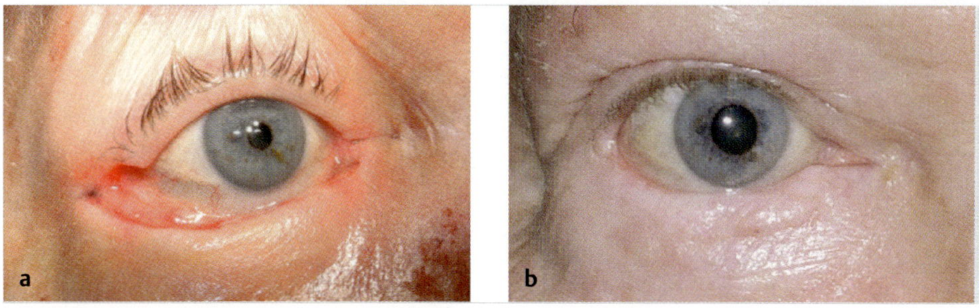

Fig. 16.19 Subtotal horizontal lower lid defect. **(a)** This subtotal horizontal lower lid defect resulted from excision of a basal cell carcinoma. **(b)** A periosteal flap from the lateral orbital rim and a Hughes plasty with a free skin graft harvested from the upper lid was used for reconstruction. This photograph shows the result 1 year postoperatively.

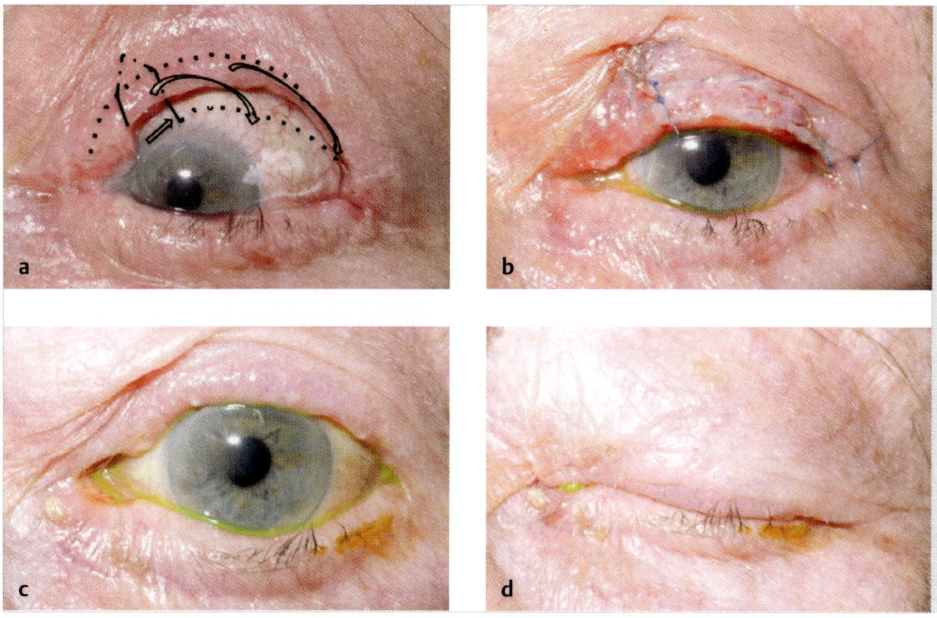

Fig. 16.20 Basal cell carcinoma of the upper lid. **(a)** Status post R0 resection and planning of the surgical procedure for reconstruction. Pentagonal excision of the anterior lamella (*dotted line*). The dotted line marks the border of the residual tarsus. In this case a transposition flap from the ipsilateral upper lid was used to reconstruct the posterior lamella and to close the pentagonal defect. The anterior lamella was created by using a free skin graft, harvested from the contralateral upper lid. **(b)** Clinical result 1 week postoperatively. **(c)** Clinical result 3 months postoperatively with eyelids open. **(d)** Clinical result 3 months postoperatively with closed eye.

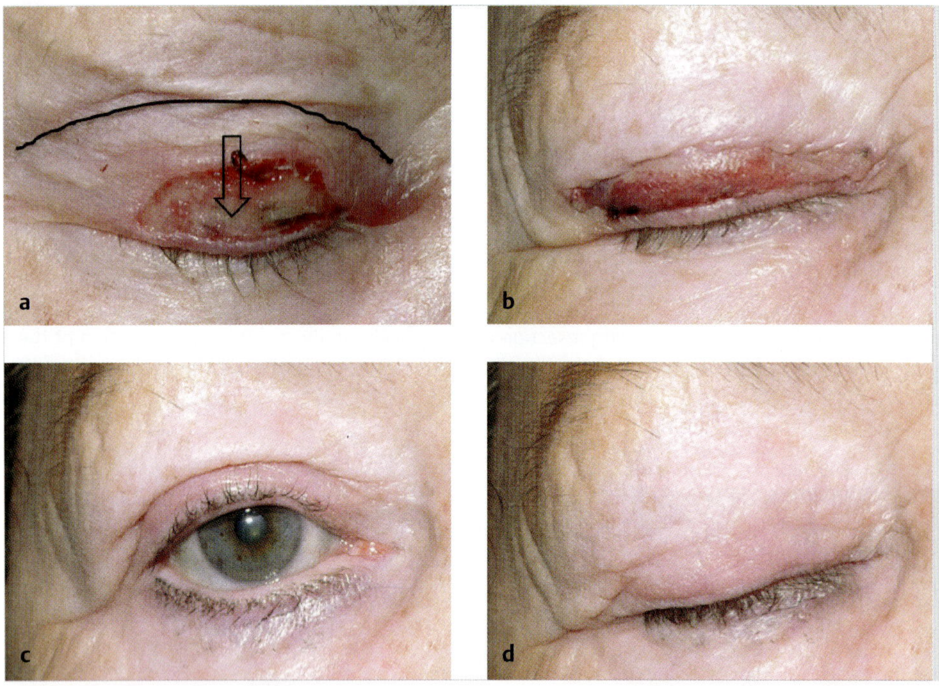

Fig. 16.21 Reconstruction of the anterior upper lid lamella using a double pedicled "bucket-handle"-transposition flap in a patient with dermatochalasis. **(a)** Status post R0 resection of an upper lid BCC. **(b)** The patient 1 week postoperatively. **(c)** The patient 3 months postoperatively with eye lids open. **(d)** The patient 3 months postoperatively with closed eyes.

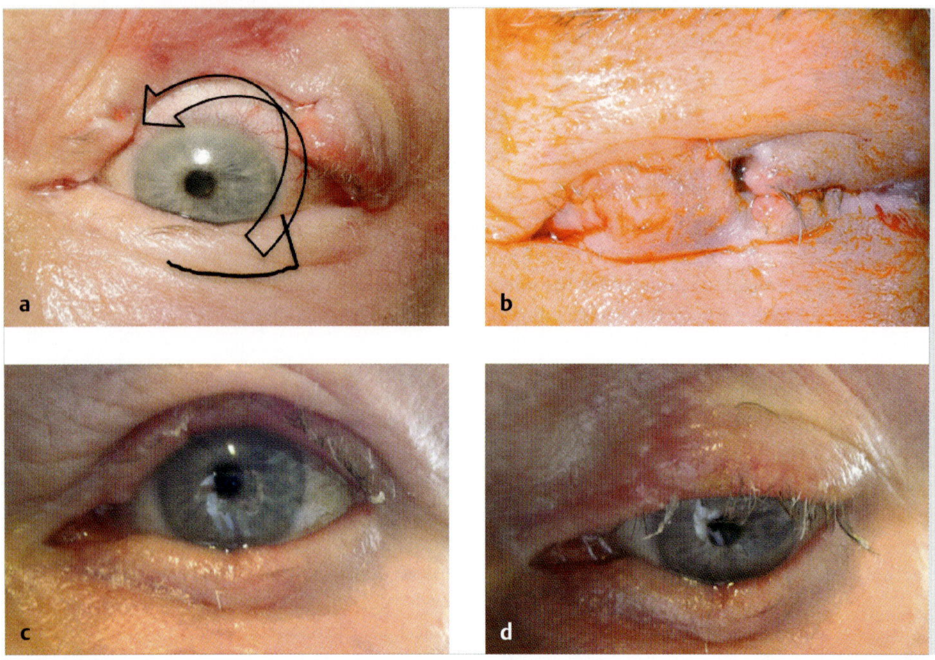

Fig. 16.22 Lower lid switch flap. **(a)** A lower lid switch flap is used for reconstruction of a mid-sized upper lid defect in a patient following R0 resection of a sebaceous gland carcinoma. There is no residual tarsus in the defect area and also a lack of lid-laxity, so that a primary wound closure is impossible, An alternative solution would be an inverse Tenzel plasty. However, the patient would lose the eyelashes with this procedure. **(b)** The patient after the first operation step. **(c)** Clinical result 2 months postoperatively, lower lid. **(d)** Clinical result 2 months postoperatively, upper lid.

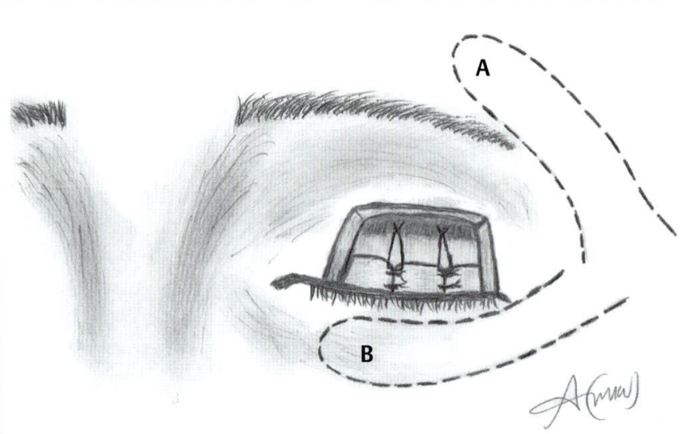

Fig. 16.23 Some options for harvesting transposition flaps with which to reconstruct the anterior upper lid lamella: A, from the temporal region. B, from the lower lid with closure of the donor site with a free skin graft (not shown). In this illustration the posterior lamella is formed by several free tarsomarginal flaps and the levator muscle is sutured to the transplants.

the laxity of the respective lids, the grafts can be taken from the contralateral upper lid and both lower lids. As these are free grafts, they have be covered with a **transposition flap** either from the temple or from the upper lid. A skin muscle flap from the ipsilateral lower lid is also an option; the secondary defect is covered with a free skin graft (▶ Fig. 16.23).

Finally, full-thickness defects of the entire upper lid can be done by the **Cutler–Beard technique**.[15] Here, the subtarsal part of the lower lid is sutured as a vascularized unit into the upper lid defect (▶ Fig. 16.24) and the flap is divided in a second stage. A disadvantage of the original procedure is possible instability with the risk of upper lid entropion due to the lack of a stabilizing tarsal plate.[16] Some authors recommend introducing ear cartilage or donor sclera[17] between the lamellae.

In upper lid reconstruction, the **levator palebrae superioris** is fixed to the tarsus or the corresponding graft with 6–0 absorbable sutures. With a significant loss of the levator due to vertically extensive defects, a corresponding repositioning of the levator is

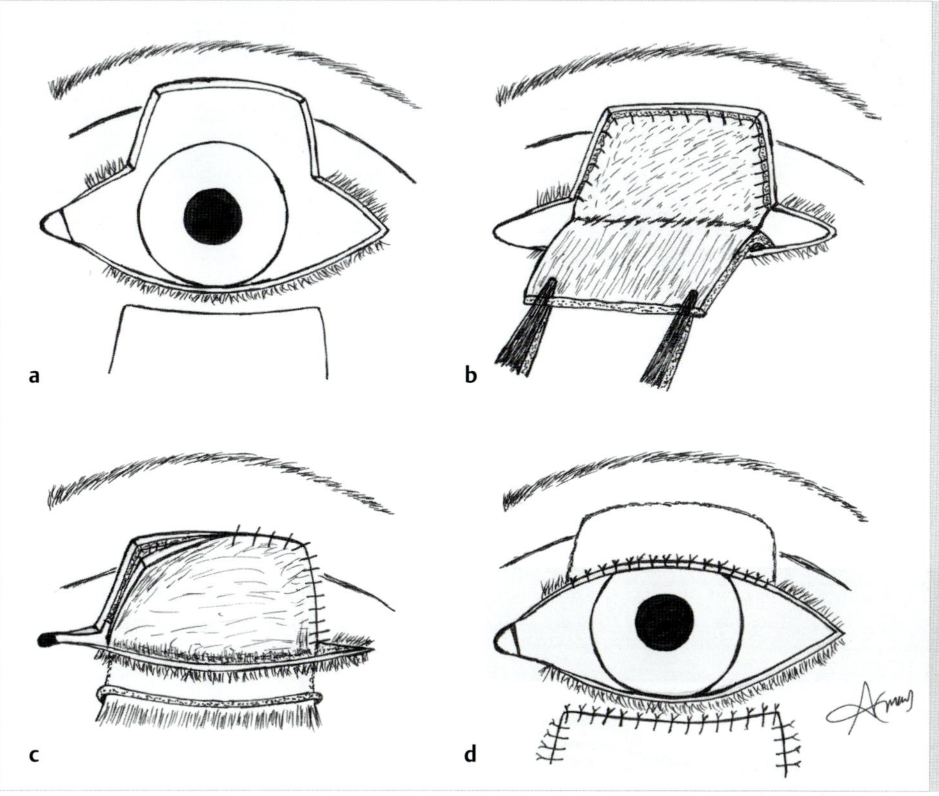

Fig. 16.24 Cutler-Beard procedure. Reconstruction of full thickness upper lid defects using infratarsal part of the lower lid. **(a)** Horizontal incision through the entire lower lid underneath the tarsus, sparing the inferior vascular cascade. Vertical inferior incisions for flap mobilizing. **(b)** Suturing of the flap into the upper lid defect (conjunctiva, orbicularis muscle, skin). A free cartilage graft harvested from the auricle, donor sclera or a bovine pericardial transplant can be used to place between the orbicularis muscle and the conjunctiva of the transplant for stabilizing and replacing the tarsus. **(c)** Suturing into the defect, layer by layer. **(d)** The eyelid is opened 3 weeks postoperatively.

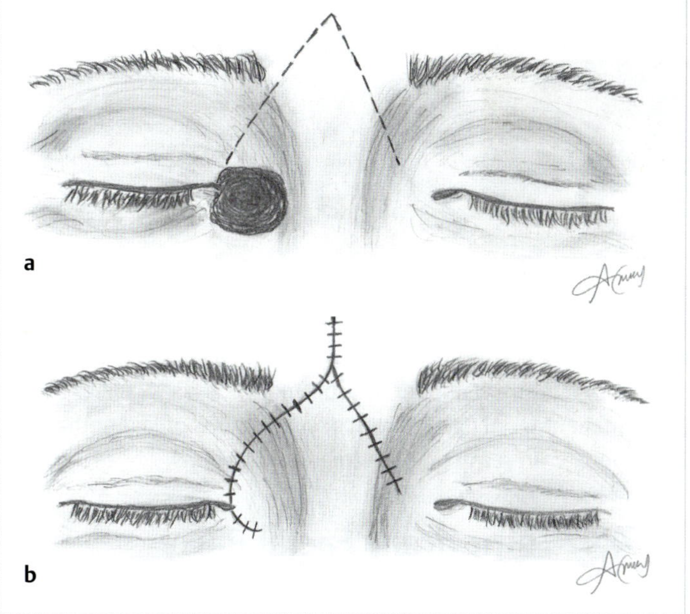

Fig. 16.25 Glabellar V-Y plasty for reconstruction of defects in the medial canthus area.

carried out or the resulting ptosis is dealt with at a later stage in order to protect the globe.

16.3.4 Reconstruction of the Lateral Canthus

In reconstructing the lateral canthal angle, the most important structure is the lateral support (lateral canthal ligament) and a pointed lateral angle. The latter is achieved by the precise adaptation of the posterior and anterior lid margins. If the LCT is spared, the reconstructing flap must be attached to it (see Tenzel flap under Chapter 16.3.2). If the wound is deeper and the LCT has been lost, it can be replaced by **periosteum** of the lateral orbital rim.[18] Skin defects here are best replaced by **local advancement flaps**. Incisions again follow the skin tension lines.[7]

16.3.5 Reconstruction of the Medial Canthus

Medial canthal reconstruction is a challenge because of its concavity. Standard approaches for covering defects in this area are the **glabella V-Y transposition flap**, the **free skin graft**, or the **"laissez faire" technique**. The latter is to allow secondary wound healing in which, due to the centripetal wound shrinkage, a deepened scar forms. This procedure can even be used with success in fairly large defects,[19] but it does have the disadvantage of a long healing time.

The **glabella flap** is a transposition flap in which skin from the glabellar area is brought into the medial canthal defect (▶ Fig. 16.25). Disadvantages are that the eyebrows can be drawn together and that existing brow hair is transposed into the medial canthal area. Harris divides the medial canthus into four aesthetic units: (1) medial upper lid, (2) medial lower lid up to the deepest point of the concavity and the areas of the nose bordering this, (3) superior, and (4) inferior to the medial canthal ligament (MCT).[20] The **reconstruction of the entire defect** is done through **reconstruction of the unit parts**, the flaps of which are fixed subcutaneously onto the MCT or the periosteum of the lateral nose. For the areas bordering the lids, horizontal **advancement flaps** are particularly suited since the skin of the lids is very mobile. The medial part of the defect is covered with simple **mobilization, rhomboid flap** (▶ Fig. 16.26), **V-Y plasty**, or **bilobar flaps**.

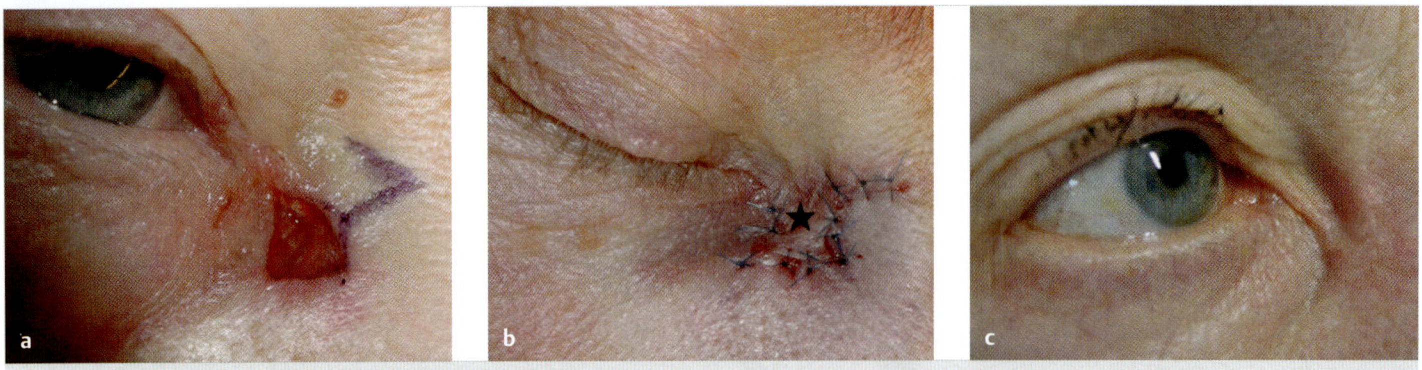

Fig. 16.26 Rhomboid flaps for medial canthus reconstruction. **(a)** A medial canthal defect status post R0 resection of a BCC. Lines are for planning the reconstruction procedure. **(b)** Flap fixation at the medial palpebral ligament is achieved using 6–0 absorbable sutures (*star*). **(c)** The patient 2 months postoperatively.

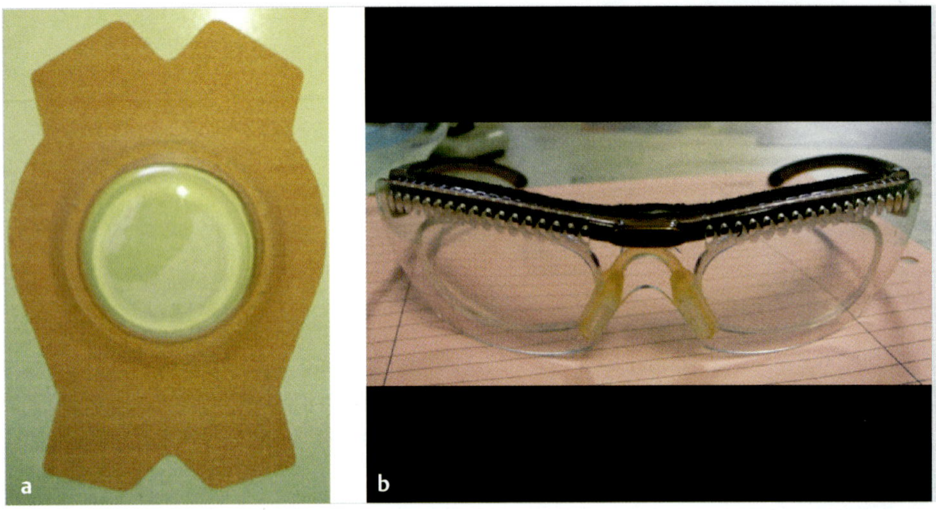

Fig. 16.27 Creating a moist chamber. **(a)** Watch glass bandage. **(b)** Eyeglasses for creating a moist chamber.

16.4 Facial Nerve Palsy

The facial nerve has five main branches, which supply the muscles of the face and the superficial neck. With a lesion of the frontal or the zygomatic branch, the functions of the orbicularis oculi muscle, which is responsible for lid closure, will be affected. Treatment depends on the degree of the paresis and its prognosis. The consequences of a paresis of the orbicularis oculi are **reduced blink frequency**, **lagophthalmos** (incomplete lid closure), **lid retraction**, and **paralytic ectropion** (lid malposition with outward rotation). The impaired lubrication of the ocular surface can result in epithelial defects and corneal ulcers. These are predominantly located in the inferior aspect of the cornea because of **Bell's phenomenon** (protective reflex of the eye; when the lids close the globe turns upward). During history taking, it is important to ask about **nocturnal lagophthalmos** from family members of the patient because, in mild cases, voluntary lid closure may be normal in an awake patient. In **blink lagophthalmos**, voluntary lid closure is possible, but, the eye remains open while blinking involuntarily.

16

Patients often complain of tearing (Chapter 15.1). Causes for **epiphora** in facial paresis are lack of orbicularis tonus and corresponding **failure of the lacrimal pump**, and **paralytic ectropion**. Causes for **lacrimation** are **corneal lesions** as well as **aberrant regeneration** ("crocodile tears").

Treatment consists of **conservative measures** such as lubrication (regular and intensive treatment with artificial tears) and, if necessary, a moist chamber and protective glasses (▶ Fig. 16.27). In permanent facial palsy, **surgical corrections** of lagophthalmos, ectropion, or lid retraction are treatment options.

16.4.1 Temporary Facial Palsy

In patients with **uncomplicated facial paresis**, in which there is the chance of spontaneous recovery (e.g., viral CN VII paresis), **lubrication** is the only treatment necessary. For more intensive lubrication, high-viscosity artificial tears and an eye ointment (vitamin A or panthenol) at night time can be given. A **moist chamber** is also recommended at night, especially when there is nocturnal lagophthalmos. Complications such as corneal ulcers, are treated with topical antibiotics and if necessary with surgical measures.

Surgical management of lagophthalmos complications are **temporary lateral** (▶ Fig. 16.28) or **central tarsorrhaphy, medial canthoplasty**, and **chemotarsorrhaphy with botulinum toxin.** In procedures that reduce the horizontal lid cleft, the assessibility of the eye and the possibility of applying drops are partly restricted. This must be taken into consideration when drawing up the indications for the procedures and when carrying them out. An alternative is the "drawstring procedure"[21], in

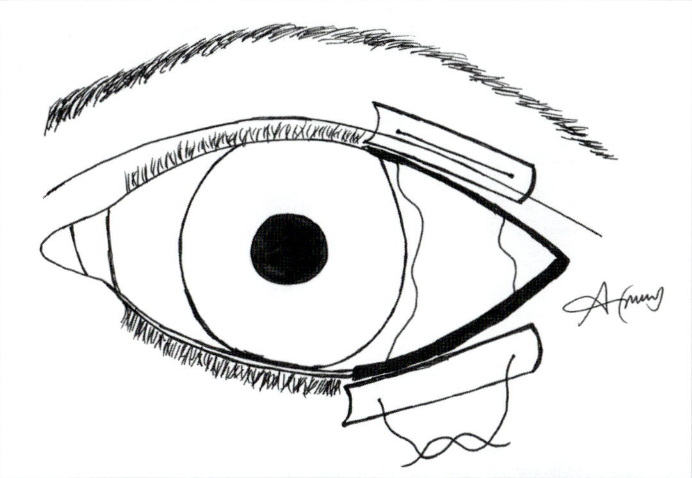

Fig. 16.28 Temporary lateral tarsorrhaphy. After debriding the lateral one-third lid margins (upper and lower), 4–0 nonabsorbable sutures are passed through both the lids over bolsters and fastened. An excision of the anterior lamella of the upper-lid and of the posterior lamella of the lower lid to a depth of 2 mm is required for permanent tarsorrhaphy, followed by suturing of the eyelid edges. The external stitches can be removed 2 weeks postoperatively.

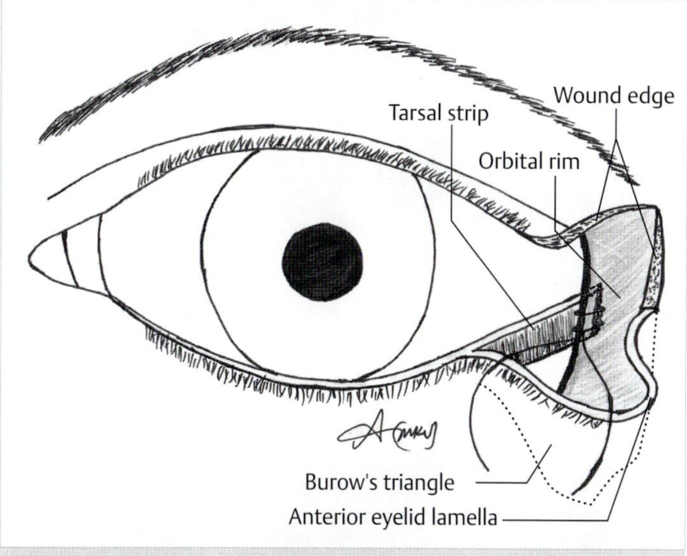

Fig. 16.29 Lateral tarsal strip. A strip is created from the lateral tarsus following lateral canthotomy and cantholysis. The lower edge of the tarsus is dissected horizontally from the conjunctiva; the covering skin along with the orbicularis muscle is excised and deepithelialized at the conjunctival side. The strip is then fixed at the inner surface of the lateral orbital rim with 5–0 polypropylene stitches, and the eyelid edges of the upper and lower lids are adapted to each other with absorbable 6–0 stitches. In cases of a short lower lid, a tissue surplus of skin and orbicularis muscle results in the upper lid, which is excised using a Burow's triangle excision to achieve smooth rounded edges.

which a complete temporary tarsorrhaphy can be opened by adjustable sutures if needed.

All the above operations have limited cosmetic effect. Therapeutic complete ptosis after botox injection to the levator muscle sets in after 2 to 3 days and lasts for 6 to 8 weeks. It can be administered transconjunctivally or transcutaneously[22] (e.g., 10 IE botox A transcutaneously) and repeated where necessary.

16.4.2 Persistent Facial Palsy

In patients with **permanent facial nerve damage**, mostly after tumor surgery of the parotid gland or of the cerebellopontine angle, that cannot be corrected by means of neuroregenerative measures, permanent solutions with acceptable cosmesis have to be found.

In uncomplicated cases, conservative treatment with lubricants and if needed a moist chamber is possible. An option for the daytime is modified sports glasses with side protection (▶ Fig. 16.27). A moist chamber is contraindicated if a corneal ulcer is present.

Correction of Ectropion

The main mechanism of **paralytic ectropion** is the lack of muscle tone in the pretarsal orbicularis fibers stabilizing the tarsal plate. In longstanding cases, there is often significant accompanying horizontal lid laxity and anterior lamellar shortening. The treatment of choice is often a **lateral tarsal strip (LTS) procedure** (▶ Fig. 16.29). With medially marked ectropion, a **tarsoconjunctival diamond excision with inverting suture** can be carried out additionally. If the LTC is stable and the ectropion is mainly medially, a **Lazy-T procedure** (the combination of horizontal lid shortening and tarsoconjunctival diamond excision) is indicated.

Longstanding, marked paralytic ectropion often has to be supported by a **canthal sling** (temporalis fascia, donor sclera or bovine pericardium are useful materials). The sling is anchored to the periosteum of the inner aspect of the lateral orbital rim and the posterior lacrimal crest with non-absorbable sutures.

Treatment of Epiphora

Despite the functional nature of the **epiphora** (not caused by a lacrimal stenosis) a **dacryocystorhinostomy** (DCR) can be done (Chapter 15.1) if no significant improvement is achieved by ectropion correction. After DCR, tear drainage functions largely independently of the lacrimal pump.

Correction of Lagophthalmos

Lagophthalmos is caused by the malposition of the lower lid and a relative upper lid retraction. With persistent lagophthalmos, despite good lower lid position, a **permanent lateral tarsorrhaphy** (▶ Fig. 16.30) can be done, though cosmesis is poor. A more elegant solution is the insertion of weights into the upper lid with **gold** or **platinum implants**. Trial weights are used preoperatively to identify the correct implant weight needed to achieve lid closure without ptosis. The implant is attached either to the anterior surface or to the upper edge of the tarsal plate.[23] Platinum chain implants are thinner and may provide a better cosmetic result[24] (▶ Fig. 16.31). Nocturnal lagophthalmos might not be corrected by the implant of weights, so that the patient might still need a moist chamber at night.

Treatment of Brow Ptosis

Brow ptosis in facial palsy is often marked so that adequate correction can best be achieved by **direct brow lift**. The skin and

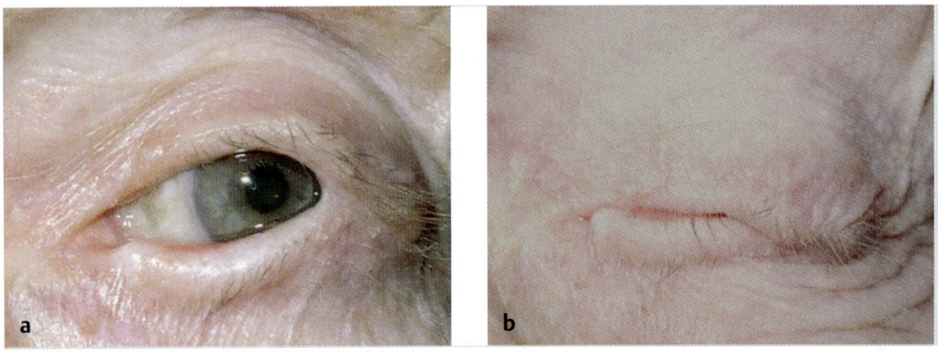

Fig. 16.30 Lateral tarsorrhaphy. **(a)** Clinical picture after lateral tarsorrhaphy of the left eye. **(b)** Complete eyelid closure is possible, but there are significant cosmetic impairments.

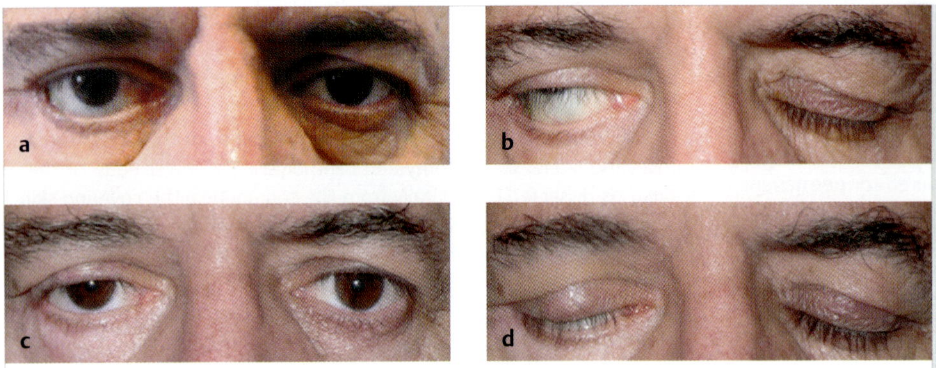

Fig. 16.31 Correction of lagophthalmos in facial nerve palsy. **(a)** In this case a lateral tarsorrhaphy had been done. The lower lid is retracted, resulting in a rounding of the lateral canthus. **(b)** Lagophthalmus. **(c)** This photograph shows the patient after a lower lid correction with a periosteal flap, lateral canthopexy, and a spacer-implant using a bovine pericardial transplant. Additionally a platinum chain has been inserted into the upper lid. This procedure resulted in a slight upper lid ptosis along with upper lid thickening. The lower lid position is favorable, as also is the configuration of the lateral canthus. **(d)** Only minor lagophthalmos.

subcutaneous tissue above the eyebrow are excised similarly to an **upper lid blepharoplasty**. The resulting scar above the eyebrow is visible and might be cosmetically impairing. In planning the surgery, the medial area above the eyebrow should be avoided as the supratrochlear and supraorbital nerves run here. An injury to these structures is associated with reduced sensitivity of the forehead up to the hairline.

An **upper lid blepharoplasty** should be carried out only sparingly as lagophthalmos and dryness can be worsened.

Treatment of Lacrimation

Gustatory hyperlacrimation through aberrant regeneration of gustatory fibers, so-called "crocodile tears," can be very debilitating for patients. The generally accepted treatment is the transcutaneous or transconjunctival **injection of botulinum toxin into the lacrimal gland**. The transconjunctival injection seems to be less often associated with ptosis as a side effect. Following topical anesthesia, the lateral upper lid is elevated while the patient is looking downward and 2.5 to 10 IE Botox A is injected directly into the palpebral part of the lacrimal gland.[25]

16

16.5 Cicatricial Ectropion, Cicatricial Entropion, Cicatricial Lagophthalmos

Surgery and trauma in the periorbital region can lead to scarring. Depending on the localization of the scar and contraction of the anterior, posterior, or both lid lamellae, the result is **cicatricial ectropion, entropion**, or **lagophthalmos**.

Correction is by lengthening the respective lamella. The excision of all scar tissue and complete correction is important.

For the correction of anterior lamellar shortening in the lower lid, a subciliary incision is made and the cutaneous and subcutaneous scar tissue is excised. Linear scars can be corrected with single or multiple **Z-plasties**. A Z-plasty alters the direction of the contraction exerted by a linear scar by 90°. The incision is marked so that the scar is excised (long arm of the "Z"). The short arms of the "Z" are drawn at 60° to this plane and parallel to each other. With short scars one "Z" is sufficient, for longer ones multiple Z-plasties are needed (► Fig. 16.32). Often a simultaneous horizontal lid shortening is necessary (wedge excision or lateral tarsal strip) to reinstate the necessary lid tension.

In case of diffuse shortening of the anterior lamella, the method of choice is a free **full-thickness skin graft** (► Fig. 16.33). A traction suture is placed to the lower lid and the subciliary incision is made across the entire length of the lid. Scar tissue is excised. Horizontal lid shortening is then performed as needed. The suborbicularis oculi fascia (SOOF) is anchored to the periosteum of the lateral orbital rim in order to generate additional support for the lid. Once the lid position is satisfactory, a vertical, slightly overcorrected template is made for the graft. The graft margins are drawn onto the donor location, the skin is infiltrated, and the graft is harvested. Any subcutaneous fat on the harvested graft is removed before suturing it to the recipient bed. The graft is sutured in place (end-to-end) with 6–0 absorbable or nonabsorbable sutures. An option is to leave every third suture longer and knot it over a bolster in order to prevent the graft from dislodging. The vascularization of the graft sets in after 5 days, and during this period it is very sensitive to friction. We recommend

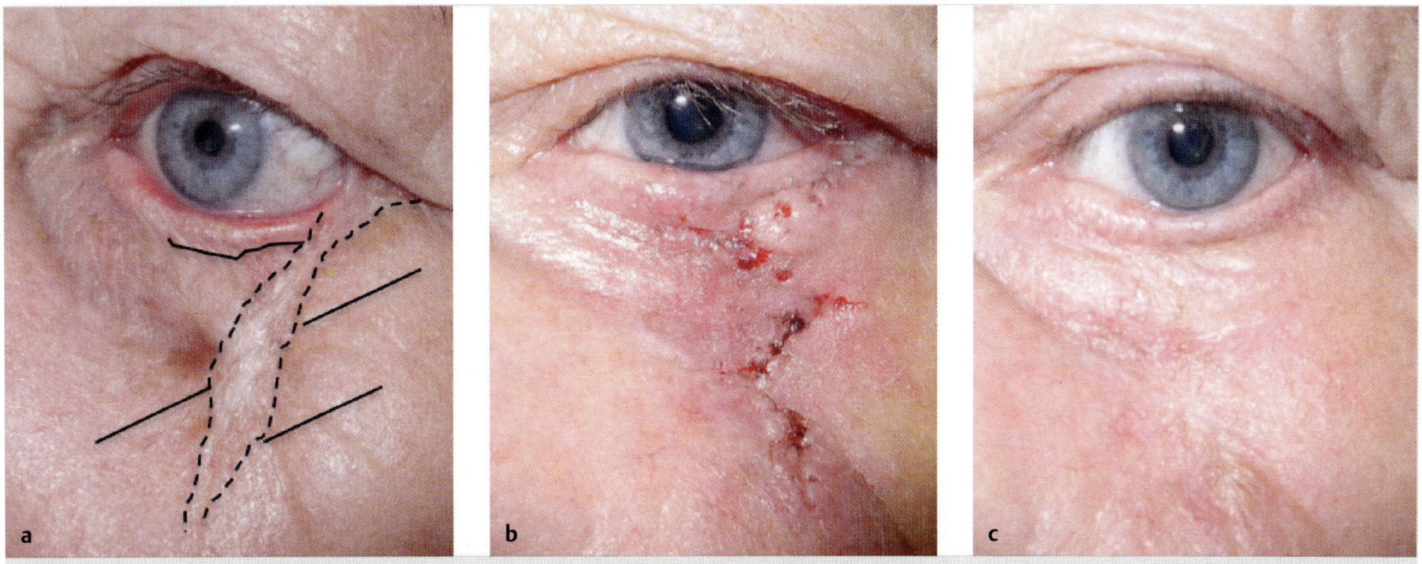

Fig. 16.32 Correction of a lower lid ectropion. **(a)** Lower lid ectropion due to scar formation in this patient following excision of a basal cell carcinoma in the left cheek. The linearly configured scar with shortening of the anterior lamella is predominant in this case. **(b)** One week postoperatively. A surgical procedure with double Z-plasty and lateral tarsal strip has been performed to correct the ectropion. **(c)** Four months postoperatively. The wound healing is completed and the lid position is favorable.

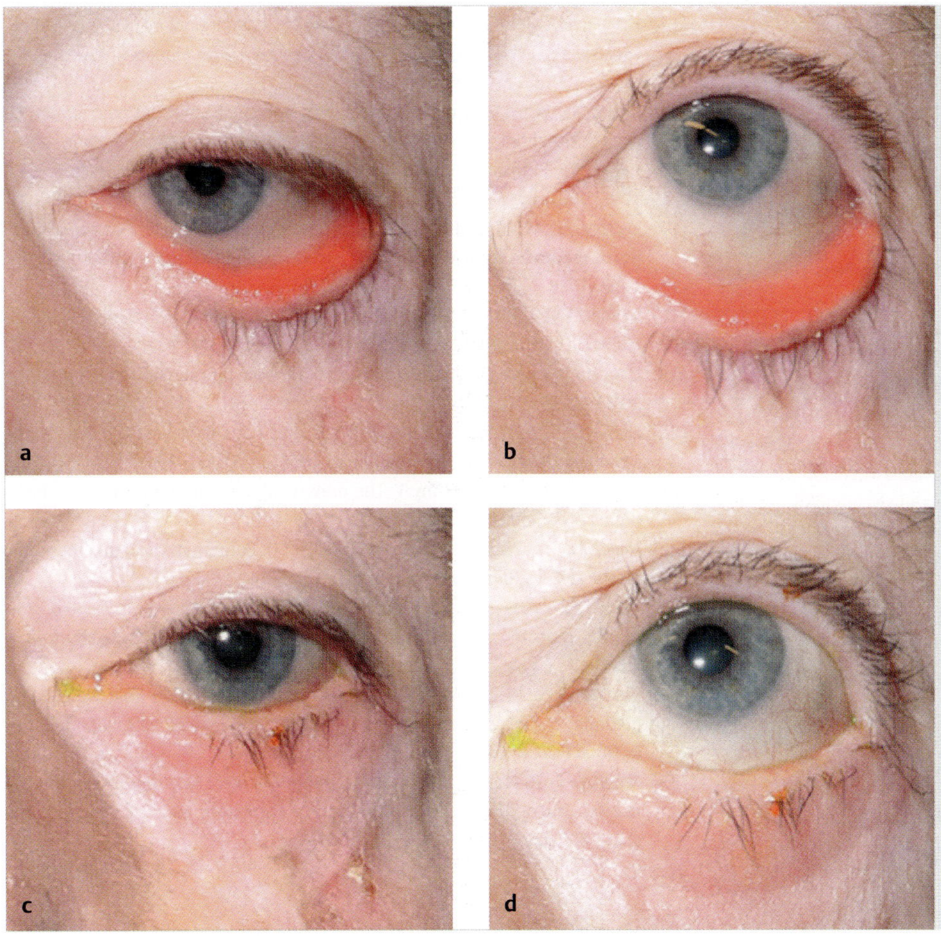

Fig. 16.33 Correction of cicatricial ectropion. **(a)** Ectropion with scar formation in the lower lid in a patient following resection of a basal cell carcinoma of the cheek. **(b)** The severity of the anterior lamellar shortening becomes obvious in upgaze. **(c)** Three months post-op picture, after ectropion correction using a retroauricular full thickness skin graft, lateral tarsal strip and reinsertion of lower lid retractors. **(d)** Good lid position in upgaze.

leaving the dressing in place for a week, if possible. The sutures are removed after 2 weeks. In larger grafts, small incisions or fixation sutures within the graft are recommended to prevent the accumulation of serum or blood.

▶ Fig. 16.34 shows the case of a lower lid retraction due to massive scarring following excision and radiotherapy for a malignant tumor. The scars were localized in the posterior as well as in the anterior lamella and there was no mobility of the lid. The conjunctival fornix was intact. Correction included recession of the lower lid retractors, use of spacer grafts (here bovine pericardium), and the replacement of the anterior lamella with a skin-muscle flap from the upper lid. In a post irradiated tissue, a vascularized flap has a better chance of survival than a free graft.

A shortening of the **posterior lamella** as the result of conjunctival scarring can be done with a Z-plasty or local advancement

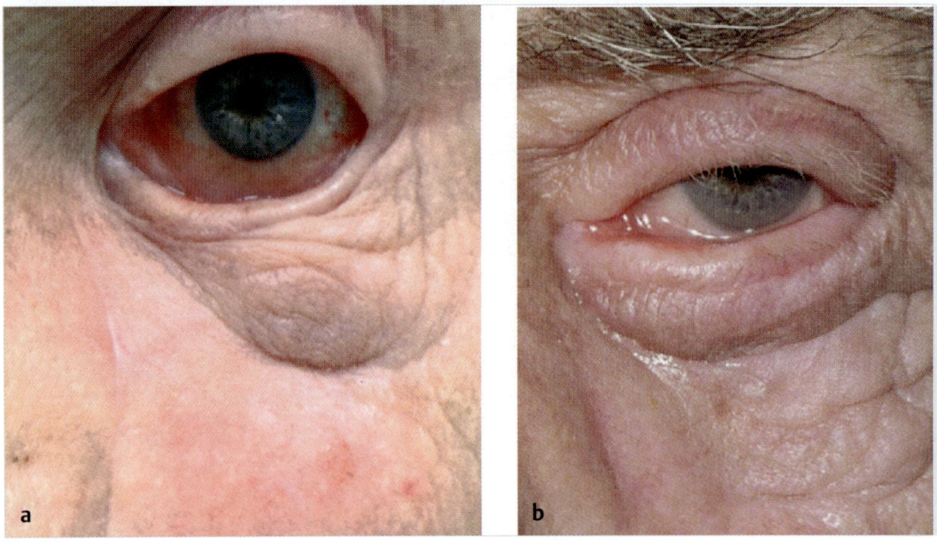

Fig. 16.34 Correction of cicatricial ectropion. (a) Ectropion along with lower lid retraction due to shortened anterior and posterior lamellae in a patient following operation and radiotherapy for a left maxillary sinus squamous cell carcinoma. Lack of lid mobility and exposure conjunctivitis. (b) This photo shows the status after surgical correction: scar tissue was completely excised. For reconstruction, a lateral tarsal strip and implantation of a bovine pericardial transplant between lower orbital rim and tarsus instead of the lower lid retractors was done. The anterior lamella, which was also shortened, was reconstructed with a laterally pedicled skin–muscle-flap harvested from the upper lid.

flaps of the conjunctiva. A free **conjunctival graft** can be taken from the ipsilateral or contralateral eye. For more pronounced defects either **amniotic membrane** or **oral mucosa** (buccal or labial) are suitable for replacing conjunctiva.

References

[1] Black EH, Nesi FA, Gladstone G, Levine MR, Calvano CJ, Eds. Smith and Nesi's Ophthalmic Plastic and Reconstructive Surgery. 3rd ed. New York, NY: Springer; 2012

[2] Yu Wai Man C, Steel D. Visual outcome after open globe injury: a comparison of two prognostic models–the Ocular Trauma Score and the Classification and Regression Tree. Eye (Lond). 2010; 24(1):84–89

[3] Kuhn F, Pieramici DJ. Ocular Trauma: Principles and Practice. New York, NY: Thieme; 2002

[4] Herzum H, Holle P, Hintschich C. [Eyelid injuries: epidemiological aspects]. [Article in German]. Ophthalmologe. 2001; 98(11):1079–1082

[5] Badia JM, Torres JM, Tur C, Sitges-Serra A. Saline wound irrigation reduces the postoperative infection rate in guinea pigs. J Surg Res. 1996; 63(2):457–459

[6] Foundation AO. Transforming Surgery—Changing Lives. Available at: https://www2.aofoundation.org/wps/portal/!ut/p/c1/04_SB8K8xLLM9MSSzPy8xBz9CP0os3hng7BARydDRwN3QwMDA08zTzdvvxBjIwN_I6B8JJK8haEFUD7U09nP2MkPqNSEgG4_j_zcVP2C3IhyADJvFMw!/dl2/d1/L2dJQSEvUUt3QS9ZQnB3LzZfQzBWUUFCMUEwRzEwMDBJNklGS05UMzIwTzI!/?showPage=startpage. Accessed September 7, 2016

[7] Harris GJ. Atlas of Oculofacial Reconstruction. Philadelphia, PA: Lippincott Williams & Wilkins; 2009

[8] Mustardé JC. Repair and Reconstruction in the Orbital Region: A Practical Guide. 3rd ed. New York, NY: Churchill Livingstone; 1991. Distributed in USA by Longman

[9] Semer NB. Practical Plastic Surgery for Nonsurgeons. Philadelphia, PA: Hanley & Belfus; 2001

[10] Patel KG, Sykes JM. Concepts in local flap design and classification. Oper Tech Otolaryngol–Head Neck Surg. 2011; 22(1):13–23

[11] Tenzel RR. Reconstruction of the central one half of an eyelid. Arch Ophthalmol. 1975; 93(2):125–126

[12] Hughes WL. Lid reconstruction. Int Ophthalmol Clin. 1964; 4:209–237

[13] Foster J. Reconstruction of the lower lid by Hughes' method. Br J Ophthalmol. 1944; 28(10):515–519

[14] Hübner H. [Modified full-lid transplants ("tarsomarginal transplants") in reconstructive eyelid surgery]. [Article in German]. Klin Monatsbl Augenheilkd. 1988; 193(6):647–650

[15] Cutler NL, Beard C. A method for partial and total upper lid reconstruction. Am J Ophthalmol. 1955; 39(1):1–7

[16] Carroll RP. Entropion following the Cutler-Beard procedure. Ophthalmology. 1983; 90(9):1052–1055

[17] Wesley RE, McCord CD, Jr. Transplantation of eyebank sclera in the Cutler–Beard method of upper eyelid reconstruction. Ophthalmology. 1980; 87(10):1022–1028

[18] Dryden RM, Edelstein JP. Lateral palpebral tendon repair for lower eyelid ectropion. Ophthal Plast Reconstr Surg. 1988; 4(2):115–118

[19] DaCosta J, Oworu O, Jones CA. Laissez-faire: how far can you go? Orbit. 2009; 28(1):12–15

[20] Harris GJ, Logani SC. Multiple aesthetic unit flaps for medial canthal reconstruction. Ophthal Plast Reconstr Surg. 1998; 14(5):352–359

[21] Kitchens J, Kinder J, Oetting T. The drawstring temporary tarsorrhaphy technique. Arch Ophthalmol. 2002; 120(2):187–190

[22] Naik MN, Soparkar CN, Murthy R, Honavar SG. Botulinum toxin in ophthalmic plastic surgery. Indian J Ophthalmol. 2005; 53(4):279–288

[23] Bladen JC, Norris JH, Malhotra R. Indications and outcomes for revision of gold weight implants in upper eyelid loading. Br J Ophthalmol. 2012; 96(4):485–489

[24] Bladen JC, Norris JH, Malhotra R. Cosmetic comparison of gold weight and platinum chain insertion in primary upper eyelid loading for lagophthalmos. Ophthal Plast Reconstr Surg. 2012; 28(3):171–175

[25] Montoya FJ, Riddell CE, Caesar R, Hague S. Treatment of gustatory hyperlacrimation (crocodile tears) with injection of botulinum toxin into the lacrimal gland. Eye (Lond). 2002; 16(6):705–709

Chapter 17

Anesthesiological Aspects of Orbit Surgery

17

17 Anesthesiological Aspects of Orbit Surgery

Jan-Peter A. H. Jantzen and Bernd Schwefler

17.1 Introduction

In the planning and conduct of anesthesiological care for surgical patients, as well as the patient's state of health, the specific nature of the operation envisaged must be taken into account. In this the anatomy and physiology of the target organ for the surgical procedure provide the focus. In this regard orbit surgery is particularly complex; in addition to the specifics of ophthalmic anesthesia, those of neuroanesthesia and ENT anesthesia have to be taken into account. This complexity derives from the anatomy and the physiological specifics of the orbit and its neighboring structures.

17.2 Clinical Anatomy

Reference should be made to Chapter 1 for an understanding of the significant clinical anatomy pertinent to anesthesiological care.

The optic nerve consists of the bundled axons of the large ganglion cells in the third neuron of the retina; unlike the other cranial nerves it is not a peripheral nerve but a continuation of the diencephalon and is surrounded by a fluid-filled sheath. The osseous channel, the dural sheath and the connective tissue bordering the chiasmatic groove—inter alia the rigid annulus of Zinn—encase the optic nerve and the ophthalmic artery. This optic sheath exhibits high elastance, whereby it is potentially at risk in the event of a mass. In this respect the optic nerve is not directly at risk from pressure; the risk is more that compression of the nutritive vessels from the pia mater will jeopardize supply (see Chapter 2).

A continually raised intracranial pressure (ICP) is transmitted into the optic sheath, where it can induce papilledema in the ocular fundus (edema of the optic nerve papilla) through the increase in the pressure of the fluid.

The orbit—the bony capsule of the eye—is a non-expandable casing, like the skull (the bony capsule of the brain). This and other analogies form the common anatomical-physiological basis of ophthalmic anesthesia and neuroanesthesia (▶ Table 17.1).

Similar aims of anesthesiological care also result from these common features (▶ Table 17.2).

17

17.3 Clinical Physiology

17.3.1 Hemodynamics

Organs close to the orbit exhibit hemodynamically relevant peculiarities. Thus the frontal brain lobe lying over the roof of the orbit has the highest oxygen requirement of the body, the choroid in the orbit the highest perfusion. Perfusion of the brain, as well as that of the retina, is subject to autoregulation; that of the choriocapillaris, owing to the absence of precapillary sphincters, is not.[1] The last-mentioned difference is clinically significant. A rise in mean arterial pressure (MAP; driving force of organ perfusion) brings about a drop in intracranial pressure (ICP), in contrast, a rise in intraocular pressure (IOP) (▶ Fig. 17.1). The cause is the autoregulatory response of the blood vessels of the brain, which respond to the rise in MAP with vasoconstriction: the consecutive drop in the cerebral blood volume (CBV) lowers the ICP. The choroidal blood volume, in contrast, rises pressure-passively, and with it so does the IOP. Awareness of these connections enables targeted control of the hemodynamics by anesthesiological measures with the aim of optimizing not only patient safety but also the surgical conditions (see also "Controlled Reduction of Blood Pressure" in Chapter 17.5.6).

17.3.2 Intracranial Pressure

The intracranial pressure (ICP) is the pressure that the contents of the skull exert on the craniodural envelope (▶ Table 17.2). ICP is position-dependent and is physiologically lower than 10 mm Hg. The pressure is built up by the blood volume expelled into the cerebral vascular bed during systole. A clearly raised ICP can affect perfusion of the brain. For the purpose of a rough assessment of cerebral perfusion, the cerebral perfusion pressure (CPP) is used, the calculated difference between mean arterial pressure and ICP (CPP =MAP – ICP). The perfusion of the brain is subject to

Table 17.1 Analogies between orbit and skull biology

	Eye	Brain
Anatomy		
Capsule	Orbit	Skull
Casing	Sclera	Dura mater
Substance	Vitreous body	Brain
Liquid	Aqueous humor	Cerebrospinal fluid
Production	Ciliary body	Choroid plexus
Fluid spaces	Anterior and posterior chamber	Ventricle system
Arterial supply	Ophthalmic artery	Carotid and vertebral arteries
Venous drainage	Jugular vein	Jugular vein
Physiology		
Perfusion barrier	Autoregulation of retinal perfusion	Autoregulation of cerebral blood flow (CBF)
Diffusion barrier	Blood–humor-barrier	Blood–brain-barrier
Internal pressure	Intraocular pressure (IOP)	Intracranial pressure (ICP)
Control parameter	Intraocular fluid balance	Cerebrospinal fluid balance
Relevant factors	Chronobiology, $PaCO_2$, AWP	Chronobiology, $PaCO_2$, AWP
Pathophysiology		
Bleeding	Vitreous hemorrhage	Intracerebral bleeding, subarachnoid bleeding
Drainage disorder	Buphthalmus	Hydrocephalus
Rise in pressure	Glaucoma	Intracranial pressure syndrome

Abbreviations: Pa, arterial partial pressure. AWP, airway pressure.

Table 17.2 Intracranial pressure: synopsis

- Intracranial pressure (ICP) is the pressure that the contents of the skull exert on the dura mater. This pressure—in line with the hydrostatic gradients and the compartmentalization of the intracranial space—is nonuniform. Under pathological conditions the regional difference can be ≥ 20 mm Hg. This is to be noted when placing a pressure sensor and interpreting the readings.
- The ICP is the "sum of the partial pressures" of the brain tissue (80%), cerebrospinal fluid (8–12%) and blood ($ICP = p_{cerebrum} + p_{fluid} + p_{blood}$). Depending on position, the ICP amounts to 0 to 15 mm Hg. Readings of 15 to 20 mm Hg/25 to 40 mm Hg show a "slightly/moderately raised" ICP; readings above 40 mm Hg show a "severely raised" ICP.
- ICP is an organ constant, which is kept constant within narrow limits under physiologic conditions. The increase in the partial pressure of one component (brain tissue, cerebrospinal fluid) is compensated by a change in the intracranial blood volume in response (Monro–Kellie hypothesis).
- The ICP is one determinant of cerebral perfusion pressure (CPP = MAP – ICP) and thus also of cerebral blood flow (CBF = CPP/CVR).
- In line with the principle "function drives metabolism, metabolism drives flow," the CPP, as the determinant of the driving force of perfusion, is a proxy variable for cerebral blood flow, which is clinically hardly measurable and in the pre-hospital setting not at all.
- A persistently elevated ICP damages the tissue of the brain not only directly (pressure damage) but also indirectly (perfusion damage). For patients with craniocerebral trauma or aneurysmal subarachnoid hemorrhage, persistently elevated ICP heralds unfavorable neurologic outcome. Pathologic ICP waves (A to E waves as per Nils Lundberg) are likewise indicators of a poor prognosis.
- Reduction of pathologically raised ICP requires it to be measured beforehand; this can only be done invasively. Established locations for measurement are the epidural space, CSF, and brain tissue. The measurement is made using the principle of communicating tubes (e.g., in the CSF space), electronically, or fiberoptically.
- Direct measurement of the pressure via a catheter in the lateral ventricle (official gold standard) enables—in addition to manometry and zero point alignment—the pressure to be reduced by draining CSF, the determination of the intracranial elastance ($\Delta P/\Delta V$), and microbiological and metabolic diagnostics. Placing the catheter is traumatizing (drill hole 4.4 mm, brain passage 4.5 cm), and the risks of bleeding (1.4%) and contamination (≤ 3%) are not trivial.
- Measurement using a fiberoptic or electronic sensor in the brain tissue is less traumatic (drill hole 2.8 mm, brain passage 1.4 cm) and burdened with fewer complications. Parenchymal pressure measurement has been established as the de facto standard in many places.
- ICP measurement should be considered if intracranial hypertension is suspected. ICP monitoring cannot be replaced by CT checks.

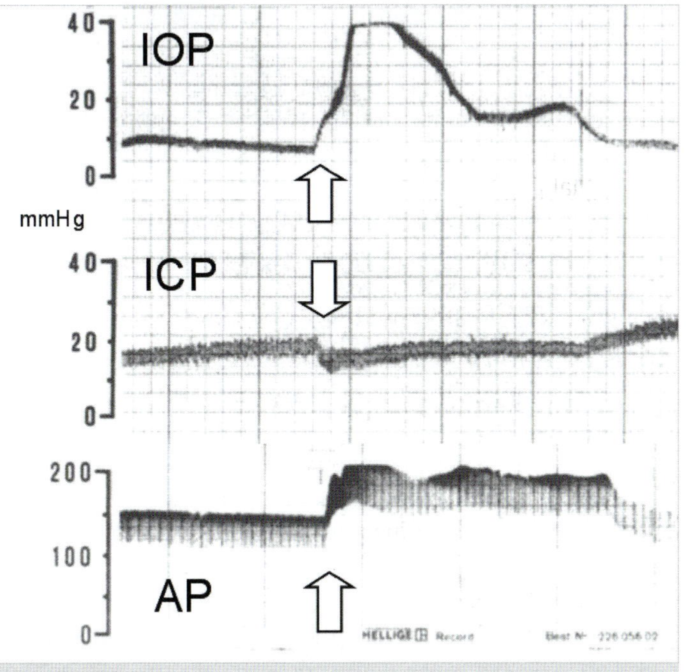

Fig. 17.1 Autoregulation. Effect of raising the cerebral and ocular perfusion pressure through angiotensin-induced arterial hypertension (arterial pressure, AP; *arrow*) on intracranial pressure (ICP) and intraocular pressure (IOP). The ICP falls as a result of autoregulation-triggered vasoconstriction; the IOP rises—due to the absence of autoregulatory competence of the choroid—in parallel with the blood pressure (pig model).[2]

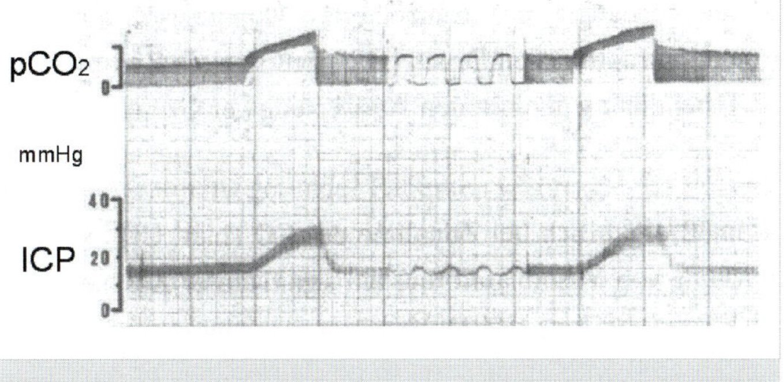

Fig. 17.2 CO_2 responsiveness. The capnographic rebreathing-induced hypercapnia causes a parallel course of the intracranial pressure (ICP) via cerebral vasodilatation (pig model).[2]

autoregulation (myogenic autoregulation, Bayliss effect); that is, it takes place for the most part independently of the systemic blood pressure and is controlled to meet metabolic requirements ($CMRO_2$: cerebral metabolic rate for oxygen). In metabolically highly active areas of the brain, CO_2 accumulates as the end product of aerobic metabolism, which dilates blood vessels and thus fosters regional substrate supply via vasodilatation. In less-active areas, relative hypocarbia results in vasoconstriction. This marked CO_2-responsiveness of the cerebral blood vessels enables the fine control required for the perfusion of the brain. Due to the same mechanism, hypoventilation-induced hypercapnia causes global cerebral vasodilatation with corresponding rise in the CBV and consequent rise of the ICP (▶ Fig. 17.2). Conversely, a raised ICP can be reduced promptly through hyperventilation. This "controlled hypocapnia" may be used only for a limited time, however, as the vasoconstriction induced is associated with the risk of cerebral ischemia.

The ICP increases in case of expansion of the intracranial compartment—for example, in hypercapnia-induced vasodilatation (see above). This rise is usually nonthreatening, though it is undesirable in supraorbital operations. All mechanisms that increase ICP with intact dura mater act as vis-a-tergo once the dura is opened, rendering ICP atmospheric. The surgeon identifies this force by the fact that brain tissue emerges over the edge of the craniotomy. This worsens surgical conditions, which is why medication and measures that would increase ICP with the dura intact should be avoided.

17

17.3.3 Intraocular Pressure

The intraocular pressure (IOP)—the pressure that the contents of the eyeball exert on the corneoscleral envelope—is a result of inner pressure and outer counterpressure. IOP is an organ constant that varies only within a narrow range. The pressure is composed of the components of the aqueous humor and perfusion balance as dynamic factors and the volume of the vitreous body and osmotic pressure gradients as predominantly static factors. The mechanical and chemical effects of controlled ventilation are further controlling or disrupting forces. Acute changes in the internal pressure of the eyes in the seconds to minutes time range result from changes in tension of the extraocular striated musculature or are produced hemodynamically. As well as effects of the preoperative medication and hydration on the IOP, the positioning of the patient is significant.

In addition to its significance for the diagnosis of glaucoma, measurement of the IOP serves as a global test that can be performed on the intact eyeball to record factors that–with the eye opened up–that is, at atmospheric IOP would act as vis-a-tergo expelling the contents of the eyeball. In most intraorbital operations, an IOP stable at a low level provides favorable operating conditions. With opening of the eyeball, especially extensive opening, one should refrain from using pharmaceuticals and measures that would increase the vis-a-tergo. The majority of anesthetics do not have a relevant effect on the IOP, or they reduce it dose dependently. As the cause of the latter phenomenon, a direct effect on an IOP control center, presumably located in the diencephalon, is assumed.[4] In contrast to anesthetics, the effects of depolarizing muscle relaxants are clinically significant (see Chapter 17.4.5).

17.4 Clinical Pharmacology

A number of well-controllable drugs with few side effects is available for the induction and maintenance of anesthesia and for neuromuscular blockade (▶ Table 17.3). The suitability of anesthetics for the goals of ophthalmic anesthesia and neuroanesthesia can be gauged from the requirements listed in ▶ Table 17.4. In addition to the desire for hemodynamic stability one should take account of the specifics of orbit surgery in relation to the pharmacodynamics with reference to the internal cranial and orbital pressures—ICP und IOP. A medication is easily controllable if it can be used with antagonists to be short-acting, or have rapid onset and offset, and be free of residual or side effects.

17.4.1 Sedatives

Sedatives and tranquillizers are administered as premedication or to deepen general anesthesia. Benzodiazepines are the most widely used. These interact with the benzodiazepine receptors in the CNS and intensify endogenous GABA-mediated inhibition mechanisms. Midazolam and diazepam inter alia are used for parenteral administration. Long-acting lorazepam is predominantly used in the United States. Midazolam is the one most suited to the aims of anesthesia in orbit surgery. In a low to moderate dose midazolam bolsters the opiate effect on the descending inhibitory pain pathway.

Midazolam can be administered as a bolus or continuously. The dosage is calculated on an individual basis according to effect, mostly in a range from 2.5 to 10 mg/h. Despite a relatively short elimination half-life of 1 to 2 hours, high lipophilia causes evident cumulation and a lengthening of the effect, particularly when administered for a longer time. For prompt termination of undesirable or intensive effects of benzodiazepines, there is specific antidote available in flumazenil.

Table 17.3 Anesthetics and adjuvants for orbit surgery in adults

Premedication	Midazolam, clonidine, dexmedetomidine
Hypnotics	Propofol, etomidate
Analgesics	Sufentanil, remifentanil, (*S*)-ketamine
Inhalational anesthetics	Sevoflurane, desflurane
Muscle relaxants	Mivacurium, cisatracurium, rocuronium
Antagonists	Sugammadex, flumazenil, naloxone

17.4.2 Hypnotics

Hypnotics and hypnoanalgesics are available for the induction of general anesthesia by injection. Ketamine and (*S*)-ketamine belong to the second group. These are used when circulatory stabilization or augmentation is desired or when hypnotics are contraindicated (see also Chapter 17.4.4). The significance of barbiturates (thiobarbiturates or hydroxybarbiturates) is in decline, due, among other causes, to their tendency to suppress the immune system. Myocardial depression is characteristic of the pharmacodynamics of barbiturates, while cumulation is significant with regard to the pharmacokinetics, so that administration by means of infusion is not indicated for lengthy interventions. Barbiturates are contraindicated in patients with porphyria; a niche still remaining for methohexital, where available, is the rectal induction of anesthesia in children.[4] When circulatory depression is a concern, etomidate is used. Etomidate is substantially circulation-neutral, short-acting, and free of cumulation potential. One disadvantage and indication-limiting feature is the suppression of cortisol synthesis.[5] An undesirable effect is myoclonus, which occurs if etomidate is administered to induce anesthesia without previous administration of opioids or benzodiazepines.

The induction hypnotic most often used is propofol. The cerebral pharmacodynamics of propofol are characterized by a decrease in $CMRO_2$, cerebral blood flow (CBF), and ICP. Cerebral autoregulation and CO_2-responsiveness remain intact. As propofol in individual cases, especially when administered quickly, lowers the blood pressure, it is often given by means of a syringe pump. This method is also selected when propofol is administered as the hypnotic component of total intravenous anesthesia (TIVA). The negligible cumulation of propofol, even when administered for a long period, is particularly advantageous when the patient is to wake up early after a lengthy operation on the orbit for neurologic assessment.

Table 17.4 Common aims of ophthalmic anesthesia and neuroanesthesia

- Intraoperative and postoperative analgesia
- Immobilization
- Orbital and/or intracranial hypotension
- Arterial normotension
- When needed, controlled arterial hypotension
- Emergence without emesis and shivering
- Early postoperative sensory assessability

17.4.3 Inhalational Anesthetics

Inhalational anesthetics are a chemically heterogeneous group of drugs, from the "simple" noble gas xenon to complex halogen-substituted hydrocarbon compounds. The only thing in common is the inhalational supply. Nitrous oxide (N_2O, "laughing gas") and diethyl ether were used in the beginning of modern anesthesiology. The importance of nitrous oxide is dwindling, not least due to the N_2O-induced inhibition of methionine synthetase. This enzyme catalyzes the conversion of homocysteine to methionine and tetrahydrofolate. Inhibition results in the accumulation of homocysteine and a lack of vitamin B_{12}. In addition to the hypovitaminosis and homocysteine-induced vascular disease, possible clinical consequences are ultimately the impairment of myelin and DNA synthesis.

The future for xenon cannot be predicted at present. Its advantages (among other things, xenon as a noble gas is biochemically inert and environmentally sustainable) are indisputable. Analgesic potency and ease of control are givens; neuroprotective properties are likely. In high-performance sports, xenon has the potential for misuse as an indirect doping medium because it increases endogenous erythropoietin synthesis without being detectable. Arguments against its widespread use in clinical anesthesiology are above all its very limited availability, with the resulting high cost, and also the lack of medical devices requisite for its administration.

The volatile inhalational anesthetics sevoflurane and desflurane are almost exclusively used now. Both are relatively easy to control and have few side effects. An absolute contraindication for both is the disposition to malignant hyperthermia (MHS). This is an autosomal dominant hereditary defect of the calcium-release channel in the sarcoplasmic reticulum of the skeletal musculature ("ryanodine receptor"). If genetically disposed patients receive a volatile inhalational anesthetic, a lasting opening of this calcium release channel can ensue. This then will result in calcium overloading of the sarcoplasm, with the consequence of a lasting activation of the contractile actin–myosin apparatus. The skeletal musculature will go into contracture, and perfusion ceases owing to vascular compression. Anaerobic metabolism brings about acidosis and hypoxia. Since several steps of the pathophysiologic cascade occur exothermally, in combination with perfusion-based limited thermal dissipation there results central hyperthermia. Blood gas analysis, which shows marked mixed respiratory–metabolic acidosis in addition to muscle rigor, hypercapnia, and hyperthermia, provides diagnostic guidance. In the further course, rhabdomyolysis occurs and the patient dies of circulatory failure. This course of events can be interrupted by the timely administration of dantrolene, which "seals" the calcium release channel.

Further contraindications to volatile agents are marked myocardial, coronary, or liver failure and—for desflurane—a history of "halothane hepatitis." When these contraindications are taken into account, both anesthetics are well tolerated, stabilize the hemodynamic profile of the anesthesia and, dose dependently, reduce cerebral oxygen consumption.[6] Sevoflurane can also be used for mask induction; desflurane is less suitable for this due to its pungent smell. Both are used as basic anesthetics, supplemented by sedatives, hypnotics, and analgesics as well as muscle relaxants where needed. The CO_2-responsiveness of the cerebral vascular system is augmented rather than damped by inhalational anesthetics. As a consequence, inhalational anesthetics can also be used when it is intended to control organ perfusion by induced hypocapnia or hypercapnia. In the in vitro model, ischemia-induced release of the excitotoxin glutamate is reduced significantly by exposure to sevoflurane.[7] This may indicate some neuroprotective potential.

17.4.4 Analgesics

The analgesic component of combination anesthesia is provided by opioids or ketamine. Fentanyl, sufentanil, alfentanil, and remifentanil are used. In terms of receptor affinity, sufentanil offers advantages in theory, but no results-relevant superiority could be demonstrated. With regard to influencing postischemic damage, opioids cannot be classified as neuroprotective or neurodestructive. With regard to controllability and (lack of) cumulation, remifentanil is far superior to the reference substances. For short-duration and diagnostic procedures on the orbit, this profile is thoroughly advantageous. With the other opioids there is the risk of an undesirably prolonged effect or of "remorphinization." This can be countered effectively and promptly with naloxone, a pure competitive opiate antagonist. The risk of a severe hemodynamic reaction and, at times, the development of a pulmonary edema must be considered.

The hypnoanalgesic ketamine, as racemate or as (*S*)-ketamine, is inherently suited to the aims of neuroanesthesia not least due to its indirect sympathomimetic properties. Earlier reservations with regard to an ICP- and $CMRO_2$-raising effect are unfounded. (*S*)-Ketamine does not raise the ICP, but can, at least in children, decrease raised ICP. Relevant "neuroprotective" properties of ketamine due to NMDA-receptor-induced anti-excitotoxic effect are suspected but have not been proven.[8]

17.4.5 Muscle Relaxants

Nondepolarizing muscle relaxants do not have any effect on ICP but they do minimally reduce intraocular pressure, probably through relaxation of the extraocular eye muscles.[9] If the surgical procedure requires intact neuromuscular transmission (e.g., facialis monitoring in ENT) the relatively short-acting nondepolarizing relaxant mivacurium is used and its effect is monitored relaxometrically. The reason for the predictable duration of the effect is the breakdown of mivacurium by pseudocholinesterase. If there is a surgical requirement for longer immobilization, cisatracurium or rocuronium are the drugs of choice. Cisatracurium is one enantiomer of racemic atracurium; both drugs are benzylisoquinolines, which are rapidly broken down chemically. Degradation pathways are Hofmann elimination and ester hydrolysis. Accordingly, offset of the neuromuscular block is predictable even with impaired liver and kidney function and also independent of the pseudocholinesterase concentration. A disadvantage is the accumulation of the metabolites monoacrylate and laudanosine, which maybe toxic or ictogenic in high concentration. Cisatracurium differs from the racemate in its slower onset, but also through producing less histamine release and laudanosine formation.

The most rapid onset of effect among nondepolarizing relaxants is provided by rocuronium, which has a medium duration of

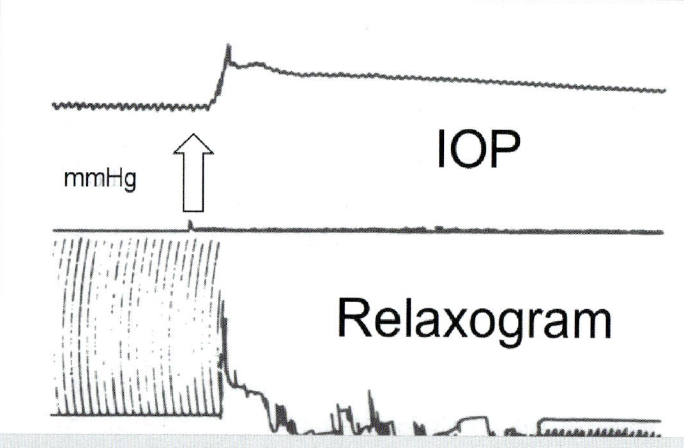

Fig. 17.3 Effect of the administration of succinylcholine (*arrow*) on the intraocular pressure (IOP). As the stimulus response fades away, the IOP rises (dog model).[16]

action. Its effect is lost through redistribution; elimination is hepatobiliary. In individual cases this limits the predictability of the action; on the other hand, only with rocuronium is there the option of rapid and complete antagonization. The modified cyclodextrin sugammadex incorporates all circulating rocuronium molecules irreversibly; the complex is excreted renally.

The very fast and short-acting depolarizing relaxant succinylcholine raises the IOP considerably (▶ Fig. 17.3), which is attributable to specific characteristics of the eye muscles. Basically, the striated muscles contain fibers with a “fibrillar structure” and others with a “field structure”[10]. The fibers with “fibrillar structure” are innervated with end plates, react quickly as well as phasically, and enable eye movements. The fibers with “field structure” are multiply innervated, have grape-shaped nerve endings, and carry out the slow, tonic fusion movements. Stimulating them with succinylcholine brings about a tonic contraction without action potential, which raises the IOP via compression of the eyeball.

17.5 Clinical Anesthesiology

The standard anesthesiological technique for operations in the area of the orbit is “balanced general anesthesia”; it is only for ophthalmic surgery on the anterior eye chamber that local anesthesia dominates. Basic anesthesia with volatile inhalational anesthetics is used extensively, where necessary supplemented with injection anesthetics, opioids, and relaxants. Alternatively, total intravenous anesthesia (TIVA) may be used (see Chapter 17.4). As inhalational anesthetics involve hydrochlorofluorocarbons (HCFCs), for reasons of environmental protection alone one must assume a reduction in usage in the long-term.

For intraorbital operations the principles of ophthalmic anesthesia apply; for retro-orbital and supraorbital operations the principles of neuroanesthesia. Infraorbital interventions and those in the interorbital area are the domains of ear nose and throat (ENT) or oro-maxillo-facial (OMF) surgery. If the surgical site in the ENT area is infiltrated with epinephrine-containing local anesthetics, it must be noted that some inhalational anesthetics sensitize the myocardium to the arrhythmogenic effects of epinephrine. With microsurgical operations predominantly in ENT, surgical field with minimal blood is an advantage, which can be obtained by induced blood pressure reduction

Table 17.5 ASA groups (according to ASA physical status classification, American Society of Anesthesiologists, 1941)

I	Normal, healthy patient
II	Patient with mild systemic disease
IIII	Patient with severe systemic disease
IV	Patient with severe systemic disease that is a constant threat to life
V	Moribund patient who is not expected to survive without the operation

(“controlled hypotension”) (see “Controlled Reduction of Blood Pressure” in Chapter 17.5.6).

17.5.1 Preoperative Preparation

Acute, space-occupying hemorrhage, septic foci, and perforating eye injury are emergencies and require prompt intervention. The majority of the other indications for surgical operations on the orbit are elective; that is, they allow for a case history to be taken and the examination of the patient. The aim of this is to assess the individual risk and to minimize it. From an anesthesiologic point of view, the cardiopulmonary case history is crucial for risk assessment, and it is likewise mandatory to take a careful history of allergies and coagulation disorders. Before strabismus surgery one should bear in mind that strabismus convergens is associated disproportionately frequently with susceptibility to malignant hyperthermia (malignant hyperthermia susceptibility, MHS). This is no indication for a preoperative malignant hyperthermia–specific contracture test, but it does justify taking a thorough family history. For older patients with a positive cardiac or medication history, additional examinations such as an ECG or a pulmonary function test can be indicated. Radiographic examination of the thorax requires a justifying indication on a case-by-case basis.

Patients are assessed on the basis of the case history and examination findings; the assessment is usually based on the classification of the *American Society of Anesthesiologists* (ASA) (▶ Table 17.5). This scale is also of interest outside anesthesiology as retrospective analyses have shown that the frequency of surgical complications also increases with the ASA class. In the physical examination the respiratory pathways are paid particular attention in order to identify a potentially “difficult airway.” In addition to craniocervical mobility, mouth opening, and the status of the teeth, also assessed and documented are the visibility of the pharyngeal structures (“Mallampati sign”) and the thyromental distance (“Patil sign”). The combined use of these tests raises sensitivity but does not protect against nasty surprises in individual cases!

If patients are on a long-term medication, this is checked and, where necessary, adapted. This applies in particular to drugs known to interfere with anesthetics, as is the case inter alia with MAO-inhibitors and metformin preparations.

17.5.2 PONV

The acronym stands for **p**ostoperative **n**ausea and **v**omiting and requires risk assessment, prevention and, where necessary, treatment. The risk of suffering from nausea postoperatively is not inconsiderable (average incidence > 10%); the risk is highest in

17

pediatric ophthalmic surgery for strabismus. PONV also occurs with above-average frequency after gynecological surgery and late postoperatively after intracranial neurosurgery. Contrary to general expectation, this complication does not always manifest itself in the recovery room (incidence < 6%) but, more often, on the first postoperative day (> 10%).[11] The individual PONV risk is assessed within the framework of the premedication interview using a score.[12] A positive case history, nonsmoker, female gender, and opiate administration are risk factors justifying prophylactic administration of corticosteroids, antikinetotics, or serotonin receptor antagonists in line with a phased approach. These drugs are administered during induction of anesthesia. The simplest and most practical form of PONV prophylaxis consists in refraining from using N_2O, opting for a high FIO_2 (fraction of inspired oxygen), and the preferred use of propofol.[13]

17.5.3 Securing the Airway

For shorter-duration orbit surgery, above all in ophthalmic surgery, endotracheal intubation can be omitted in favor of supraglottic airway devices, notably the laryngeal mask airway. With the aim of not interfering with access to the surgical site, by preference laryngeal masks are used with a spiral tube and, for long operations, mask systems that allow the stomach to be relieved. Prolonged operations as well as all supraorbital interventions require endotracheal intubation and controlled ventilation, and in individual cases neuromuscular blockade ("relaxation") as well. Direct laryngoscopy using a rigid laryngoscope is a source of great stress, the hemodynamic consequences manifest themselves in particular during prolonged intubation attempts. This can be obviated by fiberoptic intubation.[14] Alternatively, a local anesthetic can be administered intravenously (e.g., lidocaine, 1 mg/kg, 3 minutes prior to the laryngoscopy), which will prevent the laryngoscopy-induced rise in intraocular pressure.[15]

Particular requirements for the securing of the airways arise from the surgical draping of the operation field ("field avoidance"). This implies the standard use of armored tubes and their proper fixation. In this regard, fiber-endoscopic nasotracheally placed spiral tubes are particularly secure.

Succinylcholine is indicated for the intubation of nonfasted patients as its short onset allows management of the airway without the aspiration risk associated with mask ventilation. This leads to a dilemma if, for example, a perforating eye injury is to be dealt with promptly. If the patient presents with a full stomach, this requires a "crush-intubation" to avoid aspiration. This is generally done using the depolarizing relaxant succinylcholine. However, administering this would be associated with an increase in vis-a-tergo (see Chapter 17.4.5), which would destroy the outcome of surgery due to the loss of vitreous. Giving due regard to the priority of maintaining the patient's sight means that in our hospital succinylcholine is not used in open-eye surgery.[16] The risk combination "full stomach and open globe" requires a strategy. We proceed such that the patient receives an antacid (sodium citrate, 20 mL by mouth) before induction of anesthesia. Although this neither reduces the stomach contents nor hinders regurgitation and aspiration, it raises the pH of the stomach contents markedly within a very short time. This takes account of the fact that the cause of a Mendelson syndrome triggered by aspiration is not the quantity of what is aspirated but its pH.

During induction of anesthesia, a large-dimension surgical suction device (switched on and function-checked) is held ready to remove vomitus without delay. An assistant is prepared to tip the operating table into head-down position when asked to do so. This is with the aim of preventing gastric reflux from entering the trachea.

Then oxygen (fresh gas flow [FGF] > 6 L/min) is supplied to the still awake patient via a tight-fitting face mask for 3 minutes—whilst protecting the wounded eye! With this preoxygenation, the functional residual capacity (FRC; expiratory reserve capacity plus residual volume) is to a large extent denitrogenized: that is, only the obligatory alveolar gases CO_2 and H_2O remain. The pulmonary oxygen store thus set up protects the patient from hypoxia as a result of iatrogenic apnea or delays through regurgitation or airway problems. Then the anesthesia is induced intravenously, preferably with propofol and remifentanil. After loss of consciousness neuromuscular blockade is achieved with the competitive relaxant rocuronium. With the aim of the shortest onset this is administered in approximately twice the effective dosage. After ~120 seconds, laryngoscopic intubation follows; cricoid pressure (Sellick maneuver) formerly regarded as obligatory is not used anymore due to proven lack of effect.[17] If the tube cuff is blocked and the correct tube position is verified capnometrically as well as by auscultation, the stomach can be relieved using a nasogastric probe. It is not possible to suction off undigested food, but the liquid components can be removed. The resulting thickening of the residue reduces the risk of intraoperative silent regurgitation.

During the operation analgesia is maintained with remifentanil, and hypnosis with propofol. The deliberately accepted overhanging effect of the relaxant can be counteracted with the administration of the specific antagonist sugammadex. This is appropriate because the risk of aspiration persists and any residual neuromuscular block (postoperative residual curarization, PORC) would considerably enhance that risk.

If the patient provides information about a "difficult airway" this procedure is not indicated. With this, fortunately most uncommon, constellation, we would perform fiber-endoscopic nasotracheal intubation of the conscious patient.[18]

17.5.4 Positioning

Operations on the orbit are generally carried out with the patient in supine position. Slight elevation of the upper body favors venous drainage and can contribute to a "dry surgical field." However, what is more important is axially correct craniocervical alignment. Just a minimal deviation from the midline can significantly increase the internal pressures. Turning or inclination of the head can actually be more unfavorable in this regard than bilateral compression of the jugular vein (▶ Fig. 17.4)! If the head is to be positioned away from the mid-line for tactical reasons, it is recommended that the sagittal craniocervical axis be maintained, and that the operating table as a whole be rotated around the long axis.

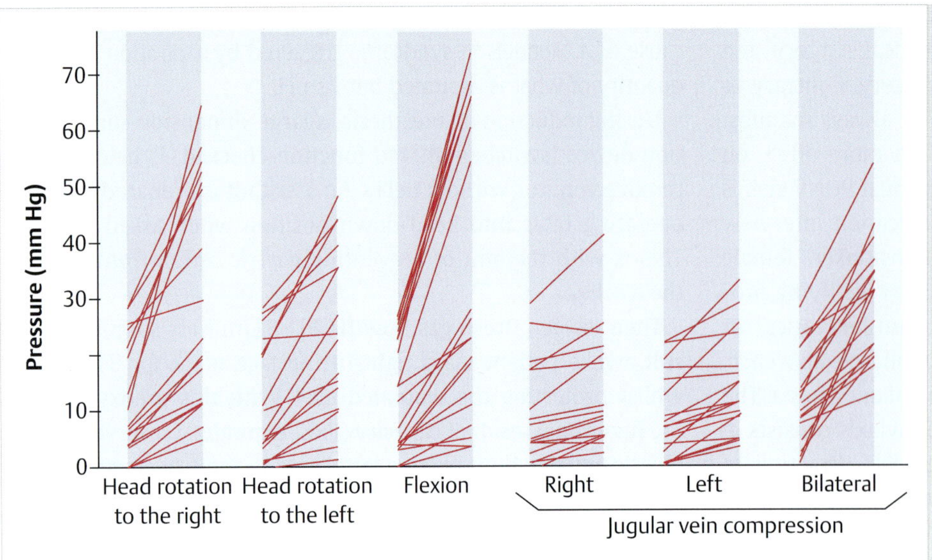

Fig. 17.4 Effect of positioning versus jugular vein compression on the intracranial pressure. (Hulme A, Cooper R. The effects of head position and jugular vein compression on intracranial pressure. A clinical study. In: Beks IWF, Bosch A, Brock M, eds. Intracranial Pressure III. Berlin: Springer; 1976: 259-263.)

17.5.5 Ventilation

The intended aim is a controlled, "lung protective" ventilation with the goal of normoxia and normocapnia. A positive end-expiratory pressure (PEEP) is obligatory; any potential undesired consequence for the internal pressures, ICP and IOP, is vastly overestimated. Nitrous oxide is not used as a carrier gas; the risk of hyperoxically induced atelectasis formation has to be kept in mind.

17.5.6 Hemodynamic Management

For the majority of orbit operations, **arterial normotension at low level** is the appropriate form of circulation control. Capillary and venous congestion is countered by appropriate positioning and ventilation. In individual cases—ENT microsurgery, skull base vascular surgery—a reduction of mean arterial pressure to subnormally low levels may be indicated. This **controlled hypotension** requires a clear indication and, where necessary, organ-specific monitoring. In view of the particular risk to the heart and the brain, monitoring of the coronary (multichannel ECG) and cerebral (cerebral oximetry) perfusion is recommended.

A hemodynamic peculiarity of ophthalmic orbit surgery is the oculocardiac reflex (Aschner–Dagnini reflex). Afference is via the trigeminal nerve; efference via the vagal nerve. When the eye muscles are stretched or pressure is applied to the eye globe, bradycardia and hypotension are elicited. As a result the heart can stop, usually reversibly. As an immediate measure all surgical manipulations are to be interrupted, where necessary a vagolytic (e.g., atropine 0.5 mg IV) is administered for secondary prophylaxis. Premedication with intramuscular atropine formerly practiced is ineffective and obsolete.

17

Controlled Reduction of Blood Pressure

Manipulation of the blood pressure serves various purposes; main priority has to be the adequate organ perfusion (primum non nocere). Sustained venous and capillary oozing as the result of congestion through, for example, unfavorable positioning or unadjusted ventilation is surgically obstructive. An uncontrolled rise in arterial blood pressure can compromise the result of intraorbital ophthalmic surgery or (supraorbitally at the skull base) allow an aneurysm to burst. In ENT microsurgery even small amounts of blood, seen microscopically, are regarded as problematic, whence arises the desire for the reduction of the blood pressure.

Harvey Cushing addressed the iatrogenic reduction of blood pressure in 1917. The experimental investigation of "controlled hypotension" was started in 1944 by Phemister, who investigated hypotension induced in rabbits. Deliberate hypotension was applied clinically in 1946 by Gardner. In 1950 Gillies employed spinal anesthesia for hypotension. He formulated the relevance of high blood flow versus that of high blood pressure:

A low head of arterial pressure associated with vasodilation and normal blood volume carries less potential danger than the illusory higher pressure which accompanies vasoconstriction and a reduced blood volume.
John Gillies, 1950[19]

At the start of the 1950s, controlled hypotension with indirect and direct vasodilators was adopted into clinical practice, supplemented by the volatile anesthetic halothane in 1956. Indications for controlled hypotension include facilitation of certain surgical interventions and the reduction of intraoperative blood loss. The first indication includes surgical treatment of intracranial aneurysms, arteriovenous malformations, and vascular tumors. The second indication applies to operations on the spine and hips, total prostate resections, and plastic surgery. A limitation of blood loss in the sense of a blood-free operating site is the indication in microsurgical operations in otosurgery and ophthalmic surgery. For certain orbit operations, such as the removal of tissue from the choroid and retina for biopsy and for the resection of uveal melanomas, a reduction of the MAP to below 75 mm Hg is recommended. At present, direct and indirect vasodilators as well as myocardial depressants are used for controlled hypotension. The drug-induced vasodilation results in **hyperdynamic hypotension**; following the afterload reduction associated with the vasodilation cardiac output increases. The administration of myocardial depressants results in **hypodynamic hypotension**. Lowering the intraocular pressure (IOP) by controlled reduction of the blood pressure is not possible.[20]

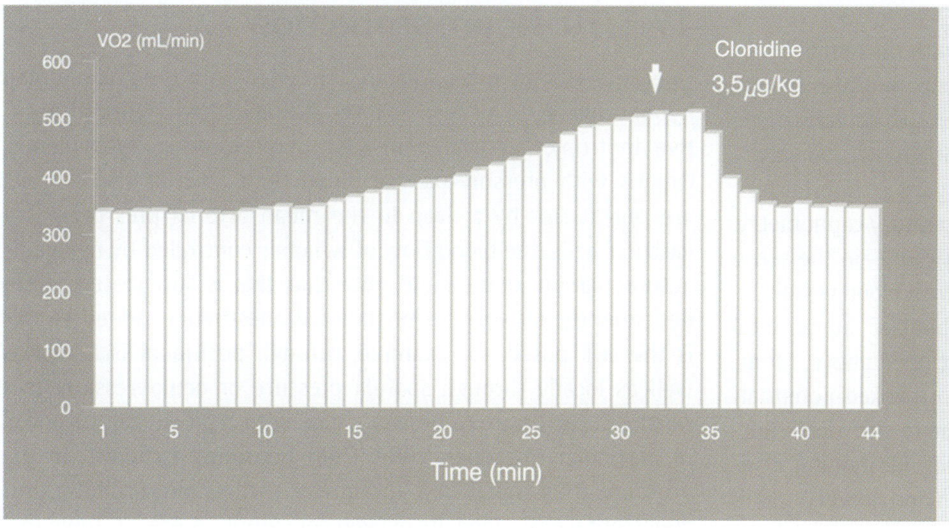

Fig. 17.5 Effect of shivering on the TM systemic uptake of oxygen (VO_2, PhysioFlex; pig model).[24]

The lower limit to which the blood pressure can be reduced without risk is unknown and is probably of great disparity between individuals. Complications are to be feared in the event of insufficient perfusion of vital organ systems. When the blood pressure is lowered, cerebral and myocardial perfusion should be monitored. The liver too is potentially at risk as its perfusion is not protected by an autoregulation mechanism. Intraorbitally, a critical drop in the perfusion pressure can cause ischemic damage to the retina and thrombosis of the ciliary arteries. The risks of controlled hypotension are not accurately quantifiable. A retrospective analysis of 1,802 otosurgical operations under deliberate hypotension revealed a morbidity of 0.11% and a mortality of 0.06%.[21] The following are regarded as relative contraindications for hypotensive anesthesia: anemia, hypovolemia, coronary and cerebrovascular perfusion disorders, hepatorenal insufficiency, and marked arterial hypertension. A prerequisite for controlled hypotension is the careful examination of the patient with the aim of identifying relative contraindications and, where applicable, removing them; auscultation of the carotids is of significance here. The induction of arterial hypotension can only be justified if the benefits outweigh the risks:

Hypotension must only be induced in the honest belief that some good to the patient will accrue.
Alex G. Larson, 1964[22]

Paying due regard to this caveat, the controlled reduction of blood pressure, particularly to very low MAP values, is not a routine measure. It maybe justified on an individual case basis, based on agreement between the anesthesiologist and the surgeon. The risk profile of the individual patient and the requirements of the planned surgery provide guidance.

17.5.7 Temperature Management

General anesthesia interferes not only peripherally (**sensor**) but also centrally (**regulator**) with temperature regulation. In combination with cool ambient temperature and cold infusions and disinfection solutions, this results in intraoperative hypothermia. Without measures to counteract this, the core body temperature will fall to a minimum after ~3 hours, after which there often follows a slow rise again. During hypothermia, reduced oxygen consumption may be assumed, associated with raised ischemia tolerance. However, the hope arising from that for a neuroprotective potential of mild hypothermia in neurovascular operations on the skull base was not confirmed in one prospective study.[23]

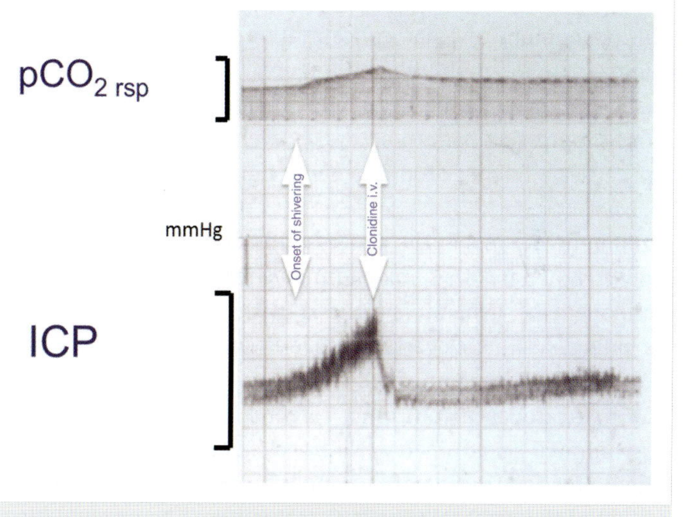

Fig. 17.6 Effect of shivering on the respiratory CO_2 concentration ($PaCO_2$, capnogram) and the intracranial pressure (ICP) (pig model).[24]

As the duration of most orbit surgery interventions is less than 3 hours, active temperature management is necessary. One should note that postoperative shivering after orbit surgery is particularly risky: it increases not only the systemic oxygen consumption but also the ICP (▶ Fig. 17.5, ▶ Fig. 17.6). Preventive measures include, primarily, the use of thermal mats and convection warmers (single-use covers connected to a fan heater). Less effective but additive in effect is the use of prewarmed infusion and disinfection solutions, as well as the use of HME (heat and moisture exchanger) breathing filters and closed-system ventilation.[24]

17.5.8 Monitoring

Patients are monitored in accordance with the recommendations of the American Society of Anesthesiology (ASA) (ASA Guidelines for patient care in Anesthesiology; last amended on October 19, 2011; http://www.asahq.org/quality-and-practice-mangement/standards-and- guidelines) as well as the Technical Requirements of the Anaesthesia Workplace (ISO 80601-2-13:2013-03). It is important to monitor the core temperature with the aim of being able to promptly counter not only hypothermia but also hyperthermia. The former would promote postoperative shivering (see above), the latter could be viewed as potentially neurodestructive. Of particular significance for orbit surgery is intermittent blood gas analysis, as well as continuous respiratory capnometry. Both take account of the marked chemosensitivity—in the sense of CO_2-responsiveness—of the cerebral and uveal blood vessels.

Organ-specific monitoring during intraorbital or supraorbital operations is not part of the standards mentioned above. Monitoring of the brain function via EEG-leads or evoked-potential-monitoring (EP) is time-consuming and prone to electrical interference in the operating theatre environment. EP monitoring is routine in selected intracranial operations in neurosurgery and in ENT operations in the proximity of peripheral pathways. Volatile inhalational anesthetics shift the EEG activity from the posterior to the anterior segments of the brain. Concentrations under 1 MAC (minimum alveolar concentration) are associated with a minimal rise in amplitude and frequency. Above 1 MAC the frequency drops while the amplitude remains raised. Over 2 MAC a burst-suppression pattern occurs. At even higher doses, sevoflurane causes a further drop in activity right through to isoelectric EEG.

Different variants of the **processed EEG** are becoming increasingly common for the semiquantitative recording of the hypnotic component of general anesthesia with the aim of not only excluding anesthetic overhangs (overdosing) but also intraoperative awareness (underdosing).

With reference to outcome, cerebral oximetry by means of near-infrared spectrometry (NIRS) has not been sufficiently validated. This is a means of continuous, non-invasive monitoring mainly of the cerebral venous O_2 saturation. The cerebral blood flow (CBF) and the $CMRO_2$ as well as the cerebral arterial oxygenation contribute to the signal. From this results an indicator, albeit unspecific, of the cerebral O_2 balance, which has a certain significance as a trend monitor.

17.5.9 Emergence and Postoperative Period

After an operation in or around the orbit, emergence from anesthesia should be accomplished as promptly as allowed by the vital functions in the interest of prompt neurologic assessability of the patient. Prolonged respiratory assistance requires a clear indication.

Prerequisites for the return of spontaneous respiration and extubation of the trachea are normothermia and recovery from the effects of anesthetics, analgesics, and muscle relaxants. Hypoventilation, hypothermia, hypoxia, and acidosis rule out extubation and require prolonged emergence.

In the early postoperative period, attention should be focused on preventing pain and shivering as well as nausea and vomiting. Pain management, where necessary as preemptive analgesia, has to be balanced so that freedom from pain is not achieved at the expense of opiate-induced hypoventilatory hypoxia. Shivering is already preempted intraoperatively by temperature management (see Chapter 17.5.7); if it nevertheless manifests, α_2-receptor agonists are administered (e.g., dexmedetomidine).

17.5.10 Neuroprotection

Operations in the orbit area are burdened with the risk of organ hypoperfusion. The cause is, inter alia, anesthetic-induced negative inotropy, aggravated in case of preexisting hypovolemia. Organs with pressure-passive blood flow, such as the choroid, are put at risk by a drop in the mean arterial pressure; with vascular beds, the blood flow of which is controlled by myogenic autoregulation, one should note that this is suppressed, dose-dependently, by volatile inhalational anesthetics. Added to this is the risk posed, for example, through positional ischemia as well as locally through spatula pressure or oculopression. This results in the desire to protect tissue with high oxygen turnover, in particular intraoperatively, from becoming ischemic. In the orbit area this affects first and foremost the supra-orbitally situated frontal brain lobe. Its oxygen consumption breaks down to ~ 60% for function, while ~40% goes to maintain the structure (▶ Fig. 17.7). The latter includes the integrity of the membranes and maintenance of the transmembrane ion gradients. The glutamate transporter systems too, which are important within the context of excitotoxicity, operate energy-intensively; when energy is in short supply they release glutamate in the extracellular space instead of accumulating it.[25] Intraoperative neuroprotection measures aim to optimize the energy balance on the one hand and, on the other, to interrupt the cascades of cerebral thanatogenesis. In terms of the first aspect, most anesthetics and hypnotics can be seen in principle as neuroprotective because they reduce $CMRO_2$. Targeted pharmacological neuroprotection measures have so far not lived up to the hopes placed in them. It remains to be seen whether the antiexcitotoxic effect of the weak noncompetitive glutamate receptor antagonist ketamine prove to have clinically relevant results.[8] Likewise, any neuroprotective potential of "therapeutic hypothermia" is not yet conclusively determined.

It has long been known that a reduction in body temperature reduces brain metabolism and this was used since the 1950s in cardiac surgery and neurosurgery. In neurosurgery the technique has been abandoned partly because of the associated bleeding complications.

A renaissance in the form of therapeutic ("mild") hypothermia occurred at the beginning of the 1990s. This proved to be surprisingly effective in animals and soon found its way into clinical

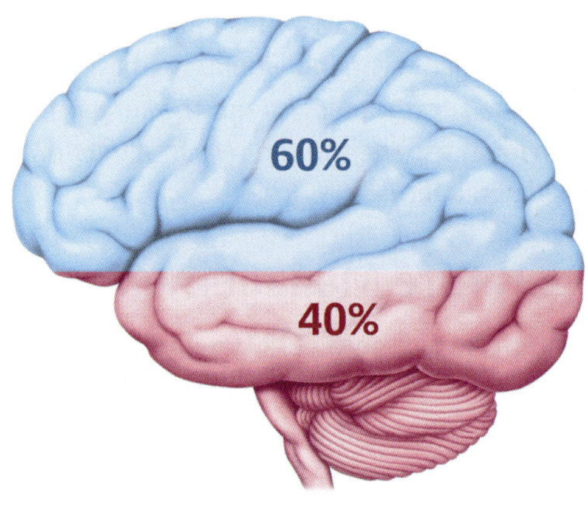

Fig. 17.7 Oxygen uptake of the brain ($CMRO_2$): function (blue) versus structure (red) metabolism.

Table 17.6 Mechanisms of potential neuroprotective effects of mild therapeutic hypothermia
Therapeutic hypothermia inhibits or alleviates • Glutamatergic ischemic response. • Intraneuronal calcium-mobilization. • Persistent activation of the glutamate receptors. • Functional disruption of the blood–brain barrier. • Proliferation of microglia. • Formation of superoxide anions and NO. And • Modulates the attachment of the AP1 transcription factor to DNA and promotes protein synthesis.

studies. A whole series of positive effects beyond the reduction of the $CMRO_2$ allows one to infer a neuroprotective potential of therapeutic hypothermia (▶ Table 17.6). For ischemic apoplectic insult[26] and in neurotraumatology,[27] however, there has not been any improvement in results with therapeutic hypothermia; intraoperative use—at least for the area of neurovascular skull base surgery—also has not demonstrated any benefit yet.[23]

The measures currently available for intraoperative neuroprotection are thus substantially limited to ensuring normoxemia as well as normoteusion, normoglycemia, normothermia, and normocapnia.

Surgery on the orbit is extremely varied and places high demands on the anesthesiological care of patients. More than in other surgical specialties, here the anesthesiologist is also challenged to be a clinical physiologist.

References

[1] Friedman E, Oak SM. Choroidal microcirculation in vivo. Bibl Anat. 1965; 7: 129–132

[2] Jantzen J-P. Untersuchung zur Auswirkung anasthesiologischer Masnahmen auf den intraokularen Druck. Eine experimentelle Studie am Schweinemodell. Wiesbaden: Wissenschaftliche Verlagsabteilung; 1990

[3] Grimes PA, Macri FJ, von Sallmann L, Wanko T. Some mechanisms of centrally induced eye pressure responses. Am J Ophthalmol. 1956; 42(4 Part 2):130–147

[4] Jantzen J-P, Tzanova I, Klein AM, Witton PK. Rectal anesthesia induction—a comparative study with methohexital and ketamine. Anasthesiol Intensivmed. 1987; 28:56–61

[5] Jantzen J-P, Korte S, Suhr D, von Gösseln HH. Etomidate vs. propofol for craniotomy: Does it make a difference? Eur J Anaesthesiol. 1998; 15(6):784

[6] Jantzen J-P, Fischer F. [Value of inhalational anesthetics in neuroanesthesia. A review of "side effects"]. Anasthesiol Intensivmed Notfallmed Schmerzther. 1993; 28:98–106

[7] Toner CC, Connelly K, Whelpton R, et al. Effects of sevoflurane on dopamine, glutamate and aspartate release in an in vitro model of cerebral ischaemia. Br J Anaesth. 2001; 86(4):550–554

[8] Jantzen J-P. Cerebral neuroprotetion and ketamine. Anaesthesist. 1994; 43 Suppl 2:S41–S47

[9] Jantzen J-P, Kleemann PP. On the effect of muscle relaxants on introcular pressure. Klin Monatsbl Augenheilk Clin Monthly Ophthalmology. 1988; 193 7:1–7

[10] Krüger P. On a possible connection between structure, function and chemical nature of the muscles. Biol Zentralbl. 1929; 49:616–620

[11] Heller J. Untersuchungen zur Effizienz der Post-Anaesthesie-Visite in Bezug auf die Ergebnisqualität am Klinikum Hannover Nordstadt. Mainz; 2003

[12] Apfel CC. Pathophysiology, risk factors and risk assessment for nausea and vomiting in the postoperative phase. Anasthesiol Intensivmed Notfallmed Schmerzther. 2005; 40(8):497–503

[13] Krüper S, Mohr OE, Patzke M, Jantzen J-P. Nausea and vomiting after gynaecological laparoscopies: propofol/sufentanil versus thiopental/isoflurane/sufentanil. Anasthesiol Intensivmed. 1997; 38:292–295

[14] Latorre F, Hofmann M, Kleemann PP, Dick WF. Fibreoptic intubation and stress. Anaesthesist. 1993; 42(7):423–426

[15] Drenger B, Pe'er J, BenEzra D, Katzenelson R, Davidson JT. The effect of intravenous lidocaine on the increase in intraocular pressure induced by tracheal intubation. Anesth Analg. 1985; 64(12):1211–1213

[16] Jantzen J-P, Hackett GH, Earnshaw G. Succinylcholine and open eye injury. Anesthesiology. 1986; 64(4):524–526

[17] Steinmann D, Priebe HJ. Cricoid pressure. Anaesthesist. 2009; 58(7):695–707

[18] Wangemann BU, Jantzen J-P. The fibreoptic intubation of neurosurgical patients. Neurochirurgia (Stuttg). 1993; 36(4):117–122

[19] Gillies J. Anaesthetic factors in the causation and prevention of excessive bleeding during surgical operations. Ann R Coll Surg Engl. 1950; 7:204–221

[20] Jantzen J-P, Hennes HJ, Rochels R, Wallenfang T. Deliberate arterial hypotension does not reduce intraocular pressure in pigs. Anesthesiology. 1992; 77 (3):536–540

[21] Pasch T, Huk W. Cerebral complications following induced hypotension. Eur J Anaesthesiol. 1986; 3(4):299–312

[22] Larson AG. Deliberate hypotension. Anesthesiology. 1964; 25:682–706

[23] Todd MM, Hindman BJ, Clarke WR, Torner JC, Intraoperative Hypothermia for Aneurysm Surgery Trial (IHAST) Investigators. Mild intraoperative hypothermia during surgery for intracranial aneurysm. N Engl J Med. 2005; 352(2):135–145

[24] Jantzen J-P, Kleemann PP. Closed circuit anaesthesia: implications for airway climate and malignant hyperthermia—experimental studies in pigs. Min Anest. 1992; 58 Suppl 1:77–78

[25] Anderson CM, Swanson RA. Astrocyte glutamate transport: review of properties, regulation, and physiological functions. Glia. 2000; 32(1):1–14

[26] Hemmen TM, Raman R, Guluma KZ, et al. ICTuS-L Investigators. Intravenous thrombolysis plus hypothermia for acute treatment of ischemic stroke (ICTuS-L): final results. Stroke. 2010; 41(10):2265–2270

[27] Clifton GL, Valadka A, Zygun D, et al. Very early hypothermia induction in patients with severe brain injury (the National Acute Brain Injury Study: Hypothermia II): a randomised trial. Lancet Neurol. 2011; 10(2):131–139

Chapter 18

Surgical Approaches to the Orbit

18 Surgical Approaches to the Orbit

18.1 Introduction

H.-J. Welkoborsky

Various surgical approaches are available for excision of a tumor or repositioning of orbital fractures. These can be subdivided into **rhinosurgical endonasal** approaches, **frontal and lateral external** approaches, and **neurosurgical extradural or intradural** approaches. The indication for the individual approaches is based to a considerable extent on the localization of the pathology and its relationship to the eye globe and the optic nerve. The approach selected should ensure the greatest possible overview of the operating area with the maximum possible protection of the adjacent structures. A useful guideline is that pathologic findings caudally to the globe or nerves are tackled via a caudal approach (e.g., transconjunctival, subciliary, infraorbital, or transmaxillary via the maxillary sinus); pathologic changes medially to the eye globe or optic nerve are tackled via an endonasal transethmoidal median orbitotomy; pathological processes laterally to the eyeball or optic nerve are tackled via a lateral orbitotomy or an orbital rim incision; and pathological processes cranially to the eyeball or the optic nerve are tackled via a transfrontal extradural or intradural approach.

In the last six decades the application of surgical approaches to the orbit has changed from more invasive approaches to ever less invasive and endoscopic approaches. There are several reasons for this development:

1. **Pathology and pathophysiology**. Knowledge of the pathology and pathophysiology of particular orbital diseases has expanded, which has considerably influenced surgical therapy.
2. **Imaging**. Latest developments in imaging techniques have led to more accurate diagnosis, for example, in identification of intraorbital tissue infiltration by a tumor.
3. **Navigation**. Computerized navigation systems permit a very precise and well-targeted operation.
4. **Endoscopy/operating microscopes**. Developments in this area have led to wider possibilities for application of microscopes or endoscopes in surgical procedures.
5. **Reconstruction**. Application of CAD-designed implants has opened new horizons for reconstruction of even very large defects.
6. **Adjuvant therapy**. Advances in radiation therapy techniques have led to the development of intensity-modulated radiation therapy (IMRT; see Chapter 14).
7. **Debulking**. Today we know that it is possible to debulk a tumor and remove it step by step. For tumor control, clear surgical margins are more decisive than the en-bloc excision of a mass. This has led to a wider indication for applying endoscopic or microscopic techniques.

With these developments, more endoscopic and minimally invasive approaches are favored.

Essentially, operations in the area of the orbit should make use of the aid of a computer-assisted navigation system for easier orientation and the greatest possible protection of the tissues.[1] Furthermore, as mentioned above, these are microsurgical interventions, in which the use of a surgical microscope or magnifying endoscope is necessary. In the following the most important surgical approaches to the orbit, their indications, procedures/techniques, and possible complications are discussed. The authors of this chapter are well aware that numerous modifications have been described of the surgical approaches under discussion. To go into all of these variations would be beyond the scope of this book: the authors restrict themselves to describing some standard approaches.

18.2 Endonasal Transethmoidal Approach (Medial Orbitotomy)

H.-J. Welkoborsky

This is a classic rhinosurgical approach.

18.2.1 Indications

The indications for this approach are peribulbar and intraconal retrobulbar space-occupying masses, abscesses, aspergillomas, or vascular malformations medially to the eyeball or the optic nerve up to the orbital apex.[2,3,4,5,6]

18.2.2 Procedure

With transethmoidal medial orbitotomy, first of all an endoscopic or microscopic **ethmoidectomy** is performed with opening of the sphenoid sinus. It is important that the approach to the ethmoid bone is made laterally to the medial nasal concha. After that the lamina papyracea is exposed in its full extent from the orbit apex right through to anterior[7] (▶ Fig. 18.1a–c.; Video 18.1). When resecting the lamina papyracea, one should make sure that the periorbita still remains intact as, otherwise, sight and orientation are affected by the prolapsing of fat tissue.[8] After resection the lamina papyracea, the incision of the periorbita is made using a curved sickle knife. The orbital adipose tissue prolapses, and is prepared with a blunt preparation instrument (e.g., curved dissectors) until the medial rectus muscle is revealed. A light pressure on the globe leads to easier exposure of the pathologic process, which can then be removed using microsurgical dissectors with the aid of an angled endoscope or of an operating microscope. If indicated, additional decompression of the optic nerve can be carried out via the same approach.[7] In this event, the nerve canal in the lateral sphenoid wall is exposed and the covering bone shell is resected. A reconstruction of the medial orbital wall is usually not necessary. The operation is terminated by the insertion of packing into the nasal cavity.

Consistent rhinological follow-up treatment is important postoperatively. As a rule, the nasal packing can be removed on the first or second day postoperatively. Any scabs and crusts forming should be endonasally suctioned away daily. Nasal oils and ointments are suitable for caring for the mucous membrane and for supporting wound healing. The healing of the endonasal wound takes between 4 and 6 weeks.

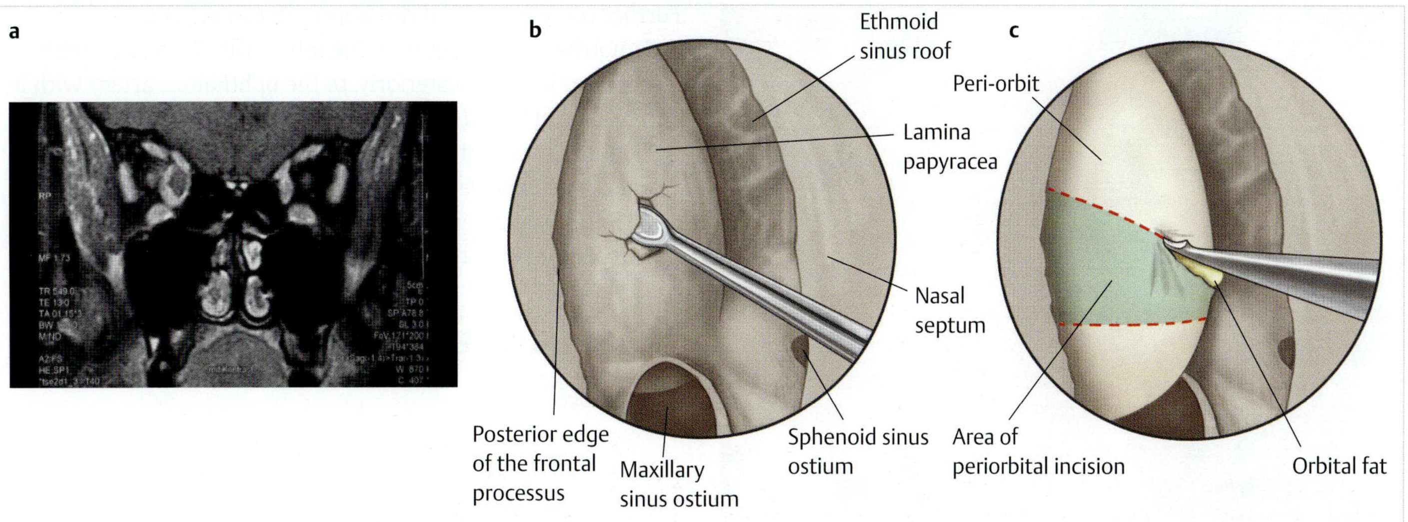

Fig. 18.1 **(a)** Orbital tumor located intraconally medial to the optic nerve. It can therefore be resected via a transethmoid medial orbitotomy. **(b)** Transethmoid medial orbitotomy: Exposure of the lamina papyracea. An ethmoidectomy has already been performed. **(c)** After the lamina papyracea has been resected the periorbita is slit with a curved sickle knife and the intraorbital space is opened. The pathological process can now be prepared and removed. Light pressure on the eyeball leads to an easier exposure of the pathologic process.

18.2.3 Complications

Possible complications of endonasal transethmoidal endoscopic orbitotomy are:

- Acute hemorrhage when the anterior or posterior ethmoid artery is injured. If the vessels run through the area of the operation without a covering of bone at the roof of the ethmoidal bone, they can be coagulated bipolarly or closed with a titanium clip to prevent bleeding.
- Injury of the skull base with subsequent liquorrhea. If liquorrhea occurs, the defect is to be closed if possible without delay, for example, with a piece of temporalis fascia.
- Injury of the optic nerve with amaurosis. This complication is rare and occurs in less than 1% of cases. To avoid damage to the nerve it is recommended to use a computerized navigation system and perform the operation with a magnifying angled endoscope or with an operating microscope. For preparation purposes it is recommended to use only blunt instruments or microinstruments that are sharp only on one side. Amaurosis caused by a nerve injury is irreversible in many cases.
- Olfactory disorders when preparation goes too far medially in the olfactory region.
- Displacement of the frontal sinus infundibulum by prolapsing orbital contents with the subsequent development of a chronic frontal sinusitis. In order to prevent this, the anterior ethmoidal cells should be opened up and resected, and a wider approach to the frontal sinus should be created.
- Injury of the medial rectus muscle with eye globe motility disorders and double vision. This complication can be avoided if, during preparation, the muscle is pushed very carefully to the side or in a cranial or caudal direction, which is only possible under direct visual control. Here one should take note that the muscle, particularly in inflammatory diseases, can often be swollen with edema, which can make its identification difficult.

18.3 Transantral Approach

H.-J. Welkoborsky

18.3.1 Indications

The transantral or transmaxillary approach (syn. transmaxillary orbitotomy) is indicated for removal of pathological processes located caudally, mediolaterally and medio-inferiorly to the eyeball or optic nerve, and also for removing lacrimal sac tumors that infiltrate the orbit from medially.[9,10] Via this approach the caudal intraconal sections of the orbit can be reached right up to the orbital apex.[6,11]

18.3.2 Procedure

The anterior wall of the maxillary sinus is exposed via a sublabial incision in the oral vestibule mucosa. When pushing the soft tissue parts of the cheek away from the bone, one should be careful not to injure the infra-orbital nerve, which exits the infra-orbital foramen in the area of the infra-orbital rim. A large fragment is then temporally removed from the anterior wall of the maxillary sinus, which is replaced at the end of the operation (osteoplastic maxillotomy). Before cutting out the bone lid, it is advantageous to adjust the microplates with which the anterior wall of the maxillary sinus will be fixed later and to create the drill holes that are necessary to receive the osteosynthesis screws. The orbital floor is then exposed, freed of mucous membrane, and the infra-orbital nerve canal is also imaged. An osseous window should be inserted in the medial maxillary sinus wall to the nasal cavity so that secretion can drain and to ensure sufficient postoperative ventilation of the sinus, which is required for complete healing. The orbit floor is resected; the periorbita lying underneath this is left intact at this time (▶ Fig. 18.2). The size of the resection is based on the position and extent of the pathologic process in the orbit. One should make sure to preserve a bony bridge with the infra-orbital canal. Other-

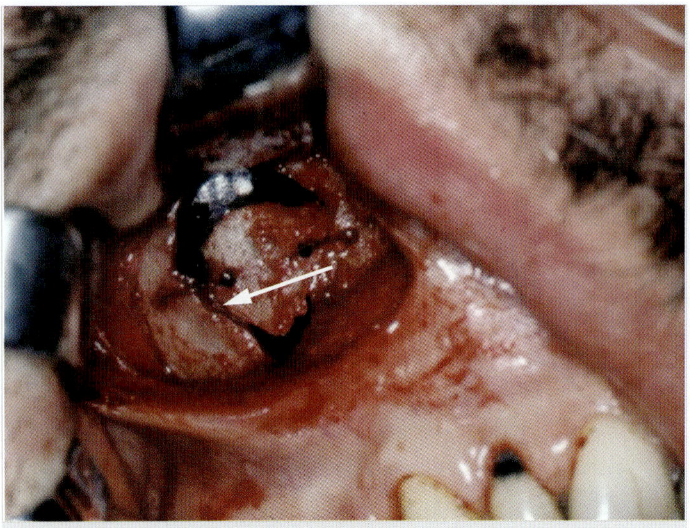

Fig. 18.2 Transantral approach to the orbit for removing a tumor localized medio-inferiorly in the orbit: after exposure of the orbital floor and the infra-orbital nerve canal (*arrow*), resection of this part of the orbital floor, which is located medially to the nerve canal. The periorbita can then be slit and the tumor removed.

wise a downward displacement of the eyeball can occur, causing double vision. In practice this means that the orbital floor can be resected laterally and medially to the nerve canal without any sequelae. The periorbita is slit using a sickle knife. One should take care of the inferior rectus muscle as well as of the inferior oblique muscle. Using microsurgical dissectors the pathological process can now be prepared and removed. The orbit floor can, if necessary, be reconstructed, for example, with a piece of temporalis fascia, a PDS (polydioxanone) plate, or titanium mesh. The operation is concluded with the reinsertion of the temporarily removed anterior wall of the maxillary sinus, which is fixed in place with the previously adjusted microplates (one plate each on the medial and lateral edge of the bone lid is usually sufficient). The closure of the mucous membrane in the oral vestibule is done with absorbable sutures (Video 18.2).

18.3.3 Complications

Possible complications of transmaxillary orbitotomy are determined by the anatomical characteristics, particularly the course of the nerves supplying the extraocular muscles[12]:

- A separation of the infra-orbital nerve or tensile or compressive stress on it, either in the course of its canal in the orbit floor or after its exit from the infra-orbital foramen, causes a hypoesthesia in the area of the cheek, the lateral nose, and the maxillary anterior teeth. For this reason too, when using retractors or isolators, one should make sure that the nerve is not touched by the instrument.
- Injury to the nerves supplying the extraocular muscles (inferior rectus, inferior oblique, possibly medial and lateral rectus muscles) results in paresis of these muscles with resulting double vision. According to anatomical investigations, nerve fibers mainly enter the muscles in the central third of the muscle belly[12] so that particular care is required during preparation. The same applies with processes located posteriorly close to the superior orbital fissure

Further complications of this approach can include:

- Hemorrhage upon injury to the infra-orbital artery or, with processes located posteriorly, to the ophthalmic artery with its infra-orbital branches.
- Enophthalmus with consequent double vision. This complication can be expected if the entire orbit floor—that is, including the infra-orbital nerve canal—has been resected. Leaving the strip of bone with the nerve canal avoids this complication.

18.4 Lateral Orbitotomy

H.-J. Welkoborsky

Lateral orbitotomy was first described by Krönlein in 1888 and since then has undergone some modifications. This is an external approach to the lateral, laterocranial and latero-inferior orbital sections.

18.4.1 Indications

Indications for a lateral orbitotomy are the removal of pathologic processes laterally to the eyeball and the optic nerve, in the region of the lacrimal glands and in the latero-inferior as well as in the laterocranial parts of the orbit, and also in the context of orbital decompression in patients with Graves's orbitopathy (balanced decompression, see Chapter 7.4.3).[3,8,13,14,15,16] Further indications are orbit reconstructions for fractures of the lateral orbital rim and wall.[17] However, processes in the area of the orbital apex are more difficult to reach via this approach due to the massive greater wing of the sphenoid bone, which represents the dorsal resection limit.[18,19]

18.4.2 Procedure

There are two possibilities available for the skin incision: an incision in the area of the lateral orbital rim, or an incision in, or dorsally, to the hairline (pterional incision). The latter has the advantage that the incision is not visible and so causes no cosmetic problem. The disadvantage of the orbital rim incision is the possibility of injury to the ramus frontalis and ramus ocularis of the facial nerve, which run through the area being operated on. If one decides on this incision, neuromonitoring of the facial nerve is recommended. Recently, methods of lateral orbitotomy via a transconjunctival endoscopic approach have been described, but this does give a significantly more restricted overview of the area of the operation compared to the external transcutaneous approaches.[20,21]

With a pterional incision, after separation of the skin and subcutaneous tissue, a skin–soft tissue flap (scalp flap) is formed and prepared far anteriorly until the lateral orbital rim is exposed (▶ Fig. 18.3; Video 18.3). One should take care to preserve the lateral palpebral ligament as, otherwise, the lateral lid angle can be obliterated. The very strong temporalis muscle overlies the lateral orbital wall and is attached by its fibers to the temporal bone. It is cranially incised and bluntly pushed away from the bony lateral orbit wall. Microplates are needed for the reconstruction later of the lateral orbital rim. It is advantageous to fit these plates and to drill the holes necessary for taking the osteosynthesis screws in

18

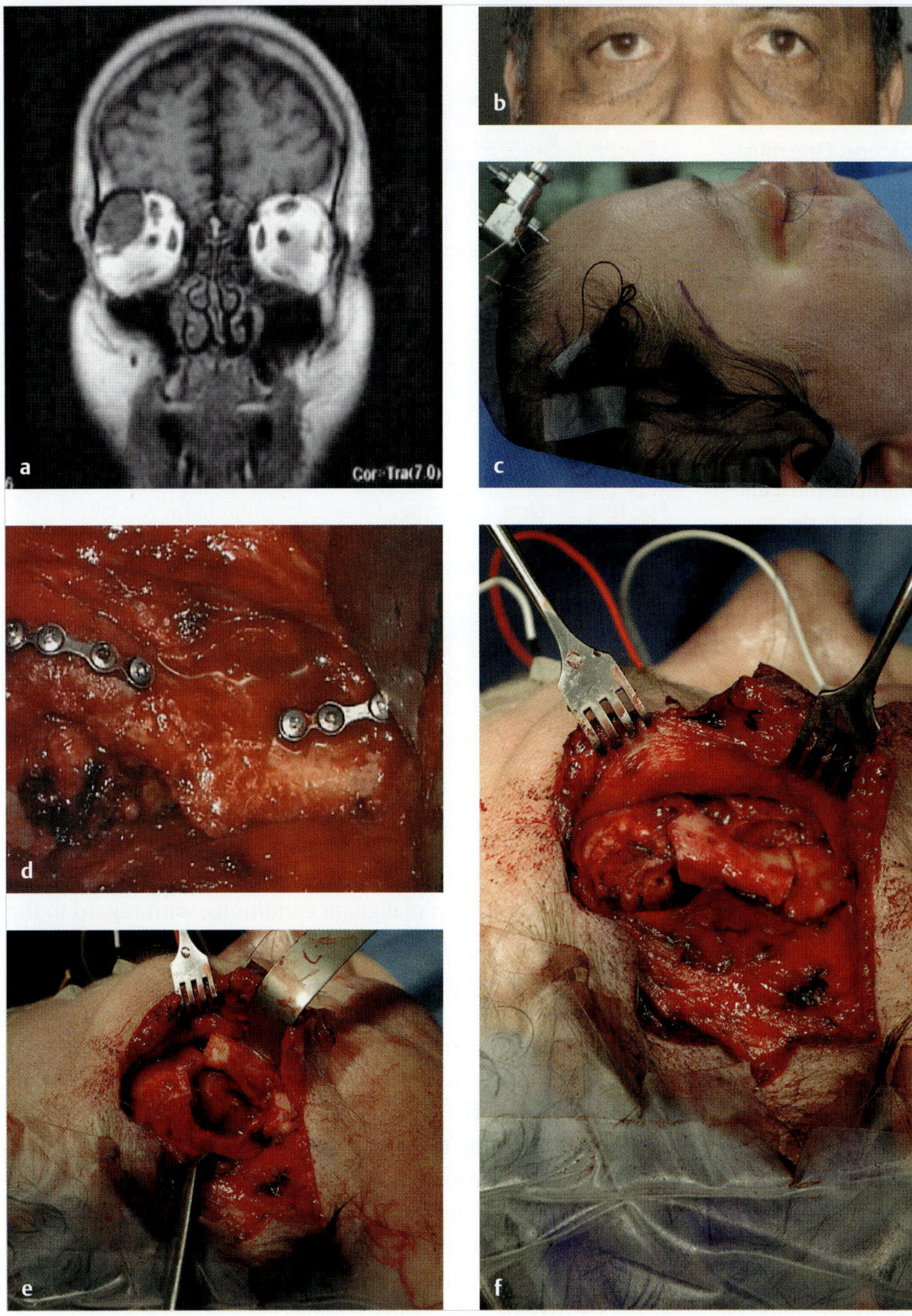

Fig. 18.3 (a) Tumor of the right sided lacrimal gland. For tumor excision a lateral orbitotomy is favorable. **(b)** Patient with a lacrimal gland tumor on the right side. The tumor led to a swelling of the laterocranial upper lid and to a displacement of the eyeball in caudal direction. **(c)** The skin incision (pterional approach) is marked in the hairline. **(d)** Lateral orbitotomy: exposition of the lateral orbital rim. The osteosynthesis plates, which are necessary for later reconstruction, are fitted before the lateral orbital rim is separated. **(e)** The bony lateral orbital rim is separated and **(f)** cut by an oscillating saw in V-shape. The lateral palpebral ligament is preserved and remains attached to the bone. The temporalis muscle is cut horizontally and displaced in caudal direction. The operation is carried out with neuromonitoring of the cranial branches of the facial nerve.

this phase of the operation. This will facilitate the later reconstruction with a perfect fit. With an oscillating saw the bone at the lateral orbital rim is now separated. Two cuts by the saw at a sagittal distance of at least 2 cm are required to temporarily separate a correspondingly large fragment temporarily. In doing this, the bone resections are arranged in a **V**-shape, which facilitates the later reconstruction (▶ Fig. 18.3; Video 18.3). One should make sure that the lateral palpebral ligament is preserved and remains attached to the bone. The sagittal distance of at least 2 cm should be adhered to as, otherwise, there will not be sufficient space for preparation in the orbit. The relatively thin lateral orbital wall can be separated with the oscillating saw parallel to the orbital roof and floor. The inferior boundary is represented by the greater sphenoid wing. At this preparation stage the periorbita remains intact. After temporary removal of the lateral orbital wall the periorbita is incised with a sickle knife. The pathologic process can now be prepared and removed using microsurgical dissectors and microscissors. One should pay attention to the lateral rectus muscle which, when the pathologic process has an intraconal site, must be displaced in the cranial or caudal direction. The periorbita can be sutured with a thin absorbable suturing material following complete resection of the pathologic process. For reconstruction of the lateral orbital wall and of the lateral orbital rim, the temporarily separated bone shell is repositioned and fixed in place by means of the already fitted microplates. The temporalis muscle is moved back and fixed. The operation is concluded with the insertion of an Easyflow drainage (alternatively, Redon drainage) and closure layer by layer of the scalp and skin layers.

18.4.3 Complications

The specific complications of the lateral approach to the orbit can be divided into intraorbital and extraorbital complications.[16,18]

- Intraorbital complications
    - Detachment of the lateral palpebral ligament from the lateral orbit rim with subsequent blunt shape of the lateral canthus. This complication can be avoided by making sure to preserve the lateral palpebral ligament on its osseous attachment.

- Injury to the lateral rectus muscle and/or the inferior rectus muscle with impairment of eye globe motility and double vision. In this connection one should once again point out the importance of conducting the operation with the aid of magnifying endoscopes or of an operation microscope. One must also take care during preparation not to exert too much pressure on the muscles and, when the site of the pathologic process being removed is located intraconally, to push the muscles very carefully in the cranial or caudal direction.
- With very extensive medial preparation there exists the risk of injuring the ciliary ganglion, located laterally to the optic nerve, with subsequent anisocoria.

• Extraorbital complications
  - Injury to the ramus frontalis or the ramus orbitalis of the facial nerve with subsequent disorder of the mimetic musculature through to an inability to close the eyelids. In order to avoid this, precedence should be given to the course of the pterional incision behind the hairline and the operation should be conducted with neuromonitoring of the facial nerve.
  - An incomplete repositioning of the temporalis muscle can result in the sinking of the tissue above the zygomatic arch.

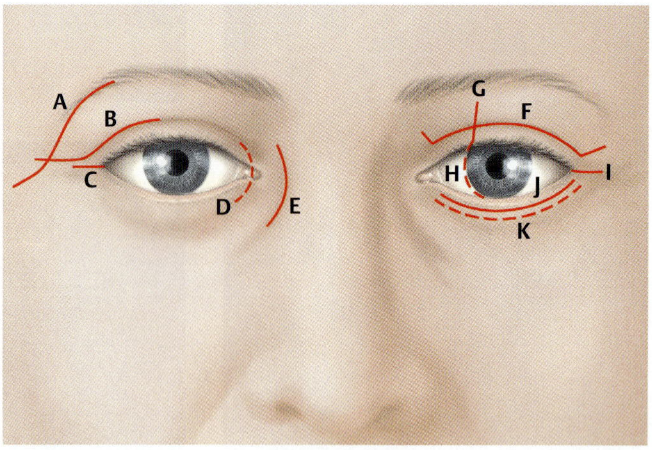

Fig. 18.4 Surgical approaches for anterior orbitotomy. A, Stallard-Wright lateral orbitotomy incision; B, lid crease with lateral extension; C, modified Berke lateral canthotomy incision; D, transcaruncular incision; H, transconjunctival (limbal) medial orbitotomy; I, lateral canthotomy incision; J, lower lid percutaneous incisions (subciliary, subtarsal, infraorbital); K, transconjunctival lower lid incision. Modified after Kersten RC, Nerad JA. Orbital Surgery. In: William Tasman, Edward A. Jaeger, eds. Duane's Ophthalmology. Philadelphia: Lippincott Williams & Wilkins; 2006.

18.5 Anterior Orbitotomy

B. Wiechens

In contrast to the approaches to the orbit described above, in this following section those approaches are described that can be summarized as "anterior orbitotomy." The majority of these approaches are used for biopsies and the removal of lesions that are palpable through the eyelids. However, processes lying deeper can also be reached via an anterior orbitotomy. The choice of which approach is appropriate is determined mainly by the location of the disease. With malignant tumors the radicality of the excision always depends on the individual case, taking into account the prognosis as well as the quality of life to be anticipated for the patient. The possibility of a complete tumor excision via an anterior orbitotomy depends considerably on how far the process extends behind the equator of the eye globe. Where necessary more invasive approaches or combinations might be recommended.

Anterior orbitotomy can be differentiated in transpalpebral and transconjunctival approaches (▸ Fig. 18.4).

Basically many interventions on small, subcutaneously located lesions in the anterior part of the orbit can easily be performed under local anesthesia. If preoperative diagnostic imaging has been inconclusive and/or if the feasibility of the operation under local anesthesia is questionable, general anesthesia is preferable as long as there are no objections due to the general situation of the patient. Thus, the operation, if necessary, can be extended without any problem, which is not possible or only to a limited extent in local anesthesia.

18.5.1 Transpalpebral Approach

When contemplating transcutaneous or transpalpebral approaches, the visibility of postoperative scars and the complication profile should also be considered. Thus, if possible, an approach should be chosen that will enable the best aesthetic result to be achieved. This manner of proceeding will of course be subject to limitations, especially in malignant conditions, with regard to the approachability of the tumor and the planned radicality.

Tumors or pathologic conditions in the upper space of the orbit can be reached either via a lateral orbitotomy in the area of the eyebrow or transpalpebrally via an incision in the upper lid groove, if necessary with lateral extension. Depending on localization, some specific potential complications should be considered: (1) injury of the trochlea superiomedially, with impairment of the levator complex and subsequent ptosis in the medial lid area; (2) damage to the lacrimal gland and its drainage system in the lateral lid area; (3) chronic edema and paresthesias following lateral extension of the incision; and (4) lesions of the lacrimal sac or lacrimal duct with medial approaches.[22]

Common tumors in the upper space of the orbit are dermoid cysts, hemangiomas, and mucoceles. Particularly with the latter, bony erosions in the area of the medial orbital wall and the orbital roof can be expected. Accordingly, careful preoperative diagnostic imaging and, where necessary, an interdisciplinary operation for resecting the tumor are recommended. Approaches to the superior orbit bear the risk of injuring in particular the supra-orbital nerve and the nerves in the medial and lateral lid angle. Thus patients must be informed preoperatively about the possibility of these complications with subsequent paresthesias/anesthesias or other functional limitations.

Preoperative assessment and marking up of the course of the incision in an erect position of the patient is necessary for all approaches. This is particularly important as anatomical conditions change in supine position of the patient. Preoperative and intraoperative photographic documentation of the findings is also recommended. In addition to the protection of anatomical structures, accurate hemostasis is important in order to reduce the risk of a postoperative orbital hematoma. Another principle is to spend as long as possible on the preparation in the extraper-

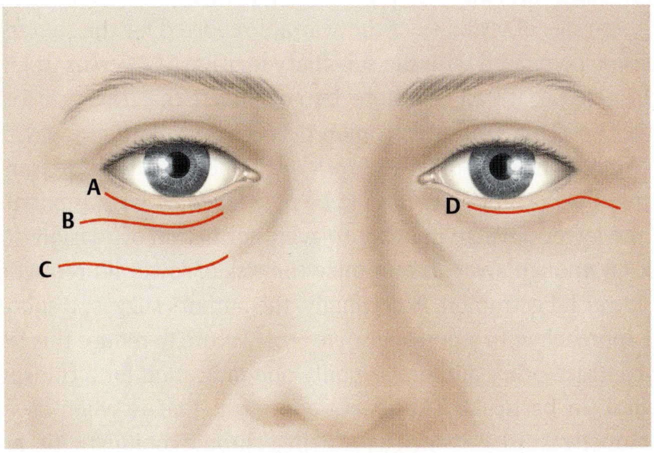

Fig. 18.5 Inferior anterior orbitotomy: transpalpebral approaches. A, subciliary incision; B, subtarsal incision; C, infraorbital incision; D, modified subciliary incision with lateral extension.

iorbital space until the lesion can be conclusively identified. This mode of procedure during the exploration significantly reduces the risk of postoperative orbital morbidity.

Upper Anterior Orbitotomy

Approaches for upper anterior orbitomy include the following.

Lateral Eyebrow Incision

Basically the approach to the superior lateral orbit via this incision is very limited due to the fact that the skin in the area of the eyebrow is very thick, the route for access to the superior lateral orbit by this approach is rather long, and the overlaying skin is not very mobile. A lateral extension of the incision, which is occasionally needed, is often associated with scarring; in contrast, an extension of the incision downward traverses important sensory nerve pathways and the relaxed skin tension lines (RSTL).

Approach via the Upper Lid Crease

This incision provides good access to the upper and lateral orbital rim and to the entire area of the upper orbit. In addition, the lid crease obscures later scar formation (AO Foundation). If necessary, this incision can be extended into the lateral canthus. After the skin incision, the approach passes through the orbicularis oculi muscle, whereby the orbital septum remains intact and, together with the orbital fat located here, protects deeper lying structures during preparation. The incision is done in a bow shape in the area of the lid crease, comparable to blepharoplasty of the upper lid, that is, ~10 mm above the lid margin medially and ~7 mm in the area of the lateral upper lid. Extraconal lesions in the upper orbit, even if they extend intraconally in part, can be reached by this approach. In the next step the orbital septum is separated. The closing of the wound is performed layer by layer (periosteum, muscle, and skin sutures) to achieve favorable cosmetic results (Video 18.4).

Inferior Anterior Orbitotomy

Many orbital conditions such as trauma, tumors, or transmitted infections occur in the inferior area of the orbit. These lesions are

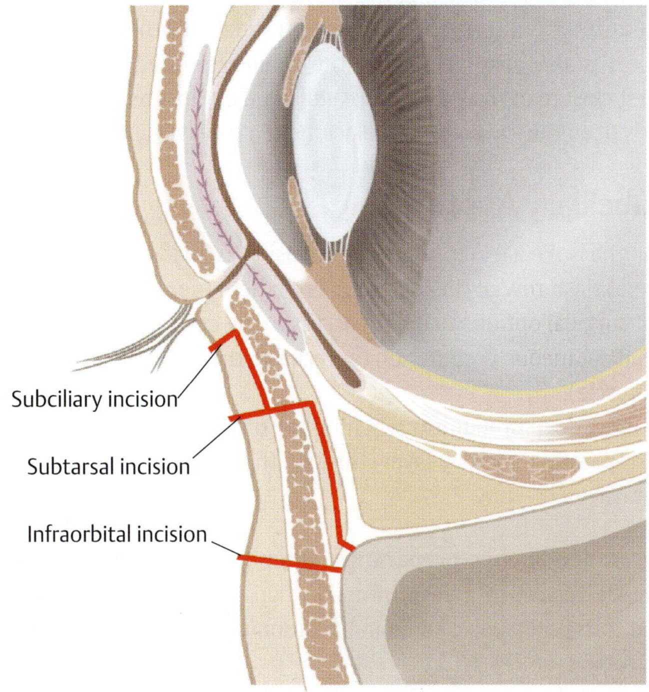

Fig. 18.6 Transpalpebral approaches. (cross section)

frequently located far anterior and so are palpable from outside. The affected regions can be easily reached via an inferior orbitotomy (▶ Fig. 18.5). Orbital processes located extraconally can usually be displayed well through this approach. Intraconal lesions can be reached through a preparation between the inferior rectus muscle and the lateral rectus muscle. Here one should pay attention to the identification and protection of the inferior oblique muscle. The medial inferior approach is more difficult due to the anatomical conditions.

Essentially, three transpalpebral incisions are possible in the area of the lower lid (▶ Fig. 18.6). Modifications to these are common and are used depending on the localization of the process and the surgical strategy.

Infra-orbital Incision

The infra-orbital incision is positioned in a transverse skin fold at the level of the infra-orbital margin. The infra-orbital rim is then exposed by means of blunt preparation between the orbicularis oculi muscle and the orbital septum, followed by a subperiostal preparation. After incision of the periosteum at the infra-orbital rim, the orbital floor is exposed subperiostally.

This approach is the shortest one to get access to the inferior orbit. However it is done in the transitional zone between the thin eyelid skin and the thicker skin of the cheek. Due to the lymph drainage pathways, this area is predisposed to postoperative edema and visible scars (AO Foundation). Because of these considerable complications, to date the infra-orbital incision is employed only in limited cases.

Subtarsal Incision

The incision is performed directly underneath the lower tarsus, medially ~2–3 mm underneath the lid rim and coursing slightly laterocaudally. After dissection of the orbicularis oculi muscle along the muscle fibers, the infra-orbital rim can finally be exposed while protecting the orbital septum. After separation of the orbital septum, a further preparation into the deeper orbit layers is also possible. Finally, the wound is closed layer by layer (first closure of the periosteum, followed by closure of the orbicularis oculi muscle, and then placement of skin suture).

Subciliary Approach

For the subciliary approach an incision is made directly under the eyelash row of the lower lid. From here there are three different surgical options to obtain access to the orbit (▶ Fig. 18.7):

- Subcutaneous preparation (anterior to the orbicularis oculi muscle).
- Direct deep preparation (behind the orbicularis oculi muscle).
- Preparation layer by layer (through the orbicularis oculi muscle).

The **subcutaneous preparation** anterior to the orbicularis oculi muscle results in a very thin skin flap, which tends to scarring and thus predisposes to lid malpositioning (in particular lower lid ectropion) (▶ Fig. 18.8).

Direct deep preparation with incision through the orbicularis muscle and subsequent preparation anterior to the orbital septum results in a combined skin–muscle flap, which postoperatively carries the risk of reduced lower lid tone with subsequent lid malposition.

Preparation in layers begins with a skin flap with subsequent horizontal separation of the orbicularis oculi muscle layer by layer.

The last two options in particular require surgical skills to ensure that the orbital septum is not injured. If preparation is inaccurate, there is risk of a postoperative contraction of the lower lid retractors with subsequent lid malposition.[23]

Basically it is possible to expose the infra-orbital rim with all three types of preparation without opening the orbital septum. If the pathological processes are located deeper in the orbit, extended preparation can take place after separation of the orbital septum.

Comparative Studies

Due to its potential complications (lower lid ectropion or lower lid retraction as well as long-lasting lid edema) the infra-orbital approach is rarely used. In this subsection only the subtarsal and subciliary approaches are discussed.

Proponents of both approaches argue that the lower orbital rim and lower orbit can be reached in its entirety.[24] Although a visible scar is created in both approaches, this can be concealed either underneath the eyelash row or in the lower lid groove—particularly in older people—and is therefore only minimally visible. One disadvantage of the inferior transpalpebral approaches is the risk of expanded eye opening in a downward direction (scleral show) or lower lid ectropion. For this reason several studies were conducted comparing the complication rates of transpalpebral (transcutaneous) approaches. The risk of lower lid retraction or ectropion with a subciliary approach lies between 12.5 and 42%,[25,26] while it is only 2.7 to 7.7% for the subtarsal approach.[26] Factors that inherently predispose to a lower lid retraction or a lower lid ectropion include the occurrence of hematomas, lid edemas, adhesions of the orbital septum, and scar contractions following treatment of an orbital floor fracture[27] (▶ Fig. 18.12). Higher rates of visibility of the scar are reported for the subtarsal incision compared with the subciliary incision (2.2 versus 0%).[28]

In general, it can therefore be concluded that the risk for a lower lid retraction or ectropion decreases the farther away the incision is made from the lower lid edge.[26] For this reason a transpalpebral approach should be positioned as close as possible to the lower lid edge in order to avoid formation of a visible scar but far enough away to minimize the risk of lower lid retraction or lower lid ectropion. Accordingly, the authors suggest a subtarsal approach with a postoperative Frost suture to reduce this risk. In contrast, other authors see only one indication for a transpalpebral (in particular subciliary) approach: that is when severe conjunctival diseases such as scarring, chronic conjunctivitis, acid burns, or severe burns are present.[29] For the reasons mentioned, to date most authors prefer the transconjunctival approach.

18.5.2 Transconjunctival Approach

The transconjunctival approach was first described by Bourguet in 1924 for the removal of an adipose tissue prolapse of the lower lid.[30] In the 1970s the transconjunctival approach was made popular for orbital surgery by McCord and Moss as well as by Tessier.[31,32] In the ensuing years, further studies confirmed a lower complication rate for this approach in relation to “classical” surgical procedures.[33,34] In addition to the lower complication rate and decreased risk for scar formation, the operation time up to the exposition of the lower orbital rim was also evaluated.[35] At about 20 minutes on average, the transconjunctival technique was the most time-consuming, while the average operation time for a subciliary approach was 15 minutes, and 5 to 8 minutes for a subtarsal approach.

In principle, the transconjunctival approach technique can be applied for operations in different areas of the orbit (▶ Fig. 18.9). The upper transconjunctival, the inferior, and **transcaruncular approaches** have been described[36] (▶ Fig. 18.10). There is still also the option of a conjunctival incision near the limbus as used in strabismus or amotio surgery.

The incision in the fornix of the superior conjunctiva can be used to reach pathological conditions located superonasally, episclerally, intraconally, and extraconally. In this, care must be taken that no damage is done to the levator palpebrae muscle, the superior oblique muscle, the trochlea, the lacrimal gland, the sensory nerves, and the blood vessels. In analogy with the transconjunctival operation for repositioning of orbital floor fractures, a transconjunctival approach via the superotemporal conjunctiva under the upper lid has been advocated for the operative care of lateral orbit rim fractures.[37,38]

The transcaruncular approach can be used either in isolation or as an expansion in the context of an inferior transconjunctival approach.[39] The incision medially to the caruncle enables an excellent display of the medial orbital area and its bony walls.[40,41] It should be made sure that the preparation route is posterior to the lacrimal duct apparatus in order to avoid damage.

The transconjunctival approach is most often used in operations in the lower orbital space, predominantly for **orbital floor fracture** repositioning. Extending the inferior incision in a lateral direction by a canthotomy and/or medially by a transcaruncular incision provides an outstanding possibility of displaying the

18

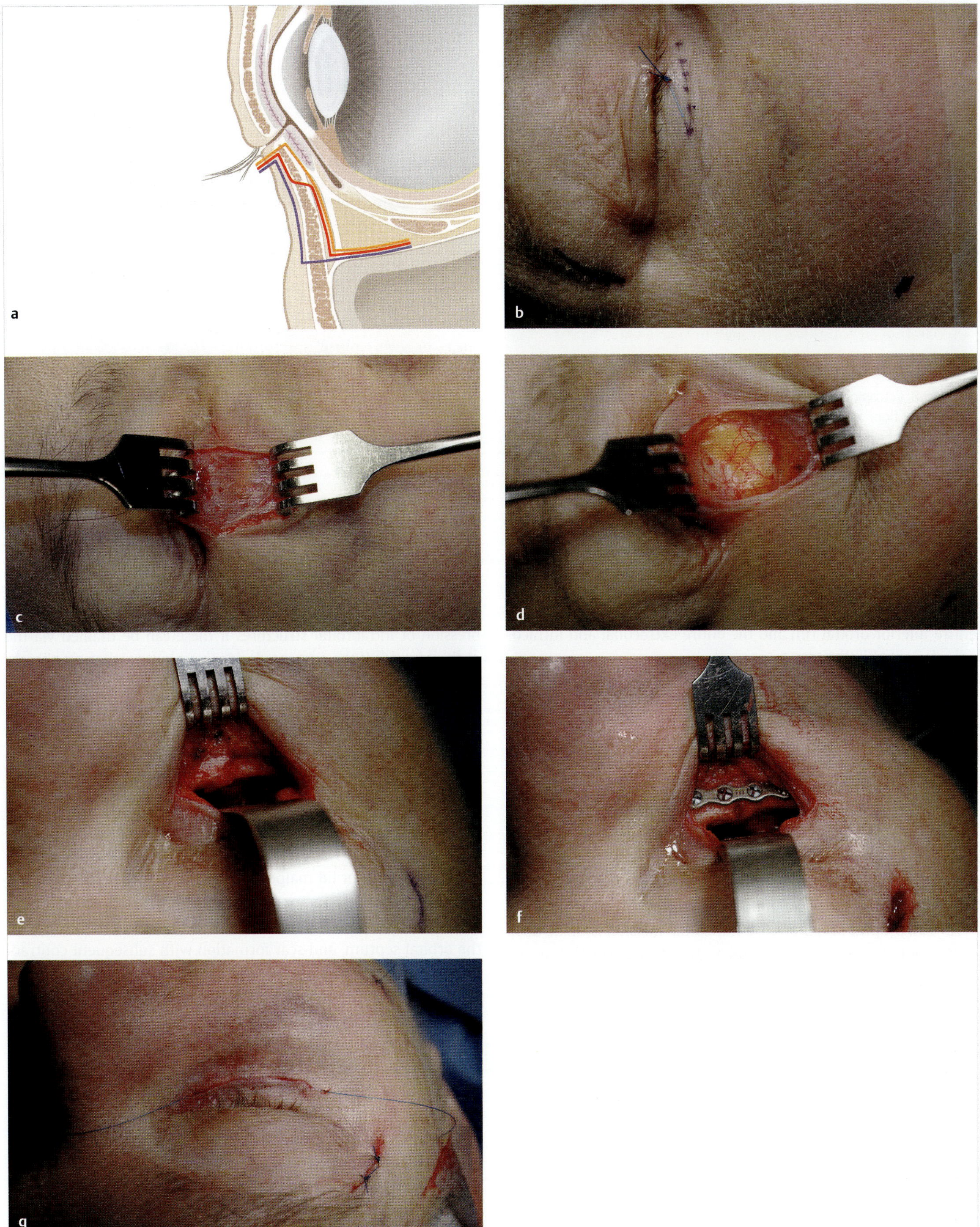

Fig. 18.7 Subciliary approach and repositioning of a zygomatic bone fracture.[23] **(a)** Possibilities for preseptal preparation routes: violet line, anterior to the orbicularis muscle; orange line, direct approach through all layers of the orbicularis muscle; red line, preparation layer-by-layer. **(b)** Subciliary approach for repositioning of a zygomatic bone fracture. The subciliary incision line is marked with a surgical pen. **(c)** The orbicularis muscle is exposed. **(d)** The orbital adipose tissue comes to the fore once the muscle is dissected. **(e)** The bony infra-orbital rim can now be exposed. **(f)** The fracture is repositioned and stabilized with an osteosynthesis plate. **(g)** This photograph shows the wound closure after the procedure has been terminated.

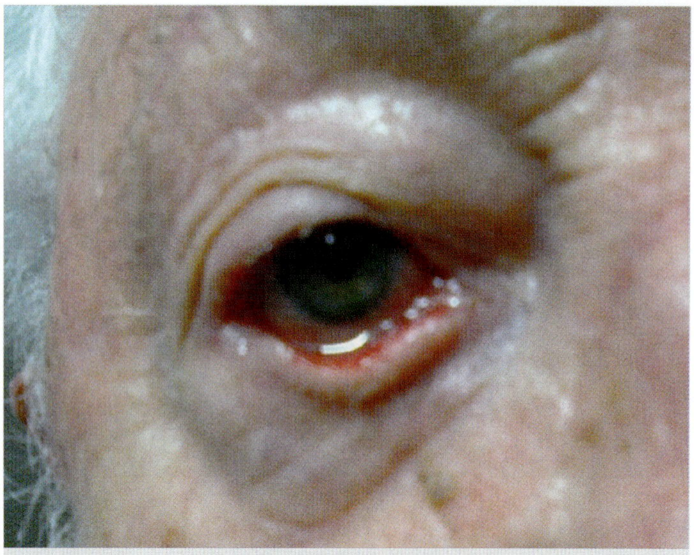

Fig. 18.8 Ectropion in an 88-year-old man, 5 months postoperatively. An orbital floor fracture has been repositioned using a polydioxanone foil via a subciliary approach.

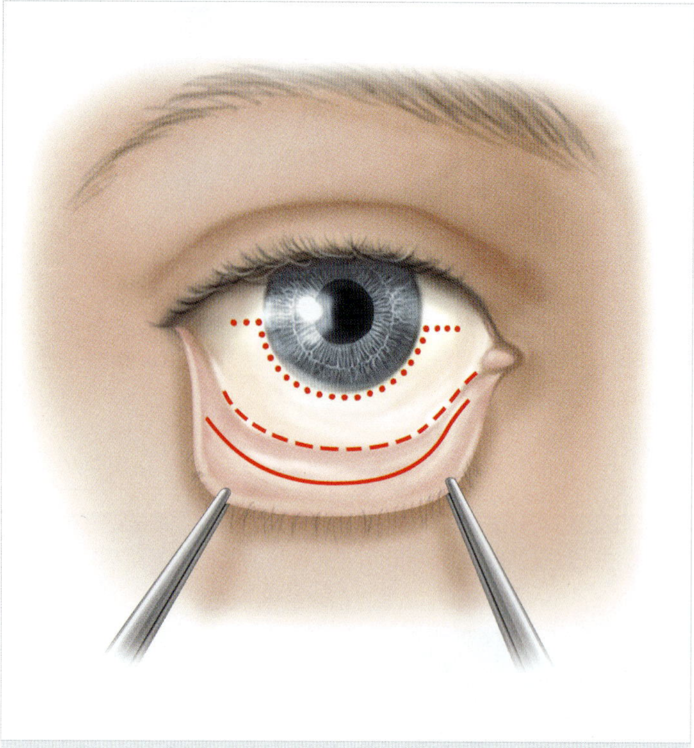

Fig. 18.9 Possible preparation routes using a transconjunctival approach. *Continuous line*, preseptal route; *dashed line*, retroseptal route; *dotted line*, limbal route.

entire inferior orbital rim and the entire extraconal and intraconal inferior orbital spaces.

Technique

There are two possibilities for exposing the inferior orbital rim and adjacent areas by a transconjunctival approach: retroseptal and preseptal preparation.

For **preseptal** preparation a conjunctival incision is made on the lower edge of the lower lid tarsus. After separation of the common attachment of the lower lid retractors and of the orbital septum, preparation is performed in the preseptal space directly behind the orbicularis oculi muscle right up to the orbital rim.[42]

For **retroseptal** preparation, a horizontal incision is made deep in the conjunctival fornix. After separation of the lower lid retractors, the infra-orbital rim is displayed directly through the orbital fat compartment.

With both techniques care should be taken that the cornea and the globe are protected and the conjunctiva is coagulated as little as possible. Particularly with retroseptal preparation, the orbital fat tissue can protrude immediately after opening and get in the way of the further preparation. In order not to disrupt the fine septation of the orbital fat and the anatomical structures found therein, and to minimize postoperative scarring, an extensive fat resection should be avoided.

18

In contrast to the retroseptal approach, with a preseptal preparation closure of the periosteum can be achieved. There is, however, disagreement about whether the conjunctiva should be sutured. Proponents argue that not only the tarsal conjunctiva but also, the fornix should be adjusted and restored in an anatomically correct position as otherwise a weakening of the lower lid retractors results in a higher rate of lower lid malpositions.[43,44] Opponents of the conjunctival suture point out that postoperative edema and hemorrhages do not lead to a compression of intraorbital structures if these can be drained via the open wound.[45] If the surgeon decides on a suture, then an absorbable running suture with a maximal thickness of 8–0 should be used and be only loosely laid and knotted.[23] This enables a sufficient adaptation of the wound; exudate or blood emerging postoperatively can drain through the gaps still present.

Complications

The advantages of the transconjunctival approach are the nonvisible scar, the better approach to the medial orbital wall, and the lower rate of lower lid malpositions compared with the transpalpebral approaches. Factors favoring a lower lid ectropion or retraction are postoperative edema, hematomas, adhesions to the orbital septum, and scar formation with subsequent contraction.[23,46] In contrast to the transpalpebral approaches, the reported complication rate for the transconjunctival technique is lower: 0%,[47,48] 1.5% (50), 2.2%,[23] 6.6%,[42] and 7.1%.[49] Most authors state that complications occur only temporarily and another operation is required only in very few cases. It must be emphasized, however, that the majority of studies have investigated the transconjunctival approach for repositioning of blow-out fractures[50] so that some of the postoperative complications are related to the underlying trauma and should be differentiated from complications deriving from the surgical technique itself.

18.5.3 Advantages and Disadvantages of the Transconjunctival vs. Transpalpebral Approach

In the past years the transconjunctival approach has established itself widely in the surgical treatment of orbital floor fractures (▶ Fig. 18.11). However the limits of this technique are a subject of discussion. While some authors deem this technique also

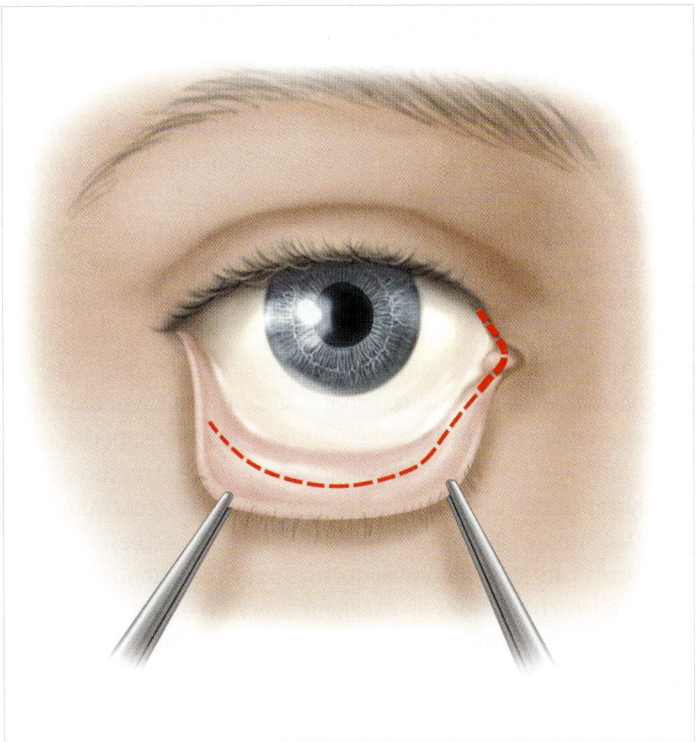

Fig. 18.10 Transconjunctival approach with possible transcaruncular extension.

suitable for large tumors,[51] others emphasize that different approaches should be preferred for removing pathologic conditions lying deep in the orbit (i.e., the orbital apex), for tumors lying extraconally,[52,53] and for tumors with firm adherence to the retrobulbar tissue or with large draining veins.

If one considers the complication rates of the transpalpebral approaches, it is striking that for the subtarsal incision these are reported to be 2.7 to 7.7% and therefore roughly coincide with those of the transconjunctival approach. The frequently mentioned disadvantage of the subtarsal incision—a visible scar—is less of a concern in older people due to existing wrinkles.

In considering whether a transpalpebral or a transconjunctival approach is preferred, Wilson and Ellis[26] pointed out that two factors should be taken into account:

- The extent of the surgical overview required.
- The surgeon's familiarity with the approach to be selected.

The overview following transconjuctival incision is very limited. For this reason in particular the incision can be combined with a lateral canthotomy or inferior cantholysis when required. However, this counteracts the actual advantage of transconjunctival approaches, namely the avoidance of a visible scar. In contrast, when expanding into the medial orbital area, transcaruncular incision can be an option.

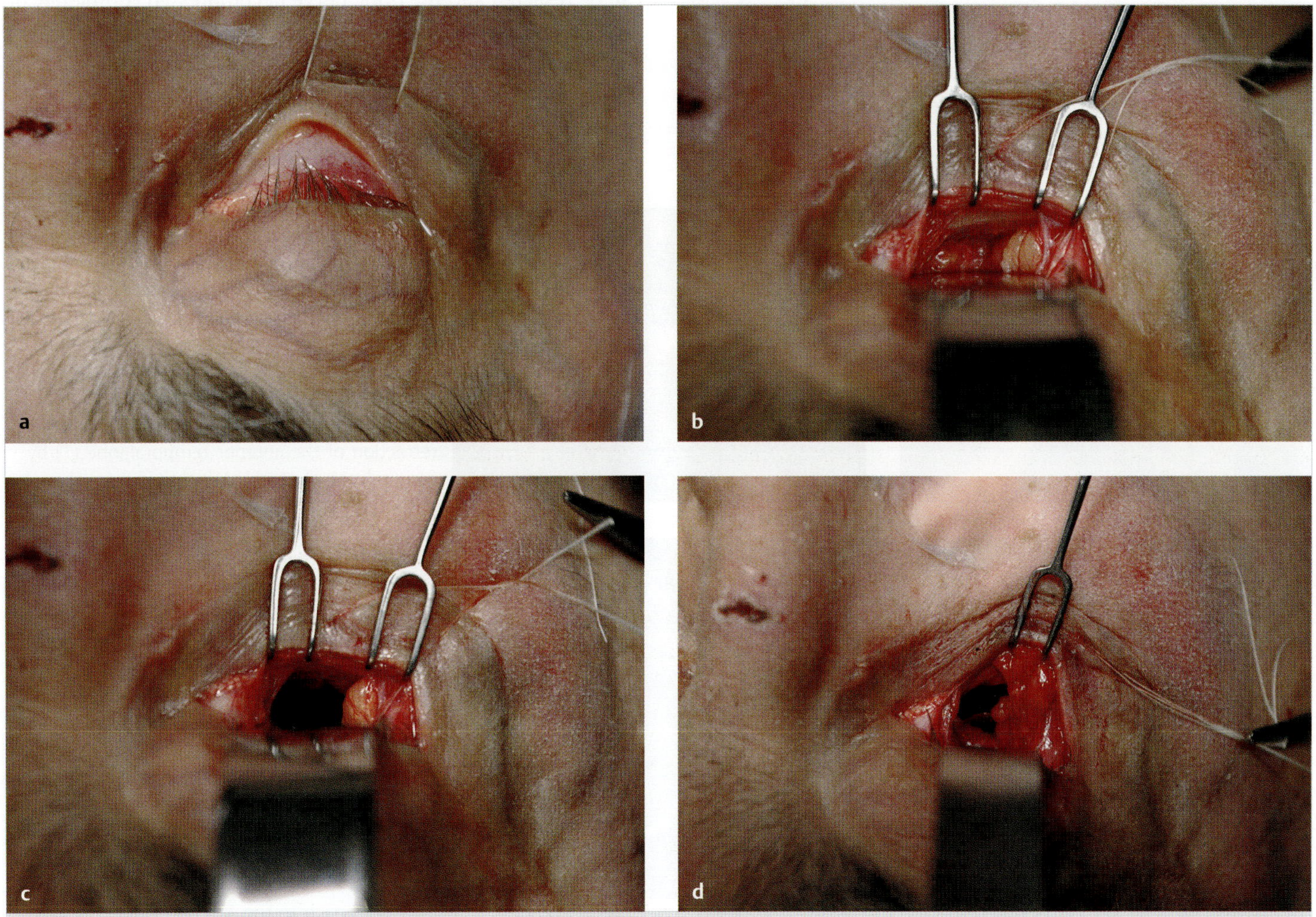

Fig. 18.11 Transconjunctival approach for repositioning an orbital floor fracture. **(a)** The conjunctival incision is located at the lower rim of the lower lid tarsus. **(b)** After the joint insertion point of the lower lid retractors is split, the orbital adipose tissue comes to the fore. **(c)** After the adipose tissue has been dissected, the orbital floor can be exposed. **(d)** The orbital floor can be reconstructed, for example, with a polydioxanone foil, following repositioning of the intraorbital content.

18

A further possible disadvantage of the transconjunctival approach is the more intense manipulation of the eye globe. Therefore, Appling et al[33] recommended refraining from the transconjunctival technique in those cases with only one seeing eye.

18.6 Transcranial Extradural and Intradural Approaches

I. E. Sandalcioglu and U. Sure

18.6.1 Introduction

Selection of the optimal surgical approach is an essential prerequisite for a good functional and cosmetic result. The goals of surgery must be defined and planned carefully and communicated to the patients in detail. Basically, complete tumor resection should be aimed for regardless of the dignity of the tumor. However, radical resection of benign and malignant tumors can be associated with significant functional limitations and risks, such as visual disturbances including blindness, increased risks for infections with cerebrospinal fluid leaks, or hypothalamic–hypophyseal disturbances. In such cases, tumor reduction with incomplete resection or optic nerve decompression for functional improvement should be considered and additional interdisciplinary treatment options with radiation and/or chemotherapy should be evaluated. Radical tumor resection with potential loss of function should be discussed in very aggressive tumors with infiltration of orbital structures, while significant improvement of the prognosis can be achieved.

18.6.2 Frontolateral Craniotomy (Pterional Craniotomy)

The frontolateral craniotomy (pterional craniotomy; ▶ Fig. 18.12) represents the standard surgical approach for most tumors, which arise from the lateral aspect of the frontal skull base.[54,55,56,57] In particular meningiomas which frequently arise from the medial and lateral sphenoid wing or meningiomas of the anterior clinoid process can be approached by this route. Due to their local mass effect, they frequently affect the optic nerve or even infiltrate the optic canal. Important osseous structures can be approached via an extradural route, such as the sphenoid wing, the anterior clinoid process, the optic canal, or the superior orbital fissure, and resected if necessary. Since these structures commonly represent the tumor attachment and consecutively their vascular supply, initial drilling and resection of these osseous structures can facilitate subsequent tumor resection. The intradural approach provides an excellent overview of important neurovascular structures, such as the optic nerve, the optic chiasm, and the internal carotid artery with corresponding branches.[56,58,59] In huge tumors, these functionally important structures are frequently visualized not before significant tumor debulking. In many cases, the entrance into the optic canal can be visualized at an early stage of the operation. After incision and separation of the dura, the complete superior osseous wall of the optic canal can be resected and the optic nerve decompressed completely on its way to the orbit.[60] Tumorous elements infiltrating the optic canal can be delineated and resected via this approach.

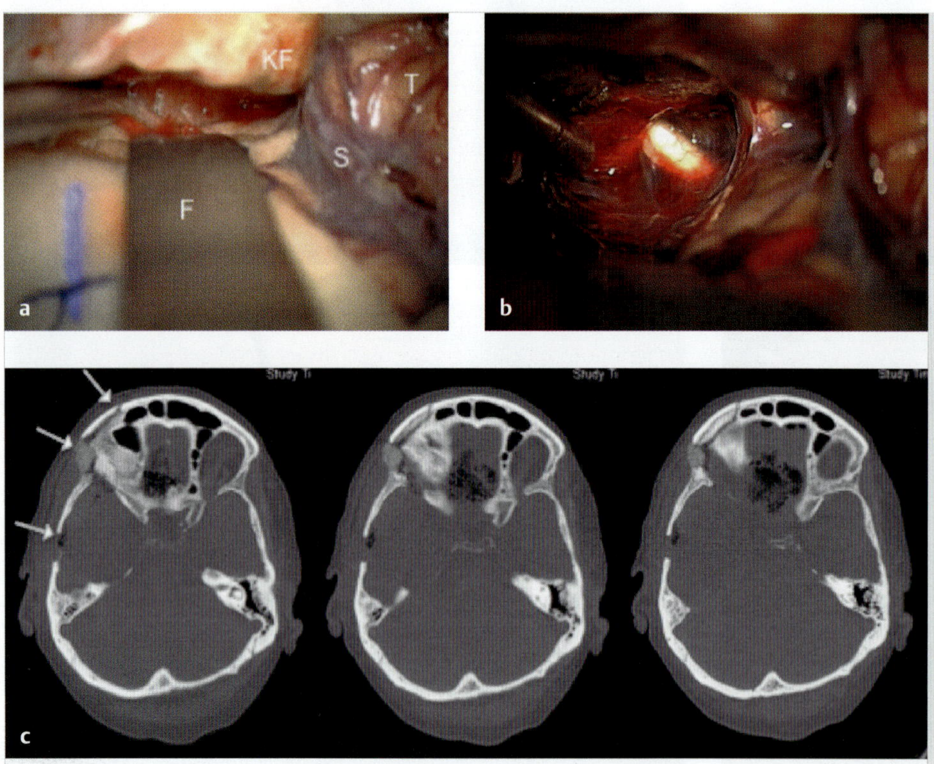

Fig. 18.12 Frontolateral approach. **(a)** Microsurgical view after right-sided frontotemporal craniotomy and subfrontal approach to the anterior cranial fossa. Meticulous extradural resection of the lateral sphenoid wing (KF) and a flat subfrontal approach to the frontal skull base are essential key points of this approach. The frontobasal skull base can be visualized without retraction of the anterior temporal lobe (T) by early release of cerebrospinal fluid from the basal cisterns, opening of the sylvian fissure (S) and gentle retraction of the frontal lobe (F). **(b)** The entire frontal skull base and the neurovascular structures at the junction to the middle fossa can be approached via this route. Both optic nerves, the entrance into the optic canals, and the basal cisterns can be exposed completely. **(c)** Opening of the frontal sinuses should be avoided in frontotemporal craniotomies. The arrows show the anterior limitation of the craniotomy without exposure of the frontal sinus and the bur holes at the keyhole (filled with bony meal) and temporobasal region. The frontobasal limitation of the craniotomy is located directly above the orbital roof and allows a flat approach to the anterior skull base.

18

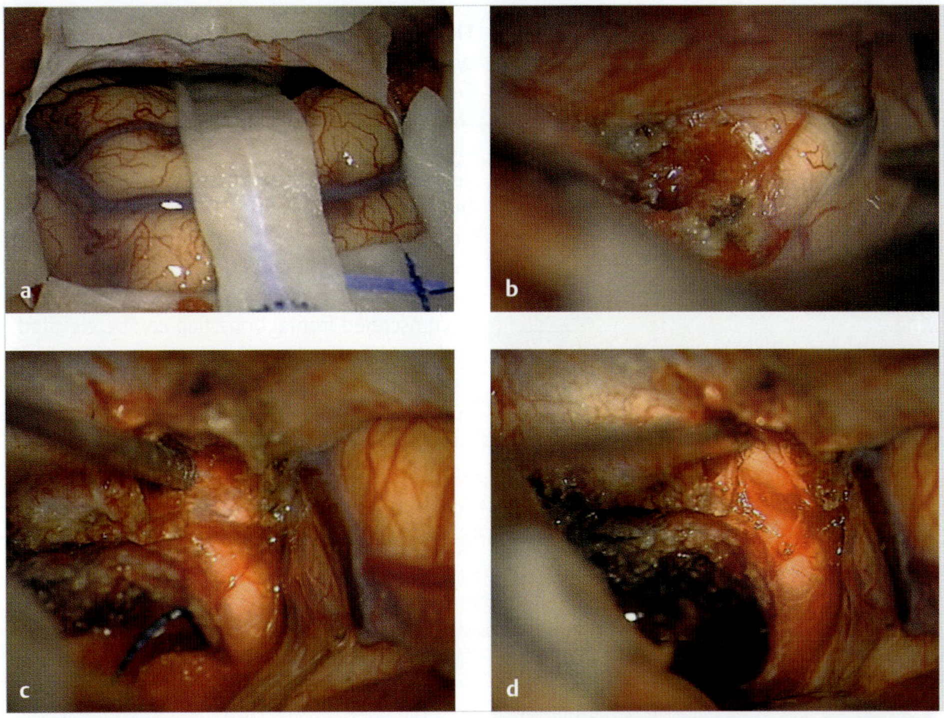

Fig. 18.13 Frontal craniotomy and subfrontal approach. **(a)** Surgical view after frontal craniotomy and dural opening. After meticulous planning and reclining of the head, the frontal lobe tilts downward by gravity. A corridor to the frontal skull base is opened. This effect can be enhanced by early release of cerebrospinal fluid from the basal cisterns. **(b)** The right-sided optic nerve is extremely compressed by the tumor in the optic canal from dorsal to ventral. In some cases it is recommendable to open the optic canal first to preserve optic nerve function before tumor resection. **(c)** After detachment of the frontobasal dura and osseous decompression of the optic canal, the dural sheet of the optic nerve is visualized. **(d)** The dural sheet of the optic nerve can be completely incised for extensive decompression of the optic nerve.

18.6.3 Frontal Unilateral Craniotomy (Subfrontal Approach)

A frontally-accentuated pterional or frontal craniotomy is needed for a subfrontal approach (▶ Fig. 18.13).[61,62,63] Similarly to other approaches, a flat approach to the anterior skull base should be planned to minimize frontal lobe retraction. This approach can be supported by optimal head reclination, leading to minimal additional retraction of the brain by making use of gravity. Special attention must be paid to the frontal sinuses because they can extend far laterally and must be meticulously supplied to avoid complications. Preoperative planning of the craniotomy should therefore always respect the anatomical details of the frontal sinuses to avoid frontal sinus opening. Especially midline tumors and tumors of the planum sphenoidale or the tuberculum sellae can be approached via this route. The orbit can be approached in the extradural way with additional osteotomy of the superior orbital rim and resection of the orbital roof. This approach is especially appropriate for tumorous processes that are localized above the optic nerve.

18.6.4 Supra-orbital "Keyhole Approach"

Similarly to the frontal craniotomy, the modified and circumscribed supra-orbital approach can be performed with an eyebrow incision, if necessary with or without resection of the superior orbital ring and the orbital roof (▶ Fig. 18.14; Video 18.5).[64,65,66] As described above, there is the possibility to delineate the superior aspects of the orbit extradurally or to demonstrate the entrance of the optic nerve into optic canal after dural incision. The advantages are circumscribed incision and minimal soft tissue mobilization, which is needed for a conventional craniotomy. The drill hole as the initiating point of craniotomy must be located at the frontozygomatic point below the attachment of the circumscribed mobilized temporal muscle. A good cosmetic result is achieved after refixation of the muscle.

18.6.5 Bifrontal Craniotomy

Bifrontal craniotomy with exposure of the entire frontal skull base is appropriate for extended processes of the anterior skull base with infiltration of the dura, the frontal cortex, the ethmoidal cells, the cranial and medial limitation of the orbits with involvement of the frontal sinuses, the sphenoid sinus, or the nasal cavity (▶ Fig. 18.15).[67] These surgeries are usually planned in terms of interdisciplinary treatment.[68,69] The approach can be adjusted to requirements with sufficient material for subsequent reconstruction being obtained with a bicoronary skin incision with preparation of a frontobasally stemmed galea-periost flap.

Via a bifrontal craniotomy and extradural approach both orbital roofs can be exposed and intradural course of the optic nerves and their entrances into the orbits can be delineated. The size of the craniotomy can be varied as necessary. Cranialization of the frontal sinuses may be needed when the osseous compartments are involved in the pathology and reconstruction is not possible. After resection of the ethmoidal cells one can approach the medial osseous walls of both orbits (lamina papyracea). Reconstruction should be very meticulous, because after extended resection of the aforementioned structures including the basal dura there is significant connection between the "sterile" intradural cerebrospinal fluid compartments and neuronal structures with the "contaminated" paranasal sinuses.

Therefore, planning of the operative approach and the preparation of an adequate galea-periost flap is essential. Also both temporal muscle fasciae can be applied as a free graft or as a stemmed graft for dural reconstruction and frontobasal revision.

A watertight closure of the dura and the frontal skull base is important. Segments of the tabula interna can be taken and applied for bony reconstruction in calvaria-split technique from the healthy portions of the craniotomy flap. Autologous tissue is

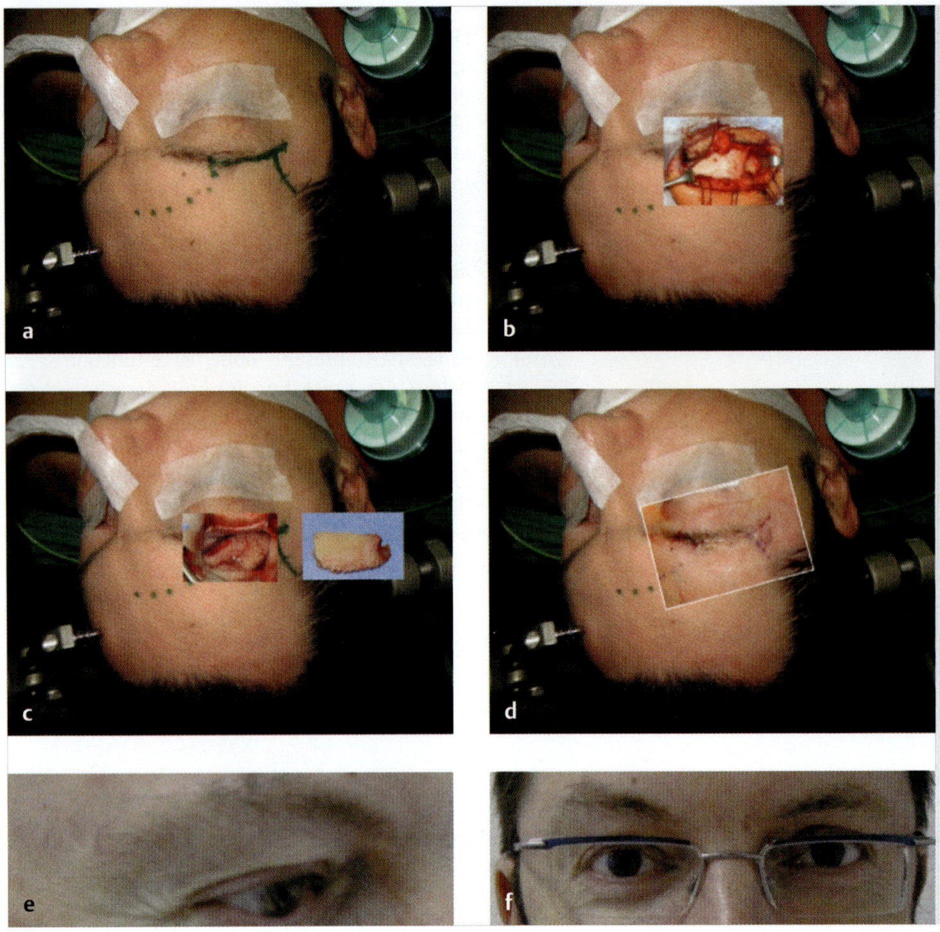

Fig. 18.14 Supra-orbital approach. **(a)** Head positioning and planning of a supra-orbital keyhole approach. The important landmarks are the frontal sinuses (*dotted line*), the marking of the eyebrow incision, and the course of the superior temporal line for the positioning of the bur hole. **(b)** Delineation of the superior orbital rim and the superior temporal line after mobilization of the attachment of the temporal muscle for the positioning of the bur hole. **(c)** A circumscribed frontal bone flap can be elevated and the dura can be opened in a basally-stemmed fashion. **(d–f)** Surgical view after complete reconstruction and subcuticular suture **(d)** with excellent cosmetic result 6 months postoperatively **(e, f)**.

usually more appropriate than exogenous dural or bony substitutes, such as titanium, PEEK, or ceramic. However, these materials can also be used for reconstruction of the superior, lateral, and medial orbital walls and the frontal skull base and are especially helpful in revision surgeries.[68]

18.7 Orbital Exenteration

H.-J. Welkoborsky

Orbital exenteration is removal and “clearing out” of the entire orbit with its adnexa. Basically, one needs to differentiate between enucleation, in which the orbital adnexa including the lid apparatus are left intact and only the eyeball is removed, and complete orbital exenteration.

18.7.1 Enucleation

18

The main indications for enucleation of the eyeball are diseases that are limited to the eyeball, such as tumors of the eyeball, severe inflammations of the eyeball, perforating eyeball injuries that cannot be treated surgically in such a way as to preserve the eyeball, or microphthalmia (e.g., after radiotherapy). A prerequisite for enucleation is the noninvolvement of the structures of the upper and lower lid as well as of the lacrimal apparatus in the pathologic process.

The surgical technique is such that the eyeball is cut around via a transconjunctival approach. It is then luxated and the intraorbital muscles are separated. If the pathologic process has not involved the outer eye muscles, they can be preserved, which is of benefit for the subsequent reconstruction and volume restoration of the orbit. If the outer eye muscles are involved in the pathologic process, these also have to be resected. After the luxation of the globe, the optic nerve and the ophthalmic artery are clamped off with a curved clamp and then tied off. The globe can then be removed. The orbit is reconstructed in line with the extent of the deformity caused. The temporal muscle, for example, is suitable for this and is incised and mobilized. A large window is then inserted into the lateral orbit, through which the muscle can be swung into the defect and fixed in the orbit.[70] The lateral border of the lateral orbital ridge must be preserved here as, otherwise, the lateral facial contour of the face would be flattened and the eyelid preserved apparatus would no longer have a sufficient hold. Free mucous membrane transplants, which can be harvested from the cheek, for example, are suitable for the mucosal lining of the new orbit. As it is possible that later a glass prosthesis will be inserted, it is advantageous to strengthen the lower lid with some cartilage (e.g., from the nasal septum or from the ear concha), as these structures to a large extent must support the weight of the prosthesis.[70] Furthermore, an eye shield already inserted during the operation improves the subsequent cosmetic result and leads to a good connection between musculature and mucous membrane so that a stable site for the prosthesis results.

18.7.2 Orbital Exenteration

The main indications for orbital exenteration are large tumors of the eyeball with infiltration of the periorbital structures; tumors of the conjunctiva, of the eyelid, or of the lacrimal apparatus with extensive infiltration of the eyeball or of the outer eye muscles; or tumors of the paranasal sinuses with infiltration of the

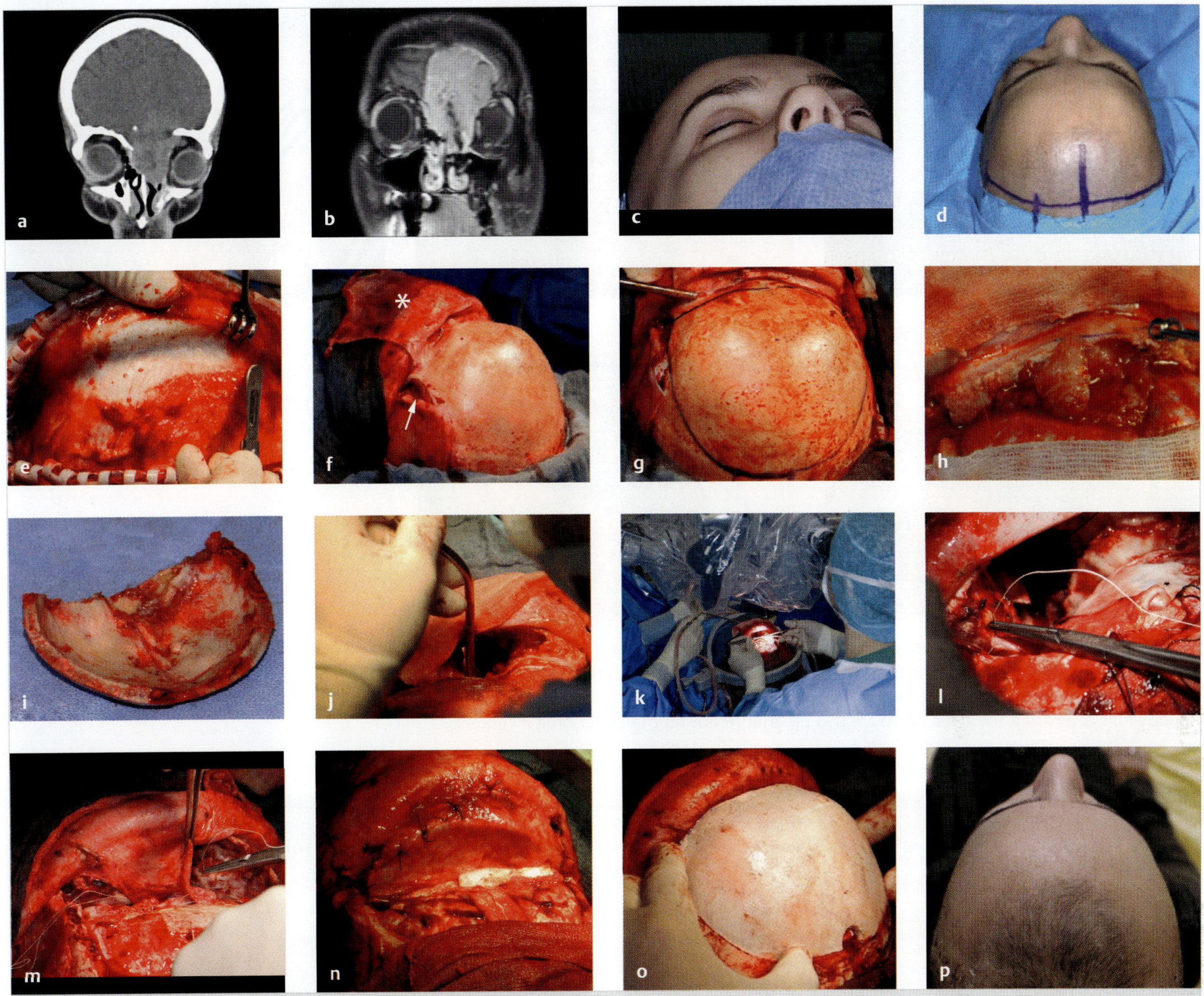

Fig. 18.15 Bifrontal approach. **(a, b)** Extended frontobasal tumor with osseous destruction of the anterior skull base and the orbit in CT scan **(a)** with infiltration of the dura and the frontal brain parenchyma with invasion into the left orbit and displacement of the intraorbital soft tissues as demonstrated on MRI scan **(b)**. The vision and bulbar motility of the 27-year-old female patient were not limited. **(c, d)** Leading symptom is bulbar protusion of the left eye with incomplete eyelid closure and left paramedian tumorous swelling of the nasal root with displacement of the ocular bulb. **(d)** Surgical positioning of the head and planning of a bicoronary skin incision. **(e)** Preparation of a separate skin and galea periost flap with exposure of sufficient autologous tissue for the dural and frontobasal reconstruction. **(f)** The galea periost flap is stemmed frontobasally (*asterisk*) and the attachment of the temporal muscle is mobilized bilaterally at the frontozygomatic point (*arrow*). Here the bur holes for the bifrontal craniotomy can be positioned. The temporalis fascia can also be prepared as a free or stemmed graft. **(g)** Planning of the dorsal extension of the craniotomy. Segments of the tabula interna can be taken and modeled from the healthy parts of the bifrontal bone flap for subsequent bony reconstruction. **(h, i)** Surgical view after bifrontal craniotomy. The tumor infiltrates the dura and has completely destroyed the dorsal wall of the frontal sinus, the anterior skull base, the orbital roof and the medial orbital wall. **(j, k)** Interdisciplinary transcranial and transnasal tumor resection. **(l)** Frontal and frontobasal reconstruction of the dura proximal to the sphenoid wing with a free graft of the temporal fascia. This graft is sutured in watertight fashion on its free ends. **(m, n)** Multilayered covering with stemmed galea-periosteum flap on the entire frontal skull base. **(o)** Reimplantation of the bifrontal bone flap. **(p)** Cosmetic result with remission of bulbar protrusion after wound healing.

intraorbital tissue, here particularly of the muscles and/or the eyeball itself.[71,72,73,74] Caution is required with retinoblastomas, rhabdomyosarcomas, and adenoid cystic carcinomas with regard to mutilating interventions. For these tumors today there are alternative treatment regimens available with chemotherapy and radiotherapy. For the tumors mentioned above and, for example, also for extensive esthesioneuroblastomas, even very extensive radical surgical procedures have not been able to improve the prognosis compared to organ-preserving tumor surgery together with adjuvant radiotherapy.[75,76] In some cases of extensive carcinomas the developments in microsurgical techniques and the increasing knowledge of tumor biology also permit a local, organ-preserving tumor resection with good oncological control.[72,74] At present, orbital exenteration is only necessary in ~8–10% of malignant orbital tumors.[77]

Basically with orbital exenteration the eyelids are cut around in a circular fashion and the periosteum of the orbital rim incised from the 12 o'clock position round to the 12 o'clock position.[70] Then the entire periorbita is bluntly separated in circular fashion from the bony orbital walls. The trochlea is ablated; the medial and lateral palpebral ligaments as well as the nasolacrimal duct are separated. After these measures, the entire orbital content is

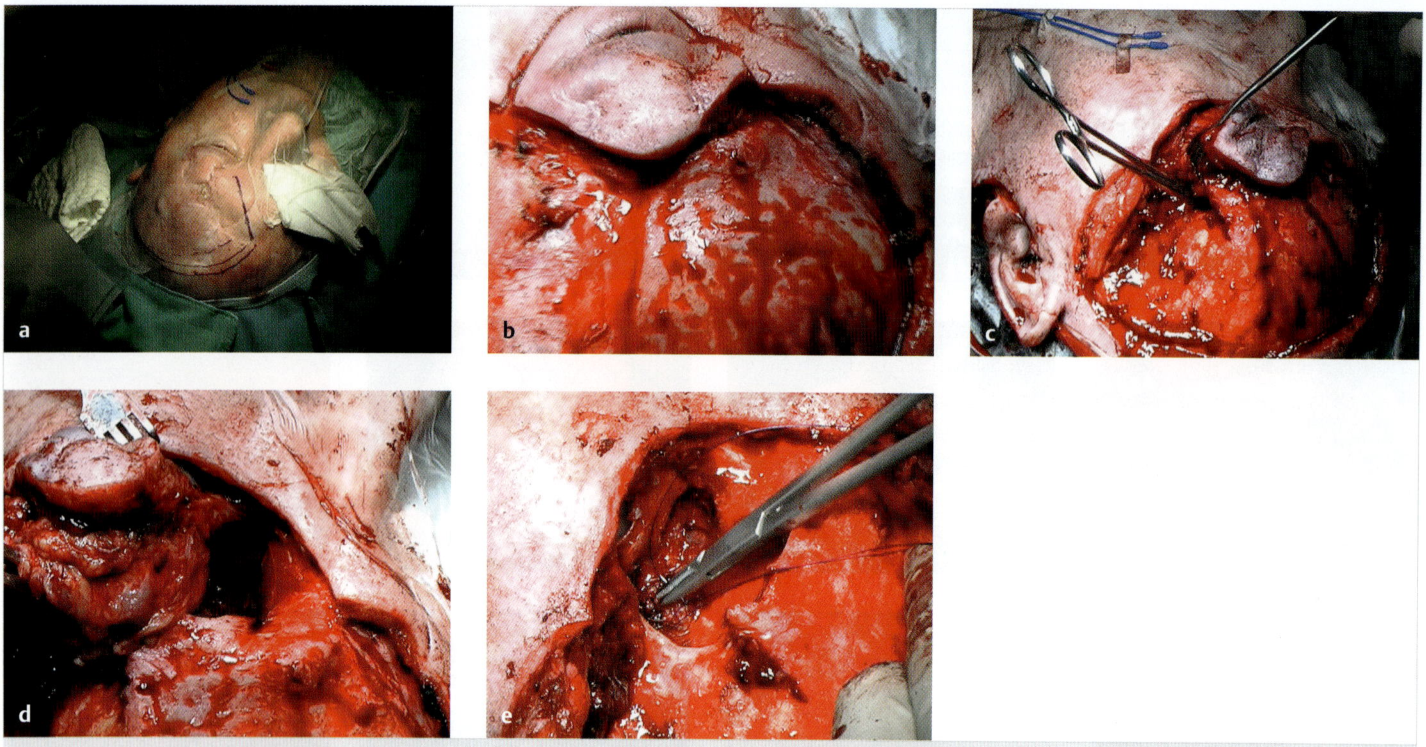

Fig. 18.16 (a) Extended tumor recurrence of a squamous cell carcinoma of the forehead skin with diffuse orbital infiltration. (b) After resection of the skin tumor, orbital exenteration is performed. (c) The ophthalmic artery and the optic nerve are grasped with a clamp after mobilization of the entire orbital contents. The tumor specimen is shown in (d); periorbital tumor parts and tumor infiltration in the cranial orbit are clearly seen. (e) The ophthalmic artery and the optic nerve are tied up after removing the entire orbital content.

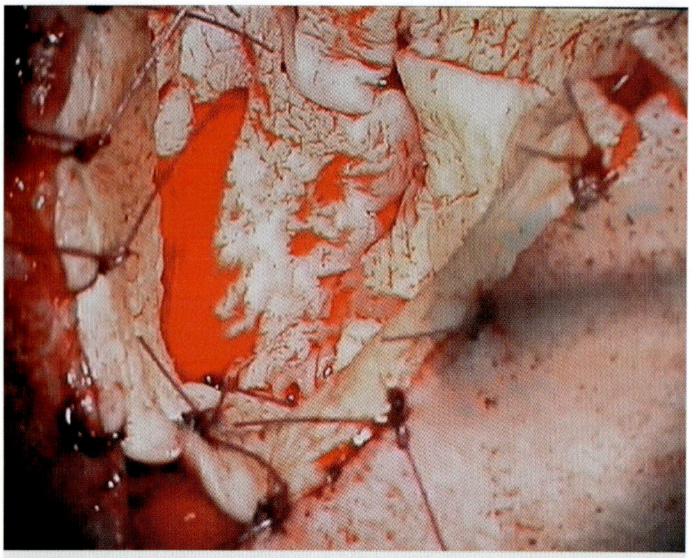

Fig. 18.17 The orbital cavity is lined with a split skin transplant.

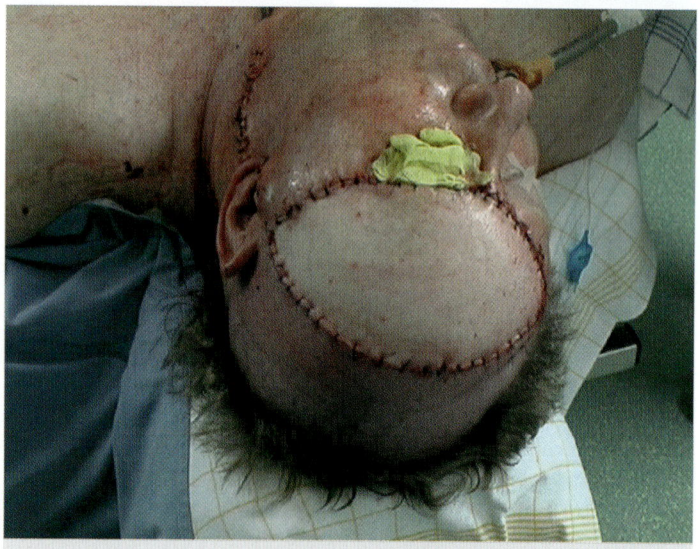

Fig. 18.18 Microvascular transplants (e.g., microvascular latissimus dorsi muscle flap as in this patient) are suitable for reconstruction of large soft tissue or skin defects. The orbit has been packed with a gauze.

mobilized and is still fixed only to the structures of the superior and inferior orbital fissure as well as to the optic nerve. The vessels in the area of the fissures are tied off. The optic nerve and ophthalmic artery are grasped with a long clamp, tied off, and separated. Smaller bleedings from other vessels can be stemmed with bipolar coagulation. The resulting orbital cavity can be lined with a wound gauze and a spontaneous epithelialization awaited. As a rule, however, this does lead to a markedly prolonged healing phase and often to wound healing disorders. It is better to line the cavity with pediculated temporal muscle fascia and split skin.[70] Alternatively microvascular flaps have been proven successful in filling the deformity (e.g., latissimus dorsi flaps) or for epithelial lining of the cavity (e.g., radial forearm flaps) (▸ Fig. 18.16, ▸ Fig. 18.17, ▸ Fig. 18.18; Video 18.6). Extensive combined deformities, which include soft tissue as well as bony structures, generally have to be treated with combined flap techniques; microvascular rectus abdominis flaps, or tensor fascia lata free flaps in combination with microvascular iliac crest grafts are available for this.[78] In the context of clinical tumor follow-up, particular attention should be paid to the flap grafts. Recurrences of the tumor often develop at the edge of the flap or under the flap grafts. Some authors therefore recommend a regular MRI scan for easier identification of tumor recurrences.[79]

With regard to a subsequent provision of a bone-anchored epithesis, great emphasis should be placed on preserving the bony orbital frame. Here one should ensure that, where possible, the bone is not exposed.

The most frequent complication of enucleation or orbital exenteration is delayed wound healing with a secondary infection of the operation cavity. Surgical reconstruction measures are available to avoid this, which have already been described above. Further complications are bleeding from the ophthalmic artery or another artery, or liquorrhea with subsequent meningitis when the optic nerve has not been sufficiently tied off.

References

[1] Enchev Y, Tzekov C, Ferdinandov D, Cekov A, Spiriev T. Neuronavigation in cranioorbital neurosurgery - do we really need it? Turk Neurosurg. 2011; 21 (2):119–126

[2] Chan JC, Yu DK, Lee DL, Abdullah VJ, Li KK. Combined lateral orbitotomy and endoscopic transnasal orbital decompression in a case of orbital aspergillosis with impending intracranial invasion. Case Rep Ophthalmol. 2012; 3(3):418–423

[3] Maier W, Ridder GJ, Kaminsky J, Grosu AL. [Therapy of posterior orbital tumors]. Ophthalmologe. 2011; 108(6):531–539

[4] Koutourousiou M, Gardner PA, Stefko ST, et al. Combined endoscopic endonasal transorbital approach with transconjunctival-medial orbitotomy for excisional biopsy of the optic nerve: technical note. J Neurol Surg Rep. 2012; 73 (1):52–56

[5] Karaki M, Akiyama K, Kagawa M, Tamiya T, Mori N. Indications and limitations of endoscopic endonasal orbitotomy for orbital lesion. J Craniofac Surg. 2012; 23(4):1093–1096

[6] Murchison AP, Rosen MR, Evans JJ, Bilyk JR. Endoscopic approach to the orbital apex and periorbital skull base. Laryngoscope. 2011; 121(3):463–467

[7] Abuzayed B, Tanriover N, Gazioglu N, Eraslan BS, Akar Z. Endoscopic endonasal approach to the orbital apex and medial orbital wall: anatomic study and clinical applications. J Craniofac Surg. 2009; 20(5):1594–1600

[8] Gigantelli JW, Gagnon MR, Arthur JA, Leopold DA. Endoscopic transethmoidal decompression of a thrombosed orbital venous malformation. Ear Nose Throat J. 2002; 81(5):346–348, 351

[9] Chhabra N, Wu AW, Fay A, Metson R. Endoscopic resection of orbital hemangiomas. Int Forum Allergy Rhinol. 2014; 4(3):251–255

[10] Alabiad CR, Weed DT, Walker TJ, et al. En bloc resection of lacrimal sac tumors and simultaneous orbital reconstruction: surgical and functional outcomes. Ophthal Plast Reconstr Surg. 2014; 30(6):459–467

[11] Gönül E, Erdogan E, Düz B, Timurkaynak E. Transmaxillary approach to the orbit: an anatomic study. Neurosurgery. 2003; 53(4):935–941, discussion 941–942

[12] Erdogmus S, Govsa F, Celik S. Innervation features of the extraocular muscles. J Craniofac Surg. 2007; 18(6):1439–1446

[13] Wang PX, Koh VT, Lun K, Sundar G. Survey on the management of orbital and intraocular tumors among oculofacial surgeons in the Asia-Pacific region. Int Ophthalmol. 2014; 34(3):723–733

[14] Halli RC, Mishra S, Kini YK, Kharkar VR, Hebbale MA. Modified lateral orbitotomy approach: a novel technique in the management of lacrimal gland tumors. J Craniofac Surg. 2011; 22(3):1035–1038

[15] Mariniello G, Maiuri F, de Divitiis E, et al. Lateral orbitotomy for removal of sphenoid wing meningiomas invading the orbit. Neurosurgery. 2010; 66(6) Suppl Operative:287–292, discussion 292

[16] Okay O, Daglioglu E, Akdemir G, et al. Lateral orbitotomy approach to orbital tumors: report of 10 cases. Turk Neurosurg. 2010; 20(2):167–172

[17] Kharkar VR, Rudagi BM, Halli R, Kini Y. Comparison of the modified lateral orbitotomy approach and modified hemicoronal approach in the treatment of unstable malunions of zygomatic complex fractures. Oral Surg Oral Med Oral Pathol Oral Radiol Endod. 2010; 109(4):504–509

[18] Kim JW, Yates BS, Goldberg RA. Total lateral orbitotomy. Orbit. 2009; 28(6): 320–327

[19] DeBattista JC, Andaluz N, Zuccarello M, Kerr RG, Keller JT. Refining the indications for the addition of orbital osteotomy during anterior cranial base approaches: morphometric and radiologic study of the anterior cranial base osteology. J Neurol Surg Rep. 2014; 75(1):e22–e26

[20] Shimizu Y, Nagasao T, Sakamoto Y, Kishi K. Inferolateral marginal orbitectomy: a simple adjuvant technique for orbital decompression. Int J Oral Maxillofac Surg. 2014; 43(10):1211–1215

[21] Park SJ, Yang JW. The transconjunctival approach a minimally invasive approach to various kinds of retrobulbar tumors. J Craniofac Surg. 2013; 24(6): 1991–1995

[22] Behrendt S. Proceedings of the German Society of Otorhinolaryngology, Head and Neck Surgery, 1998. Berlin, Germany: Springer; 1998:1–21

[23] Rhim CH, Scholz T, Salibian A, Evans GR. Orbital floor fractures: a retrospective review of 45 cases at a tertiary health care center. Craniomaxillofac Trauma Reconstr. 2010; 3(1):41–47

[24] Fleiner B, Hoffmeister B, Eickbohm JE, Dreesen W. [The subciliar incision as an infraorbital approach in caring for midface fractures]. Dtsch Zahn Mund Kieferheilkd Zentralbl. 1991; 79(5):381–386

[25] Ridgway EB, Chen C, Colakoglu S, Gautam S, Lee BT. The incidence of lower eyelid malposition after facial fracture repair: a retrospective study and meta-analysis comparing subtarsal, subciliary, and transconjunctival incisions. Plast Reconstr Surg. 2009; 124(5):1578–1586

[26] Wilson S, Ellis E, III. Surgical approaches to the infraorbital rim and orbital floor: the case for the subtarsal approach. J Oral Maxillofac Surg. 2006; 64(1): 104–107

[27] Appling WD, Patrinely JR, Salzer TA. Transconjunctival approach vs subciliary skin-muscle flap approach for orbital fracture repair. Arch Otolaryngol Head Neck Surg. 1993; 119(9):1000–1007

[28] Bähr W, Bagambisa FB, Schlegel G, Schilli W. Comparison of transcutaneous incisions used for exposure of the infraorbital rim and orbital floor: a retrospective study. Plast Reconstr Surg. 1992; 90(4):585–591

[29] Goldberg RA. Anterior orbitotomy. In: Thot BA, Keating RR, Stewart WB, eds. An Atlas of Orbitocranial Surgery. Martin Dunitz London; 1999:45–55

[30] Bourget J. Les hernies graisseuses de l'orbite. Notre traitement chirurgical. Bull Acad Med Paris. 1924; 92:1270–1271

[31] McCord CD, Jr, Moses JL. Exposure of the inferior orbit with fornix incision and lateral canthotomy. Ophthalmic Surg. 1979; 10(6):53–63

[32] Tessier P. The conjunctival approach to the orbital floor and maxilla in congenital malformation and trauma. J Maxillofac Surg. 1973; 1(1):3–8

[33] Appling WD, Patrinely JR, Salzer TA. Transconjunctival approach vs subciliary skin-muscle flap approach for orbital fracture repair. Br J Plast Surg. 1977; 30 (2):142–145

[34] Wray RC, Holtmann B, Ribaudo JM, Keiter J, Weeks PM. A comparison of conjunctival and subciliary incisions for orbital fractures. Arch Otolaryngol Head Neck Surg. 1993; 119(9):1000–1007

[35] Holtmann B, Wray RC, Little AG. A randomized comparison of four incisions for orbital fractures. Plast Reconstr Surg. 1981; 67(6):731–737

[36] Garcia GH, Goldberg RA, Shorr N. The transcaruncular approach in repair of orbital fractures: a retrospective study. J Craniomaxillofac Trauma. 1998; 4 (1):7–12

[37] Langsdon PR, Knipe TA, Whatley WS, Costello TH. Transconjunctival approach to the zygomatico-frontal limb of orbitozygomatic complex fractures. Facial Plast Surg. 2005; 21(3):171–175

[38] Langsdon PR, Rohman GT, Hixson R, Stumpe MR, Metzinger SE. Upper lid transconjunctival versus transcutaneous approach for fracture repair of the lateral orbital rim. Ann Plast Surg. 2010; 65(1):52–55

[39] Rodriguez J, Galan R, Forteza G, et al. Extended transcaruncular approach using detachment and repositioning of the inferior oblique muscle for the traumatic repair of the medial orbital wall. Craniomaxillofac Trauma Reconstr. 2009; 2(1):35–40

[40] Moe KS. The precaruncular approach to the medial orbit. Arch Facial Plast Surg. 2003; 5(6):483–487

[41] Oh JY, Rah SH, Kim YH. Transcaruncular approach to blowout fractures of the medial orbital wall. Korean J Ophthalmol. 2003; 17(1):50–54

[42] Santosh BS, Giraddi G. Transconjunctival preseptal approach for orbital floor and infraorbital rim fracture. J Maxillofac Oral Surg. 2011; 10(4):301–305

[43] Goldberg RA, Lessner AM, Shorr N, Baylis HI. The transconjunctival approach to the orbital floor and orbital fat. A prospective study. Ophthal Plast Reconstr Surg. 1990; 6(4):241–246

[44] Mullins JB, Holds JB, Branham GH, Thomas JR. Complications of the transconjunctival approach. A review of 400 cases. Arch Otolaryngol Head Neck Surg. 1997; 123(4):385–388

[45] Ho VH, Rowland JP, Jr, Linder JS, Fleming JC. Sutureless transconjunctival repair of orbital blowout fractures. Ophthal Plast Reconstr Surg. 2004; 20(6): 458–460

[46] Westfall CT, Shore JW, Nunery WR, Hawes MJ, Yaremchuk MJ. Operative complications of the transconjunctival inferior fornix approach. Ophthalmology. 1991; 98(10):1525–1528

[47] Baumann A, Ewers R. Use of the preseptal transconjunctival approach in orbit reconstruction surgery. J Oral Maxillofac Surg. 2001; 59(3):287–291, discussion 291–292

[48] De Riu G, Meloni SM, Gobbi R, Soma D, Baj A, Tullio A. Subciliary versus swinging eyelid approach to the orbital floor. J Craniomaxillofac Surg. 2008; 36(8): 439–442

[49] Novelli G, Ferrari L, Sozzi D, Mazzoleni F, Bozzetti A. Transconjunctival approach in orbital traumatology: a review of 56 cases. J Craniomaxillofac Surg. 2011; 39(4):266–270

[50] Raschke GF, Rieger UM, Bader RD, Schaefer O, Guentsch A, Schultze-Mosgau S. Transconjunctival versus subciliary approach for orbital fracture repair–an anthropometric evaluation of 221 cases. Clin Oral Investig. 2013; 17(3):933–942

[51] Harders A, Schmieder K, Grönemeyer U, et al. Der transkonjunktivale Zugang zu retrobulbären Tumoren. In: Rochels R, Behrendt S, eds. Orbitachirurgie. Reinbek, Germany: Einhorn; 1997:226–229

[52] Cheng JW, Wei RL, Cai JP, Li Y. Transconjunctival orbitotomy for orbital cavernous hemangiomas. Can J Ophthalmol. 2008; 43(2):234–238

[53] Hejazi N, Hassler W. The transconjunctival microsurgical approach to the orbit: recent experience in 22 cases. Br J Neurosurg. 1997; 11(4):310–317

[54] Yasargil MG, Antic J, Laciga R, Jain KK, Hodosh RM, Smith RD. Microsurgical pterional approach to aneurysms of the basilar bifurcation. Surg Neurol. 1976; 6(2):83–91

[55] Yaşargil MG, Reichman MV, Kubik S. Preservation of the frontotemporal branch of the facial nerve using the interfascial temporalis flap for pterional craniotomy. Technical article. J Neurosurg. 1987; 67(3):463–466

[56] Hassler W, Zentner J. Surgical treatment of olfactory groove meningiomas using the pterional approach. Acta Neurochir Suppl (Wien). 1991; 53:14–18

[57] Pamir MN, Ozduman K, Belirgen M, Kilic T, Ozek MM. Outcome determinants of pterional surgery for tuberculum sellae meningiomas. Acta Neurochir (Wien). 2005; 147(11):1121–1130, discussion 1130

[58] Schaller C, Rohde V, Hassler W. Microsurgical removal of olfactory groove meningiomas via the pterional approach. Skull Base Surg. 1994; 4(4):189–192

[59] Sandalcioglu IE, Gasser T, Mohr C, Stolke D, Wiedemayer H. Spheno-orbital meningiomas: interdisciplinary surgical approach, resectability and long-term results. J Craniomaxillofac Surg. 2005; 33(4):260–266

[60] Mariniello G, de Divitiis O, Bonavolontà G, Maiuri F. Surgical unroofing of the optic canal and visual outcome in basal meningiomas. Acta Neurochir (Wien). 2013; 155(1):77–84

[61] Markakis E, Kolenda H, Behnke J, Mühlendyck H. [Frontobasal osteoplastic orbitotomy in surgical treatment of intraorbital processes]. [Article in German]. Neurochirurgia (Stuttg). 1990; 33(3):73–77

[62] Gorman CA, DeSanto LW, MacCarty CS, Riley FC. Optic neuropathy of graves's disease. Treatment by transantral or transfrontal orbital decompression. N Engl J Med. 1974; 290(2):70–75

[63] Donald PJ. Frontobasal approach for trauma and tumor. Minim Invasive Neurosurg. 1994; 37(2):37–41

[64] Wiedemayer H, Sandalcioglu IE, Wiedemayer H, Stolke D. The supraorbital keyhole approach via an eyebrow incision for resection of tumors around the sella and the anterior skull base. Minim Invasive Neurosurg. 2004; 47(4):221–225

[65] Hassler W, Schick U. The supraorbital approach–a minimally invasive approach to the superior orbit. Acta Neurochir (Wien). 2009; 151(6):605–611, discussion 611–612

[66] Reisch R, Stadie A, Kockro RA, Hopf N. The keyhole concept in neurosurgery. World Neurosurg. 2013; 79(2) Suppl:17.e9–17.e13

[67] Rochels R, Beigel A, Mehdorn HM. [Coronal incision as the surgical approach to the orbits]. [Aticle in German]. Ophthalmologe. 1995; 92(2):212–214

[68] Hoffmann TK, El Hindy N, Müller OM, et al. Vascularised local and free flaps in anterior skull base reconstruction. Eur Arch Otorhinolaryngol. 2013; 270(3): 899–907

[69] Jimbo H, Kamata S, Miura K, et al. Operative management of skull base malignant tumors arising from the nasal cavity and paranasal sinus: recent strategies used in 25 cases. Neurol Med Chir (Tokyo). 2010; 50(1):20–26, discussion 26

[70] Strutz J, Welkoborsky HJ. Zugangswege zur Orbita. In: Strutz J, Mann WJ, eds. Praxis der HNO-Heilkunde, Kopf- und Halschirurgie. 2nd ed. Stuttgart: Thieme; 2010:785–789

[71] Klufas MA, Wolden SL, Bohle GC, III, Wexler LH, Abramson DH. Exenteration and custom implant brachytherapy as a treatment for recurrent primary and extraskeletal orbital ewing sarcoma. Ophthal Plast Reconstr Surg. 2015; 31 (4):e89–e91

[72] Miller CV, Wolf A, Klingenstein A, et al. Clinical outcome of advanced squamous cell carcinoma of the conjunctiva. Eye (Lond). 2014; 28(8):962–967

[73] Wong JC, Thampy R, Cook A. Life expectancy following orbital exenteration. Br J Ophthalmol. 2015; 99(1):1–4

[74] Sakashita T, Hayashi R, Homma A, et al. Multi-institutional retrospective study for the evaluation of ocular function-preservation rates in maxillary sinus squamous cell carcinomas with orbital invasion. Head Neck. 2015; 37(4): 537–542

[75] Herr MW, Gray ST, Erman AB, Curry WT, Deschler DG, Lin DT. Orbital preservation in patients with esthesioneuroblastoma. J Neurol Surg B Skull Base. 2013; 74(3):142–145

[76] Weizman N, Horowitz G, Gil Z, Fliss DM. Surgical management of tumors involving the orbit. JAMA Otolaryngol Head Neck Surg. 2013; 139(8):841–846

[77] Tang W, Hei Y, Xiao L. Recurrent orbital space-occupying lesions: a clinicopathologic study of 253 cases. Chin J Cancer Res. 2013; 25(4):423–429

[78] Joseph ST, Thankappan K, Mathew J, Vijayamohan M, Sharma M, Iyer S. Defect components and reconstructive options in composite orbitomaxillary defects with orbital exenteration. J Oral Maxillofac Surg. 2014; 72(9):1869.e1–1869.e9

[79] Lee PS, Sedrak P, Guha-Thakurta N, et al. Imaging findings of recurrent tumors after orbital exenteration and free flap reconstruction. Ophthal Plast Reconstr Surg. 2014; 30(4):315–321

Suggested Further Readings

Pelton RW, Patel BC. Superomedial lid crease approach to the medial intraconal space: a new technique for access to the optic nerve and central space. Ophthal Plast Reconstr Surg. 2001; 17(4):241–253

Scolozzi P. [A combined transcaruncular transconjunctival approach to orbital medial wall fractures. Surgical technique]. Rev Stomatol Chir Maxillofac. 2010; 111(5–6):302–307

Chapter 19

Reconstructive Orbital Surgery

19 Reconstructive Orbital Surgery

N. C. Gellrich and M. Rana

19.1 Introduction

Reconstructive orbital surgery has the mission of restitution of a basically normally configured orbit (for example, in trauma cases), or of reconstructing the morphology of the orbit such that the association of intraorbital soft tissues, bony orbital walls, and periorbital soft tissues achieve a favorable functional and cosmetic outcome.

Hardly any other surgical field in maxillofacial surgery has undergone such intense changes over recent years as has reconstructive orbital surgery. The developments in this field have been influenced strongly by the improvement of three-dimensional imaging, the advances in computer techniques, the optimization of biomaterials that are available for reconstructive surgery, and modern manufacturing techniques along with development of autoclavable orbital implants that can be adapted preoperatively to the individual patient's anatomy.

19.2 Principles of Orbital Reconstruction

Both congenital and acquired orbital deformities can necessitate reconstructive treatment of the orbit. However, this does not mean that functional impairments, such as diplopia, are always clinically evident. Due to posttraumatic primary treatments of large bony orbital wall defects with bioresorbable materials, for example, a slow volume change of the orbital content can occur although the orbital content itself remains constant. As a consequence, hypoglobus and enophthalmos can occur without apperception of diplopia. This is a typical example of a shift of orbital content developing slowly (over months) that nevertheless, due to the plasticity of the brain, will not necessarily result in functional impairment. On the other hand, when these intraorbital volume shifts take place very rapidly, the consequence is usually an impairment of vision—typically accompanied by diplopia.

From the outset of a chapter on reconstructive orbital surgery it seems reasonable to assume that right and left orbits in the same patient are basically homologous and virtually symmetrical (with the exception of congenital malformations with disturbance of orbital growth and microphthalmos). However, particular pathology in a patient could be a reason not only to try to reestablish this symmetry as an operative aim when contemplating orbital reconstruction procedures, but also to apply corrections according to the volume requirement of the orbit—for example, an extension of the bony orbit (e.g., in cases of Graves's disease) or reduction of orbital volume (e.g., in posttraumatic enophthalmos) (▶ Fig. 19.1).

The authors of this chapter are not aware of the existence of any considerable orbital deformities that do not have a correlate in a voxel-based dataset. That means that CT scans, MRI scans, and digital volume tomography scans usually show the morphologic correlate of a visible orbital wall deformity, such as hypoglobus, hyperglobus, enophthalmos, or exophthalmos. This is especially evident in posttraumatic or tumor-associated orbital deformities. Orbital volume–associated aspects, such as posttraumatic atrophy of orbital fat tissue, are only mentioned in passing here, with the intention to indicate that they are considered subordinate to the more important issues already mentioned. The authors regard orbital volume–associated aspects not as a primary issue of a volume difference but as a side aspect that should, nevertheless, be included in consideration.

19.3 Summary History of the Development Reconstructive Orbital Surgery

The history of modern orbital surgery is inalienably connected with **Paul Tessier** (1917–2008), who developed surgical approaches to the orbit along with the understanding necessary for the complex and stable reconstruction of the orbit. Tessier advocated and achieved detailed three-dimensional reconstruction. These ideas were transposed to the present time by various surgeons—Joseph Gruss (Seattle, WA, U.S.A.), and Paul Manson (Baltimore, MA, U.S.A.). **Beat Hammer** (Aarau, Switzerland) has the reputation of being currently the foremost European pioneer of the concept of modern three-dimensional orbital reconstruction. Hammer took the so called "key areas" of the orbit into consideration for reconstruction and optimized the use of form-stable materials, particularly autogenous bone.[1] Hammer recognized the necessity for and importance of complex reconstruction of the three-dimensionality of the orbit and periorbital structures even before computer-assisted planning was available. His reconstruction concepts have been shown to be feasible and

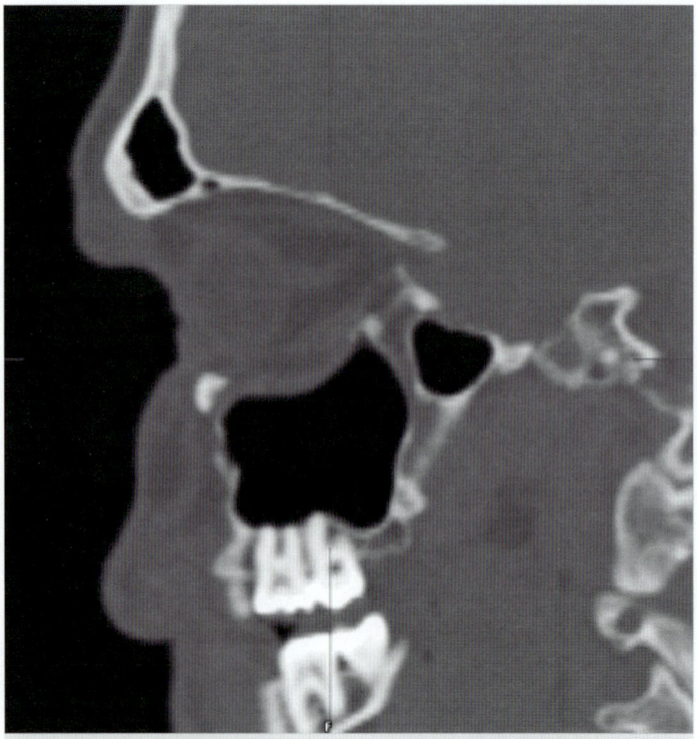

Fig. 19.1 Sagittal oblique plane image before secondary orbital reconstruction. The primary reconstruction of the orbital floor using absorbable implants had been performed some years before.

19

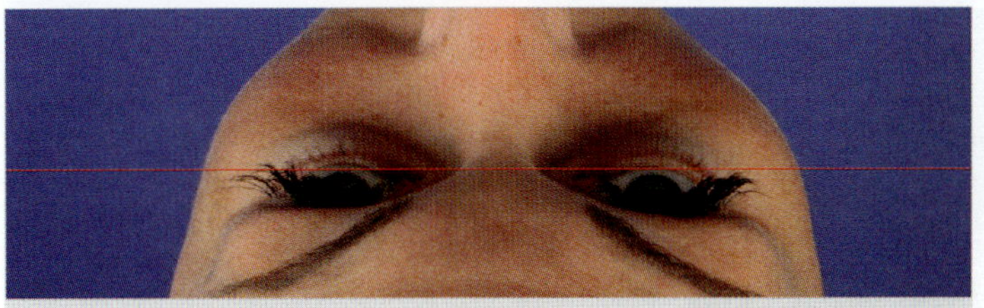

Fig. 19.2 Cranial view before secondary reconstruction of a right-sided enophthalmos following primary posttraumatic reconstruction using an absorbable implant.

effective even under most difficult circumstances (e.g., post trauma, post radiation therapy, and in congenital malformations), wherein he perfected the reconstruction the bony orbit and periorbital structures. This is demonstrated, for example, by the particular reconstruction of the medial ligament, which he inaugurated. Transnasal medial ligament repositioning and fixation was long the standard procedure for reducing the intercanthal distance. Nowadays this technique has been shown ineffective in cases of complex medial ligament malpositioning, and has been replaced by the so called "Hammer technique," which allows not only a transversal reduction but also a vertical, and—more importantly—a sagittal repositioning of the medial ligament region, with results that are predictable preoperatively. Hammer's turn around technique, with particular consideration of structural positioning of the medial ligament, is described in detail later in this chapter.

It was **Paul Manson** in his important paper "Deep orbital reconstruction for correction of post-traumatic enophthalmos"[2], who pointed out the influence of posttraumatic problems in cases with shape and volume changes of the orbit, and the consequences for the long-term result of enophthalmos, which was then hard to correct (▶ Fig. 19.2). His surgical concept involved an extended dissection of the orbit and the reconstruction of the bony orbital walls using bone transplants (calvaria split bone grafts), which were precisely positioned and adapted to the individual patient. In 1989 **Joe Gruss** published a critical analysis on the results of primary treatment of complex posttraumatic orbital defects using bone transplants. He pointed out that enophthalmos was the most frequent orbital deformity, which in his opinion was essentially attributable to non-form-stable biomaterials used for reconstruction; he related the volume problem of the orbit due to lack of form-stable materials to other problems, such false positioning of intraconal or extraconal adipose tissue, scar formation, or incarceration of the supporting ligament system of the orbit.[3]

In 2004 **Edward Ellis** III and **E. Messo** investigated the usage of nonresorbable alloplastic implant materials for reconstruction of the bony orbital walls.[4] In their validation of solid, nonpermeable alloplastic materials—silicone and Teflon, but also biomaterials—they focused on titanium mesh–based reconstruction materials as the material of first choice for reconstructing the inner orbit. Teflon and Vitallium mesh were reported in the literature as reconstruction material before the currently accepted first choice of titanium grade IV.

One of the first titan mesh–based orbital reconstruction was described by Adrian Sugar (Swansea, Wales, U.K.),[5] who as early as 1991 published the use of titanium mesh for form-stable orbital reconstruction. However, the form specificity of the metallic and other form-stable mesh materials was missing from these early reports. In most cases a non-patient-specific preformed mesh was used, which was adapted to the patient intraoperatively according to the surgeon's experience. Later Sugar and colleagues developed the idea of patient-specific individualized orbital implants, which were first processed out of cold deformed titanium sheets. Porous polyethylene was also described as a form-stable material. However, like other biomaterials (bioabsorbable materials, fascia, etc.) it has one disadvantage: they all have only minor radiolucency so that these materials are not directly visible in postoperative control CT scans or CBCT datasets, but only indirectly after a time interval by constrasting the paranasal sinuses.[6,7]

19.4 Shape and Volume Reconstruction of the Orbit

The purpose of primary (especially posttraumatic) reconstruction of the orbit is the exact anatomical restoration of shape and volume of the orbit. Any reconstruction procedure, particularly for dimension-relevant orbital wall defects, must have the aim of long-term form stability. Otherwise secondary deformities might occur, which—although sometimes not functionally relevant—are morphologically adverse, and which cannot preserve the stability of the primary reconstruction result. In addition to this, reconstructions in orbital surgery must be visualized, which means that the materials used must have radiopacity. Accordingly it is the authors' opinion that neither polyethylene-based materials nor polyether ether ketone (PEEK) implants are materials of first choice.[8]

▶ Fig. 19.3 shows a typical manifestation of an orbital deformity that occurred several months following primary posttraumatic reconstruction. The material used initially (in this case PDS foil) did not maintain the form stability and revision surgery with secondary orbital reconstruction was required.

The necessity of a successful primary reconstruction with the aim of restoration of the natural anatomy using form-stable materials emphasizes the importance of a competent primary reconstruction as summarized by Paul Manson: "You never get a second chance."

The need for reconstruction of the complex three-dimensional shape and volume of the orbit is to provide the ability for quantification of both planning and the intraoperative transformations implemented, and also for postoperative evaluation. Thus three-dimensional imaging with thin slices (CT scans are ideal; axial planes, minimum slice thickness 1 mm, dataset in soft tissue kernel, and saved in DICOM format) is required for preoperative analysis and planning, as well as for postoperative three-dimensional image analysis. This allows evaluation of the morphologic reconstruction of the inner orbital structures.

There are basically two anatomical structures that are important with respect to the evaluation of a deformity and also for evaluation of a reconstruction result: (1) the transition zone between medial orbital wall and orbital floor, and (2) the oblique sagittal plane of the orbit,[8] which is the view in the course of the optic nerve or from the optic nerve canal entrance to the midline of the infraorbital ridge. These structures represent the most important elements and key areas that, according to Hammer, are critical for a successful orbital reconstruction (▶ Fig. 19.4, ▶ Fig. 19.5, ▶ Fig. 19.6).

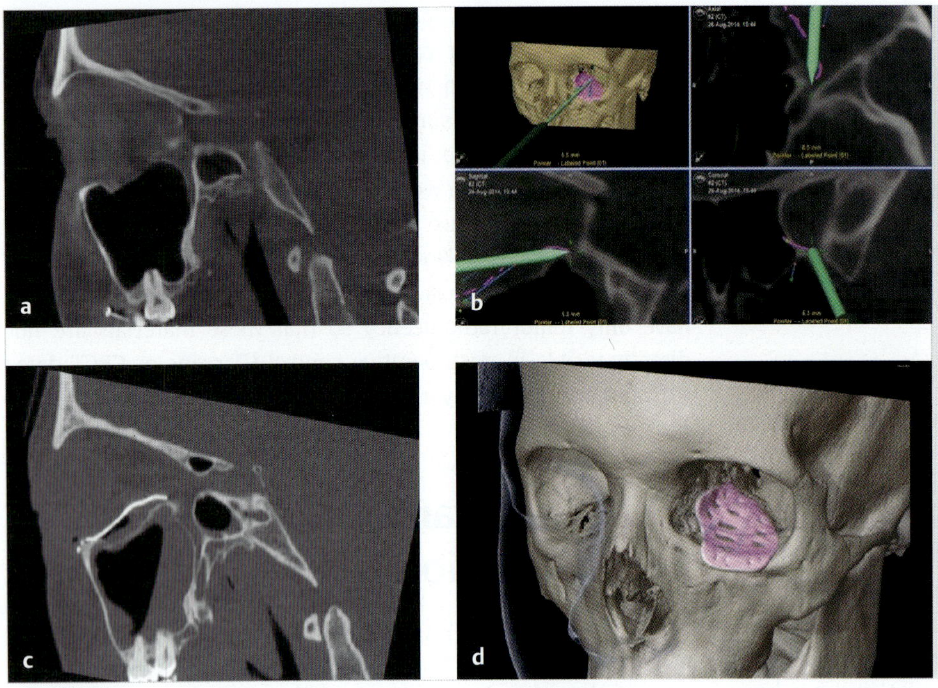

Fig. 19.3 Defect of the left orbit before secondary reconstruction. The primary surgical procedure had been performed using a bioabsorbable implant. **(a)** Sagittal view and **(b)** multiplanar view of the intraoperative navigation; (c, d) postoperative control visualization of the final secondary reconstruction.

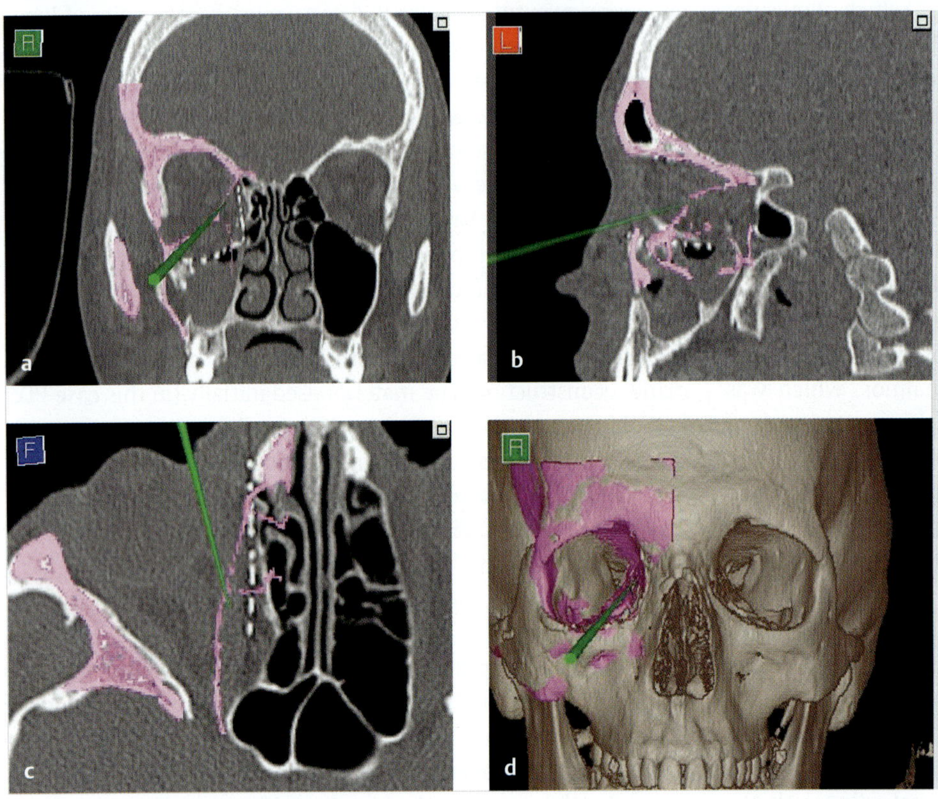

Fig. 19.4 Visualization of the intraoperative navigation of a CAD model (pink) during secondary correction of a malpositioned primary reconstruction of the right-sided orbital floor and median orbital wall region. The initial reconstruction typically differs more from the ideal model the more posteriorly the reconstruction extends into the orbit. **(a)** Coronal. **(b)** Sagittal. **(c)** Axial. **(d)** 3D volume reconstruction.

19.5 Digital 3D Analysis and Virtual Models

Interactive image analysis in combination with clinical examination (e.g., exophthalmometry using a Naugle exophthalmometer) and standardized image documentation (photographic, 3D photographic, video, surface face scan) allows a high grade of quantification of findings that can be the basis for a complete digital workflow, for example, to produce patient-specific orbital implants by computer-aided design and computer aided manufacturing (CAD/CAM-technology). To date it is also possible to digitally set up preoperative ideal plans based on virtual models (e.g., reflection; segment shifting; deformation models), so that they can be used intraoperatively as blueprints by navigation systems to correlate these data with the real situation in the particular patient. Gellrich, Schramm, and Schmelzeisen did pioneering work on this in the late 1990s and introduced this workflow into clinical routine.[9] ▶ Fig. 19.7 shows an example of such a consistent digital workflow scheme for reconstructive orbital surgery.

Further, postoperative imaging is already possible in the operating room by the use of modern intraoperative imaging techniques (e.g., intraoperative CBCT or 3D C-arm x-ray unit). With this equipment it is possible to perform additional corrections if required (e.g. to optimize the positioning of an orbital implant) before anesthesia terminates.

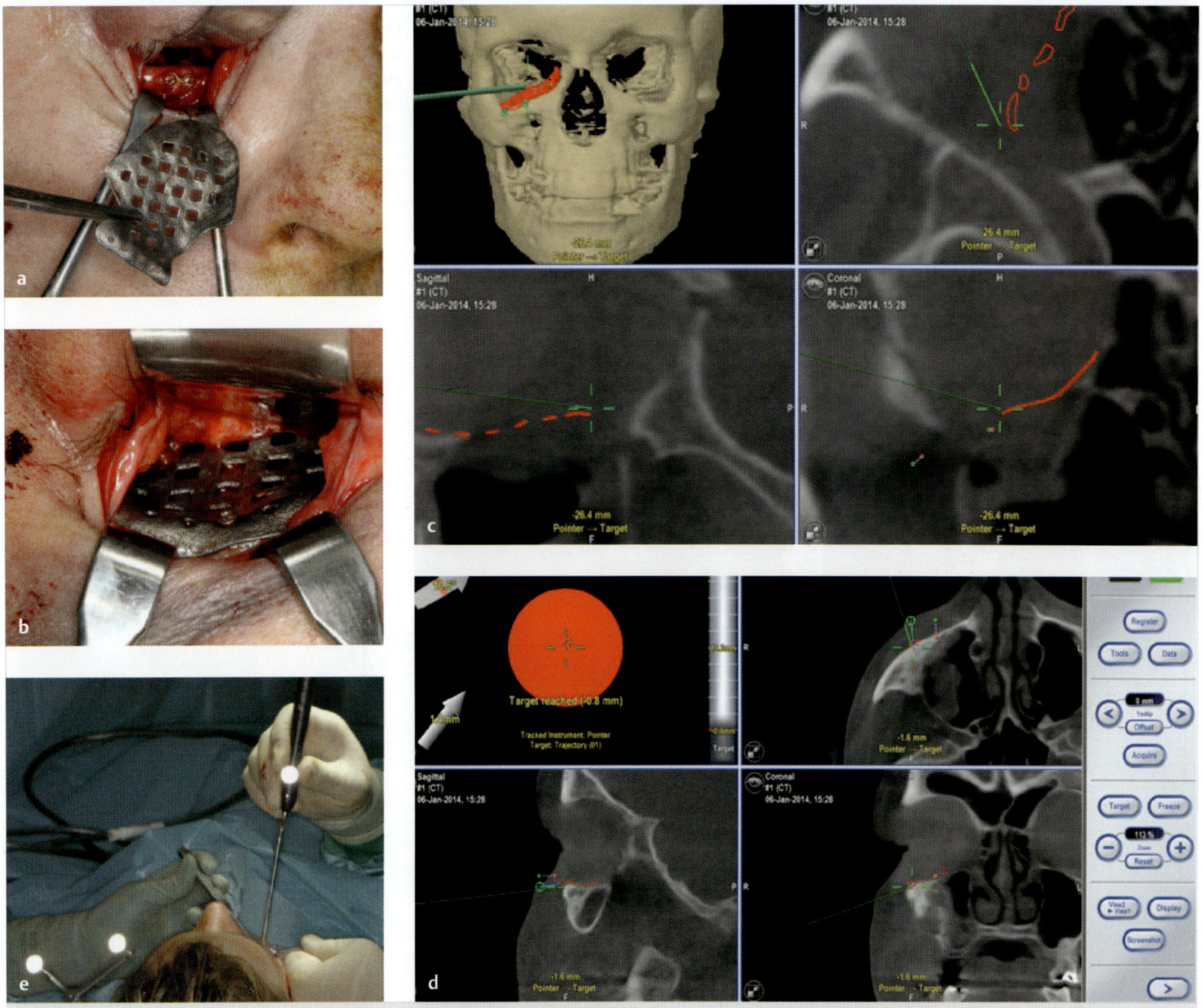

Fig. 19.5 Primary reconstruction of the right orbit and medial orbital wall using a patient-specific implant (PSI), produced by a selective laser melting (SLM) procedure. **(a)** Insertion of the orbital implant via a retroseptal transconjunctival approach. **(b)** Fixation of the PSI with a mini screw. **(c)** Control of the incorporated PSI using a computerized navigation system. The multiplanar view (3D, axial, coronal, sagittal) is demonstrated in this figure. The virtually planned PSI is displayed in red. The pointer position on the implant is represented by the green lines. **(d)** Another multiplanar view. The upper left panel shows the distance to the intended target in millimeters. The gray arrow represents the direction and angle of the pointer. **(e)** The first incision of the navigational pointer and the navigational star is shown in this figure.

Although the 3D C-arm x-ray units currently available for intraoperative use have only limited image quality compared with digital volume tomography machines, it can be considered adequate for this purpose. The challenge is for industrial companies to improve image quality and scan fields.

Computer-based techniques allow superimposition initial preoperative conditions with the digital ideal plan and the actual achieved postoperative result so that significant differences can be detected without any additional radiation exposure. The authors have long-term clinical experience using planning and navigation systems (BrainLab, Feldkirchen, Germany, and IVS Solutions, Chemnitz, Germany) in more than 1000 patients. While the VOXIM software by IVS Solutions is readily adaptable for rapid quantitative analysis of orbital deformities, and can be adjusted for all deformities independently of the anatomical region, the i-Plan planning software together with the navigation system by Brainlab encompasses the entire workflow including intraoperative navigation and connection with intraoperative imaging. With STL import and export and DICOM export even a virtual planning is possible.

The introduction of standard orbital implants based on and computed from average values by Marc Metzger, Brad Strong, and Rainer Schmelzeisen led to a considerable improvement in the anatomical reconstruction of posttraumatic orbital wall defects. This method enables the surgeon to compare the geometry of the entire orbital implant (computed and constructed based on average values) to the individual defect geometry of the particular patient by STL import in a planning system. The surgeon is then able to choose the appropriate dimension of the implant for the actual intraoperative implementation (► Fig. 19.8).

The international AO Foundation has recently conducted a study (the "Orbital-3 study") to scrutinize the precision and accuracy of orbital wall reconstruction using radiopaque biomaterials.

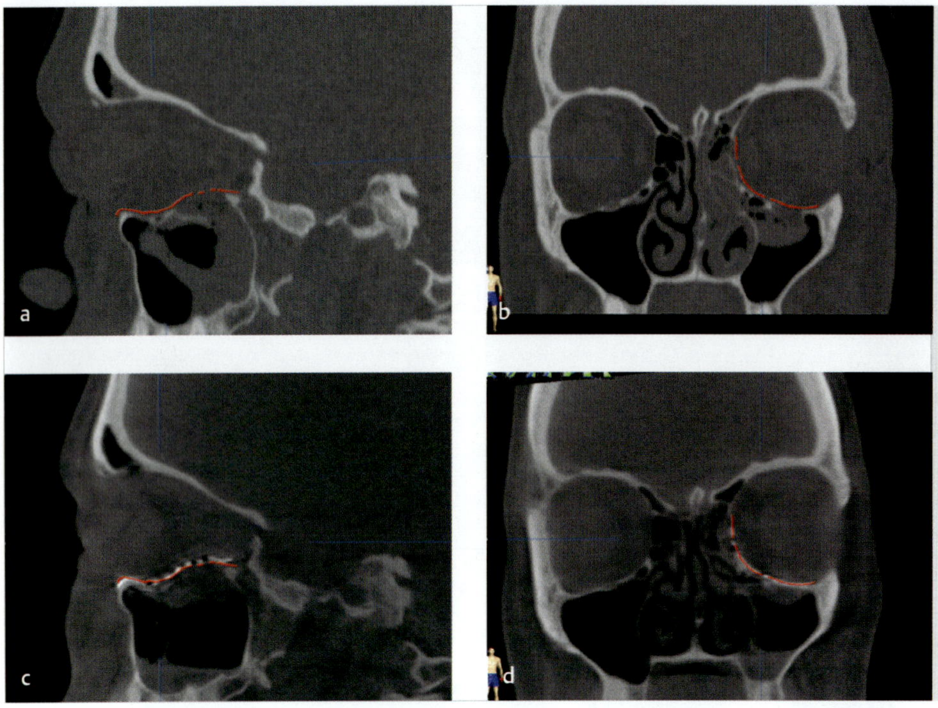

Fig. 19.6 Virtual planning of a CAD implant of the left orbit in sagittal **(a)** and coronal **(b)** views. Analogous postoperative dataset **(c, d)** compared to previous planning (red).

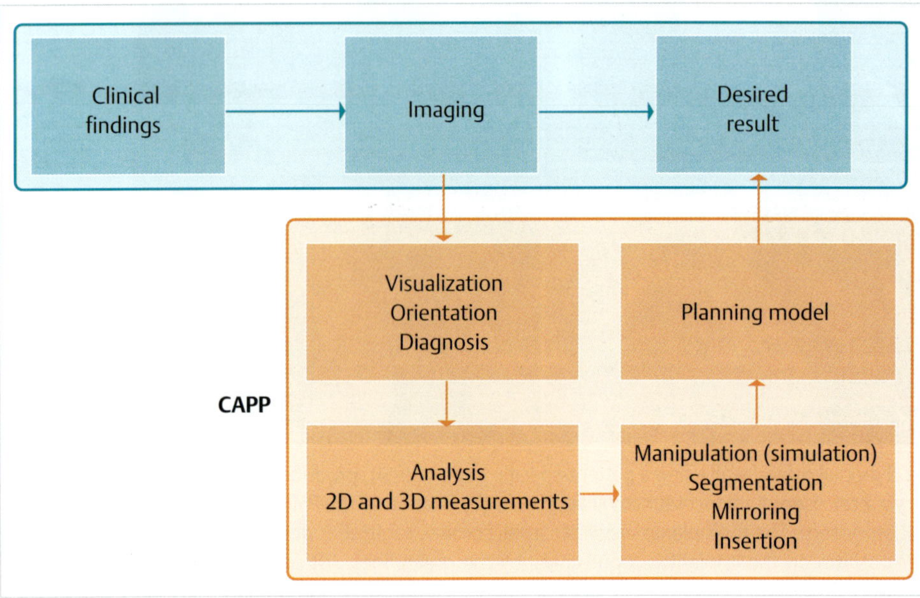

Fig. 19.7 Workflow of the computer-assisted preoperative planning process (CAPP).

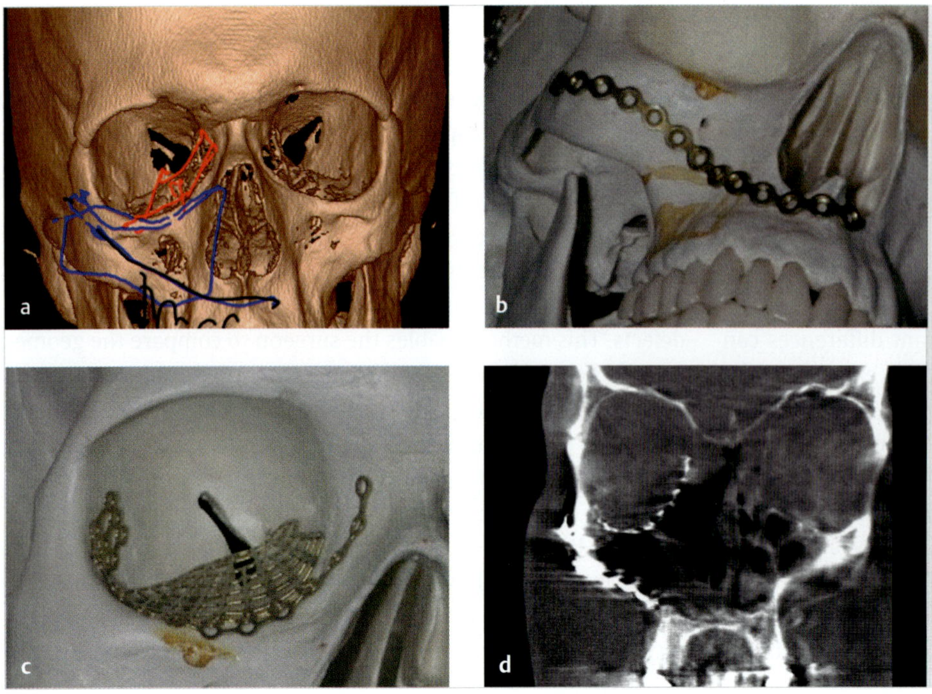

Fig. 19.8 **(a)** Schematic presentation of the midface region, which has to be resected due to a malignant tumor of the maxillary sinus (blue). The planned orbital two-wall reconstruction is displayed in red. The position of the planned implant for the right mid face is represented by the black line. **(b)** Prebending of the right midface implants as a hard tissue support from the right zygomatic column to the opposite side subnasally. **(c)** Prebending of the two-wall orbital implant at the cranial reference. **(d)** Postoperative coronal digital volume tomography view after primary reconstruction of the orbit and midface.

This international prospective multicenter study will investigate and compare the use of preformed and nonpreformed radiopaque orbital implants for primary posttraumatic reconstructions will be investigated.

In contrast to posttraumatic orbital deformities, which require a reconstructive orbital surgical procedure, the aim with tumor-related deformations, and also many congenital orbital deformations along with secondary posttraumatic orbital reconstruction, is not the restoration of some preexisting state but a reconstruction that is esthetically acceptable by balancing consideration of the tissues as found, the adjuvant therapy already performed and that still necessary, the total status, the patient's health condition, and the therapeutic strategy. It may therefore be reasonable to choose, say, just an eye patch or an anchored epithesis as a simple reconstruction method instead of an extended operation in cases of extensive midface resections due to a tumor when, for example, the prognosis of a particular patient is poor or the necessity for many operative procedures for reconstruction of the orbital region is unacceptable. Description of all the details and variations of orbital reconstruction would occupy more than chapter of such a book as this, so the intention is here to describe only the fundamentals of reconstructive orbital surgery.

Because the orbit is a paired organ, the orbit that is not affected can serve as a reference—for reflection, shifting, or deforming—and can therefore be used for a computer-aided modeling of an orbit affected by tumor, trauma, or congenital deformities. The technique of elastic deformation models, developed by H. Essig and H. Shin, can be used for complete computation of an orbit or a midface, using one CT reference dataset in cases of deformities of both orbits extending the midline. To achieve this, essentially only a few intact subvolumes of a patient's dataset are required. The iPlan software by Brainlab in combination with auto-segmenting and atlas functions affords an effective virtual reconstruction technique for the surgeon. This virtual reconstruction technique considers mainly the bony orbit. However, additional functionality and soft tissue orbital contents along with their contextual relationships to other periorbital structures, particularly eyelids and lacrimal apparatus, must be considered. Shifting of a reflected orbit (coarse function) or elastic deformation by the digital smart shaper are additional important functions provided by this software. An existing or clinically accepted disproportion between orbital soft tissue and bony orbit must be taken into consideration preoperatively when surgical therapy planning is undertaken. An example of this is a posttraumatic anophthalmic enophthalmos. In such cases the eyeball is removed but is reconstructed with an ocular prosthesis with or without an orbital implant. Later dorsal tilt of the prosthesis in the upper part occurs in nearly all of cases along with changes in the supratarsal fold, because the positional support of an ocular prosthesis is fundamentally different from the highly complex suspension of the original globe (▶ Fig. 19.9). In these cases a secondary contraction of the anterior orbital rim by 8 to 10 mm might be required to secure the vertical support of the prosthesis and to counter the dorsal tipping of the upper pole of the prosthesis. In these orbital reconstructions there might be a need for narrowing and deformation of the small orbit using autogenous or alloplastic materials; for example, plastic deformation of the lower lid by transposition of a skin-muscle-flap from the upper to the lower lid or insertion of a so called "Tenzel flap" as a support in the ipsilateral lower lid might be required. It should be stressed that the variety of injuries that can lead to an orbital deformity (burns, gunshot wounds, intrusion of foreign bodies, tissue loss) necessitate individual treatment approaches and do not allow the possibility of a universally applicable therapy plan.

19.6 Individualization of Implant Materials for Orbital Reconstruction

There are direct and indirect procedures available for producing patient-specific orbital implants. In indirect procedures a digitally stored virtual construction plan created with computer-assisted planning is transformed into a physical model (e.g., in polyamide) that serves as a blueprint for three-dimensional attachment of a non-individualized profiled implant. In direct techniques, a digital plan created by computer-assisted planning is transformed directly into a patient-specific individually adapted implant without intermediate steps. The latest techniques to achieve this include the laser melting procedure, using titanium powder, which is suitable for producing patient-specific implants of any geometry and internal structure for orbital and midface reconstructions as well as for any other anatomical region. These digital plans can alternatively control CNC (computer numerical control) milling cutters or can be used to produce implants by spraying or molding techniques.

The most recent developments by the authors have extended the functionality of patient-specific orbital implants and have perfected their shapes. Vector implementations are possible for the form and internal structure of a particular patient's orbit; for example, for control of the implant position and trajectory based on a navigation system with no radiation exposure. This innovation allows reproduction of completely form-stable patient-specific orbital implant geometry. Furthermore, the insertion and intraoperative positioning of these implants can be controlled using this technique, with which quality of the entire pathway of preoperative defect analysis, patient specific production of implants, and insertion of implants can be assured. In addition, aids to the positioning of implants (e.g., in relation to the bony orbital frame) can be accommodated in these laser-sintered orbital implants by integration of important anatomical landmarks such as the infraorbital ridge or new target positions for the infraorbital ridge into the implant geometry (▶ Fig. 19.10).

19.7 Restitution of the Medial Telecanthus Using the Hammer Technique

The malpositioned medial ligament leads to a visible deformity of the affected palpebral fissure, even when the dislocation is minor. These are most often caused by trauma, especially following naso-orbital ethmoidal fractures, in which the palpebral ligament might be with or without bony contact. Generally this leads to posttraumatic telecanthus. The aim of reconstruction in these cases is to achieve a transversal reduction, and the classical transnasal wire extrusion might be suitable for this. However,

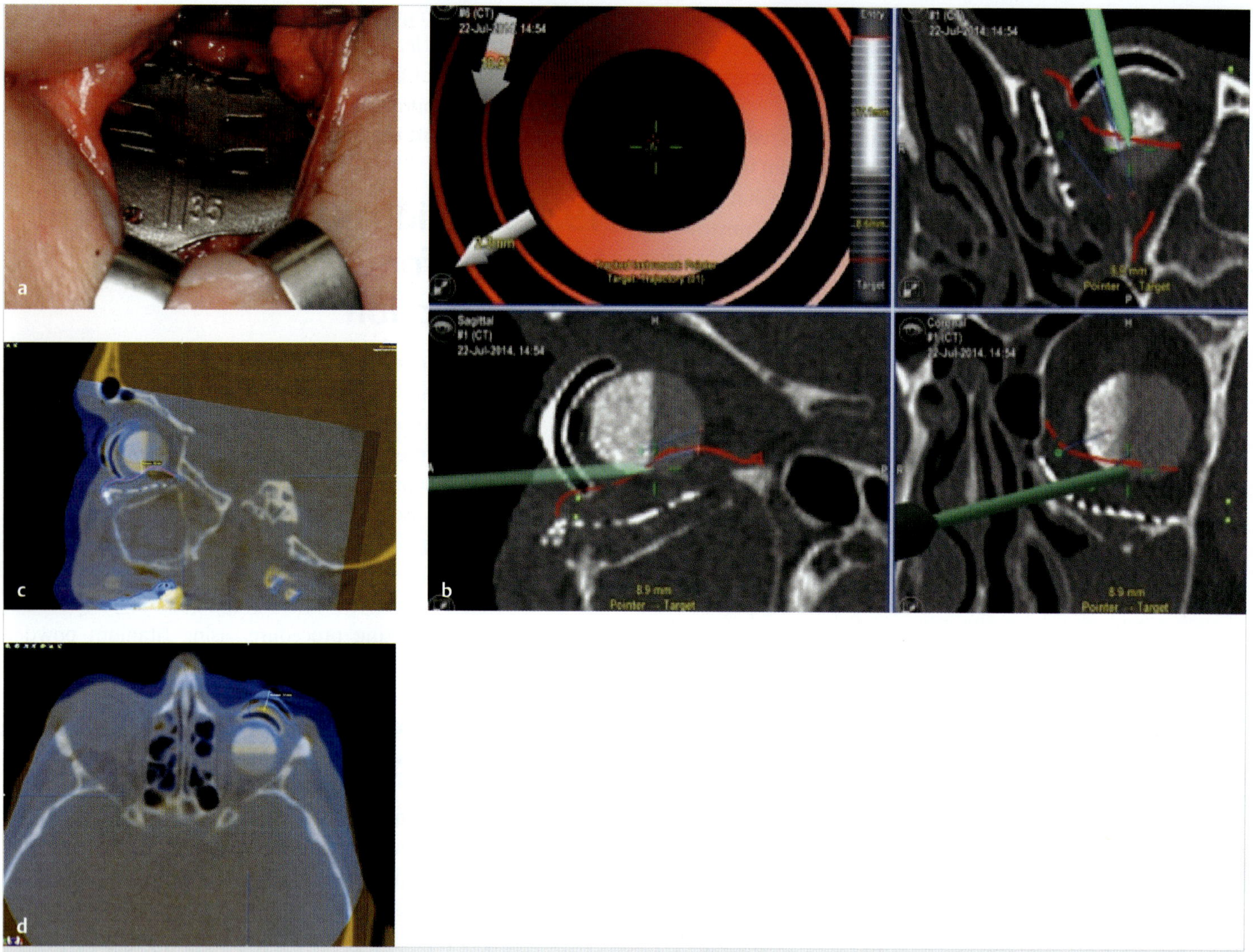

Fig. 19.9 **(a)** Intraorbital view of the patient-specific implant (PSI). The oblique sagittal main vector for positioning of the implant is demonstrated. The length of the implant is represented by the numbers. **(b)** The achieved planned overcorrection over the entire orbital floor is shown by the multiplanar view. **(c, d)** Image fusion before preoperative (orange) and postoperative imaging (blue): **(c)** sagittal; **(b)** axial.

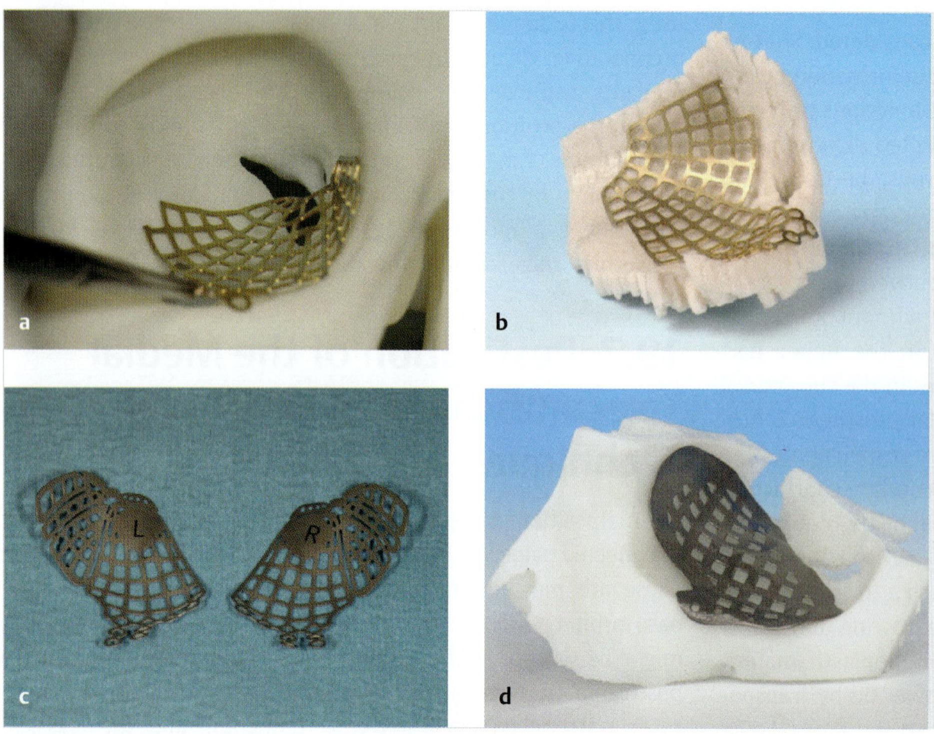

Fig. 19.10 **(a)** Prebending of a three-wall orbital implant using a reference orbital model based on average values. **(b)** The CAD biomodel of a patient-selective two-wall orbital implant. **(c)** Prebent average-value two-wall orbital implants for the right and left orbits, produced by Depuy-Synthes Cie., West Chester, PA, U.S.A. **(d)** Patient specific left-sided two-wall orbital implant, which was produced using the selective laser melting process in CAD/CAM (KLS Martin, South Jacksonville, FL, U.S.A.) and the corresponding polyamide model.

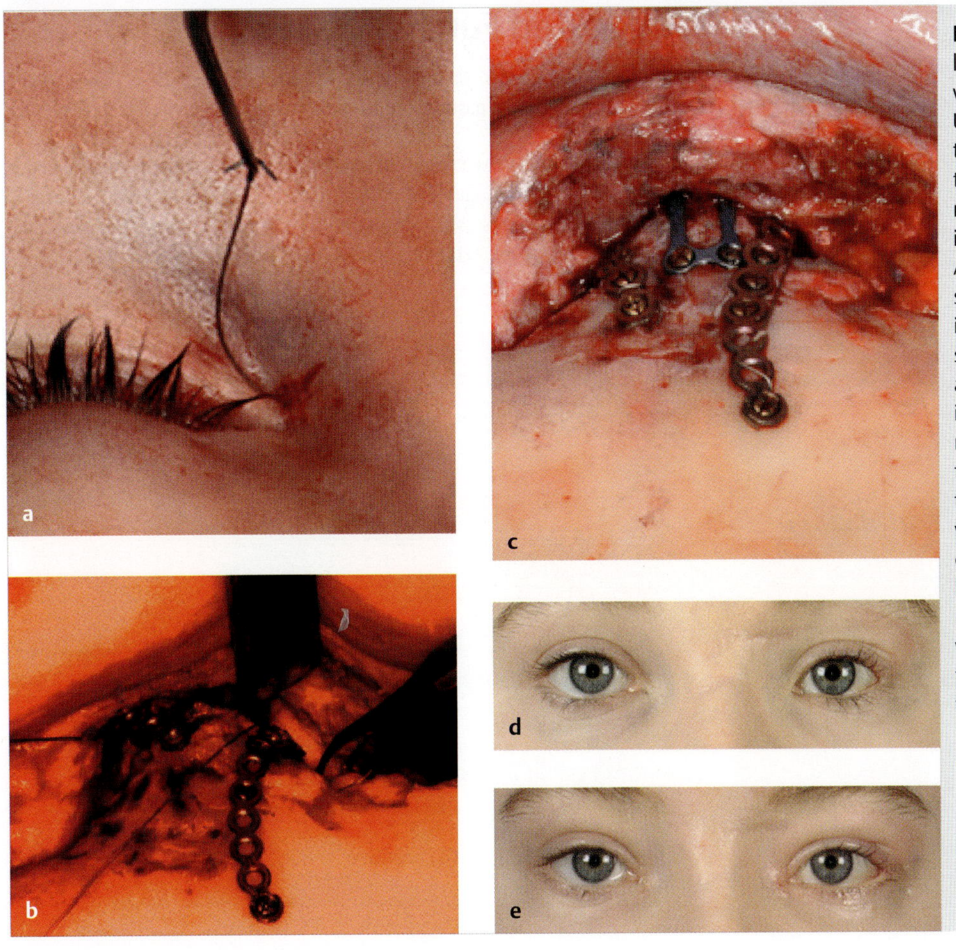

Fig. 19.11 **(a)** Sectional view from above with left sided insertion of an anchor-armed titanium wire (Depuy-Synthes Cie, West Chester, PA, U.S.A.) via a stab incision directly underneath the median lid region. **(b)** Titanium wire passed transnasally from the median palpebral ligament region on the right side following shifting via the inferior plate hole of the right sided orbit (wire A). Titanium wire passed transnasally at the left sided median palpebral ligament region following shifting via the posterior plate hole in the left sided orbit (wire B). **(c)** Situation after wrapping and clipping of each contralateral titanium wire in the osteosynthesis plate in the glabellar region. The right-angled blue-gray osteosynthesis plate serves for fixation of the dorsum of the nose at the glabella. **(d, e)** En-face views with a broadened dorsum of the nose, hypoglobus, and exophthalmos on the left side before **(d)** and after **(e)** secondary orbital reconstruction. The median palpebral ligaments were newly repositioned using the Hammer technique and the lateral left tarsorrhaphy and the lateral left canthopexy were abolished.

malposition of the medial palpebral ligament involves not only transversal but also vertical and sagittal malposition in most cases, so that the resulting dimensional contraction has to be treated in all three planes. The posterior and sagittal reduction cannot be achieved satisfactorily using the classic transnasal reduction method; the Hammer technique is the solution for precisely this issue. The fundamental principle of this technique is an ipsilateral fulcrum function of a nonabsorbable strand or wire. A wire is then guided to the opposite side, and is usually anchored in the glabellar region (by overcross knotting under the osteosynthesis plate (▶ Fig. 19.11); 2.0-mm or 1.5-mm mini plates have been shown to be suitable as fulcrum (hypomochlion) structures. Nevertheless, care must be taken that the ~2 cm long intraorbitally extended part does not dislocate into the orbital content. The plate should therefore be over-bent medially, and the nonabsorbable strand or wire should be guided in such a way so that a rather medial plate load traction results.

The repositioning of the medial ligament is quite often accompanied by an osteotomy in the naso-ethmoidal region, either unilaterally (in cases with unilateral deformities) or bilaterally (in cases with bilateral deformities). It is reasonable therefore to adopt a coronal approach when this technique is employed. Preoperative evaluation on the basis of voxel-based datasets has proved to be suitable for planning the osteotomies,. In general, the reduction should be performed with an overcorrection.

Suture/wire guidance is suitable for positioning the planned new medial ligament, which takes up the tissue directly below the dislocated median palpebral ligament transcutaneously from without. The nonabsorbable suture or wire should then be guided on the inner side of the coronal flap, then turned around in the area of the posterior of the above-mentioned osteosynthesis plate, and finally led out transversally on the reverse side. This procedure can obviously also be performed on the opposite side in cases of bilateral medial ligament repositioning. It is important to note that in medial ligament repositioning, whether unilaterally or bilaterally, the final fixation should be performed as the last step of the operation, before repositioning of the coronal flap. This means that any simultaneously necessary intraorbital reconstructions must be performed prior to the medial ligament correction. ▶ Fig. 19.11 shows an example of posttraumatic enophthalmos correction.

References

[1] Hammer B. Orbital Fractures: Diagnosis, Operative Treatment, Secondary Corrections. Kirkland, WA: Hogrefe and Huber Publications; 1995

[2] Manson PN, Ruas EJ, Iliff NT. Deep orbital reconstruction for correction of post-traumatic enophthalmos. Clin Plast Surg. 1987; 14(1):113–121

[3] Antonyshyn O, Gruss JS, Galbraith DJ, Hurwitz JJ. Complex orbital fractures: a critical analysis of immediate bone graft reconstruction. Ann Plast Surg. 1989; 22(3):220–233, discussion 234–235

[4] Ellis E, III, Messo E. Use of nonresorbable alloplastic implants for internal orbital reconstruction. J Oral Maxillofac Surg. 2004; 62(7):873–881

[5] Sugar AW, Kuriakose M, Walshaw ND. Titanium mesh in orbital wall reconstruction. Int J Oral Maxillofac Surg. 1992; 21(3):140–144

[6] Schubert W, Gear AJ, Lee C, et al. Incorporation of titanium mesh in orbital and midface reconstruction. Plast Reconstr Surg. 2002; 110(4):1022–1030, discussion 1031–1032

[7] Gear AJ, Lokeh A, Aldridge JH, Migliori MR, Benjamin CI, Schubert W. Safety of titanium mesh for orbital reconstruction. Ann Plast Surg. 2002; 48(1):1–7, discussion 7–9

[8] Rake PA, Rake SA, Swift JQ, Schubert W. A single reformatted oblique sagittal view as an adjunct to coronal computed tomography for the evaluation of orbital floor fractures. J Oral Maxillofac Surg. 2004; 62(4):456–459
[9] Schramm A, Gellrich NC, Schmelzeisen R. Navigational Surgery of the Facial Skeleton. Berlin, Germany: Springer; 2007

Suggested Further Readings

Gellrich NC, Schramm A, Hammer B, et al. Computer-assisted secondary reconstruction of unilateral posttraumatic orbital deformity. Plast Reconstr Surg. 2002; 110(6):1417–1429

Rana M, Essig H, Rücker M, Gellrich NC. Development and demonstration of a novel computer planning solution for predefined correction of enophthalmos in anophthalmic patients using prebended 3D titanium-meshes–a technical note. J Oral Maxillofac Surg. 2012; 70(11):e631–e638

Index

Note: Page numbers set **bold** or *italic* indicate headings or figures, respectively.

D

E

F

G

H

I

N

O

T